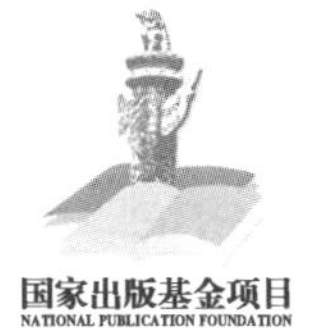

An Intensively Compiled Practical English-Chinese Library of Traditional Chinese Medicine

(英汉对照)精编实用中医文库

Chief General Compilers CHEN Kaixian LI Qizhong(Executive) HE Xinghai

总主编 陈凯先 李其忠(执行) 何星海

Chief General Translators SHI Jianrong HU Hongyi XU Yao(Executive)

总主译 施建蓉 胡鸿毅 徐 瑶(执行)

Chinese Acupuncture and Moxibustion

中国针灸

Chief Compilers ZHANG Haimeng SHEN Xueyong

Chief Translators XIAO Yuanchun XU Jingren

主编 张海蒙 沈雪勇

主译 肖元春 许敬人

上海浦江教育出版社(原上海中医药大学出版社)

Shanghai Pujiang Education Press (Former Shanghai University of TCM Press)

An Intensively Compiled Practical English-Chinese Library of Traditional Chinese Medicine

Compilation Board of the Library

Compilation and Translation Committee of the Library

Chinese Acupuncture and Moxibustion

Chief Compilers	ZHANG Haimeng	SHEN Xueyong
Vice Chief Compilers	ZHAO Ling	XU Jianmin
	DENG Haiping	CHENG Ke
Members	WANG Lizhen	WU Fan
	GUO Menghu	CAO Hongping
Chief Translators	XIAO Yuanchun	XU Jingren

《(英汉对照)精编实用中医文库》

编纂委员会

总　主　编　陈凯先　李其忠(执行)　何星海

编　　　委(按姓氏笔画为序)

马烈光　何建成　余小萍　沈雪勇

张婷婷　陈红风　陈德兴　赵　毅

郭　忻　黄　平　虞坚尔　詹红生

缪晚虹

编译委员会

总　主　译　施建蓉　胡鸿毅　徐　瑶(执行)

编　译　者(按姓氏笔画为序)

朱爱秀　杨　渝　肖元春　张亿萍

诸建民　黄国琪　董　晶　韩丑萍

《中国针灸》

主　编　张海蒙　沈雪勇

副主编　赵　玲　许建敏　邓海平　程　珂

编　委　王丽祯　吴　凡　郭梦虎　曹红平

主　译　肖元春　许敬人

Foreword
前　言

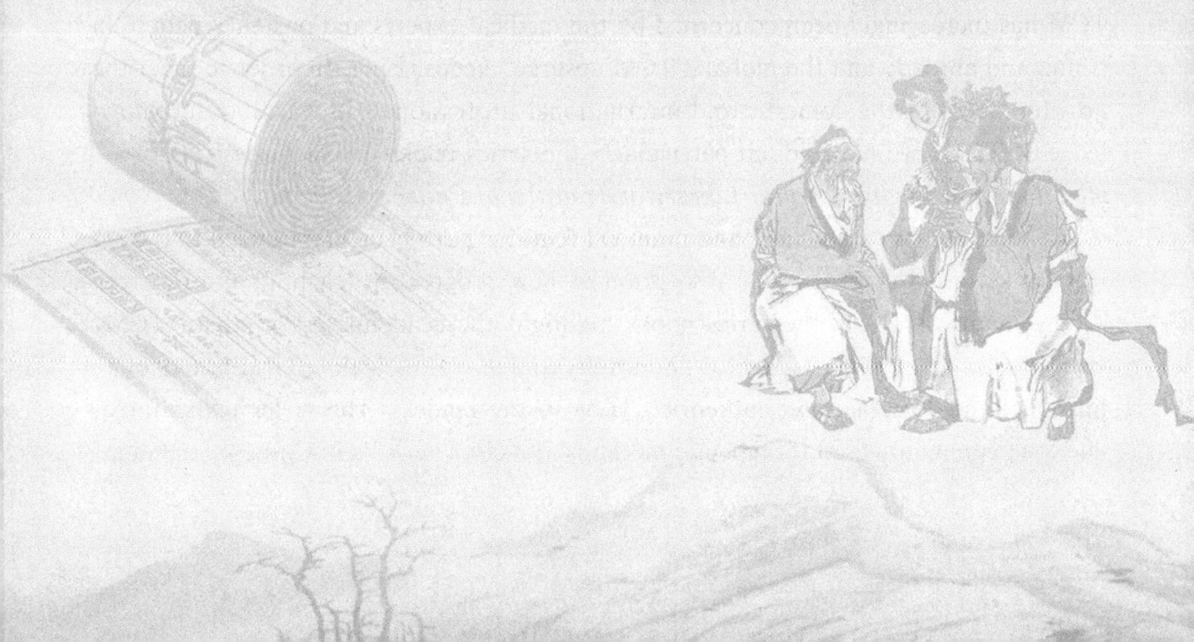

With the traditional medical philosophy and clinical experience as the principal body, the science of Traditional Chinese Medicine (TCM) is a comprehensive subject to study the rules of life activities and the disease prevention, diagnosis, treatment, rehabilitation as well as healthcare. The science of TCM has a long history of development and belongs to a summary of experiences that Chinese nation has fought against diseases for over several thousand years, is also an important component part of Chinese outstanding traditional culture and has contributed greatly to the healthcare undertaking and development of Chinese nation.

By increasing enhancement of modern living standard, change of living modes and acceleration of ageing process, the chronic diseases represented by tumors, cardiovascular diseases and diabetes become gradually the important factors in impacting the health of mankind, but TCM presents the better therapeutic effects. Nowadays, the modern medical mode of "society-psychology-biology" has been advocated in medical science, changing from the medical idea of "disease treatment" to "health promotion". The more and more patients in China and abroad have chosen natural and low side-effect Chinese herbal medicine for their problems. With the changes in medicine modes and in spectrum of diseases in the recent several dozens of years, TCM has increasingly been concerned by the medical experts and ordinary people in China and abroad, and the global " TCM upsurge" keeps rising. In order to meet the growing needs of the domestic and international professionals in learning the knowledge of TCM, we have edited particularly the series books of *An Intensively Compiled Practical English-Chinese Library of Traditional Chinese Medicine*.

The scientific, systematic and practical features have been emphasized in the series books. Based upon the full absorption of new progress in teaching and research achievements of TCM, the series books highlight the academic essentials of TCM, with precise exposition of medical philosophy and down-to-earth clinical practice, to introduce the "original and authentic" TCM to the readers. The series books introduce the commonly used therapeutic methods and clinical skills in Chinese medicine, by the clinically encountered and frequently seen diseases and the relevant ailments predominantly effective by Chinese medical therapies.By studying the series books, the readers can learn the knowledge and techniques of TCM on gradual progress and become proficient gradually in TCM.

The series books highlight "the precise features in three aspects" —capable in authors, refined in contents and accurate in translation. The majority of the authors of the series books are senior experts from the related faculties of Shanghai University of Traditional Chinese Medicine. The translator team is composed of the senior teachers with plentiful expertise in translation of TCM from international education college and foreign language center of Shanghai University of Traditional Chinese Medicine. In order to meet the needs of the readers in China and abroad, the basic and clinical core contents are selected and the latest research achievements are consulted based upon the principle "to seek its essentials but its completion" in the series books.

The series books can satisfy the beginners with certain knowledge of English language in studying TCM systematically and can also be used as the textbooks for education of TCM and pharmacy for foreign students. We sincerely hope the publication of the series books plays its promoting role for TCM going to the world.

Editors

June, 2017

中医学是以传统医学理论与实践经验为主体，研究人体生命活动规律和疾病预防、诊断、治疗、康复以及保健的一门综合性学科。中医学历史悠久，源远流长，是中华民族几千年来同疾病作斗争的经验总结，也是中国传统文化的重要组成部分，长期以来为中国人民的健康保健事业和民族繁衍作出了巨大的贡献。

随着现代生活水平的不断提高、生活方式的改变以及老龄化进程的加快，以肿瘤、心血管疾病和糖尿病等为代表的慢性病日渐成为影响人类健康的重要因素，而中医药显示了良好的治疗效果。当今的医学倡导"社会—心理—生物"的现代医学模式，医学理念从"疾病治疗"向"健康促进"转变，国内外越来越多的患者选择天然、毒副作用低的中医药治疗疾病。近几十年来，随着医学模式的转变和疾病谱的改变，中医学日益引起越来越多的海内外医学专家和普通民众的关注，全球性的"中医热"正在持续升温。为了满足海内外人士日益高涨的学习中医学知识的需求，我们特地编撰了《（英汉对照）精编实用中医文库》丛书。

本丛书注重"三性"——科学性、系统性、实用性。丛书在充分吸取近年中医教学、科研进展的基础上，突出中医学术精华，理论阐述准确、临床切合实际，向读者介绍"原汁原味"的中医学；丛书介绍中医学常用的治疗方法和临床技能，所涉及的病证均为临床常见病、多发病和中医优势病种。丛书的13个分册涵盖了中医基础与临床的主干课程，通过阅读本丛书，读者可以由浅入深、循序渐进地学习中医药知识和技能。

本丛书突出"三精"——作者精干、内容精炼、翻译精准。丛书的中文作者绝大部分为上海中医药大学各相关教研室的资深专家，翻译团队由上海中医药大学国际教育学院和外语中心具有丰富的中医药学翻译经验的骨干教师组成。为了适合海内外读者的需求，丛书本着"求其精而不求其全"的原则，选取了基础和临床的核心内容，翻译上参考了最新的研究成果。

本丛书既可满足具有一定英语水平的初学中医者系统学习中医所用，也可供中医药留学生教育作为教材使用，衷心希望本丛书的出版在中医药走向海外进程中发挥应有的推动作用。

编者

2017年6月

Note for Compilation

编写说明

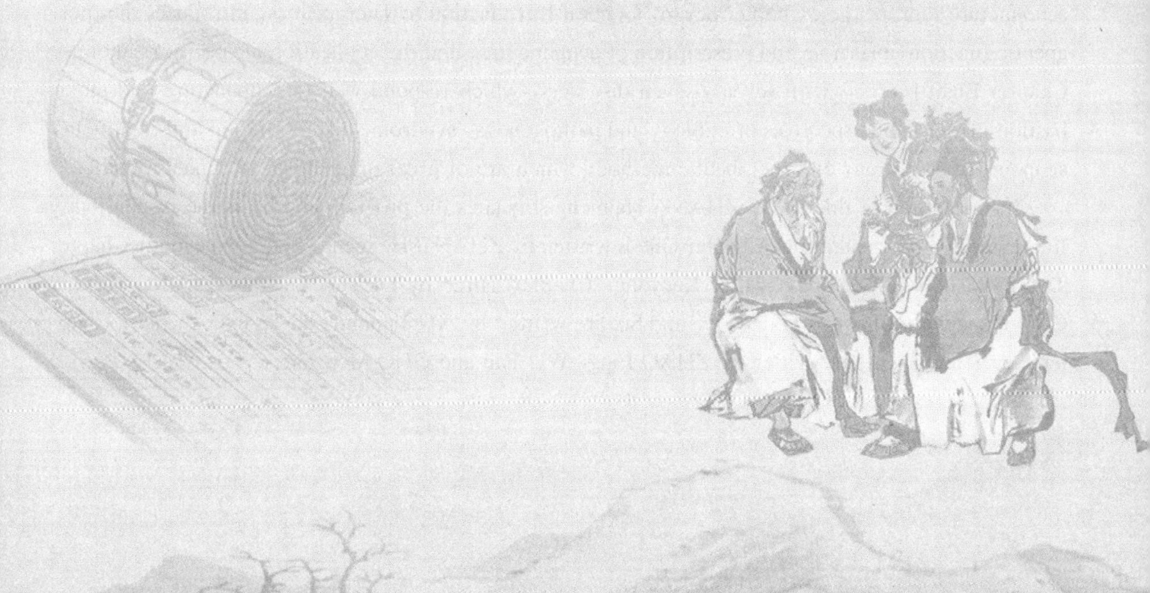

Acupuncture and moxibustion is an distinctive external therapy in Chinese medicine. Meridian theory in acupuncture and moxibustion is also an important component of Chinese medical theory, involves its physiology, pathology, diagnostics and therapeutics, and thus greatly helps clinical practice in acupuncture and Chinese medicine as well.

To meet oversea students' requirements of learning and applying Chinese acupuncture and moxibustion, this book attempts, with concise and accurate words and illustrations, to systematically introduce the basic knowledge, theory and techniques of acupuncture and moxibustion and its therapies for common diseases, which enables the readers to learn the elementary and comprehensive theory of acupuncture and moxibustion.

This book is comprised of three parts. The First Part deals with the meridians and acupoints. Chapter One, General Introduction to Meridians, systematically presents with the composition of meridian system, functions of meridians and its clinical application; Chapter Two, General Introduction to Acupoints, introduces the categorization, nomenclature, location, action and indication laws of acupoints, and the concept of specific acupoints and their application; Chapter Three first describes the running course and distribution of the meridians, and then introduces the location, indication, and needling and moxibustion methods of the acupoints. The Second Part deals with acupuncture and moxibustion methods. Chapter Four introduces the needling methods, needling manipulation, reinforcing and reducing techniques, and needling precautions; Chapter Five presents with the techniques and application of moxibustion; Chapter Six introduces other acupuncture therapies, such as electroacupuncture, scalp acupuncture, ear acupuncture and cupping. The Third Part deals with acupuncture therapeutics. Chapter Seven, General Introduction to Therapeutics, introduces the therapeutic function, principle and prescription of acupuncture, and the application of specific acupoints; Chapter Eight presents with seventy-seven disorders, which respond well to acupuncture and moxibustion, from the perspectives of etiology and pathogenesis, syndrome differentiation and treatment, acupoint combination, and therapeutic method, which are of great pragmatism in clinical practice.

In the edition of this book, ZHANG Haimeng stipulates the program and bears the responsibility for reviewing the manuscripts. Chapter One is written by ZHANG Haimeng, SHEN Xueyong; Chapter Two by ZHANG Haimeng, SHEN Xueyong; Chapter Three by DENG Haiping, CHENG Ke and CAO Hongping; Chapters Four, Five and Six are written by XU Jianmin and WANG Lizhen; Chapters Seven and Eight are written by ZHAO Ling, WU Fan and GUO Menghu.

针灸是中医学的特色外治法，其中的经络学说又是中医基础理论的重要组成部分，内容非常广泛，涉及中医学的生理、病理、诊断和治疗等各个方面，对针灸学及中医其他临床各科均有重要指导意义。

为适应海外读者学习和运用中国针灸疗法的需要，本书的编写力争以简明准确的语言，配以图表，系统地介绍针灸学的基本知识、基本理论、基本技能，及临床常见病的针灸疗法，使读者通过学习能够对针灸学有一个初步而又较完整的了解。

本书分上、中、下三篇。上篇为经络腧穴学。第一章“经络总论”，阐述经络系统的主要组成内容、经络的作用及其理论的临床应用；第二章“腧穴总论”，介绍腧穴的分类、命名、定位方法、作用和主治规律及特定穴的概念和应用等；第三章为经络腧穴各论，先论述经络的循行和分布，再介绍腧穴的定位、主治、刺灸方法等。中篇是刺法灸法学。第四章着重介绍针刺方法、行针手法、针刺补泻及注意事项；第五章介绍各种灸法的操作应用；第六章介绍电针、头针、耳针、火罐等多种疗法。下篇为针灸治疗学。第七章“针灸治疗总论”，介绍针灸治疗作用、针灸治疗原则、针灸处方以及特定穴的应用；第八章“针灸治疗各论”，精选临床上针灸疗效肯定、适合海外临床实际的内外妇儿伤科的 77 个病种，介绍病因病机、辨证治疗、配伍用穴及操作方法，具有很强的临床实用性。

本书由张海蒙草拟编写大纲，并负责全书中文稿的统稿工作。上篇第一章由张海蒙、沈雪勇撰写，第二章由张海蒙、沈雪勇撰写，第三章由邓海平、程珂、曹红平撰写；中篇第四、第五、第六章由许建敏、王丽祯撰写；下篇第七、第八章由赵玲、吴凡、郭梦虎撰写。

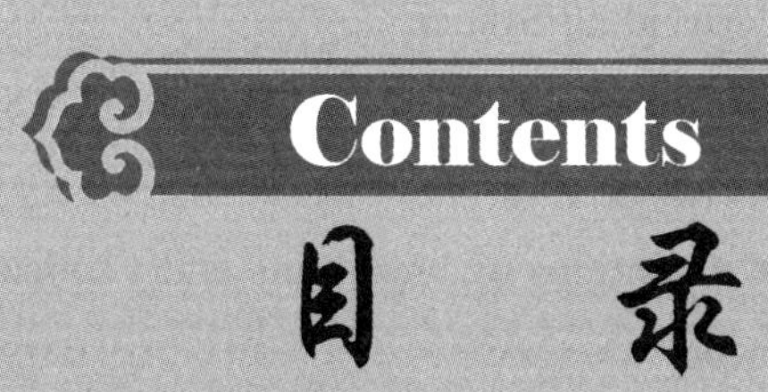

Contents
目　录

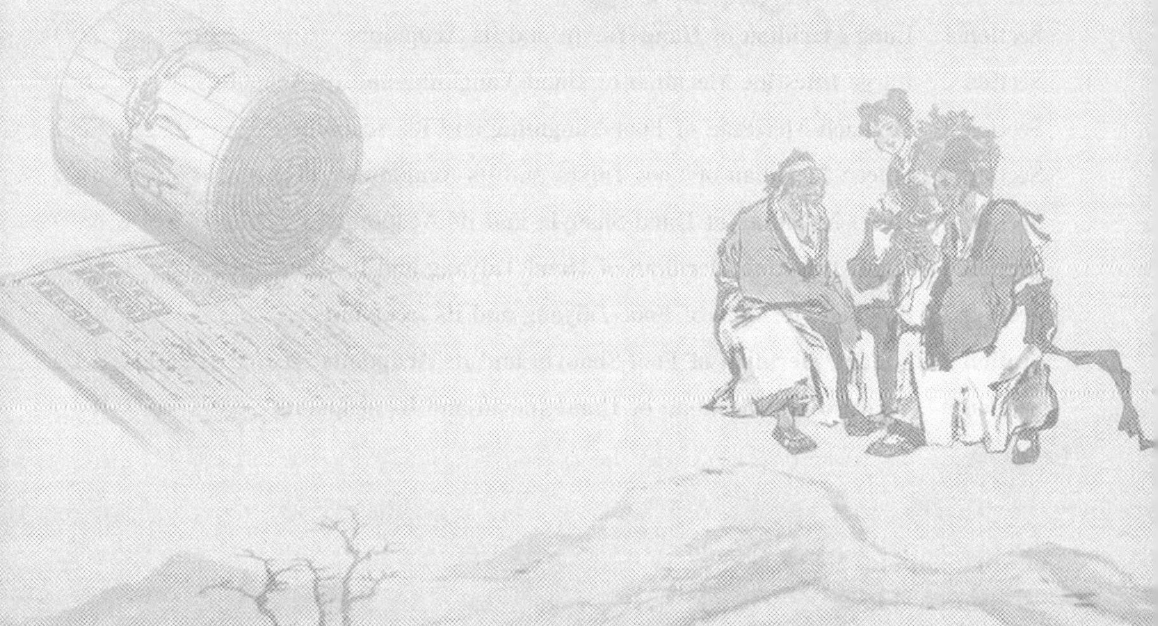

Part One Basics of Acupuncture and Moxibustion

上篇 针灸基础

下篇 针灸临床

Part One
Basics of Acupuncture and Moxibustion

上 篇
针 灸 基 础

Chapter 1 Introduction to Meridian System

第1章 经络总论

Meridian (*Jing* in Chinese) and collateral(*Luo* in Chinese) are pathways that longitudinal conduct qi and blood, connect the internal zang-fu organs with the body surface, and unify all parts of the body. *Jing,* originally meaning the longitudinal line and route, is the major trunk of the meridian system, running longitudinally and interiorly within the body. *Luo,* on the other hand, is the collaterals, which represent the branching network, running transversely and superficially from, and interlocking with, the *jing*.

经络是运行气血、联系脏腑和体表及全身各部的通道。经,原意是"纵丝",有路径的含义,就是直行主线的意思,是经络系统中的主干,深而在里,贯通上下,沟通内外;络,有网络的含义,是经脉别出的分支,浅而在表,纵横交错,遍布全身。

The meridian theory studies the pathway distribution, physiological functions, and pathological changes of the meridians and collaterals in the human body, as well as the interrelationship with internal zang-fu organs. It is the foundation of acupuncture and moxibustion science and also an important component of the basic theories of traditional Chinese medicine. Moreover, the meridian theory provides an essential basis for understanding the various physiological, pathological, diagnostic and therapeutic aspects of traditional Chinese medicine, and has been of the great significance in guiding Chinese medical practice.

经络理论是阐述人体经络的循行分布、生理功能、病理变化及其与脏腑的相互关系的一门学说,是针灸学科的基础,也是中医基础理论的重要组成部分,贯穿于中医的生理、病理、诊断和治疗等各个方面,对中医各科的临床实践有重要指导意义。

Section 1 Overview of Meridian System

第1节 经络系统概述

Meridian system comprises twelve main meridians, eight extra meridians, twelve meridian divergences, fifteen collateral vessels, twelve meridian sinews and twelve cutaneous regions. Among them, the twelve main meridians are the major trunk in the meridian system, and "connect internally with the vital organs and externally with the body surface and extremities" [*Spiritual Pivot* (Ling Shu)], thus integrating all the body's internal and external parts into an organic whole. The twelve meridian divergences branch off from the twelve main meridians and travel internally through the chest, the abdomen and the head. The fifteen collateral vessels consist of twelve collaterals from the regular meridians on the limbs, one collateral from the conception vessel on the anterior trunk, one collateral from the governor vessel on the posterior trunk and one collateral from the spleen on the lateral trunk. The eight extra meridians are eight meridians with particular pathways and functions in the meridian system. Besides, the muscles and tendons along the twelve main meridians are called twelve meridian sinews; the skin areas along with the twelve main meridians are named twelve cutaneous regions.

经络系统，包括十二经脉、奇经八脉、十二经别、十五络脉、十二经筋和十二皮部。十二经脉是经络系统的主干，“内属于府藏(腑脏)，外络于支节”(《灵枢·海论》)，将人体内外联结成一个有机的整体。十二经别是十二经脉在胸、腹及头部的内行支脉。十五络脉是十二经脉在四肢部及躯干前、后、侧三部的外行支脉。奇经八脉是具有特殊分布和作用的经脉。此外，经络的外部，筋肉也受经络支配分为十二经筋，皮部也按经络的分布分为十二皮部。

The circulation of qi and blood in the meridians follows the sequence: lung meridian→large intestine meridian→stomach meridian→spleen meridian→heart meridian→small intestine meridian→bladder meridian→kidney meridian→pericardium meridian→triple energizer meridian→gallbladder meridian→

十二经脉按其流注次序分别为手太阴肺经、手阳明大肠经、足阳明胃经、足太阴脾经、手少阴心经、手太阳小肠经、足太阳膀胱经、足少阴肾经、手厥阴心包经、手少阳三

liver meridian. The twelve meridians are the major trunk of the meridian system, and are therefore called "main meridian".

1　Twelve meridians

1.1　Nomenclature and connotation of the twelve meridians

The complete name of each of the main meridians is composed of three parts. The first part reflects whether, in its external course on the limbs, the meridian transverses the arm or leg. The second part is the organ to which the meridian pertains internally, for example, the lung meridian pertains to the lung. The third part describes the meridian's affiliation with either yin or yang, and the amount of yin qi or yang qi. The yin and yang are then further divided into three yin and three yang categories according to the amount of yin or yang of the meridian. The meridian that carries the most abundant yin qi is called taiyin meridian; the one that carries less amount of yin qi is called shaoyin meridian; while the one carries the least yin qi is called jueyin meridian. Similarly, the meridian that carries the most abundant yang qi is called yangming meridian, and the one that carries less amount of yang qi is called taiyang meridian, while the one that carries the least amount of yang qi is named shaoyang meridian. According to the amount of yin/yang qi in the meridians, the three yin and three yang meridians are coupled with their corresponding yang or yin meridians to make three interior-exterior pairs. The names of three yin and three yang are widely used in the nomenclature of the meridian system, such as meridian divergences, collateral vessels and meridian sinews.

焦经、足少阳胆经和足厥阴肝经。十二经脉是经络系统的主体，故又被称为"正经"。

1　十二经脉

1.1　十二经脉的名称和含义

十二经脉的名称由手足、阴阳和脏腑三部分组成。手足表示经脉的外行路线分布于上肢或下肢。脏腑表示经脉的脏腑属性，如肺经表示该经脉属肺脏。阴阳表示经脉的阴阳属性及阴阳气的多寡。一阴一阳衍化为三阴三阳，以区分阴气和阳气的盛衰（多少）：阴气最盛为太阴，其次为少阴，再次为厥阴；阳气最盛为阳明，其次为太阳，再次为少阳。根据阴气和阳气的多少，三阴三阳之间组成对应的表里相合关系。三阴三阳的名称广泛应用于经络的命名，经别、络脉、经筋也是如此。

1.2 Distribution of the twelve main meridians

1.2.1 External course On the body surface, the twelve main meridians are placed over the limbs, head and trunk. On the limbs, the three yin meridians of the hand are distributed on the medial aspect of the upper limbs, and the three yang meridians of the hand on the lateral aspect of the upper limbs, the three yin meridians of the foot on the medial aspect of the lower limbs, and the three yang meridians of the foot on the lateral aspect of the lower limbs (Fig. 1-1～Fig. 1-3). The body position is described with the thumb forwards and the little finger backwards, thus the twelve main meridians on the limbs are distributed as follows: the taiyin meridians and yangming meridians are distributed along the anterior border of the limbs, the jueyin meridians and shaoyang meridians along the middle region of the limbs, and the shaoyin meridians and taiyang meridians along the posterior border of the limbs(Fig. 1-4). Exceptionally, below 8 cun above the internal malleolus, the liver meridian of foot jueyin travels in front of the spleen meridian of foot taiyin. At 8 cun above the internal malleolus, the jueyin meridian backwards crosses the taiyin meridian and then runs between the taiyin meridian and shaoyin meridian. On the head and trunk, the three yin meridians of the hand connect with the chest; the three yin meridians of the foot connect with the abdomen and chest; the yang meridians of both hand and foot connect with the head, which is hence called "meeting place of yang meridians". Similarly, the yangming meridian travels along the front trunk, the shaoyang meridian along the lateral trunk and the taiyang meridian along the back trunk. So do they travel on the head.

1.2 十二经脉的分布

1.2.1 外行部分 在外部，十二经脉分布于四肢、头面和躯干。在四肢部，手三阴经分布于上肢的内侧，手三阳经分布于上肢的外侧，足三阴经分布于下肢的内侧，足三阳经分布于下肢的外侧(图 1-1～1-3)。以大指向前、小指向后的体位描述，十二经脉在四肢的分布规律是：太阴、阳明在前，厥阴、少阳在中(侧)，少阴、太阳在后(图 1-4)。在小腿下半部及足部，足厥阴有例外的分布情况而排列于足太阴之前，至内踝上 8 寸处再交叉到足太阴之后而循行于足太阴和足少阴之间。在头和躯干部，大致是手三阴经联系胸；足三阴经联系腹及胸；手足三阳经联系头，故称"头为诸阳之会"。阳经在头和躯干部的分布大致是阳明行于身前，少阳行于身侧，太阳行于身后，在头部也是如此。

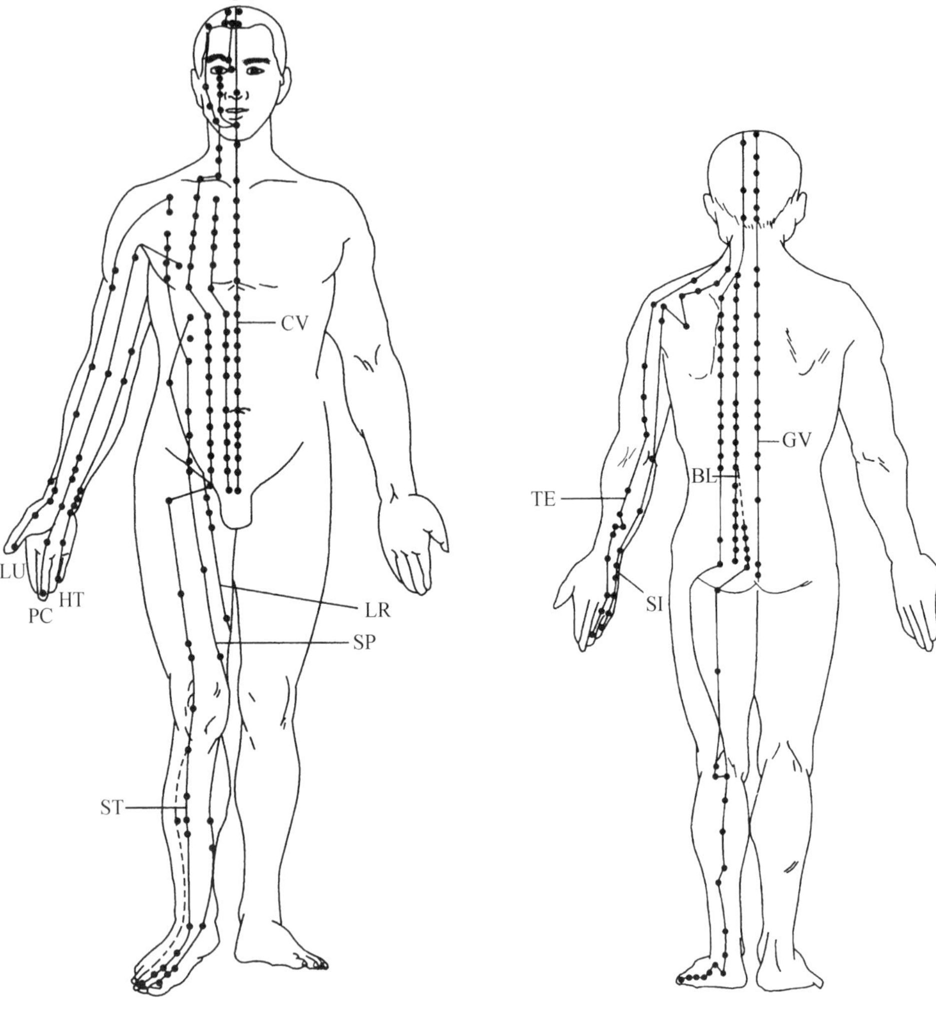

CV　Conception Vessel 任脉
GV　Governor Vessel 督脉
HT　Heart Meridian of Hand-Shaoyin 手少阴心经
LR　Liver Meridian of Foot-Jueyin 足厥阴肝经
LU　Lung Meridian of Hand-Taiyin 手太阴肺经
PC　Pericardium Meridian of Hand-Jueyin 手厥阴心包经
SP　Spleen Meridian of Foot-taiyin 足太阴脾经
ST　Stomach Meridian of Foot-Yangming 足阳明胃经

Fig.1-1　Distribution of fourteen meridians in front side

图 1-1　十四经分布概况(正面)

BL　Bladder Meridian of Foot-Taiyang 足太阳膀胱经
GV　Governor Vessel 督脉
SI　Small Intestine Meridian of Hand-Taiyang 手太阳小肠经
TE　Triple Energizer Meridian of Hand-Shaoyang 手少阳三焦经

Fig.1-2　Distribution of fourteen meridians in back side

图 1-2　十四经分布概况(背面)

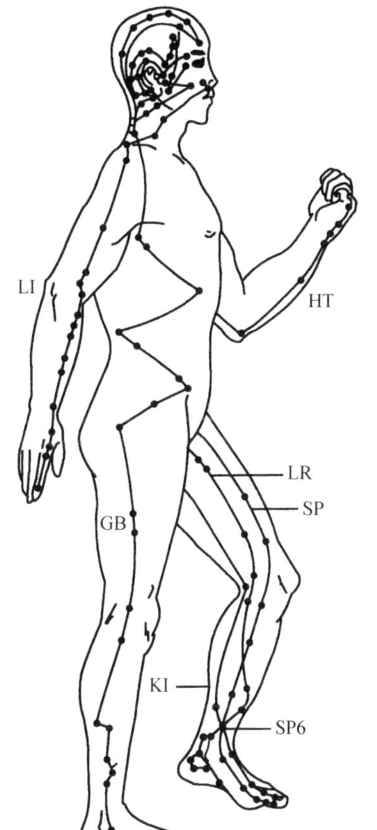

GB Gallbladder Meridian of Foot-Shaoyang 足少阳胆经
HT Heart Meridian of Hand-Shaoyin 手少阴心经
KI Kidney Meridian of Foot-Shaoyin 足少阴肾经
LI Large Intestine Meridian of Hand-Yangming 手阳明大肠经
LR Liver Meridian of Foot-Jueyin 足厥阴肝经
SP Spleen Meridian of Foot-taiyin 足太阴脾经
SP6 Sanyinjiao 三阴交

Fig.1-3 Distribution of fourteen meridians in lateral side

图 1-3 十四经分布概况(侧面)

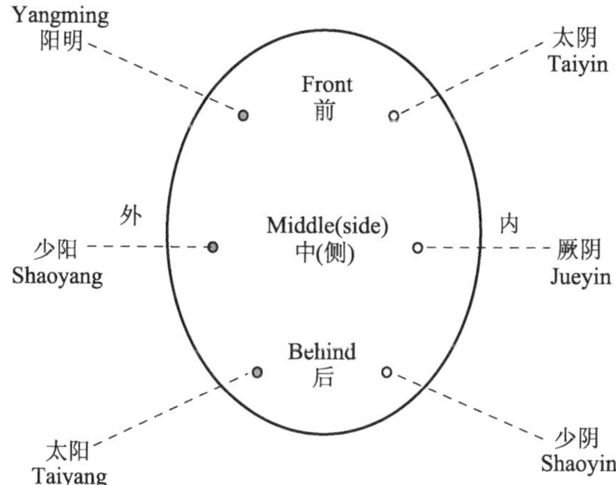

Fig.1-4 Distribution rules of fourteen meridians in cross section of the four limbs

图 1-4 十四经脉在四肢的分布规律(截面)

1.2.2 Internal course Inside the body, the twelve main meridians pertain to or communicate with the zang-fu organs. As regards the attribution of zang-fu organs, the zang-organs are attributed to yin, and the fu-organs to yang. The three yin meridians of the hand are associated with the chest and respectively pertain to the lung, pericardium and heart; the three yin meridians of the foot are associated with the abdomen and respectively pertain to the spleen, liver and kidney. The yang meridians connect with the fu-organs; the three yang meridians of the foot respectively pertain to the stomach, gallbladder and urinary bladder, and the three yang meridians of the hand respectively pertain to the large intestine, triple energizer and small intestine.

1.2.2 内行部分 在内部，十二经脉隶属于脏腑。脏腑中，脏为阴，腑为阳。手三阴经联系胸部，内属于肺、心包、心；足三阴经联系腹部，内属于脾、肝、肾。阳经属于腑，足三阳经内属于胃、胆、膀胱；手三阳经内属于大肠、三焦、小肠。

1.3 Exterior-interior relationship of the twelve main meridians

All the twelve main meridians internally pertain to the zang-fu organs; the yin meridians, attributed to the interior, pertain to the zang-organs and communicate with the fu-organs; the yang meridians, attributed to the exterior, pertain to the fu-organs and communicate with the zang-organs. The exterior-interior yin meridians and yang meridians are inter-related via "pertaining to" and "communicating with" relationship. For instance, the lung meridian of hand-taiyin pertains to the lung and communicates with the large intestine, whilst the large intestine meridian of hand yangming pertains to the small intestine and communicates with the lung. Thus six pairs of exteriorly-interiorly related meridians are formed: the lung meridian of hand-taiyin pairs with the large intestine meridian of hang yangming, the pericardium meridian of hand jueyin with

1.3 十二经脉的表里属络

十二经脉内属于脏腑，其中阴经为里，属脏络腑，阳经为表，属腑络脏。互为表里的阴经与阳经在体内有属络关系，如手太阴肺经属肺络大肠、手阳明大肠经属大肠络肺。十二经脉如此构成六对表里属络关系：手太阴肺经与手阳明大肠经，手厥阴心包经与手少阳三焦经，手少阴心经与手太阳小肠经，足太阴脾经与足阳明胃经，足厥阴肝经与足少阳胆经，足少阴肾经与足太阳膀胱经。经脉的表里关系还通过经别和络脉的表里沟通而得到加强。

the triple energizer meridian of hand shaoyang, the heart meridian of hand shaoyin with the small intestine meridian of hand shaoyang, the spleen meridian of foot taiyin with the stomach meridian of foot yangming, the liver meridian of foot jueyin with the gallbladder meridian of foot shaoyang, the kidney meridian of foot shaoyin with the bladder meridian of foot taiyang. The links between the exteriorly-interiorly related meridians can still be enhanced via the meridian divergencies and collaterals in the limbs.

1.4 Flow of the twelve main meridians

The twelve main meridians travel in a fixed order: The three yin meridians of the hand run from the chest to the hands, the three yang meridians of the hand from the hands to the head, the three yang meridians of the foot from the head to the feet, and the three yin meridians of the foot from the feet to the abdomen or chest. The circulation of qi and blood starts from the lung meridian of hand-taiyin, then to subsequent meridians, and finally comes to the liver meridian. The qi and blood again reach into the lung meridian from the liver meridian, restarting a new circulation. The twelve main meridians thus link up with one another to form a constant and cyclical flow of qi and blood, circulating with out a break. Furthermore, the twelve main meridians also connect with the governor vessel and conception vessel. The circulating order of qi and blood is shown in Table 1-1.

1.4 十二经脉的走向和流注

十二经脉的循行走向规律是:手三阴经从胸走手,手三阳经从手走头,足三阳经从头走足,足三阴经从足走腹(胸)。气血运行始于手太阴肺经,然后依次运行到肝经,自肝经上注肺,再返回至肺经,重新开始循环。十二经脉之间由此就可连贯起来,构成"如环无端"的气血流注关系,而且与前后正中的督脉和任脉也相通。这种流注关系如表 1-1 所示。

Table 1-1　The cyclical flow of qi in the fourteen meridians

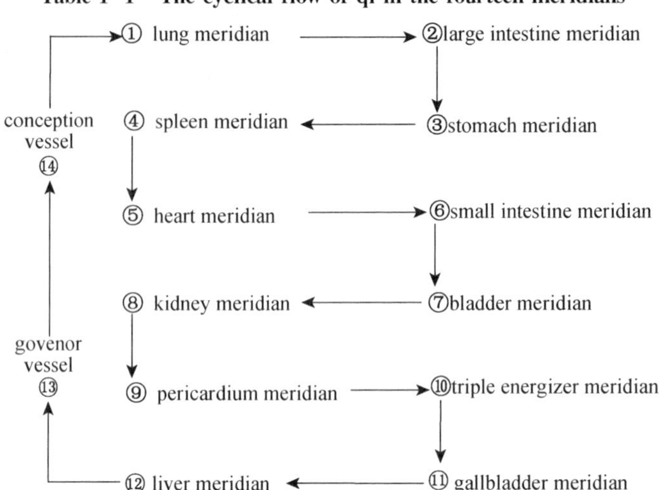

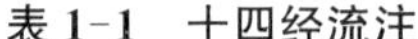

表 1-1　十四经流注

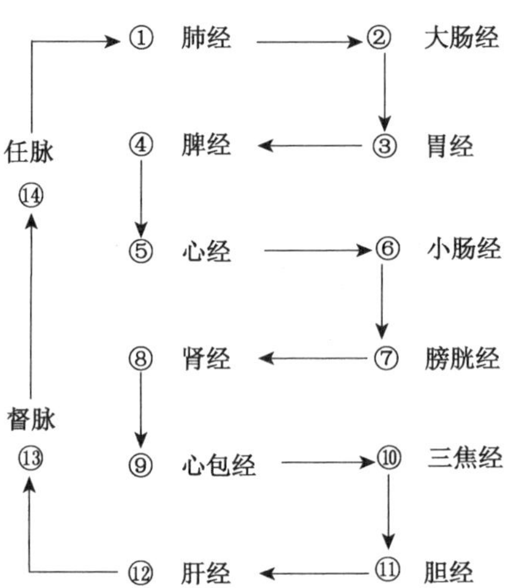

1.5　Connection of the twelve main meridians

The twelve main meridians meet and connect in following three fashions. See Table 1-2.

1.5　十二经脉的衔接

十二经脉之间通过以下三种形式相互衔接(表 1-2)。

Table 1-2 Meeting and connection of the twelve main meridians

lung
① lung meridian of Hand-Taiyin
index finger
nasal sides
② large intestine meridian of Hand-Yangming
③ stomach meridian of Foot-Yangming
big toe(medial aspect)
heart
④ spleen meridian of Foot-taiyin
⑤ heart meridian of Hand-Shaoyin
little finger
inner canthus
⑥ small intestine meridian of Hand-Taiyang
⑦ bladder meridian of Foot-Taiyang
little toe
chest
⑧ kidney meridian of Foot-Shaoyin
⑨ pericardium meridian of Hand-Jueyin
ring finger
outer canthus
⑩ triple energizer meridian of Hand-Shaoyang
⑪ gallbladder meridian of Foot-Shaoyang
big toe(lateral aspect)
lung
⑫ liver meridian of Foot-Jueyin

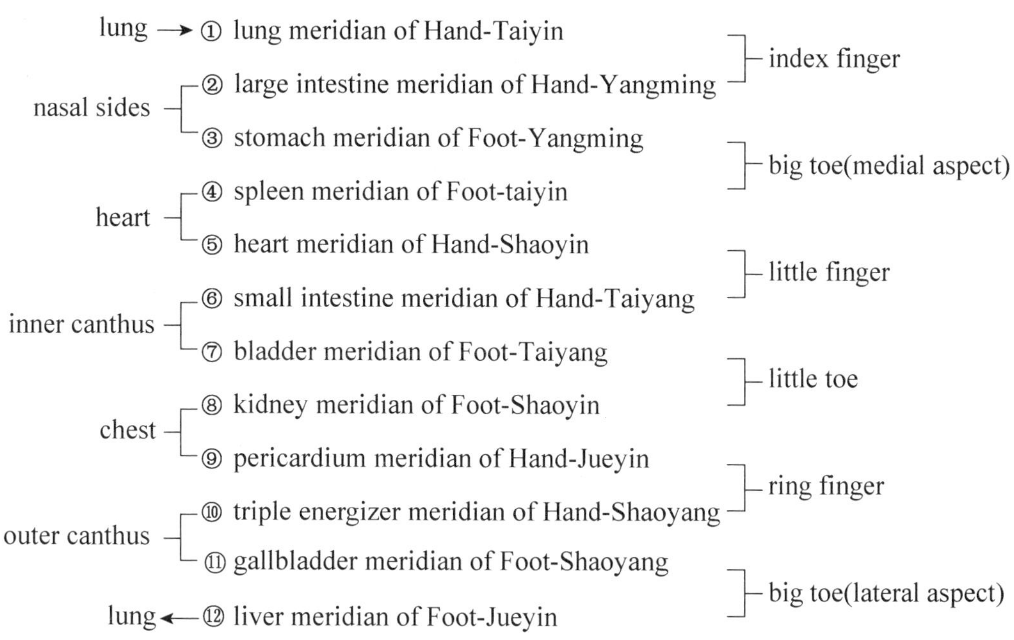

表 1-2 十二经脉的衔接

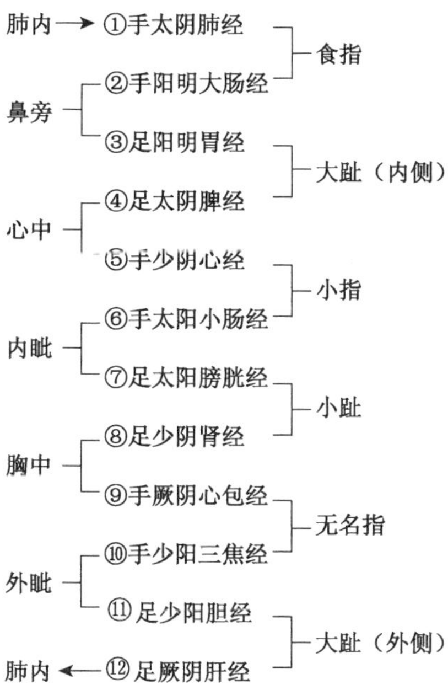

1.5.1 Yin meridians and yang meridians with exteriorly-interiorly relationship meet on the four limbs The lung meridian of hand-taiyin meets the large intestine meridian of hand yangming at the index finger; the heart meridian of hand shaoyin meets the small intestine meridian of hand taiyang at the little finger; the pericardium meridian of hand jueyin meets the triple energizer meridian of hand shaoyang at the ring finger; the stomach meridian of foot yangming meets the spleen meridian of foot taiyin at the medial aspect of the big toe; the bladder meridian of foot taiyang meets the kidney meridian of foot shaoyin at the little toe; the gallbladder meridian of foot shaoyang meets the liver meridian of foot jueyin at the lateral aspect of big toe.

1.5.1 阴经与阳经(表里经)在手足部衔接　手太阴肺经在食指与手阳明大肠经交接，手少阴心经在小指与手太阳小肠经连接，手厥阴心包经在无名指与手少阳三焦经衔接，足阳明胃经在足大趾(内侧)与足太阴脾经相接，足太阳膀胱经在足小趾与足少阴肾经相连，足少阳胆经在足大趾(外侧)与足厥阴肝经连接。

1.5.2 Yang meridians meet yang meridians bearing the same name on the head and face The large intestine meridian of hand yangming and the stomach meridian of foot yangming meet at the sides of the nose; the small intestine of hand taiyang and the bladder meridian of foot taiyang meet at the inner canthus; the triple energizer meridian of hand shaoyang and the gallbladder meridian of foot shaoyang meet at the outer canthus.

1.5.2 阳经与阳经(同名阳经)在头面部衔接　手阳明大肠经和足阳明胃经在鼻旁连接，手太阳小肠经与足太阳膀胱经在目内眦交接，手少阳三焦经和足少阳胆经在目外眦衔接。

1.5.3 Hand yin meridians and foot yin meridian meet in the chest The spleen meridian of the hand-taiyin meets the heart meridian of hand shaoyin at the heart; the kidney meridian of foot shaoyin meets the pericardium meridian of hand jueyin in the chest; the liver meridian of foot jueyin meets the lung meridian of hand-taiyin the lung.

1.5.3 阴经与阴经(手足阴经)在胸部衔接　足太阴脾经与手少阴心经交接于心中，足少阴肾经与手厥阴心包经交接于胸中，足厥阴肝经与手太阴肺经交接于肺中。

2 Eight extra meridians

2 奇经八脉

The eight extra meridians are governor vessel,

奇经八脉，包括督脉、任

conception vessel, thoroughfare vessel, belt vessel, yang heel vessel and yin heel vessel, yang link vessel and yin link vessel. They are unlike the twelve main meridians as none of them pertains to a zang-organ or fu-organ, or communicates with a zang-organ or fu-organ, and they are not exteriorly-interirorly related, with their particular pathways. These meridians, with special functions, act to govern and link other meridians, and regulate qi and blood.

The eight extra meridians crisscross with and are distributed among the twelve main meridians. The governor vessel runs along the midline of the back, and the conception vessel runs along the front midline. The governor vessel and conception vessel have their own acupoints, so these two vessels and twelve main meridians are collectively called "fourteen meridians". The acupoints of the thoroughfare vessel, belt vessel, heel vessels and link vessels are on the fourteen meridians. The thoroughfare vessel, communicating with the kidney meridian of foot shaoyin, runs along the first line lateral to the midline on the abdomen. The conception vessel, governor vessel and thoroughfare vessel all originate in the uterus and emerge from the perineum, therefore they are termed "three branches from the same origin". The belt vessel runs transversely around the waist like a belt and communicates with the acupoints of foot shaoyang meridian. The yang heel vessel runs along the lateral aspect of foot and shoulder to the head, and communicates with the acupoints of the foot taiyang meridian. The yin link vessel runs along the medial aspect of the foot up to the eyes, and communicates with the foot shaoyin meridian. The yang link vessel travels along the lat-

脉、冲脉、带脉、阳蹻脉和阴蹻脉、阳维脉和阴维脉，共八条经脉。它们与十二正经不同，既不直属脏腑，又无表里配合关系，"别道奇行"。这是具有特殊作用的经脉，对其余经络起统率、联络和调节气血盛衰的作用。

奇经八脉的分布部位与十二经脉纵横交互。督脉行于后正中线，任脉行于前正中线，任脉和督脉各有本经所属穴位，故与十二经相提并论，合称为"十四经"。其余的冲、带、蹻、维六脉的穴位均交会于十二经和任、督脉中。冲脉行于腹部第一侧线，交会足少阴肾经穴。任、督、冲三脉皆起于胞中，同出会阴而异行，称为"一源三歧"。带脉横斜地行于腰腹，交会足少阳经穴。阳蹻行于下肢外侧及肩、头部，交会足太阳等经穴。阴蹻行于下肢内侧及眼，交会足少阴经穴。阳维行于下肢外侧、肩和头项，交会足少阳等经及督脉穴。阴维行于下肢内侧、腹第三侧线和颈部，交会足少阴等经及任脉穴。

eral aspect of the leg up to the shoulder and nape, and communicates with the acupoints of the foot shaoyang meridian and the governor vessel. The yin link vessel travels along the medial aspect of the leg and the third line lateral to the front midline up to the neck, and communicates with the acupoints of foot shaoyin meridian and the conception vessel.

3　Fifteen collaterals

Each of the twelve main meridians, as well as the governor and conception vessels, has a collateral, and, along with the major collateral of the spleen, they are known collectively as "fifteen collaterals". The twelve collaterals of the twelve main meridians branch off from its luo-connecting and run towards their exteriorly-interiorly related meridians. The collaterals of the conception vessel, governor vessel and thoroughfare vessel respectively disperse in the abdomen, the head and lateral trunk. The twelve collaterals on the limbs have the functions of strengthening the relationship between exteriorly-interiorly related meridians, and make up for the limited course of their meridians; the other three collaterals function to accumulate and regulate qi and blood.

3　十五络脉

十二经脉在四肢部各分出一络，再加躯干前的任脉络、躯干后的督脉络及躯干侧的脾之大络，共十五条，称"十五络脉"。十二络脉在四肢部从相应络穴分出后均走向相应的表里经，躯干部三络则分别分布于身前、身后和身侧。四肢部的十二络，主要起沟通表里两经和补充经脉循行不足的作用；躯干部的三络，起渗灌气血的作用。

4　Twelve meridian divergencies

The twelve meridian divergencies branch off from the main meridians and run deep into the body. In its distribution, the twelve meridian divergencies have their own features, separating, entering, resurfacing and joining. Separating refers to the branching from the twelve main meridians; entering means the entrance of the meridian divergencies into the thoracic and abdominal cavities; resur-

4　十二经别

十二经别，是十二经脉别行深入体腔的支脉，又称"别行之正经"。十二经别有"离、入、出、合"的分布特点。从十二经脉分出称"离"；进入胸腹腔称"入"；在头项部浅出体表称"出"；出于头颈部后，阳经经别合于原经脉，

facing refers to the coming-out of the meridian divergencies to the body surface on the face and neck; joining means that the meridian divergencies of the yang meridians connect with its yang meridians, while the meridian divergencies of the yin meridians connect with its exteriorly-interiorly related yang meridians, for instance, the meridian divergency of hand yangming joins with the hand yangming meridian and the meridian divergency of hand-taiyin also joins with the hand yangming meridian. Thus the twelve meridian divergencies, six yin meridian divergencies and six yang meridian divergencies, can be paired in light of their interior-exterior relationship into six convergences. By the course of separating, entering, resurfacing and joining, these meridian divergencies strengthen the linkage between the exteriorly-interiorly related meridians as well as between the meridians and zang-fu organs. They make closer relationship between the twelve main meridians and the heart and head, extend the pathways of the main meridians, and widen the indications of meridians and acupoints.

阴经经别合于相表里的阳经经脉称"合",如手阳明经别合于手阳明经脉,手太阴经别也合于手阳明经脉。手足三阴三阳经别,按阴阳表里关系组成六对,称为"六合"。经别通过离、入、出、合的分布,加强了表里两经及经脉与脏腑的联系,突出了心和头的重要性,扩大了经脉的循行联系和经穴的主治范围。

Both the collaterals and meridian divergencies are branches from the main meridians to strengthen the interrelationship between the exterior-interior meridians. The meridian divergencies govern the interior of the body, and have no acupoints and indications; while the collaterals control the exterior of the body, each of which has one luo-connecting acupoint and its indications. Apart from the fifteen collaterals, other collaterals are named in accordance with its shape, thickness and distribution depth; those which run superficially are known as "superficial collaterals", their minute branches are

络脉和经别都是经脉的分支,均有加强表里两经的作用。但经别主内,无所属穴位,也无所主病证;络脉则主外,各有一络穴,并有所主病证。络脉按其形状、大小、深浅等的不同又有不同的名称,浮行于浅表的络脉称"浮络",最细小的络脉称"孙络",细小的血管称"血络"。

known as "minute collateral", and those small vessels are known as "blood collaterals".

5 Twelve meridian sinews

The twelve meridian sinews are the peripheral connecting parts of the twelve main meridians at muscles, tendons and joints, and generally follow the external courses of the twelve main meridians. Accordingly, the meridian sinews are classified, as the distribution of the twelve main meridians, into three yin meridian sinews of hand, three yin meridian sinews of foot, three yang meridian sinews of hand and three yang meridian sinews of foot. The meridian sinews originate from the extremities of the limbs, gather at the bones and joints; some of them enter into the thoracic and abdominal cavities, but they do not directly connect with the internal organs as the main meridians do. The meridian sinews of the yang meridians gather at the head, the meridian sinews of the three yin meridians of hand at the chest, and the meridian sinews of the three yin meridians of foot at the genital region. The meridian sinews possess the function of controlling the bones and joint movements to ensure the normal motion and posture of the human body.

5 十二经筋

十二经筋，是指与十二经脉相应的筋肉部分，其分布范围与十二经脉大体一致。全身筋肉按经络分布部位同样分成手足三阴三阳。经筋均起于四肢末端，结聚于骨骼和关节部位，有的进入胸腹腔，但不像经脉那样属络脏腑。手足三阳之经筋都到达头面，手三阴之经筋到胸膈，足三阴之经筋到阴部。经筋的作用是约束骨骼，活动关节，保持人体正常的运动功能，维持人体正常的体位姿势。

6 Twelve cutaneous regions

The twelve cutaneous regions are the skin portion within the domains of the twelve main meridians, where the twelve main meridians and their collaterals distribute. The cutaneous regions are also categorized into three yin cutaneous regions of hand, three yin cutaneous regions of foot, three yang cutaneous regions of hand and three yang cutaneous regions of foot. The cutaneous regions are the

6 十二皮部

十二皮部，是指与十二经脉相应的皮肤部分，属十二经脉及其络脉的散布部位。体表皮肤也按手足三阴三阳划分。这是十二经脉在体表的功能活动部位，也是络脉之气散布之所在。皮部位于人体最外层，是机体的

sites through which the functional activities of the twelve main meridians manifest and the collateral qi distributes. Since the cutaneous regions are the most superficial part of the body tissues, they bear the protective function of the organism. In *Essential Questions*(Su Wen), it is said that the exo-genous pathogens may penetrate the skin into zang-fu organs through meridians and result in diseases, and that the diseases in the zang-fu organs and meridians may also reflect on the cutaneous regions. Thereby, surface examination and treatment may infer and treat the diseases inside the body. The cutaneous regions function to protect the body from external pathogens, reflect diseases and help diagnosis. Skin acupuncture, collateral-needling therapy and ointment application are the clinical application of cutaneous regions.

卫外屏障。《素问·皮部论》指出，邪气可经皮→络→经→腑→脏的途径入侵机体而致病；脏腑、经络的病变也可反映到皮部。因此通过外部的诊察和施治可推断和治疗内部的疾病。皮部具有抗御外邪、保卫机体和反映病候、协助诊断的作用。临床上皮肤针、刺络、敷贴等疗法，就是皮部理论的应用。

Section 2 Origin and Termination, Root and Branch, Qi Street and Four Seas in Meridian Theory

第2节 经络的根结、标本、气街和四海

Origin and termination, root and branch, qi street and four seas are some theories that describe the vertical or horizontal relationship of meridians to clarify the rules in common, consequently to guide clinical syndrome differentiation and acupoint selection. The origin-termination and root-branch theories analyze the vertical relationships between the meridians, while the qi-street and four-sea theories analyze the horizontal relationships of meridians from a wider range. These four theories are in-

根结、标本、气街和四海是关于经络纵横关系的理论，它是从各经的纵向或横向方面阐述若干规律性的认识，以指导临床辨证和用穴。根结和标本，主要分析经络的纵向关系，气街和四海主要从大范围分析经络的横向关系，其间又是相互联系的。

ter-related.

1 Origin and termination

Origin and termination, *gen* and *jie* in Chinese, refer to the originating and gathering sites of the qi of the twelve main meridians. Origin, meaning the starting place, lies in the Jing-Well points at the extremities of the limbs; termination, meaning the gathering and accumulating place, lies in certain parts of the head, chest and abdomen. The origin and termination of the six foot meridians are presented in Table 1-3.

1 根结

"根"和"结",是指十二经脉之气起始和归结的部位。根,有起始的含义,此指四肢末端的井穴;结,是结聚、归结的意思,在头、胸、腹部。足六经根结部位见表1-3。

Table 1-3　The origin and termination of the six foot meridians

Meridian	Root	Termination
Foot-Taiyang meridian	Zhiyin (BL 67)	Mingmen(eye)
Foot-Yangming meridian	Lidui(ST 45)	Hangsang(nasal pharynx)
Foot-Shaoyang meridian	Qiaoyin (GB 44)	Chuanglong(ear)
Foot-Taiyin meridian	Yinbai(SP 1)	Taicang(stomach)
Foot-Shaoyin meridian	Yongquan (KI 1)	Lianquan(beneath the tongue)
Foot-Jueyin meridian	Dadun(LV 1)	Yuying(yutang), connecting Danzhong

表1-3　足六经根结部位表

经名	根	结
足太阳	至阴	命门(目)
足阳明	厉兑	颃颡(鼻咽)
足少阳	窍阴	窗笼(耳)
足太阴	隐白	太仓(胃)
足少阴	涌泉	廉泉(舌下)
足厥阴	大敦	玉英(玉堂),络膻中

The origin-termination theory, illustrating the relationship of meridian qi movement between the upper and lower bodies, regards the extremities of

根结理论说明了经气活动的上下联系,强调以四肢末端为出发点,着重经气循

limbs as the starting places of meridian qi, and concentrates on the gathering places of meridian qi circulation. This theory stresses the vital role of the limb acupoints on the head, chest and abdomen from the therapeutic perspectives.

行的根源与归结,强调四肢腧穴对于头、胸、腹部的重要作用。

2 Root and branch

Root and branch, *ben* and *biao* in Chinese, signify the correspondent relationship of meridians between the upper and lower parts. Branch, originally meaning the tip of trees, refers to such upper body as head, chest and back; root, originally meaning the part of plant in the soil, refers to the limbs. The root and branch of the twelve main meridians are presented in Table 1-4.

2 标本

"标"和"本",是指经脉的上下对应关系。"标",原意指树梢,此指人体上部的头面胸背部位。"本",原意指树根,此指人体下部的四肢部。十二经标本部位见表1-4。

Both root-branch theory and origin-termination theory detail the mutual relationship between the limbs and the head and trunk. The limbs are taken as the origin and root, and the head and trunk as the termination and branch. The origin specifically refers to the Jing-Well acupoint, and the root refers to some places below the elbows and knees; the termination refers to the head, chest and abdomen, and the branch covers the acupoints of the back. In *Inner Classic*(Nei Jing), the origin and termination are described just for the six foot meridians, and the root and branch are described for all the twelve meridians, with a wider range in the latter.

标本与根结两者都是论述四肢与头面躯干之间的相互关系,以四肢为"根"、为"本",以头面躯干为结、为标。"根"专指井穴,"本"则扩及四肢肘膝以下的一定部位;"结"在头、胸、腹部,"标"扩及背部的背俞。《内经》论根结仅以足六经为代表,论标本则有手足六经,范围更为广泛。

Origin-termination theory and root-branch theory are similar in connotation. Both theories hold that the meridian qi originates from the limbs, which are regarded as the origin and root; that the meridian qi reaches the head and trunk, which are regarded as the termination and branch. Both the

根结和标本理论在意义上大体是一致的,都是强调经气之"源"在四肢,以此为"根"、为"本";而其"流"在头面躯干,以此为"结"、为"标"。根结、标本理论主要

theories principally detail the therapeutic effects of the acupoints below the elbows and knees on the distant head and trunk, which helps clinical acupoint selection.

阐明四肢肘膝以下的经穴对头面躯干远隔部位的重要治疗作用，从而指导临床取穴。

Table 1-4　The root and branch of the twelve main meridians

Meridian	Root	Acupoint	Branch	Acupoint
Foot-Taiyang	5 cun superior to heel	Fuyang (BL 59)	Mingmen(eye)	Jingming (BL 1)
Foot-Shaoyang	Zuqiaoyin (GB 44)	Zuqiaoyin (GB 44)	Chuanglong (anterior ear)	Tinghui (BL 2)
Foot-Yangming	Lidui(ST 45)	Lidui(ST 45)	Renying (ST 9), cheek, hangsang	Renying(ST 9), Dicang(ST 4)
Foot-Taiyin	4 cun anterior and Superior to Zhongfeng(LR 4)	Sanyinjiao(SP 6)	Back-Shu acupoints, Tongue root	Pishu (BL 20), Lianquan(CV 23)
Foot-Shaoyin	2 cun superior to the medial malleolus	Jiaoxin (KI 8)	Back-Shu acupoints, sublingual veins	Shenshu (BL 23), Lianquan(CV 23)
Foot-Jueyin	5 cun superior to Xingjian (LR 2)	Zhongfeng(LR 4)	Back-Shu acupoints	Ganshu (BL 18)
Hand-Taiyang	Posterior to the lateral malleolus of the hand	Yanglao(SI 6)	1 cun superior to eyes	Cuanzhu (GB 2)
Hand-Shaoyang	2 cun superior to the interspace of the little and ring fingers	Zhongzhu(TE 3)	Posterior-anterior corner of the ear, inferior to the outer canthus	Sizhukong(TE 23)
Hand-Yangming	Near the elbow, up to bie yang	Quchi(LI 11) Binao(LI 14)	Inferior to cheek and superior to he qian	Futu(LI 18)
Hand-Taiyin	Wrist pulse	Taiyuan(LU 9)	Arteries in the armpit	Zhongfu(LU 1)
Hand-Shaoyin	Top of the pisiform bone of the hand	Shenmen (HT 7)	Back-Shu points	Xinshu (GB 15)
Hand-Jueyin	2 cun posterior to the wrist and between the two tendons	Neiguan (PC 6)	3 cun inferior to the armpit	Tianchi (PC 1)

表 1-4 十二经标本部位表

经 名	本 部	相应穴	标 部	相应穴
足太阳	足跟上 5 寸	跗阳	命门(目)	睛明
足少阳	足窍阴之间	足窍阴	窗笼(耳前)	听会
足阳明	厉兑	厉兑	人迎、颊、颃颡	人迎、地仓
足太阴	中封前上 4 寸	三阴交	背俞、舌本	脾俞、廉泉
足少阴	内踝上 2 寸	交信	背俞、舌下两脉	肾俞、廉泉
足厥阴	行间上 5 寸	中封	背俞	肝俞
手太阳	手外踝之后	养老	命门(目)上一寸	攒竹
手少阳	小指次指间上 2 寸	中渚	耳后上角,下外眦	丝竹空
手阳明	肘骨中,上至别阳	曲池、臂臑	颊下合钳上	扶突
手太阴	寸口之中	太渊	腋内动脉处	中府
手少阴	锐骨之端	神门	背俞	心俞
手厥阴	掌后两筋间 2 寸中	内关	腋下三寸	天池

3 Qi street

Qi street is the pathway where the meridian qi flows and spreads over the head and trunk. In Ling shu, it states that, "there exists a passage for the qi in the chest, a passage for the qi in the abdomen, a passage for the qi in the head and a passage for the qi in the shin. The qi in the head converges at the brain; the qi in the chest converges at the greater pectoral muscles and Back-Shu points; the qi in the abdomen converges at the Back-Shu points, the thoroughfare vessel and the arteries beside the navel; the qi in the shin converges at the major passage inferior to Chengshan(BL 57) and above the ankle."

Qi street, the common pathway for meridian qi circulation in the head, chest, abdomen and shin, signifies the transverse linkage between the meridians and is the passage where the meridian qi transversely pours and the zang-fu-organ qi spreads for-

3 气街

气街是经气在头面躯干部横斜扩散的通路。《灵枢·卫气》记载:"胸气有街,腹气有街,头气有街,胫气有街。故气在头者,止之于脑;气在胸者,止之膺与背俞;气在腹者,止之背俞与冲脉于脐左右之动脉者;气在胫者,止之于气街与承山踝上以下。"

气街,主要说明头、胸、腹、胫这些部位是经气循行的共同通道,说明了经络的横向联系,是经气横向输注及脏腑之气前后布散的路

wards and backwards, which provides theoretical evidences for clinical acupoints combination.

径，为临床处方配穴提供了理论依据。

4　Four seas

The four seas are the collective term for the seas of the marrow, the blood, the qi and the foodstuffs. In Ling Shu, it states that, "The stomach is the sea of the foodstuffs, and the stomach qi flows upwards to Qichong(ST 30) and downwards to Zusanli(ST 36); the thoroughfare vessel is the sea of the twelve main meridians, and its qi flows upwards to Dazhu(BL 11) and downwards to Shangjuxu(ST 37) and Xiajuxu(ST 39); Danzhong is the sea of qi, and its qi flows upwards to Dazhui(GV 14) and forwards to Renying(ST 9); the brain is the sea of the marrow, and its qi flows upwards to Baihui(GV 20) and downwards to Fengfu(GV 16)." Ling Shu also describes the conditions due to the excess and insufficiency of the four seas, which provides an important guidance in acupuncture practice.

4　四海

四海，即髓海、血海、气海、水谷之海的总称。《灵枢·海论》指出："胃者，水谷之海，其输上在气街（气冲），下至三里；冲脉者，为十二经之海，其输上在于大杼，下出于巨虚之上下廉（上、下巨虚）；膻中者，为气之海，其输上在于柱骨之上下（大椎），前在于人迎；脑为髓之海，其输上在于盖（百会），下在风府。"《灵枢·海论》还描述了四海有余、不足的有关病候，对针灸临床有重要指导意义。

There is some consistency among the four seas, qi street, termination and branch. The meridian qi starts from the origin and root, and gathers at the termination and branch, and spreads through qi street to form the four seas.

四海与"气街""结""标"有其一致性。经气从"根""本"部汇集到"结""标"部时，通过气街的弥散形成四海。

Section 3　Physiological Functions of Meridians and Clinical Application of Meridian Theory

第 3 节　经络的作用及经络理论的临床应用

The meridian theory not only places an important role in the basic theory of Chinese medicine, and its significance also manifests in the clinical ap-

经络学说不仅在中医基础理论中居重要地位，经络理论的意义还体现在中医各

plication of Chinese medical subjects. The meridian theory and clinical practice complement with each other, specifically, the meridian theory can guide the clinical practice, and the clinical practice can improve and develop the meridian theory.

1 Physiological functions of the meridians

In Ling Shu, it states that, "the meridian can be applied to judge whether one is healthy or dying, manage hundreds of diseases, and regulate deficiency and excess conditions of the body. Therefore, the meridian theory must be mastered." This statement generalizes the importance of meridian system in physiology, pathology and therapeutics. Judgment of whether one is healthy or dying depends on meridian's functions to connect the exterior with the interior, and to transport qi and blood; management of diseases depends on meridian's functions to protect exogenous influences and reflect the symptoms and signs of diseases; regulation of excess and deficiency conditions depends on meridian's functions to conduct the needling sensation.

1.1 Linking zang-organs with fu organs, and connecting interior with exterior

All tissues such as internal organs, limbs and joints, sense organs and orifices, skin and tendons have different physiological functions. However, they are mutually related and cooperated to form an holistic organism and maintain coordination. This is accomplished primarily by the connecting functions of the meridian system. The twelve main meridians and meridian divergencies primarily connect the body surface with internal organs, and connect zang-organs with fu-organs; the twelve main meridi-

科的临床应用中。经络理论与临床实践是相互结合的，经络理论可指导临床实践，而临床实践可不断完善、发展经络理论。

1 经络的作用

《灵枢·经脉》指出："经脉者，所以决死生，处百病，调虚实，不可不通。"这概括地说明了经络系统在生理、病理和疾病防治等方面的重要性。其所以能决定人的生和死，是因为其具有联系人体内外和运行气血的作用；处治百病，是因其具有抗御病邪、反映证候的作用；调整虚实，是因其具有传导感应而起补虚泻实的作用。

1.1 联系脏腑，沟通内外

人体的五脏六腑、四肢百骸、五官九窍、皮肉筋骨等组织器官，虽有各自不同的生理功能，但又互相联系，互相配合，使人体构成一个有机的整体，保持协调统一。这主要是依靠经络系统的联络沟通而实现的。十二经脉及经别着重于人体体表与脏腑，以及脏腑间的联系；十二

ans and fifteen collaterals primarily strengthen the connection between the parts on body surface, and between the body surface and zang-fu organs; the eight extra meridians strengthen the relationship between the twelve main meridians; the origin and termination, root and branch of the twelve main meridians, qi street and four seas strengthen the relationship between the front and back parts of the head and trunk.

经脉和十五络脉,着重于体表与体表,以及体表与脏腑间的联系;十二经脉通过奇经八脉,加强了经与经之间的联系;十二经的根结、标本、气街和四海,则加强了人体头面躯干之前后腹背的分段联系。

1.2 Transporting qi and blood, harmonizing yin and yang

In Ling Shu, it states that, "meridian serves to conduct qi and blood, functioning to nourish yin and yang, strengthening tendons and bones, and lubricating the joints." This statement shows that the meridians function to conduct qi and blood to nourish the human body and to harmonize yin and yang. Qi and blood, the material foundation for all activities of the human body, are transported to all parts of the body through meridians. And, the organs and tissues can exert their physiological functions only after they are nourished by qi and blood. Through meridians, qi and blood come internally to the organs and externally to the body surface(Ling Shu). Via the linkage of meridians, the amount of qi and blood and the body functions are maintained to be in a dynamic balance, as Su Wen states, "when yin and yang are in balance, the body spirit maintains excellent".

1.2 运行气血,协调阴阳

《灵枢·本藏》指出,"经脉者,所以行血气而营阴阳,濡筋骨,利关节者也",说明经络具有运行气血、濡养周身和协调阴阳的作用。气血是人体生命活动的物质基础。气血在全身各部的输布有赖于经络的运行。人体各个脏腑组织器官得气血的濡养后才能发挥其正常生理作用,而气血必须经过经络输布于周身内外,"内溉脏腑,外濡腠理"(《灵枢·脉度》)。在经络的联系下,气血盛衰和机能动静保持相对平衡,使人体"阴平阳秘,精神乃治"(《素问·生气通天论》)。

1.3 Fighting pathogenic factors and manifesting symptoms

Meridians function to fight the pathogenic factors and manifest the symptoms of diseases. The minor collaterals of meridians distribute extensively

1.3 抗御病邪,反映证候

经络具有抗御病邪、反映证候的作用。经络中的孙络分布广而浅表,是机体的

and superficially, and serve as the barrier to protect the body. Meridians are also approaches of pathogenic factors to the body. The pathogenic factors invade the body gradually from the minor collaterals to collaterals, meridians and zang-fu organs. Su Wen: "When the pathogenic factors attack the body, they first invade the skin, then the collaterals, meridians, zang-fu organs and finally spread into the stomach and intestine." The pathological changes of zang-fu organs can be manifested on the body surface via the meridians, which is of great value in clinical diagnosis.

卫外屏障。经络又是外邪入侵的途径,外邪可经孙络、络脉、经脉、脏腑之途径由表及里,逐步深入。《素问·缪刺论》说的"夫邪之客于形也,必先舍于皮毛,留而不去,入舍于孙脉,留而不去,入舍于络脉,留而不去,入舍于经脉,内连五脏,散于肠胃",即是此意。脏腑的病理变化也可经经络途径由内而外地反映到体表,这对临床诊断有重要应用价值。

1.4 Transmitting sensation and regulating deficiency and excess

In needling, such phenomena as qi arrival, qi movement and qi transmission to the affected areas are the manifestations of the meridians, transmitting sensation. Needling sensation is crucial to achieve good clinical efficacy in acupuncture treatment, while the needling sensation is transmitted through the meridians, hence the needling sensation to the affected areas can regulate the deficiency and excess.

1.4 传导感应,调整虚实

针刺时的"得气""行气"和"气至病所"现象是经络传导感应的表现。针刺感应是针刺取得疗效的关键,而针感是通过经络传导的,针感循经络通路最终到达病变部位而起调整虚实的作用。

2 Clinical application of meridian theory

Clinically, meridian theory is used in diagnosis and treatment. In diagnosis, the meridian theory is employed in meridian examination and meridian differentiation; and in treatment it is employed in acupoint selection along the meridians and herbal tropism to meridians.

2 经络理论的临床应用

经络理论的临床应用可体现在诊断和治疗两个方面。诊断方面包括经络诊法和分经辨证;治疗方面包括循经取穴和分经用药。

2.1 Meridian examination

The methods of examining meridians consist of inspecting, nailing, stroking, pressing, observing the changes of local areas and the excess of qi and blood. In disease diagnosis, the skin appearance and color, or marked positive objects such as nodes and streaks along the pathways of meridians help diagnose the diseases. Recently, some objective detection methods were introduced, such as skin temperature, skin electrical resistance and infrared thermal detection. These detection methods are diversified, objectified and modernized.

Pulse taking along the meridians is previously the main content of meridian examination. For example, In Ling Shu, pulse in Cunkou was employed to judge the excess and deficiency of the yin meridians, and pulse in Renying to judge the excess and deficiency of the yang meridians. Because of abundant qi in the yangming meridian, its conditions can be judged by taking Fuyang pulse; the conditions of kidney qi can be judged by taking Taixi pulse.

Regional collateral examination is to observe the color of skin blood vessels, hence to differentiate the pain, blockage, cold and heat conditions. Recently-developed rash differentiation is also a collateral examination.

Tenderness examination is particularly important in acupuncture practice. In Ling Shu, it states, “pressure at the tenderness points can relieve pain.” Taking the tenderness points as acupoints is actually

2.1 经络诊法

对经络部位进行诊察的方法，包括审查、指切、推循、扪摸、按压，以及对局部寒温和气血盛衰现象的观察。经络外诊多用直接的检查。在诊察某些疾病的过程中，常可发现在经络循行路线上有皮肤形态、色泽的变化，或有明显的结节、条索状物等阳性反应物，这些都有助于对疾病的诊断。近代又采用一些客观的检测方法，如皮肤温度、皮肤电阻、红外热象等检测，使探测方法更趋于多样化、客观化和现代化。

分经切脉，原是经络诊法的主要内容。例如：《灵枢》以寸口脉诊候阴经病证的虚实，人迎脉诊候阳经病证的虚实。又以阳明脉气最盛，其下部可诊候冲阳（趺阳）脉，肾气盛衰则可诊候太溪脉。

分部诊络，是诊察皮部血络的色泽，以辨痛、痹、寒、热等。近人的皮疹辨证，也属诊络法。

压痛的检查，对临床取穴尤为重要。《灵枢·背腧》说：“按其处，应在中而痛解（懈）。”这种以痛为腧的取穴方法，实

meridian examination.

际上也是一种经络诊法。

2.2 Meridian differentiation

The acupoints of the twelve main meridians can treat the disorders in association with the main meridians. The indications of each meridian include the disorders along the pathways of meridians and those related to their zang-fu organs. Besides, the collaterals and muscle sinews have their own indications; and the manifestations along the cutaneous regions are actually the external symptoms of meridian disorders. Intersecting with the main meridians, the eight extra meridians have their particular indications. In clinical practice, the disorders are differentiated to a meridian in accordance with meridian pathways and relevant zang-fu organs. Meridian differentiation principally focuses on the twelve main meridians and the eight extra meridians.

Meridian differentiation to observe the excess or deficiency, and adversity or depletion of meridian qi helps determine the focus and judge the nature, severity, development and prognosis of a disease, which is of great significance in clinical diagnosis and treatment.

2.2 分经辨证

十二经穴能主治其所发生的病证，这就是经脉的主病。各经脉既有其循行所过部位的外经病（证），又有其有关的脏腑病（证）。此外，络脉、经筋也各有主病；皮部病证实际上是经络病候的综合反映。奇经八脉与各经相交会，其所主病证又有其特殊性。临床上可根据所出现的病证，结合经络循行部位及所联系的脏腑进行辨证归经。分经辨证，主要分十二经（合为六经）和奇经八脉。

通过分经辨证对经气虚实、经气厥逆甚或经气终厥等证候的观察，可明确病位，了解疾病的性质、程度、发展和预后，对疾病的诊断和治疗有重要意义。

2.3 Acupoint selection along meridians

Acupoint selection along meridians, a common and essential acupoint-selecting method, is to select the distal acupoints of related meridians on the basis of meridian theory and meridian differentiation. In *Ode to Four Acupoints* (Si Zong Xue Ge), it states, "abdominal disorders can be treated with Zusanli (ST 36), back disorders with Weizhong (BL 40), head and neck disorders with Lieque (LU 7), and face disorders with Hegu (LI 4)." These are typical of acupoint selec-

2.3 循经取穴

循经取穴，是以经络理论为指导，通常是在分经辨证的基础上，选用病变相关经脉的远道经穴，是针灸临床上的常用和基本取穴方法。《四总穴歌》所说的"肚腹三里留，腰背委中求，头项寻列缺，面口合谷收"，是典型的循经取穴。

tion along meridian.

2.4 Herbal tropism to meridians

In Chinese materia medica, each herb is thought to enter one or several meridians in light of its actions and indications, which is simplified as herbal tropism to meridian theory. This theory is developed on the basis of meridian differentiation. Since a disorder can be differentiated and attributed to some meridians, the herb effective against the disorder can be thought to enter one or several meridians. *Medical Origin and Development* (Yi Xue Yuan Liu Lun), by Xu Lingtai in the Qing Dynsaty, recorded that "an herb is considered to enter one meridian on account of its effectiveness for the disorders of one meridian". As matter of fact, herbal tropism to meridians signifies that one herb can treat the disorders in relation to one or several meridians, and is the result of analyzing and categorizing the herbal indications on meridian theory.

Meridians and collaterals not only exert vital role in regulating the physiological functions of human body, but also illustrate the pathological changes and guide meridian differentiation and acupuncture treatment.

2.4 药物归经

药物按其主治性能归入某经或某几经,简称药物归经。此说是在分经辨证的基础上发展而来,因病证可以分经,主治某些病证的药物也就成为某经或某几经之药。清代徐灵胎《医学源流论》说:"因其能治何经之病,后人即指为何经之药。"可见,药物归经实际上是指某药能主治某经或某几经所属的病证,是运用经络理论对药物性能进行的分析和归类。

经络不仅在人体生理功能的调控上具有重要作用,而且是临床上说明人体病理变化,指导辨证归经和针灸治疗的重要理论依据。

Chapter 2 General Introduction to Acupoints

第 2 章 腧穴总论

Acupoints, *shu* and *xue* in Chinese characters, are specific sites through which the qi of zang-fu organs and meridians is transported to the body surface. *Shu* means transportation and *xue* means hole. In Nei Jing, acupoint is also named as "joining site", "meeting site", "qi hole", "qi house" and "bone valley". Acupoints are the sites where disorders manifest, and also the places where acupuncture and moxibustion are applied for treatment. Acupoints are in close relationship to zang-fu organs and meridians. Acupoints are on meridians, and meridians link with the zang-fu organs, hence the acupoints are associated with the internal zang-fu organs.

腧穴是人体脏腑经络之气血输注于体表的特殊部位。腧，又作"俞"，通"输"，有输注、转输的意思；穴，指孔隙、空窍。腧穴在《内经》中又有"节""会""气穴""气府""骨空"等名称。腧穴既是疾病的反映处，也是针灸的施术部位。腧穴与脏腑、经络有密切关系。腧穴归于经络，经络属于脏腑，所以腧穴与脏腑内外相通。

Section 1 Classification and Nomenclature of Acupoints

第 1 节 腧穴的分类和命名

1 Classification of acupoints

Acupoints fall into three categories: meridian acupoints, extraordinary acupoints and Ashi acupoints.

1 腧穴的分类

腧穴通常分为经穴、奇穴和阿是穴三类。

1.1 Meridian acupoints

Acupoints of the twelve main meridians, conception vessel and governor vessel are collectively termed "fourteen meridian acupoints", simply called "meridian acupoints". These acupoints are on the pathways of the fourteen meridians, and have definite name, fixed location and specific indications. In Nei Jing, it mentioned 365 acupoints, but there were about 160 acupoints with the names; 349 acupoints were recorded in *A-B Canon of Acupunture and Moxibustion*(Zhen Jiu Jia Yi Jing) and *Supplement to Thousand Ducat Prescriptions*(Qian Jin Yi Fang); 354 acupoints were recorded in *Illustraled of Acupuncture and Bronze Points on the Bronze Model* (Tong Ren Shu Xue Zhen Jiu Tu Jing) and *Elucidation of the Fourteen Meridians* (Shi Si Jing Fa Hui) in the Song Dynasty; 359 acupoints were recorded in *Great Compendium of Acupuncture and Moxibustion* (Zhen Jiu Da Cheng) in the Ming Dynasty; till the Qing Dynasty, acupoints were up to 361 in *Complement to Acupuncture and Moxibustion*(Zhen Jiu Feng Yuan), which is the total number today.

1.1 经穴

凡归属于十二经脉和任脉、督脉的腧穴，亦即归属于十四经的穴位，总称"十四经穴"，简称"经穴"。经穴都有具体的穴名和固定的位置，分布在十四经循行路线上，有明确的针灸主治病证。《内经》多处提到"三百六十五穴"之数，但实际其载有穴名者约160穴；经穴专书《针灸甲乙经》载古代《明堂孔穴针灸治要》共349穴（《千金翼方》所载相同）；宋代《铜人腧穴针灸图经》（《十四经发挥》同）穴数有所增加，穴名数达354个；明代《针灸大成》载有359穴；至清代《针灸逢源》，经穴总数才达361个，目前经穴总数即以此为准。

1.2 Extraordinary acupoints

The extraordinary acupoints (or extra points) are the empirical points with specific names and definite locations, but not as yet assigned into the fourteen meridians. Extraordinary acupoints originate from Ashi acupoints, and have fewer indications but excellent therapeutic effects in treating certain diseases; for instance, Bailao(EX-HN 15) is quite effective for scrofula, and Sifeng(EX-UE 10) for infantile malnutrition. Some extraordinary acupoints are not single point but the combination of several acupoints, such as Shixuan(EX- UE 11),

1.2 奇穴

凡未归入十四经穴范围，而有具体的位置和名称的经验效穴，统称"经外奇穴"，简称"奇穴"。奇穴是在"阿是穴"的基础上发展起来的，这类腧穴的主治范围比较单一，多数对某些病证有特殊疗效，如百劳穴治瘰疬、四缝穴治小儿疳积等。有的奇穴并不是指一个穴位，而是多个穴位的组合，如十宣、

Baxie(EX-UE 9), Bafeng(EX-LE 10) and Huatuo Jiaji(EX-B 2). Some extraordinary acupoints are actually meridian acupoints; for example, Baomen (EX) and Zihu(EX) are actually Shuidao(ST 38), Sihua(EX) are actually Danshu(BL 19) and Geshu (BL 17), Jiulao(EX) is actually Xinshu(BL 15).

八邪、八风、华佗夹脊等；有些虽名为奇穴，但实际上就是经穴，如胞门、子户，实际就是水道穴，四花就是胆俞、膈俞四穴，灸痨穴就是心俞二穴。

1.3 Ashi acupoints

Ashi acupoints are also variously called "reactive points" and "unfixed points". Usually, they are neither meridian acupoints nor extraordinary acupoints, just as the tender sites. Ashi acupoints have no specific names and locations, and they are just the tender spots or reactive points for acupuncture and moxibustion treatment. Ashi acupoints are often situated near the affected sites, nevertheless they may also be far from the affected sites. The name of Ashi acupoints was first seen in *Thousand Ducat Prescriptions for Emergencies* (Bei Ji Qian Jin Yao Fang) in the Tang Dynasty, however, this acupoints-locating method was derived from the "tender sites as acupoints" in Nei Jing.

1.3 阿是穴

阿是穴，又称天应穴、不定穴等，通常是指该处既不是经穴，又不是奇穴，只是按压痛点取穴。这类穴位既无具体名称，又无固定位置，而是以压痛或其他反应点作为刺灸的部位。阿是穴多位于病变附近，也可在与其距离较远处。"阿是"之名见于唐代《备急千金要方·灸例》，其取穴方法，实即出自《内经》所说之"以痛为腧"。

2 Nomenclature of acupoints

Acupoints have their own locations and names. The names of acupoints have some significance, as *Supplement to Thousand Ducat Prescriptions* (Qian Jin Yi Fang) stated that "the names of acupoints have their meanings, and each is of profound significance". The names of acupoints were explained in ancient literature. The nomenclature of acupoints by ancient doctors was based upon a variety of subjects ranging from astronomy, geography, daily life, natural objects and anatomy, as well as the distribution, actions and indications. The nomencla-

2 腧穴的命名

腧穴各有一定的部位和命名。腧穴的名称都有一定的意义，故孙思邈《千金翼方·针灸下》说："凡诸孔穴，名不徒设，皆有深意。"有关腧穴命名含义的解释在古代文献中早有记载。古人对腧穴的命名，取义很广，可谓上察天文，下观地理，中通人事，远取诸物，近取诸身，结合腧穴的分布特点、作用、主治等

ture of acupoints is presented as follows.

内容赋予一定的名称。现将腧穴命名归纳介绍如下。

2.1 Nomenclature bearing analogue to astronomy and geography

2.1 天象地理类

2.1.1 Acupoints named after sun, moon or stars Riyue(GB 24), Shangxing(GV 23), Xuanji(CV 21), Huagai(CV 20), Taiyi(ST 23), Taibai(SP 3), and Tianshu(ST 25).

2.1.1 以日月星辰命名 如日月、上星、璇玑、华盖、太乙、太白、天枢等。

2.2.2 Acupoints named after mountains, hills or valleys Chengshan(BL 57), Hegu(LI 4), Daling(PC 7), Liangqiu(ST 34) and Qiuxu (GB 40).

2.2.2 以山、谷、丘、陵命名 如承山、合谷、大陵、梁丘、丘墟等。

2.2.3 Acupoints named after water stream Houxi (SI 3), Zhigou(TE 6), Sidu(TE 9), Shaohai(HT 3), Chize(LU 5), Quchi(LU 11), Ququan(LR 8), Jingqu(LU 8) and Taiyuan(LU 9).

2.2.3 以大小水流命名 如后溪、支沟、四渎、少海、尺泽、曲池、曲泉、经渠、太渊等。

2.2.4 Acupoints named after traffic pass Qichong (ST 30), Shuidao(ST 28), Guanchong(TE 1), Neiguan(PC 6) and Fengshi(GB 31).

2.2.4 以交通要冲命名 如气冲、水道、关冲、内关、风市等。

2.2 Nomenclature bearing analogue to animals, plants or utensils

2.2 人事物象类

2.2.1 Acupoints named after animals and plants Yuji(LU 10), Jiuwei(CV 15), Futu(ST 32), Dubi (ST 35), Cuanzhu (BL 2) and Heliao(LI 9).

2.2.1 以动植物名称命名 如鱼际、鸠尾、伏兔、犊鼻、攒竹、禾髎等。

2.2.2 Acupoints named after building Tianjing(TE 10), Yutang(CV 18), Juque(CV 14), Quyuan(SI 13), Kufang(ST 14), Fushe(SP 13), Tianchuang(SI 16), Dicang(ST 4), Liangmen(ST 21), Zigong(CV 19), Neiting(ST 44) and Qihu(St 13).

2.2.2 以建筑居处命名 如天井、玉堂、巨阙、曲垣、库房、府舍、天窗、地仓、梁门、紫宫、内庭、气户等。

2.2.3 Acupoints named after utensils Dazhu (BL 11), Diji(SP 8), Yangfu (GB 38), Quepen(ST 12), Tianding(LI 17) and Xuanzhong (GB 39).

2.2.3 以生活用具命名 如大杼、地机、阳辅、缺盆、天鼎、悬钟等。

2.2.4 Acupoints named after human activities Renying(ST 9), Baihui(GV 20), Guilai(ST 29) and Zusanli(ST 36).

2.2.4 以人事活动命名 如人迎、百会、归来、足三里等。

2.3 Nomenclature bearing anatomy and functions

2.3.1 Acupoints named after anatomy Wangu(SI 4), Wangu (GB 12), Dazhui(GV 14), Qugu(CV 20), Jinggu (BL 64) and Jugu(LI 16).

2.3.2 Acupoints named after zang-fu organ functions Back-Shu acupoints, Shentang(BL 44), Pohu (BL 42), Hunmen (BL 47), Yishe(BL 49) and Zhishi (BL 52).

2.3.3 Acupoints named after yin and yang Sanyinjiao(SP 6), Sanyangluo(TE 8), Yindu(KI 19), Yanggang(BL 48), Yinlingquan(SP 9) and Yanglingquan(GB 34).

2.3.4 Acupoints named after their functions Chengjiang(CV 24), Chengqi(ST 1), Tinghui (GB 2), Yingxiang(LI 20), Lianquan(CV 22), Laogong (PC 9), Qihai(CV 6), Xuehai(SP 10), Guangming (GB 37) and Shuifen(CV 9).

2.3 形态功能类

2.3.1 以解剖部位命名 如腕骨、完骨、大椎、曲骨、京骨、巨骨等。

2.3.2 以脏腑功能命名 如脏腑背俞、神堂、魄户、魂门、意舍、志室等。

2.3.3 以经络阴阳命名 如三阴交、三阳络、阴都(腹)、阳纲(背)、阴陵泉、阳陵泉等。

2.3.4 以穴位作用命名 如承浆、承泣、听会、迎香、廉泉、劳宫、气海、血海、光明、水分等。

Section 2 Therapeutic Properties and Rules of Acupoints

第2节 腧穴的主治特点和规律

1 Therapeutic properties of acupoints

Acupoints act to receive external stimulation to prevent and treat diseases. Acupoints are the places where the qi and blood pour in and the pathogenic factors invade the body, and they are also the stimulating sites for acupuncture and moxibustion in the prevention and treatment of diseases. Stimulation at the acupoints by acupuncture and moxibustion can unblock the meridians and regulate qi and blood to balance yin and yang, harmonize the zang-fu or-

1 腧穴的主治特点

腧穴有接受刺激、防治疾病的作用。腧穴是气血输注的部位,也是邪气所客之处,又是针灸防治疾病的刺激点。通过针刺、艾灸等对腧穴的刺激可通其经脉、调其气血,使阴阳归于平衡,脏腑趋于和调,从而达到扶正祛邪的目的。腧穴的主治作

gans, as a result to achieve the purpose of reinforcing the healthy qi and eliminating the pathogenic factors. The therapeutic properties of acupoints fall into three aspects.

用有以下三个方面的特点。

1.1 Local therapeutic function

Local therapeutic function is a common feature of the meridian acupoints, extraordinary acupoints and Ashi acupoints; in other words, all acupoints can treat the disorders around or adjacent to the acupoints. For instance, Zhongwan(CV 12), Jianli (CV 11) and Liangmen(ST 21) around the stomach can treat the stomach disorders; Jingming(BL 1), Chengqi(ST 1) and Sibai(ST 2) are around the eyes and all can be used to treat eye diseases; Tinggong(SI 19), Tinghui(TE 21) and Yifeng(TE 11) are all around the ears and can be employed to treat the ear diseases. Local and adjacent actions may extend to a larger range; for example, treatment of the intercostal segments by the Back-Shu acupoint and Front-Mu acupoints on the trunk is a kind of adjacent actions.

1.1 近治作用

这是经穴、奇穴和阿是穴所共有的主治作用特点，即腧穴都能治疗其所在部位及邻近部位的病证，如胃部的中脘、建里、梁门等穴，均能治胃病；眼区的睛明、承泣、四白各穴，均能治眼病；耳区的听宫、听会、翳风诸穴，均能治耳病。邻近作用还可包括较大的范围，如躯干部俞募穴的分段选穴，即出于腧穴的邻近作用。

1.2 Distal therapeutic function

Distal therapeutic function of the acupoints is an essential feature of the meridian acupoints, especially those acupoints below the elbow and knee joints. These acupoints are indicated not only for local disorders but also for distal disorders along the courses of the meridians, just as a saying goes, "an acupoint is indicated for the disorders which happen along the course of its pertaining meridian". For example, Hegu(LI 4) is indicated not only for the disorders of the upper limbs, but also for the disorders of the nape, head and face; Zusanli(ST 36) is indicated not only for the disorders of the lower limbs, but also for the gastrointestinal disorders.

1.2 远治作用

这是经穴，尤其是十二经脉在四肢肘膝关节以下的腧穴的主治特点。这些穴位不仅能治局部病证，而且能治本经循行所到达的远隔部位的病证。这就是常说的“经络所过，主治所及”。如合谷穴，不仅能治上肢病证，而且能治颈部和头面部病证；足三里穴不但能治下肢病证，而且能治胃肠及更高部位的病证。

1.3 Special therapeutic function

Apart from the local and distal therapeutic functions, some acupoints can exert biphasic and holistic regulatory effects, and have a relative therapeutic specificity. Many acupoints have biphasic regulatory effects; for instance, in the case of constipation, needling Tianshu(ST 25) can relieve constipation, while in the case of diarrhea, needling Tianshu(SR 25) can check diarrhea. Puncturing Neiguan(PC 6) can slow down heart beat in the case of tachycardia, and can quicken heart beat in the case of bradycardia. Some acupoints, particularly the acupoints of the yangming meridians and the governor vessel, are effective for the general disorders. For instance, Hegu(LI 4), Quchi(LI 11) and Dazhui(GV 14) can treat exogenous fever; Zusanli (ST 36), Guanyuan(CV 4) and Gaohuangshu(BL 43) act to strengthen the body and enhance healthcare. Some acupoints have relative therapeutic specificity; for instance, Zhiyin(BL 67) can correct a breech presentation, and Lanwei(EX - LU) can treat appendicitis.

1.3 特殊作用

除了上述近治和远治作用外,腧穴还具有双向调整、整体调整和相对的特异治疗作用。很多腧穴都有双向调整作用,如天枢穴,便秘时针刺能通便,泄泻时针刺则可止泻;内关穴,心动过速时针刺能降低心率,心动过缓时针刺则可提高心率。有些穴位还能调治全身性的病证,这在手足阳明经穴和任督脉经穴中更为多见,如合谷、曲池、大椎可治外感发热;足三里、关元、膏肓俞具有强壮保健作用。有些穴位的治疗作用还具有相对的特异性,如至阴穴可矫正胎位、阑尾穴可治阑尾炎等。

2 Rules of acupoint indications

Each acupoint has a wide variety of indications, which is associated with its pertaining meridian and location. Both the local and distal therapeutic functions of acupoints are based on the meridian theory. The rules of acupoint indications can be understood from the perspectives of its pertaining meridian and location.

2 腧穴的主治规律

每个腧穴都有较广泛的主治范围,这与其所属经络和所在部位的不同有直接关系。无论腧穴的远隔治疗作用,还是局部治疗作用,都以经络学说为依据。要掌握腧穴的主治规律,一般可以从腧穴的分经、分部两方面来分析、总结。

2.1 Rules of acupoint indication along meridians

The twelve meridian acupoints on the limbs, such as the Five-Transport acupoints, Yuan-Source acupoints, Luo-Connecting acupoints and Xi-Cleft acupoints, have special therapeutic effects on the disorders of the head, trunk and zang-fu organs. These are the foundations of acupoint indications along the meridians, and also the origin of the therapeutic rules of so-called "Four Roots and Three Tips" summarized by ancient doctors. The limbs are the "Roots" and "*Ben*" of the meridians, so the acupoints of the limbs exert distal therapeutic effects on the disorders of the head and trunk. Each meridian has its own indications, and its adjacent meridians have similar indications, two or three adjacent meridians have the same indications. These are the therapeutic commonality of the three yin or yang meridians on the limbs. The rules of the indications on limb meridians are summed up in following tables (Table 2-1～2-4).

2.1 分经主治规律

十二经脉在四肢部的五输、原、络、郄穴对于头身部及脏腑病证有特殊治疗作用，这是腧穴分经主治的基础，也是古人所总结的"四根三结"主治规律的由来。四肢是经脉的"根"和"本"部，对于头身的"结"和"标"部有远道主治作用。各经有各自的主治病证，邻近的经脉又有类似作用，或两经相同，或三经相同，这是"三阴""三阳"在治疗作用上的共性。现将手足三阴三阳经穴主治归纳成表(表2-1～2-4)，因腧穴的局部治疗作用很好理解，表中只列远道主治病证而省略四肢部病证。

Table 2-1　Indications of three yin meridians of the hand

Meridians	Indications of one meridian	Commonality of two meridians	Commonality of three meridians
Hand-Taiyin meridian	Lung and throat diseases		Chest disorders
Hand-Jueyin meridian	Heart and stomach diseases	Mental diseases	
Hand-Shaoyin meridian	Heart disorders		

表2-1　手三阴经穴主治病证

经名	本经主病	二经相同	三经相同
手太阴经	肺、喉病		胸部病
手厥阴经	心、胃病	神志病	
手少阴经	心病		

Table 2-2 Indications of three yang meridians of the hand

Meridians	Indications of one meridian	Commonality of two meridians	Commonality of three meridians
Hand-Yangming meridian	Diseases of front head, nose and teeth		Diseases of the eyes and throat, fever
Hand-Shaoyang meridian	Diseases of lateral head and flanks	Ear disorders	
Hand-Taiyang meridian	Diseases of back head, shoulder and in mind		

表 2-2 手三阳经穴主治病证

经名	本经主病	二经相同	三经相同
手阳明经	前头、鼻、口齿病		眼病、咽喉病、热病
手少阳经	侧头、胁肋病	耳病	
手太阳经	后头、肩胛、神志病		

Table 2-3 Indications of three yang meridians of the foot

Meridians	Indications of one meridian	Commonality of two meridians	Commonality of three meridians
Foot-Yangming meridian	Diseases of front head, mouth, teeth, throat, stomach and intestine		Mental disorders and fever
Foot-Shaoyang meridian	Diseases of lateral head, ears, neck, flank and gallbladder	Eye diseases	
Foot-Taiyang meridian	Diseases of back head, nape, back and anus		

表 2-3 足三阳经穴主治病证

经名	本经主病	二经相同	三经相同
足阳明经	前头、口、齿、咽喉、胃肠病		神志病、热病
足少阳经	侧头、耳病、项、胁肋、胆病	眼病	
足太阳经	后头、项、背腰、肛肠病		

Table 2-4 Indications of three yin meridians of the foot

Meridians	Indications of one meridian	Commonality of two meridians	Commonality of three meridians
Foot-Taiyin meridian	Stomach and intestine diseases		Abdominal disorders
Foot-Jueyin meridian	Liver diseases	External genitalia disorders	
Foot-Shaoyin meridian	Diseases of kidneys, lungs and throat		

表 2-4　足三阴经穴主治病证

经名	本经主病	二经相同	三经相同
足太阴经	脾胃病		腹部病
足厥阴经	肝病	前阴病	
足少阴经	肾、肺、咽喉病		

2.2 Rules of indications on location

The head, chest, abdomen and back are the parts of "Four Seas" "Qi Street" "Termination" and "Branch" of the twelve meridians. The qi of the zang-fu organs is communicable with the abdomen and back. This is the rule of indications on location, showing that there is a transverse relationship among the body apart from its vertical pathways. See Table 2-5 and Table 2-6.

2.2 分部主治规律

头身部从上而下分为头、胸、上下腹，各与背腰部前后对应，这是四海、气街及十二经脉"结"和"标"的所在部位。"脏腑腹背，气相通应"，这是分部主治的规律，体现经脉在纵行分经的基础上又有横行分部的关系。各部经穴主治见表 2-5～2-6。

Table 2-5　Indications of acupoints on the head and neck

Parts	Indications
Front and lateral head	Diseases of the eyes and nose
Back head	Mental and head disorders
Nape	Mental, throat, eye and head diseases
Eyes	Eye diseases
Nose	Nose diseases
Neck	Diseases of tongue, throat, trachea and neck

表 2-5　头面颈项部经穴主治病证

分　部	主治病证
前头、侧头区	眼、鼻病
后头区	神志、头部病
项区	神志、咽喉、眼、头项病
眼区	眼病
鼻区	鼻病
颈区	舌、咽喉、气管、颈部病

Table 2-6 Indications of acupoints on chest, abdomen and back

Front	Back	Indications
Chest	Upper back	Diseases of the lungs and heart
Flank	Lower back	Diseases of the liver, gallbladder, spleen and stomach
Lateral abdomen	Waist	Diseases of genitalia, anus, kidney, intestine and bladder

表 2-6 胸腹背腰部经穴主治病证

前	后	主治病证
胸膺部	上背部	肺、心(上焦病)
胁腹部	下背部	肝、胆、脾、胃(中焦病)
少腹部	腰尻部	前后阴、肾、肠、膀胱(下焦病)

For example, the acupoints on the neck and scapular areas are indicated for the local and adjacent disorders; the nape acupoints are indicated for the throat diseases, fever and upper limb disorders; the flank acupoints are indicated for the liver and gallbladder diseases; the acupoints on the lateral abdomen are indicated for the spleen and stomach diseases; the acupoints on the waist are indicated for the disorders of the lower limbs, and the zang-fu organs in the lower abdomen as well.

再如颈项和肩胛区,主局部病证,颈项当头与背之间,还主咽喉、热病和上肢病证;侧胁部对于肝胆,侧腹对于脾胃,与中焦范围相类;腰髋部对下焦脏腑之外,主要用于下肢病证。

Section 3 Specific Acupoints

第3节 特定穴

Specific acupoints, the points of the fourteen meridians, have special therapeutic functions and are grouped under separate classifications. These acupoints not only make up a considerable proportion of the fourteen meridian acupoints, but also play a vital role in the basic theory and clinical application in acupuncture and moxibusiton.

十四经穴中具有特殊治疗作用,并按特定称号归类的腧穴,称特定穴。特定穴在十四经穴中不仅在数量上占有相当的比例,而且在针灸学的基本理论和临床应用方面也有着非常重要的意义。

1　Five transport acupoints

The five transport acupoints are five groups of acupoints of the twelve main meridians below the elbows and knees, namely the Jing-Well, Ying-Spring, Shu-Stream, Jing-River and He-Sea. They were first recorded in Ling Shu. Ling Shu detailed the names and locations of these acupoints.

The ancients described the circulation of meridian qi as the stream of flowing water, representing the volume of the qi in the meridians and the depth of the qi flowing within the body. Thus the five transport acupoints are named the Jing-Well acupoint, Ying-Spring acupoint, Shu-Stream acupoint, Jing-River acupoint and He-Sea acupoint from the tips of the limbs to the elbows or knees. The Jing-Well acupoint is mostly located at the tips of the limb, from which meridian qi wells up just like water coming out, hence named the Jing-Well acupoint; the Ying-Spring acupoint is located before the metacarpal-phalangeal joint or the metatarsophalangeal joint, where meridian qi starts to rush just like a spring, hence named the Ying-Spring acupoint; the Shu-Stream acupoint is located after metacarpal-phalangeal joint or the metatarsophalangeal joint, where meridian qi flows and pours in, just like a stream, hence named Shu-Stream acupoint; the Jing-River acupoint is located around the wrist or ankle, where meridian qi passes on through in abundance, just like a river, hence named Jing-River acupoint; the He-Sea acupoint is located near the elbow or knee joints, where meridian qi enters

1　五输穴

五输穴，是十二经脉分布在肘膝关节以下的“井、荥、输、经、合”五类腧穴。五输穴的记载首见于《灵枢·九针十二原》，《灵枢·本输》详细载述了各经井、荥、输、经、合各穴的名称和具体位置。

古人把经气运行过程用自然界的水流由小到大、由浅入深的变化来形容，把五输穴按井、荥、输、经、合的顺序，从四肢末端向肘膝方向依次排列。“井”穴多位于手足之端，喻作水的源头，是经气所出的部位，即“所出为井”。“荥”穴多位于掌指或跖趾关节之前，喻作水流尚微，萦迂未成大流，是经气流行的部位，即“所溜为荥”。“输”穴多位于掌指或跖趾关节之后，喻作水流由小而大、由浅注深，是经气渐盛，由此注彼的部位，即“所注为输”。“经”穴多位于腕踝关节以上，喻作水流变大，畅通无阻，是经气正盛、运行经过的部位，即“所行为经”。“合”穴位于肘膝关节附近，喻作江河水流汇入湖海，是经气由此深入，进而会合于脏腑的部位，即“所入为合”。

the body to the zang-fu organs, just like water converging into the sea, hence named He-Sea acupoint.

2 Yuan-Source acupoint

The twelve main meridians all have their own Yuan-Source acupoints around the ankle or wrist joints, where the yuan(source)qi of the zang-fu organs pours in and retains, 12 Yuan-Source acupoints in total. "Yuan", meaning source or original qi, is the vital motive of living activities. The name of the Yuan-Source acupoint was first mentioned in Ling Shu. The Yuan-Source acupoints of the yin meridians are the same acupoints as the Shu-Stream acupoints of the meridians; the qi of the yang meridians is more vigorous than that of the yin meridians, thereby their Yuan-Source acupoints are additionally established.

2 原穴

十二经脉在腕踝关节附近各有一个腧穴,是脏腑原气留止的部位,称为"原穴",合称"十二原"。"原"即本原、原气之意,是人体生命活动的原动力。原穴名称首载于《灵枢·九针十二原》。阴经之原穴,即是五输穴中的输穴。阳经的脉气较阴经盛长,故于输穴之外另立一原穴。

3 Luo-Connecting acupoint

The Luo-Connecting acupoints are the sites where the meridian divergencies branch off from the main meridians. Luo means connection. The name of Luo-Connecting acupoint was first mentioned in Ling Shu. The twelve main meridians have their own Luo-Connecting acupoints below the elbow and knee joints, together with the Luo-Connecting acupoints of the conception vessel, governor vessel and the great collateral of the spleen, there are fifteen Luo-Connecting acupoints in all.

3 络穴

络脉由经脉分出之处各有一穴,称"络穴"。"络",是联络的意思。络穴名称首载于《灵枢·经脉》。十二经在肘膝关节以下各有一络穴,加上躯干前的任脉络穴、躯干后的督脉络穴和躯干侧的脾之大络,合称"十五络穴"。

4 Xi-Cleft acupoint

The Xi-Cleft acupoints are the sites where the qi of the meridians is deeply converged in the limbs. Xi means cleft or hollow. The name and location of Xi-Cleft acupoints were recorded in Zhen Jiu Jia Yi Jing. The Xi-Cleft acupoints are mostly located be-

4 郄穴

郄穴是各经脉在四肢部经气深聚的部位。郄与"隙"通,是空隙、间隙的意思,其名称和位置首载于《针灸甲乙经》。郄穴大多分布于四

low the elbow and knee joints. Each of the twelve main meridians and four extraordinary meridians (yin heel vessel, yang heel vessel, yin link vessel and yang link vessel) has a Xi-Cleft acupoint, amounting to 16 acupoints in all.

肢肘膝关节以下。十二经脉、阴阳蹻脉和阴阳维脉各有一郄穴，合为十六郄穴。

5　Back-Shu acupoints

The Back-Shu acupoints are places on the back where the qi of the zang-fu organs is infused. Back-Shu acupoints were first mentioned in Ling Shu. The Back-Shu acupoints are on the first lateral line of the bladder meridian of foot taiyang and arranged downwards in accordance with the anatomical positions of the zang-fu organs. Each of the zang-fu organs have one Back-Shu acupoint, totally twelve acupoints, which are named after their respective zang or fu organs.

5　背俞穴

背俞穴是脏腑之气输注于背腰部的腧穴。背俞穴首见于《灵枢·背腧》。背俞穴位于背腰部足太阳膀胱经的第一侧线上，大体依脏腑位置而上下排列。六脏六腑各有一相应的背俞穴，共十二个，分别冠以脏腑之名。

6　Front-Mu acupoint

The Front-Mu acupoints are the places on the chest and abdomen where the qi of the zang-fu organs converges. The Front-Mu acupoints were first mentioned in Su Wen. Mu means convergence or gathering. Each of the zang and fu organs have its Front-Mu acupoint, twelve acupoints in all, which is anamitcally near its corresponding zang-fu organ.

6　募穴

脏腑之气结聚于胸腹部的腧穴，称“募穴”。募穴始见于《素问·奇病论》。“募”，有聚集、汇合之意。六脏六腑各有一相应的募穴，共十二个，其部位都接近其相应的脏腑。

7　Lower He-Sea acupoints

The Lower He-Sea acupoints are six acupoints on the three foot yang meridians, where the qi of the six-fu organs pours down. The Lower He-Sea acupoints were first mentioned in Ling Shu. There are six Lower He-Sea acupoints in all. The Lower He-Sea acupoints of the stomach, gallbladder and bladder are actually the He-Sea acupoints of its own meridian; while the Lower He-Sea acupoints of the

7　下合穴

下合穴，即六腑下合穴，是六腑之气下合于足三阳经的六个腧穴。下合穴首见于《灵枢·邪气藏府病形》。下合穴共六个，其中胃、胆、膀胱三腑的下合穴，即本经五输穴中的合穴，而大肠、小肠、三焦三腑在下肢另有合

large intestine and small intestine are on the stomach meridian, and that of the triple energizer is on the bladder meridian.

穴。大肠、小肠下合于胃经，三焦下合于膀胱经。

8 Eight Influential acupoints

The eight Influential acupoints are the sites for the convergence of zang-organs, fu-organs, qi, blood, tendons, vessels, bones and marrow respectively. The eight Influential acupoints were first mentioned in *Canon of Perplexities* (Nan Jing). These acupoints are distributed on the limbs and trunk, among which the Influential acupoints of zang-organs, fu-organs, qi, blood and bones are on the trunk, whereas those of the tendons, vessels and marrow are on the limbs.

8 八会穴

八会穴，是指脏、腑、气、血、筋、脉、骨、髓所会聚的八个腧穴。八会穴首载于《难经·四十五难》。“会”，是聚会的意思。八会穴分散在躯干部和四肢部，其中脏、腑、气、血、骨之会穴位于躯干部，筋、脉、髓之会穴位于四肢部。

9 Eight Confluent acupoints

The eight Confluent acupoints are the eight acupoints on the limbs through which the eight extraodinary meridians communicate with the twelve main meridians. The eight Confluent acupoints were first mentioned in *Guide to Acupunctare Canon* (Zhen Jing Zhi Nan). These acupoints are all distributed below the elbow and knee joints.

9 八脉交会穴

八脉交会穴是指与奇经八脉相通的十二经脉在四肢部的八个腧穴，原称“交经八穴”“流注八穴”和“八脉八穴”。八脉交会穴首见于窦汉卿《针经指南》。八脉交会穴均分布于肘膝关节以下。

10 Crossing acupoints

The Crossing acupoints are those at the intersection of two or more meridians. The Crossing acupoints were first recorded in Zhen Jiu Jia Yi Jing. Crossing acupoints are principally situated on the head and trunk.

10 交会穴

交会穴是指两经或数经相交会合的腧穴。交会穴的记载始见于《针灸甲乙经》。交会穴多分布于头面、躯干部。

Section 4　Methods of Locating Acupoints

第4节 腧穴定位法

The method of locating acupoints is the essential method in determining the location of acupoints. The precise location of acupoints mainly depends on the anatomical landmarks. To locate the acupoints far from the anatomical landmarks, the distance between two anatomical landmarks should be first converted into several proportional units, which are termed as "bone-length proportional cun", thus the "cun" is used to express the distance between the acupoint and the anatomical landmark. In locating acupoints, fingers are utilized to express the distance away from the landmarks. Principally, there are four methods of loating acupoints: anatomical reference points, bone-length proportional units, finger meansurement and convenient location.

腧穴定位法，又称取穴法，是指确定腧穴位置的基本方法。确定腧穴位置，要以体表标志为主要依据，在距离标志较远的部位，则于两标志之间折合一定的比例"寸"，即"骨度分寸"，用此"寸"表示上下左右的距离。取穴时，用手指比量这种距离，则有手指"同身寸"的应用。以下就分体表标志、骨度分寸、手指同身寸和简便取穴四法进行介绍。

1　Anatomical landmarks on body surface

Measurement with anatomical landmarks on body surface is an acupoint-locating method in accordance with the anatomical landmarks on the body surface, which is also known as natural landmark method. The anatomical landmarks, including the bone landmarks and muscle landmarks throughout the body surface, fall into fixed landmarks and movable landmarks.

1　体表标志定位法

体表标志定位法，是以人体的各种体表标志为依据来确定穴位位置的方法，又称自然标志定位法。体表标志，主要指分布于全身体表的骨性标志和肌性标志，又可分固定标志和活动标志两类，分述如下。

1.1　Fixed landmarks

Fixed landmarks are those which do not change with body movement, such as the five sense organs, hair, nail, nipple, umbilicus, and the prominence

1.1　固定标志

固定标志定位，是指利用五官、毛发、爪甲、乳头、脐窝、骨节凹凸及肌肉隆起等

and depression of the muscles and bones. These landmarks are usually used in the location of acupoints. For example, Suliao(CV 25) is situated on the tip of the nose; Yintang(EX-HN 3) is located at the midpoint between the eyebrows; Danzhong (CV 17) is located at the midpoint between the two nipples; Tianshu(ST 25) is located at the points 2 cun lateral to the umbilicus; Yanglingquan(GB 34) is located anterior and inferior to the capitulum fibulae; Dazhui(GV 14) is located below the seventh spinous process. Some acupoints are located at the bifuration of two bones; for instance, Jugu(LI 16) is located at the bifurcation of the scapular extremity of the clavicle and the scapular spine; and Zhongting(CV 16) is located at the bifurcation of the costal cartilage and the lower border of the xiphoid bone. Furthermore, the scapular spine is on the same level as the third thoracic spinous process; the inferior angle of the scapula is on the same level as the seventh thoracic spinous process; the iliac crest is on the same level as the fourth lumbar spinous process. These landmarks are frequently used to locate the acupoints on the back.

固定标志来取穴的方法。比较明显的标志,如:鼻尖取素髎;两眉中间取印堂;两乳中间取膻中;脐旁二寸取天枢;腓骨小头前下缘取阳陵泉;俯首显示最高的第七颈椎棘突下取大椎等。在两骨分歧处,如:锁骨肩峰端与肩胛冈分歧处取巨骨;胸骨下端与肋软骨分歧处取中庭等。此外,肩胛冈内侧端平第三胸椎棘突,肩胛骨下角平第七胸椎棘突,髂嵴平第四腰椎棘突,这些可作背腰部穴的取穴标志。

1.2 Movable landmarks

Movable landmarks refer to those which appear only when a certain part of the body is kept in a specific position, such as a crease or fold of the skin, a depression or prominence formed out of the movement of the joints, muscles and skin. For example, Ermen(TE 21), Tinggong(TE 19) and Tinghui (GB 2) are located when the mouth opens, while Xiaguan(ST 7) is located when the mouth closes; Quchi(LI 11) is located at the lateral end of the transverse crease when the elbow is bent; Jianyu(LI

1.2 活动标志

活动标志定位,是指利用关节、肌肉、皮肤随活动而出现的孔隙、凹陷、皱纹等活动标志来取穴的方法。如:耳门、听宫、听会等应张口取;下关应闭口取。又如:曲池宜屈肘于横纹头处取之;外展上臂时肩峰前下方的凹陷中取肩髃;取阳溪穴时应将拇指翘起,当拇长、短伸肌腱

15) is located in the depression anterior and inferior to the acromial process when the arm abducts; Yang xi(LI 5) is located in the depression between the muscle tendons of the extensor pollicis longus and the extensor pollicis brevis when the thumb erects; Yanglao(SI 6) is located in the bone cleft radial to the capitulum ulnae when the forearm adducts with the palm facing the chest.

之间的凹陷中取之;取养老穴时,应正坐屈肘,掌心向胸,当尺骨小头桡侧骨缝中取之。

The anatomical landmarks on the body surface, especially the fixed landmarks, do not change. Therefore, acupoints location based on these fixed landmarks is the most accurate method, and remains the essential method for locating acupoints. However, only a part of acupoints are situated near these landmarks, thus this method also has certain limitations.

人体体表标志,尤其是固定标志的位置恒定不变,用这些标志定穴是准确性最高的取穴法,故此法是确定腧穴位置的主要依据。但由于全身腧穴中分布于体表标志处的仅限于部分穴位,所以此法也有一定的局限性。

2 Bone-length proportional measurement

2 骨度分寸定位法

Bone-length proportional measurement, known as "Bone Measurement" in ancient time, is an acupoints-locating method in which the width or length of various portions of the human body is divided into definite numbers of equal units, each unit being termed one cun. Bone Measurement is first found in Ling Shu. The proportional unit depends on the build of the individuals. In locating acupoints, the length between two landmarks are divided into certain units, which are taken as the standards of measurement, applicable to any patients, of any sex, age or body weight. See Table 2-7, Fig.2-1.

骨度分寸法,古称"骨度法",即以骨节为主要标志测量周身各部的大小、长短,并依其尺寸按比例折算作为定穴的标准。骨度法最早见于《灵枢·骨度》篇。分部折寸以患者本人的身材为依据。取用时,将设定的骨节两端之间的长度折成为一定的等分,每一等分为一寸。不论男女老幼,肥瘦高矮,均以此标准折量作为量取腧穴的依据。现将全身各部骨度折量寸列表、图示如下(表2-7,图2-1)。

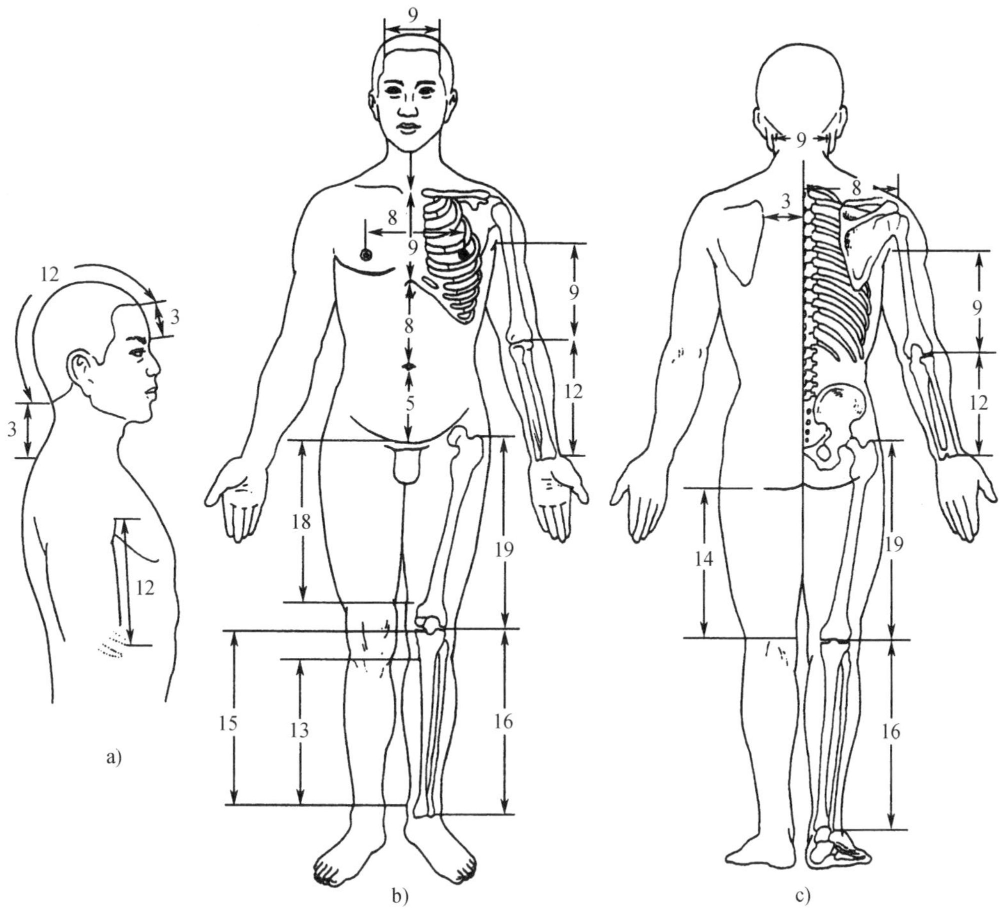

a) bone measurement(head) b) bone measurement(front side) c) bone measurement(lateral side)

a) 头部骨度分寸 b) 正面骨度分寸 c) 背面骨度分寸

Fig.2-1 common bone measurement units(unit: cun)

图 2-1 常用骨度分寸示意图(单位:寸)

Bone-length proportional measurement is applied to measure the length or width of all parts of the body on the basis of the anatomical landmarks of body surface. Actually, this measurement is the extended application of anatomical landmarks measurement and can make up its limitations, it is hence

骨度分寸法通常是以体表标志为基准,测量全身各部的长度或宽度,实际上是体表标志定位法应用的扩大,可补充体表标志定位法的局限性,是临床常用、适用

considered to be a frequently-used, widely applicable and more accurate acupoint-locating method.

3 Finger measurement

Finger measurement is an acupoint-locating method in which the length and width of the patients' fingers is taken as the standard for acupoint location. This method may be practised in three ways: middle-finger measurement, thumb measurement and four-finger measurement.

3.1 Middle-finger measurement

In this measurement, when the patients' middle finger is flexed, the distance between the two medial ends of the creases of the interphalangeal joints is taken as one *cun* (Fig. 2-2). This measurement unit *cun* is a bit longer than that in bone measurement, which should arouse clinical attention.

3.2 Thumb measurement

In this measuremwnt, the width of the interphalangeal joint of the patients' thumb is taken as one *cun* (Fig. 2-3). In comparison with the middle finger measurement, the thumb measurement is clear in landmarks and convenient in application, thus it is more commonly used in acupoint location.

3.3 Four-finger measurement

In this measurement, the width of the four fingers (the index, middle, ring and little) when paralleled together, at the level with the dorsal skin crease of the proximal interphalangeal joint of the middle finger, is taken as three *cun* (Fig. 2-4). This measurement is also a common method for acupoint location.

穴位多、准确性较高的腧穴定位法。

3 手指同身寸定位法

手指同身寸定位法，是指以患者本人的手指为尺寸折量标准来量取穴位的定位方法，又称“手指比量法”和“指寸法”。此法常用的有中指同身寸、拇指同身寸和横指同身寸三种。

3.1 中指同身寸

中指同身寸是以患者中指屈曲时中节桡侧两端纹头之间的距离为1寸(图2-2)。这种“同身寸”法与骨度分寸相比略为偏长，临床应用时应予注意。

3.2 拇指同身寸

拇指同身寸是以患者拇指指间关节之宽度为1寸(图2-3)。与中指同身寸比较，拇指同身寸标志清晰，应用方便，故是指寸法中较为常用的一种。

3.3 横指同身寸

横指同身寸是当患者第2～5指并拢时中指近侧指间关节横纹水平的4指宽度为3寸(图2-4)。四横指为一夫，合3寸，故此法又称“一夫法”。横指同身寸也是指寸法中较为常用的一种。

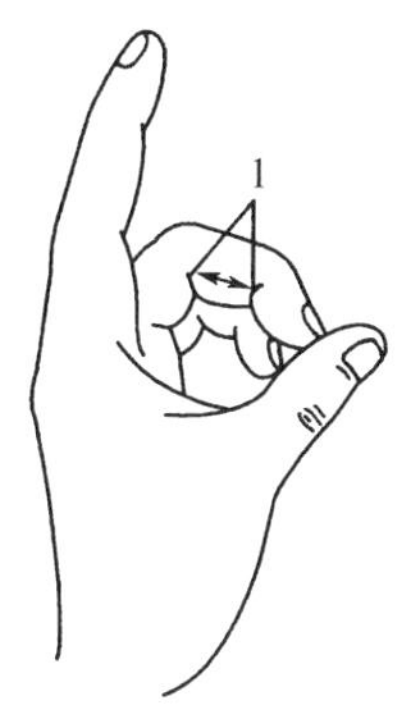

Fig.2-2 Middle-finger measurement

图 2-2 中指寸

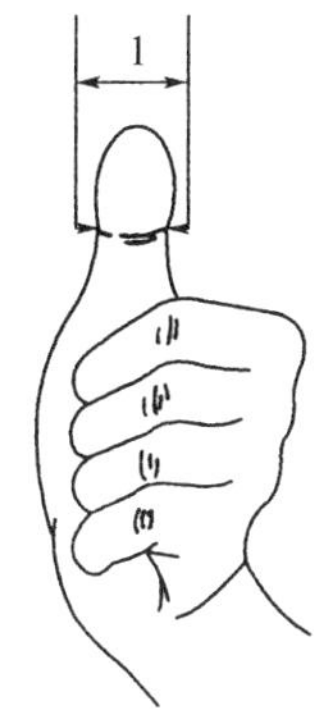

Fig.2-3 Thumb measurement

图 2-3 拇指寸

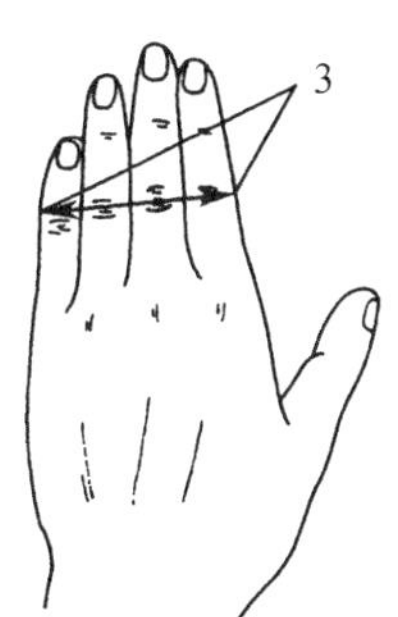

Fig.2-4 Four-finger measurement

图 2-4 横指寸(一夫法)

Finger measurement for acupoint location is based upon the anatomical landmarks and the bone-length proportional measurement. But it cannot be applied in all parts of the body, or the measurement units fail to locate acupoints precisely.

手指同身寸定位法是在体表标志和骨度法的基础上应用的,不能以指寸悉量全身各部,否则长短失度。

4 Simple measurement

This is an acupoint-locating method by means of simple ways. For example, Lieque(LU 7) is located by asking the patient to cross the index fingers and the thumbs of both hands, with the index finger of one hand placed on the styloid process of the radius of the other; the acupoint is right under the tip of the index finger. Laogong(PC 8) is located by making a fist loosely, where the middle finger touching the palm is the acupoint. Fengshi(GB 31) is located by asking the patient to stand upright with the hands close to the sides and the acupoint is at the site where the tip of the middle finger touches. Zhangmen(LR 13) is located by asking the patient to drop the shoulder and bend the elbow and the acupoint is at the site where the tip of elbow tou-

4 简便定位法

简便定位法是一种简便易行的腧穴定位方法。常用的简便定位方法有:两手伸开,于虎口交叉,当食指端处取列缺;半握拳,当中指端所指处取劳宫;两手自然下垂,于中指端处取风市;垂肩屈肘于平肘尖处取章门;两耳角直上连线中点取百会;等。

ches. Baihui(GV 20) is located at the midpoint of the line connecting the two ear apexes.

This simple measurement is just taken as a reference and complemented method for acupoint location.

简便定位法通常仅作为取穴法的参考和补充。

Table 2-7　Common bone measurements

Portion	Starting and ending sites	*Cun*	Direction	Notes
Head	Anterior hairline → Posterior hairline	12	longititude	For measuring the longititude distance on the head
	Yintang(EX 2) → Anterior hairline	3	longititude	For measuring the longititude distance from the anterior hairline to the head
	Between acupoints Touwei(ST 8)	9	transverse	For measuring the transverse distance on the frontal head
	Between acupoints Wangu (GB 12)	9	transvese	For measuring the transverse distance on the back head
Chest and abdomen	From Tiantu(CV 22) → xiphoid	9	longititude	For measuring the longititude distance of the conception vessel on the chest
	Xiphoid → navel	8	longititude	For measuring the longititude distance on the upper abdomen
	Navel → the upper border of symphysis	5	longititude	For measuring the longititude distance on the lower abdomen
	Between the internal borders of scapular coracoid process	12	transverse	For measuring the transverse distance on the chest
	Between two nipples	8	transverse	For measuring the transverse distance on the chest
Back	Internal border of scapula→ posterior midline	3	transverse	For measuring the transverse distance on the back
Upper limb	The end of axillary fold→ transverse cubital crease	9	longititude	For measuring the longititude distance on the upper limbs
	Transverse cubital crease→ transverse wrist crease	12	longititude	For measuring the longititude distance on the forearm
Lower limb	The upper border of symphysis pubis→medial epicondyle of femur	18	longititude	For measuring the longititude distance on the thigh
	Medial epicondyle of femur→ tip of patella	2	longititude	
	Tip of patella→tip of medial malleolus	15	longititude	For measuring the longititude distance on the medial aspect of leg
	Prominence of greater trochanter→ transverse popliteal crease	19	longititude	For measuring the longititude distance on the frontal and lateral aspect of the thigh

(continued)

Portion	Starting and ending sites	*Cun*	Direction	Notes
Lower limb	Transverse gluteal crease → transverse popliteal crease	14	longititude	For measuring the longititude distance on the back of the thigh
	Transverse popliteal crease→ tip of the lateral malleolus	16	longititude	For measuring the longititude distance on the lateral aspect of the leg
	Tip of medial malleolus→sole	3	longititude	For measuring the longititude distance on the internal side of the foot

表 2-7 常用骨度表

部位	起止点	折量寸	度量法	说明
头面部	前发际正中→后发际正中	12	直寸	用于确定头部腧穴的纵向距离
	眉间(印堂)→前发际正中	3	直寸	用于确定前发际及其头部腧穴的纵向距离
	两额角发际(头维)之间	9	横寸	用于确定头前部腧穴的横向距离
	耳后两乳突(完骨)之间	9	横寸	用于确定头后部腧穴的横向距离
胸腹胁部	胸骨上窝(天突)→剑胸结合中点(歧骨)	9	直寸	用于确定胸部任脉穴的纵向距离
	剑胸结合中点(歧骨)→脐中	8	直寸	用于确定上腹部腧穴的纵向距离
	脐中→耻骨联合上缘(曲骨)	5	直寸	用于确定下腹部腧穴的纵向距离
	两肩胛骨喙突内侧缘之间	12	横寸	用于确定胸部腧穴的横向距离
	两乳头之间	8	横寸	用于确定胸腹部腧穴的横向距离
背腰部	肩胛骨内侧缘→后正中线	3	横寸	用于确定背腰部腧穴的横向距离
上肢部	腋前、后纹头→肘横纹(平尺骨鹰嘴)	9	直寸	用于确定上臂部腧穴的纵向距离
	肘横纹(平尺骨鹰嘴)→腕掌(背)侧远端横纹	12	直寸	用于确定前臂部腧穴的纵向距离
下肢部	耻骨联合上缘→髌骨底	18	直寸	用于确定大腿部腧穴的纵向距离
	髌骨底→髌骨尖	2	直寸	
	髌骨尖(膝中)→内踝尖(胫骨内侧髁下方阴陵泉→内踝尖为 13 寸)	15	直寸	用于确定小腿内侧部腧穴的纵向距离
	股骨大转子→腘横纹(平髌骨尖)	19	直寸	用于确定大腿部前外侧部腧穴的纵向距离
	臀沟→腘横纹	14	直寸	用于确定大腿后部腧穴的纵向距离
	腘横纹(平髌尖)→外踝尖	16	直寸	用于确定小腿外侧部腧穴的纵向距离
	内踝尖→足底	3	直寸	用于确定足内侧部腧穴的纵向距离

Chapter 3 Meridians and Acupoints

第3章 经络腧穴各论

Section 1 Lung Meridian of Hand-Taiyin and its Acupoints

第1节 手太阴肺经及其腧穴

1 Distribution course

The lung meridian of hand-taiyin originates from the middle energizer and runs downwards to connect with the large intestine. Turning back, it follows the upper orifice of the stomach and passes through the diaphragm to enter the lungs, the organ it pertains to. From the lung system (where the lungs communicate with the throat), the meridian comes out transversely to the body surface under the clavicle. Descending along the medial aspect of the upper arm, it then runs in front of the heart meridian of hand-shaoyin and the pericardium meridian of hand-jueyin, and reaches the elbow crease. From there, it runs continuously along the anterior border of the forearm and enters cunkou, close to the radial artery at the wrist where the pulse is palpated; passing through the thenar eminence, it goes along the radial side of the tip of the thumb. A branch

1 经脉循行

手太阴肺经，起始于中焦，向下联络大肠，回过来沿着胃上口，穿过膈肌，上属于肺脏。从肺系——气管、喉咙部横出腋下，向下循上臂内侧，行于手少阴经、手厥阴经之前，经过肘，沿前臂内侧桡骨下缘，进入寸口（桡动脉搏动处），经大鱼际部，沿其边缘，出于大指的桡侧端。其支脉，从腕后分出走向食指桡侧，出于末端，连接手阳明大肠经（图3-1）。

splits from the lung meridian just above the wrist and runs directly to the radial side of the tip of index finger, where it links with the large intestine meridian(Fig. 3-1).

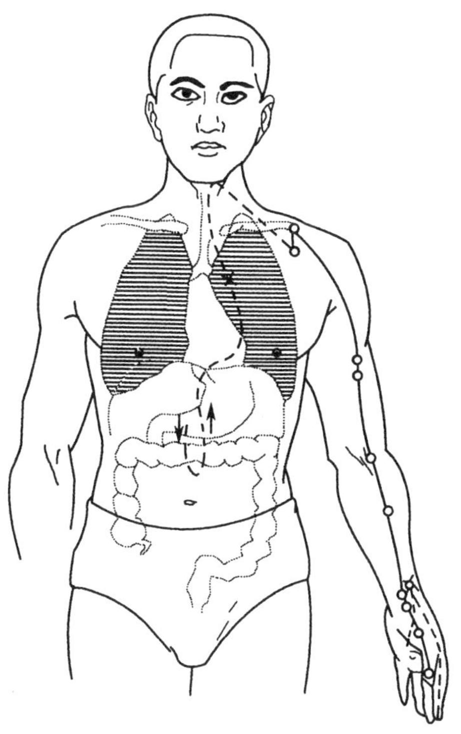

Fig.3-1 The distribution course of lung meridian of hand-taiyin

图 3-1 手太阴肺经循行示意图

—— Course of lung meridian with acupoints; ------- course of lung meridian without acupoints; ○ acupoints of lung meridian; △ acupoints of other meridians

图例：—— 本经有穴通路；------- 本经无穴通路；○ 本经腧穴；△ 他经腧穴

2 Location of acupoints

The starting acupoint of the lung meridian is Zhongfu(LU 1) and the ending one is Shaoshang (LU 11), totally 11 acupoints on each side. The location of lung meridian acupoints is presented in Table 3-1 and Fig. 3-2～3-5.

2 腧穴定位

本经首穴为中府，末穴为少商，左右各 11 穴。腧穴定位见表 3-1、图 3-2～3-5。

Table 3-1　Location of acupoints of the lung meridian of hand-taiyin

Name		Location	Specific Features
LU 1*	Zhongfu	At the same level with the first intercostal space, outside the infraclavicular fossa, 6 cun lateral to the anterior midline	Front-Mu acupoint of the lung, Crossing acupoint of hand and foot-taiyin meridians
LU 2	Yunmen	In the depression of the infraclavicular fossa, the medial border of coracoid process of scapula, 6 cun lateral to the anterior midline	
LU 3	Tianfu	3 cun distal to the end of the anterior axillary fold, on the lateral border of the biceps brachialis muscle	
LU 4	Xiabai	4 cun distal to the end of the anterior axillary fold, on the lateral border of the biceps brachialis muscle	
LU 5*	Chize	On the cubital crease, in the depression on the lateral border of the biceps brachialis muscle	He-Sea acupoint
LU 6*	Kongzui	7 cun proximal to the wrist crease, on the line connecting Chize(LU 5) and Taiyuan(LU 9)	Xi-Cleft acupoint
LU 7*	Lieque	1.5 cun proximal to the palmar wrist crease, between short extensor tendon of thumb and long abductor tendon of thumb, in the depression of long abductor tendon groove of thumb	Luo-Connecting acupoint, Confluent acupoint of the thoroughfare vessel
LU 8	Jingqu	1.5 cun proximal to the palmar wrist crease, between the styloid process and radial artery	Jing-River acupoint
LU 9*	Taiyuan	On the radial aspect of the palmar wrist crease, the lateral side of the radial artery	Shu-Stream acupoint, Yuan-Source acupoint, Influential acupoint of vessel
LU 10*	Yuji	At the midpoint of the palmar border of the first metacarpal bone	Ying-Spring acupoint
LU 11*	Shaoshang	On the thumb, 0.1 cun from the radial corner of the nail	Jing-Well acupoint

note: * Labelled as commonly used acupoints in the whole book.

表 3-1　手太阴肺经的腧穴定位

腧穴		定位	特定穴属性
中府*	Zhōngfǔ	横平第 1 肋间隙,锁骨下窝外侧,前正中线旁开 6 寸	肺募穴;手足太阴经交会穴
云门	Yúnmén	锁骨下窝凹陷中,肩胛骨喙突内缘,前正中线旁开 6 寸	
天府	Tiānfǔ	腋前纹头下 3 寸,肱二头肌桡侧缘处	

（续表）

腧穴		定位	特定穴属性
侠白	Xiábái	腋前纹头下 4 寸，肱二头肌桡侧缘处	
尺泽*	Chǐzé	在肘横纹上，肱二头肌腱桡侧缘凹陷中	合穴
孔最*	Kǒngzuì	腕掌侧远端横纹上 7 寸，尺泽（LU 5）与太渊（LU 9）连线上	郄穴
列缺*	Lièquē	腕掌侧远端横纹上 1.5 寸，拇短伸肌腱与拇长展肌腱之间，拇长展肌腱沟的凹陷中	络穴；八脉交会穴（通任脉）
经渠	Jīngqú	腕掌侧远端横纹上 1 寸，桡骨茎突与桡动脉之间	经穴
太渊*	Tàiyuān	在腕掌侧横纹桡侧，桡动脉搏动处	输穴；原穴；八会穴（脉会）
鱼际*	Yújì	第 1 掌骨桡侧中点赤白肉际处	荥穴
少商*	Shàoshāng	拇指末节桡侧，指甲根角侧上方 0.1 寸（指寸）	井穴

注：* 为常用穴位。全书同。

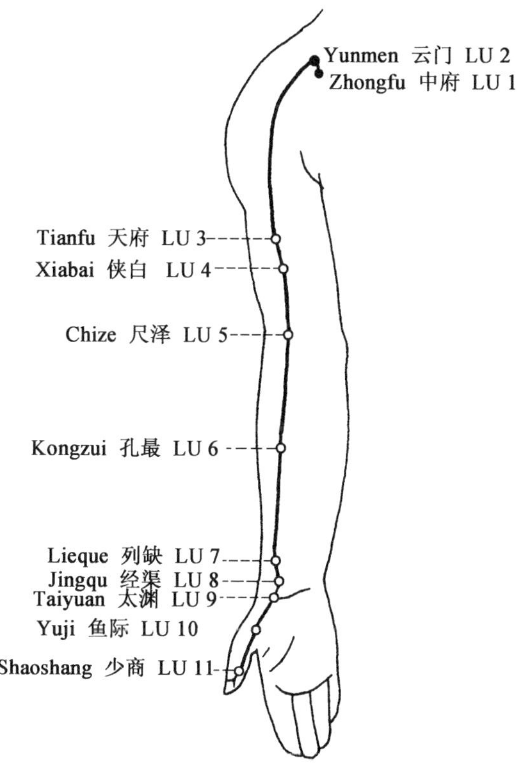

Fig.3-2 Acupoints of lung meridian of hand-taiyin

图 3-2 手太阴肺经腧穴总图

3 Indications of acupopints

The acupoints of lung meridian of hand-taiyin are indicated for the conditions in relation to the throat, chest, lung and the areas where the lung meridian goes along. Acupoints Zhongfu(LU 1), Taiyuan(LU 9) and Yuji(LU 10) act to relieve cough and asthma; Kongzui(LU 6) acts to relieve blood-coughing; Shaoshang(LU 11) and Yuji(LU 10) act to relieve sore throat; Chize(LU 5) acts to treat excess lung-heat disorders; Lieque(LU 7) acts to relieve headache and nape pain. The indications and needling manipulations of common acupoints are presented as follows.

3 腧穴主治

本经腧穴主要用于治疗咽喉、胸、肺以及经脉所过部位的病证。治疗咳喘常用中府、太渊、鱼际；治疗咯血常用孔最；治疗咽喉痛常用少商、鱼际；治疗肺实热证常用尺泽；治疗头项痛常用列缺。临床常用腧穴的主治及针刺操作如下。

3.1 Zhongfu (LU 1) Front-Mu acupoint of the lung; Crossing acupoint of hand and foot-taiyin meridians

Indications: ① Cough, breathlessness, chest distress, chest pain; ② shoulder and back pain.

Needling: Puncture obliquely or horizontally 0.5～0.8 cun in a lateral direction towards the coracoid process. Since the lungs are beneath the acupoint, the needle should not be inserted too deeply to prevent lung injury and ensuing pneumothorax.

3.1 中府 Zhōngfǔ 肺募穴；手足太阴经交会穴

主治：①咳嗽，气喘，胸闷，胸痛；②肩背痛。

操作：向外斜刺或平刺0.5～0.8寸。因穴位深部有肺脏，故针尖不可向内深刺，以免伤及肺脏，导致气胸。

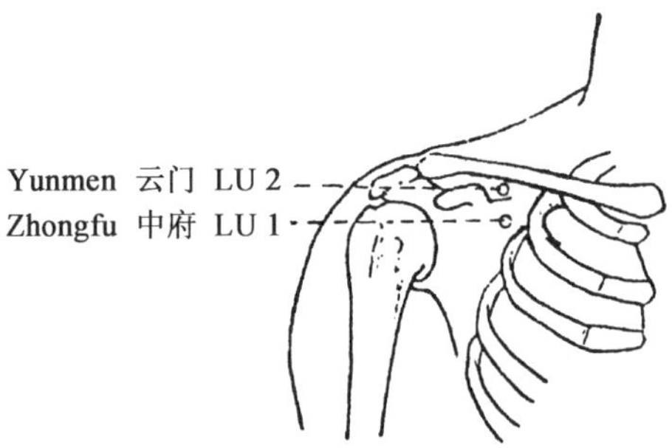

Fig.3-3 Chest acupoints on the lung meridian of hand-taiyin

图3-3 手太阴肺经胸部经穴图

3.2 Chize (LU 5) He-Sea acupoint

Indications: ① Cough, breathlessness, bloody coughing; ② sore throat, fever; ③ acute vomitting and diarrhea; ④ infantile convulsion; ⑤ spasm and pain of the elbow and arm.

Needling: Puncture vertically 0.8～1.2 cun; or prick to bleed.

3.2 尺泽 Chǐzé 合穴

主治: ①咳嗽,气喘,咳血;②咽喉肿痛,发热;③急性吐泻;④小儿惊风;⑤肘臂挛痛。

操作: 直刺0.8～1.2寸;或点刺出血。

3.3 Kongzui (LU 6) Xi-Cleft acupoint

Indications: ① Bloody coughing, cough, breathlessness; ② nasal bleeding, sore throat; ③ hemorrhoidial bleeding; ④ spasm and pain of the elbow and arm.

Needling: Puncture vertically 0.5～1.0 cun.

3.3 孔最 Kǒngzuì 郄穴

主治: ①咯血,咳嗽,气喘;②鼻衄,咽喉肿痛;③痔血;④肘臂挛痛。

操作: 直刺0.5～1.0寸。

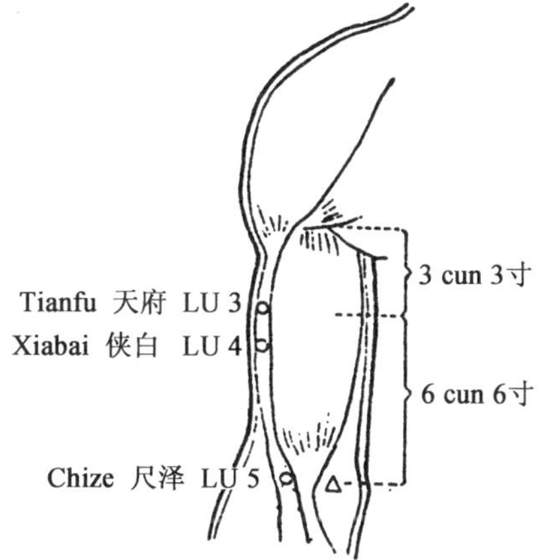

Fig.3-4 Upper arm acupoints on the lung meridian of hand-taiyin

图3-4 手太阴肺经上臂部经穴图

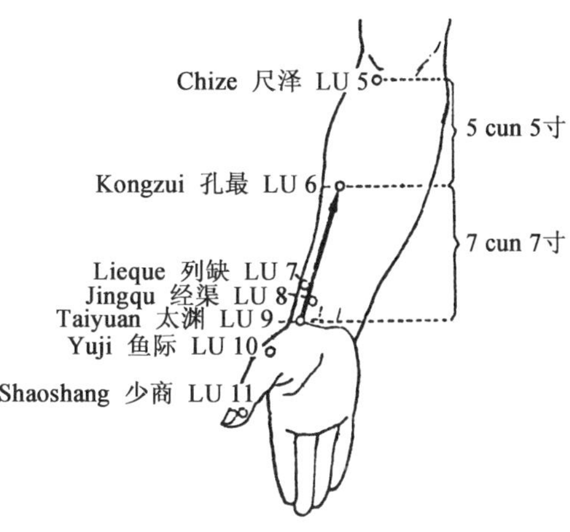

Fig.3-5 Forearm acupoints on the lung meridian of hand-taiyin

图3-5 手太阴肺经前臂部经穴图

3.4 Lieque (LU 7) Luo-Connecting acupoint; Confluent acupoint of the thoroughfare vessel

Indications: ① Cough, breathlessness; ② headache, nape stiffness, toothache, sore throat, facial

3.4 列缺 Lièquē 络穴;八脉交会穴(通任脉)

主治: ①咳嗽,气喘;②头痛,项强,齿痛,咽喉肿

palsy; ③ wrist pain.

Needling: Puncture proximally 0.5～0.8 cun.

痛，口眼歪斜；③手腕痛。

操作： 针尖向上斜刺0.5～0.8寸。

3.5 Taiyuan (LU 9) Shu-Stream acupoint; Yuan-Source acupoint; Influential acupoint of vessel

3.5 太渊 Tàiyuān 输穴；原穴；八会穴（脉会）

Indications: ① Cough, breathlessness, bloody coughing, chest pain; ② sore throat; ③ absent pulse; ④ hand and wrist pain.

Needling: Puncture vertically 0.3～0.5 cun, avoid radial artery.

主治： ①咳嗽，气喘，咳血，胸痛；②咽喉肿痛；③无脉症；④手腕痛。

操作： 避开桡动脉，直刺0.3～0.5寸。

3.6 Yuji (LU 10) Ying-Spring acupoint

3.6 鱼际 Yújì 荥穴

Indications: ① Cough, breathlessness, bloody coughing; ② sore throat, aphonia; ③ fever.

Needling: Puncture vertically 0.5～1.0 cun.

主治： ①咳嗽，气喘，咳血；②咽喉肿痛，失音；③发热。

操作： 直刺0.5～1.0寸。

3.7 Shaoshang (LU 11) Jing-Well acupoint

3.7 少商 Shàoshāng 井穴

Indications: ① Sore throat, nasal bleeding; ② fever, coma, mania; ③ cough; ④ arm numbness.

Needling: Puncture shallowly 0.1 cun; or prick to bleed.

主治： ①咽喉肿痛，鼻衄；②高热，昏迷，癫狂；③咳嗽；④手臂麻木。

操作： 浅刺0.1寸；或点刺出血。

Section 2 Large Intestine Meridian of Hand-Yangming and its Acupoints

第2节 手阳明大肠经及其腧穴

1 Distribution course

The large intestine meridian of hand-yangming

1 经脉循行

手阳明大肠经，起始于

begins at the radial side of the tip of the index finger and proceeds upwards along the radial side of the index finger between the first and second metacarpal bones of the hand. It passes through the interspace between the tendons of long and short extensor muscles of thumb, and follows upwards along the anterior border of the lateral aspect of the forearm to the lateral side of the elbow. From there, it ascends along the anterior border of the upper arm to the highest point of the shoulder, and meets the governor vessel on the nape. On the top of the shoulder, the meridian enters the chest cavity from supraclavicular fossa, and connects with the lungs before descending across the diaphragm to the large intestine, the organ it pertains to. A branch separates from the meridian at supraclavicular fossa, ascends externally along the neck, passes through the cheek, and enters internally the lower teeth and gums. From there, it curves around the upper lip and intersects the same meridian coming from the opposite side of the body at the philtrum. The branch finally terminates at the side of the nose to connect with the stomach meridian of foot yangming(Fig.3-6).

食指末端，沿食指桡侧缘，经第一、二掌骨间，进入两筋（拇长伸肌腱和拇短伸肌腱）之间，沿前臂外侧前缘，上肘外侧，经上臂外侧前缘，上肩，出肩峰部前边，上行颈部交会督脉，从缺盆部进入胸腔，联络于肺脏，通过横膈，属于大肠。颈部支脉，从缺盆部上行颈旁，上面颊，进入下齿，出来挟口旁，交会于人中部——左脉向右，右脉向左，上挟鼻翼两旁，连接足阳明胃经（图 3-6）。

2 Location of acupoints

The starting acupoint of the large intestine meridian is Shangyang(LI 1) and the ending acupoint is Yingxiang(LI 20), totally 20 acupoints in each side. The location of acupoints is presented in Table 3-2 and Fig.3-7～3-11.

2 腧穴定位

本经首穴为商阳，末穴为迎香，左右各 20 穴。腧穴定位见表 3-2、图 3-7～3-11。

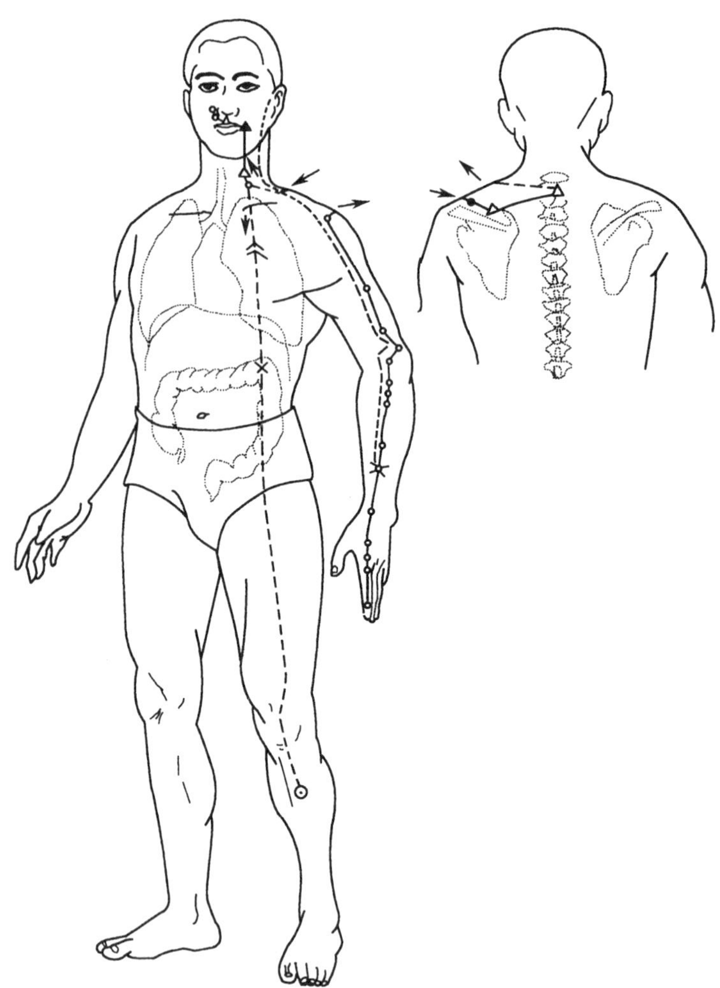

Fig.3-6　The distribution course of large intestine meridian of hand-yangming

图 3-6　手阳明大肠经循行示意图

Table 3-2　Location of acupoints of the large intestine meridian of hand-yangming

Acupoint		Location	Specific Features
LI 1*	Shangyang	On the distal end of the index finger, 0.1 cun from the radial corner of the nail	Jing-Well acupoint
LI 2	Erjian	On the radial aspect of the index finger, distal to the metacarpophalangeal joint, at the junction of the shaft and the head of the second metacarpal bone	Ying-Spring acupoint

(continued)

Acupoint		Location	Specific Features
LI 3*	Sanjian	On the radial aspect of the index finger, proximal to the metacarpophalangeal joint, at the junction of the shaft and the head of the second metacarpal bone	Shu-Stream acupoint
LI 4*	Hegu	On the radial aspect, between the first and second metacarpal bones, closer to the second metacarpal bone and approximately at its midpoint	Yuan-Source acupoint
LI 5*	Yangxi	With the thumb abducted, in a depression between the tendons of the extensor pollicis longus and brevis muscles(anatomical snuff box), on the redial aspect of the wrist	Jing-River acupoint
LI 6*	Pianli	3 cun proximal to the wrist crease, on the line between LI 5 and LI 11	Luo-Connecting acupoint
LI 7	Wenliu	5 cun proximal to the wrist crease, on the line between LI 5 and LI 11	Xi-Cleft acupoint
LI 8	Xialian	On the line connecting LI 5 and LI 11, 4 cun distal to LI 11	
LI 9	Shanglian	On the line connecting LI 5 and LI 11, 3 cun distal to LI 11	
LI 10*	Shousanli	On the line connecting LI 5 and LI 11, 2 cun distal to LI 11	
LI 11*	Quchi	At the midpoint of the line between Chize(LU 5) and the lateral epicondyle of the humerus	He-Sea acupoint
LI 12	Zhouliao	Upper border of the lateral epicondyle of the humerus and the anterior border of the humerus	
LI 13	Shouwuli	3 cun above the cubital transverse crease, on the line connecting Quchi(LI 11) and Jianyu(LI 15)	
LI 14*	Binao	7 cun above Quchi(LI 11), at the anterior border of deltoid muscle	
LI 15*	Jianyu	With the arm abducted or leveled, in the anterior depression inferior to acromioclavicular joint	Crossing acupoint of hard-yangming meridian and yang heel vessel
LI 16	Jugu	In the depression between the acromial extremity of the clavicle and the scapular spine	Crossing acupoint of hard-yangming meridian and yang heel vessel
LI 17	Tianding	At the level with the laryngeal prominence and the posterior border of the sternocleidomastoid muscle	
LI 18	Futu	At the level with the laryngeal prominence and between the sternal and clavicular heads of the sternocleidomastoid muscle	

(continued)

Acupoint		Location	Specific Features
LI 19	Kouheliao	At the level with the crossing point of upper one-third and lower two-thirds of philtrim, right below the lateral margin of the nostril	
LI 20*	Yingxiang	In the nasolabial groove, at the level with the midpoint of the lateral border of ala nasi	Crossing acupoint of the hand and foot-yangming meridians

表 3-2　手阳明大肠经的腧穴定位

腧穴		定位	特定穴属性
商阳*	Shāngyáng	食指末节桡侧，指甲根角侧上方 0.1 寸(指寸)	井穴
二间	Erjiān	第 2 掌指关节桡侧远端赤白肉际处	荥穴
三间*	Sānjiān	第 2 掌指关节桡侧近端凹陷中	输穴
合谷*	Hégǔ	第二掌骨桡侧的中点处	原穴
阳溪*	Yángxī	腕背侧远端横纹桡侧，桡骨茎突远端，解剖学“鼻咽窝”凹陷中	经穴
偏历*	Piānlì	腕背侧远端横纹上 3 寸，阳溪(LI 5)与曲池(LI 11)连线上	络穴
温溜	Wēnliū	腕背侧远端横纹上 5 寸，阳溪(LI 5)与曲池(LI 11)连线上	郄穴
下廉	Xiàlián	肘横纹下 4 寸，阳溪(LI 5)与曲池(LI 11)连线上	
上廉	Shànglián	肘横纹下 3 寸，阳溪(LI 5)与曲池(LI 11)连线上	
手三里*	Shǒusānlǐ	肘横纹下 2 寸，阳溪(LI 5)与曲池(LI 11)连线上	
曲池*	Qūchí	尺泽(LU 5)与肱骨外上髁连线的中点处	合穴
肘髎	Zhǒuliáo	肱骨外上髁上缘，髁上嵴的前缘	
手五里	Shǒuwǔlǐ	肘横纹上 3 寸，曲池(LI 11)与肩髃(LI 15)连线上	
臂臑*	Bìnào	曲池(LI 11)上 7 寸，三角肌前缘处	
肩髃*	Jiānyú	臂外展或向前平伸时肩峰前下方凹陷中	手阳明经、阳蹻脉交会穴
巨骨	Jùgǔ	锁骨肩峰端与肩胛冈之间凹陷中	手阳明经、阳蹻脉交会穴
天鼎	Tiāndǐng	横平环状软骨，胸锁乳突肌后缘	
扶突	Fútū	横平喉结，胸锁乳突肌前后缘中间	
口禾髎	Kǒuhéliáo	横平人中沟上 1/3 与下 2/3 交点，鼻孔外缘直下	
迎香*	Yíngxiāng	鼻翼外缘中点旁，鼻唇沟中	手足阳明经交会穴

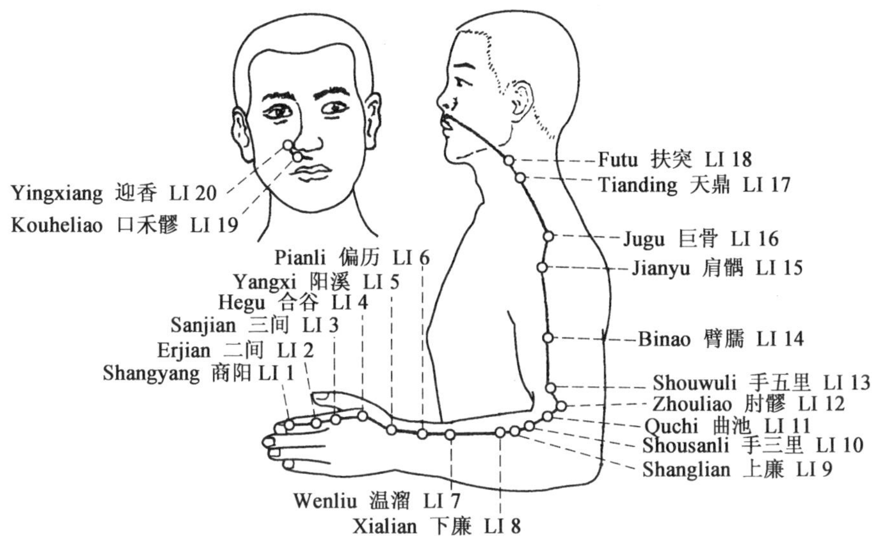

Fig.3-7 Acupoints of the large intestine meridian of hand-yangming

图 3-7 手阳明大肠经腧穴总图

3 Indications of acupoints

The meridian acupoints are indicated for diseases of the head and face, five sense organs, febrile disorders and other disorders of the places where the meridian supplies. For the diseases of the head, face and five sense organs, Hegu(LI 4) is applied; for nose diseases, Hegu(LI 4) and Yingxiang(LI 20) are used; for throat diseases, Shangyang(LI 1) and Hegu(LI 4) are selected; for febrile disorders, Shangyang(LI 1), Hegu(LI 4) and Quchi(LI 11) are selected; for shoulder and arm pain, Hegu(LI 4), Quchi(LI 11), Shousanli(LI 13), Binao(LI 14) and Jianyu(LI 15) are used. In addition, Hegu(LI 4) and Quchi(LI 11) are indicated for gastrointestinal disorders. The clinical indications and needling methods are presented as follows.

3 腧穴主治

本经腧穴主要用于治疗头面五官疾病、热病以及经脉所过部位的病证。治疗头面五官疾病常用合谷;治疗鼻疾常用合谷、迎香;治疗咽喉病可用商阳、合谷;治疗热病常用商阳、合谷、曲池;治疗肩臂痛常用合谷、曲池、手三里、臂臑和肩髃。另外,合谷、曲池亦可治疗胃肠病。临床常用腧穴的主治及针刺操作如下。

3.1 Shangyang (LI 1) Jing-Well acupoint

Indications: ①Sore throat, toothache; ② coma, sunstroke; ③ febrile diseases.

Needling: Puncture superficially 0.1 cun; or prick to bleed.

3.1 商阳 Shāngyáng 井穴

主治: ①咽喉肿痛,齿痛;②昏迷,中暑;③热病。

操作: 浅刺 0.1 寸,或点刺放血。

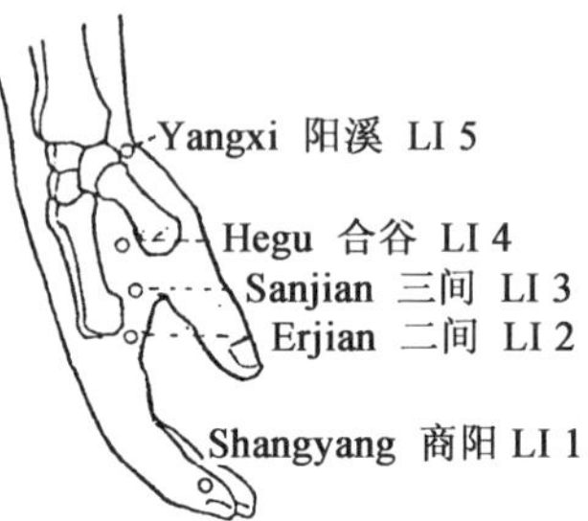

Fig.3-8 Hand acupoints on the large intestine meridian of hand-yangming

图 3-8 手阳明大肠经手部经穴图

3.2 Sanjian (LI 3) Shu-Stream acupoint

Indications: ① Toothache, sore throat; ② general feverishness.

Needling: Puncture vertically 0.3～0.5 cun.

3.3 Hegu (LI 4) Yuan-Source acupoint

Indications: ① Headache, deviation of the mouth and eyes, toothache, redness, swelling and pain in the eyes, nasal bleeding, deafness; ② fever and chills, profuse sweating, absence of sweating; ③ amenorrhea, delayed labor; ④ flaccidity, paralysis and inability to move of the upper limbs, finger convulsion and pain.

Needling: Puncture 0.5～1.0 cun; this acupoint is contraindicated for pregnant women.

3.4 Yangxi (LI 5) Jing-River acupoint

Indications: ① Wrist pain; ② headache, tooth-

3.2 三间 Sānjiān 输穴

主治: ① 齿痛,咽喉肿痛;②身热。

操作: 直刺 0.3～0.5 寸。

3.3 合谷 Hégǔ 原穴

主治: ①头痛,口眼㖞斜,齿痛,目赤肿痛,鼻衄,耳聋;②发热恶寒,多汗,无汗;③经闭,滞产;④上肢痿痹不遂,手指挛痛。

操作: 直刺 0.5～1.0 寸;孕妇禁针。

3.4 阳溪 Yángxī 经穴

主治: ① 手腕痛;② 头

ache, and sore throat.

Needling: Puncture 0.5～0.8 cun.

痛，齿痛，咽喉肿痛。

操作：直刺 0.5～0.8 寸。

3.5 Pianli (LI 6) Luo-Connecting acupoint

Indications: ① Nasal bleeding, tinnitus, deafness; ② aching and painful arms; ③ edema.

Needling: Puncture vertically or obliquely 0.5～0.8 cun.

3.5 偏历 Piānlì 络穴

主治：①鼻衄，耳鸣，耳聋；②手臂酸痛；③水肿。

操作：直刺或斜刺0.5～0.8 寸。

3.6 Shousanli (LI 10)

Indications: ① Paralysis of upper limbs, painful elbow and arms; ② toothache, swollen cheeck; ③ abdominal pain and diarrhea.

Needling: Puncture vertically 0.5～0.8 cun.

3.6 手三里 Shǒusānlǐ

主治：①上肢不遂，肘臂痛；②齿痛，颊肿；③腹痛，腹泻。

操作：直刺 0.8～1.2 寸。

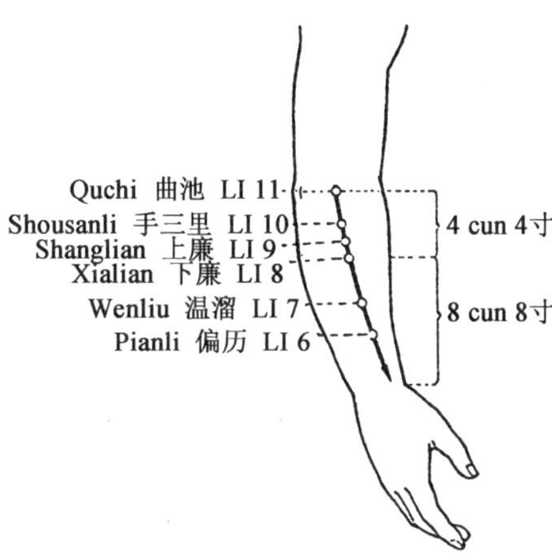

Fig.3-9 Forearm acupoints on the large intestine meridian of hand-yangming

图 3-9 手阳明大肠经前臂部经穴图

3.7 Quchi (LI 11) He-Sea acupoint

Indications: ① Sore throat, toothache, redness and pain of the eyes; ② febrile diseases; ③ rashes, eczema; ④ hypertension; ⑤ paralysis of upper limbs, painful weak elbow and arms; ⑥ psychosis; ⑦ abdominal pain and diarrhea.

3.7 曲池 Qūchí 合穴

主治：①咽喉肿痛，齿痛，目赤痛；②热病；③风疹，湿疹；④高血压；⑤上肢不遂，肘臂疼痛无力；⑥癫狂；⑦腹痛，腹泻。

Needling: Puncture vertically 0.8～1.5 cun.

操作: 直刺0.8～1.5寸。

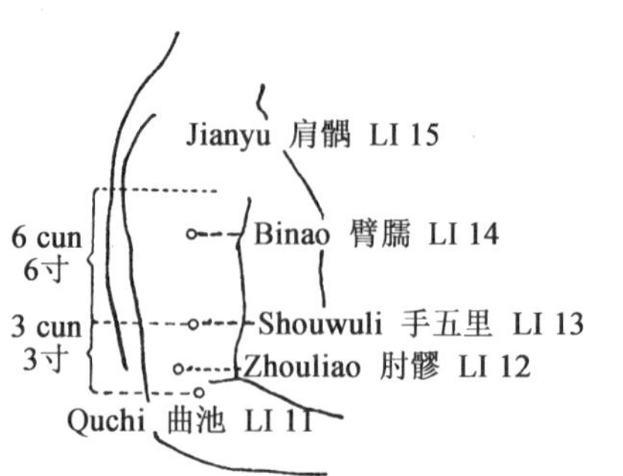

Fig.3-10 Upper arm acupoints on the large intestine meridian of hand-yangming

图3-10 手阳明大肠经上臂部经穴图

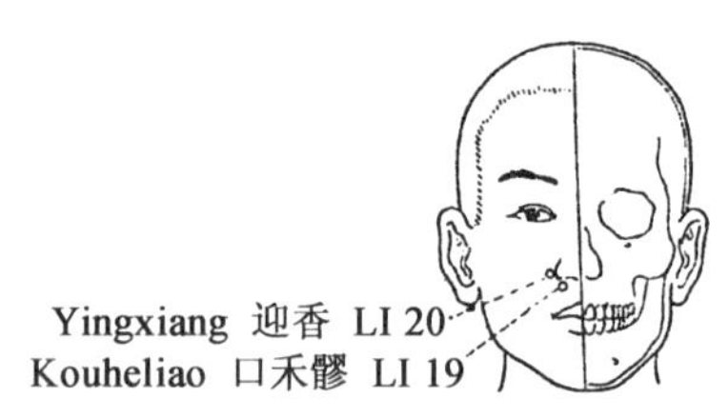

Fig.3-11 Head and face acupoints on the large intestine meridian of hand-yangming

图3-11 手阳明大肠经头面部经穴图

3.8 Binao (LI 14)

Indications: ① Painful shoulder and arm, paralysis of the upper limbs; ② eye disorders.

Needling: Puncture 0.8～1.5 cun vertically or obliquely with the needle tip upwards.

3.8 臂臑 Bìnào

主治: ①肩臂痛,上肢不遂;②目疾。

操作: 直刺或向上斜刺0.8～1.5寸。

3.9 Jianyu (LI 15) Crossing acupoint of hand-yangming meridian and yang heel-vessel

Indications: Painful shoulder failing to rise, paralysis of the upper limbs.

Needling: Puncture 0.8～1.5 cun vertically or obliquely with the needle tip downwards.

3.9 肩髃 Jiānyú 手阳明经、阳蹻脉交会穴

主治: 肩痛不举,上肢不遂。

操作: 直刺或向下斜刺0.8～1.5寸。

3.10 Yingxiang (LI 20) Crossing acupoint of the hand and foot-yangming meridians

Indications: ① Nasal stuffiness, nasal bleeding, sinusitis; ② deviated mouth, facial itching.

Needling: Puncture obliquely or horizontally 0.3～0.5 cun.

3.10 迎香 Yíngxiāng 手足阳明经交会穴

主治: ①鼻塞,鼻衄,鼻渊;②口㖞,面痒。

操作: 斜刺或平刺0.3～0.5寸。

Section 3 Stomach Meridian of Foot-Yangming and its Acupoints

1 Distribution course

The stomach meridian of foot-yangming begins from the lateral side of the ala nasi, and ascends to the bridge of the nose, where it meets the bladder meridian at the inner canther of the eyes, Jingming (GB 1). Descending along the lateral side of the nose, it enters the upper gum and curves around the lips, descending to meet the conception vessel at Chengjiang(CV 24) in the mentolabial groove. Then it runs posteriorly along the facial artery, winding along the angle of the mandible, it then ascends in the front of the ear and transverses along the upper border of zygomatic arch; then it follows the anterior hairline from the corner of the forehead to the middle part of the forehead. A branch descends in front of Daying(ST 12) and runs along the neck artery and throat to enter supraclavicular fossa; it descends through the diaphragm and enters the stomach, the organ it pertains to, and connects with the spleen. Another branch arising from the supraclavicular fossa runs downwards passing through the nipple(4 cun lateral to the anterior midline); then it descends by the umbilicus(2 cun lateral to the anterior midline) and terminates in the groin. A branch from the lower orifice of the stomach descends inside the abdomen to join the previous branch in the groin. From this point, the meridian runs downwards over the front of the thigh to the outer side of the knee, and continues along the lat-

第3节 足阳明胃经及其腧穴

1 经脉循行

足阳明胃经，从鼻旁开始，上行鼻根处，与足太阳经交会于睛明，向下沿鼻外侧，入上齿，出来挟口旁，环绕口唇，向下交会于颏唇沟的承浆穴；向后沿下颌面动脉部，经下颌角，上耳前，经颧弓上部，沿额角发际，至额前中部。颈部支脉，从大迎前向下，经颈动脉，沿喉咙，进入锁骨上窝，通过膈肌，属于胃，络于脾。胸腹部主脉，从锁骨上窝向下，经乳中（在胸部旁开前正中线4寸），向下挟脐两旁（在腹部旁开前正中线2寸），进入腹股沟。腹内支脉，从胃下口向下，沿腹里，至腹股沟与前外行脉会合。由此下行经髋关节前，到股四头肌隆起处，下入膝关节中，沿胫骨外侧，下行足背，进入足中趾内侧趾缝至足第二趾外侧端。小腿部支脉，从膝下3寸处分出，向下进入中趾外侧趾缝，出中趾末端。足部支脉，从足背部分出，进入大趾内侧，出大趾末端，连接足太阴脾经（图3-12）。

eral aspect of the tibia to the dorsum of the foot, and reaches the lateral side of the tip of the second toe. A branch emerges from the stomach meridian three cun below the knee and ends at the lateral side of the middle toe. A branch arises from the dorsum of the foot and terminates at the medial side of the big toe to connect with the spleen meridian of foot taiyin(Fig. 3-12).

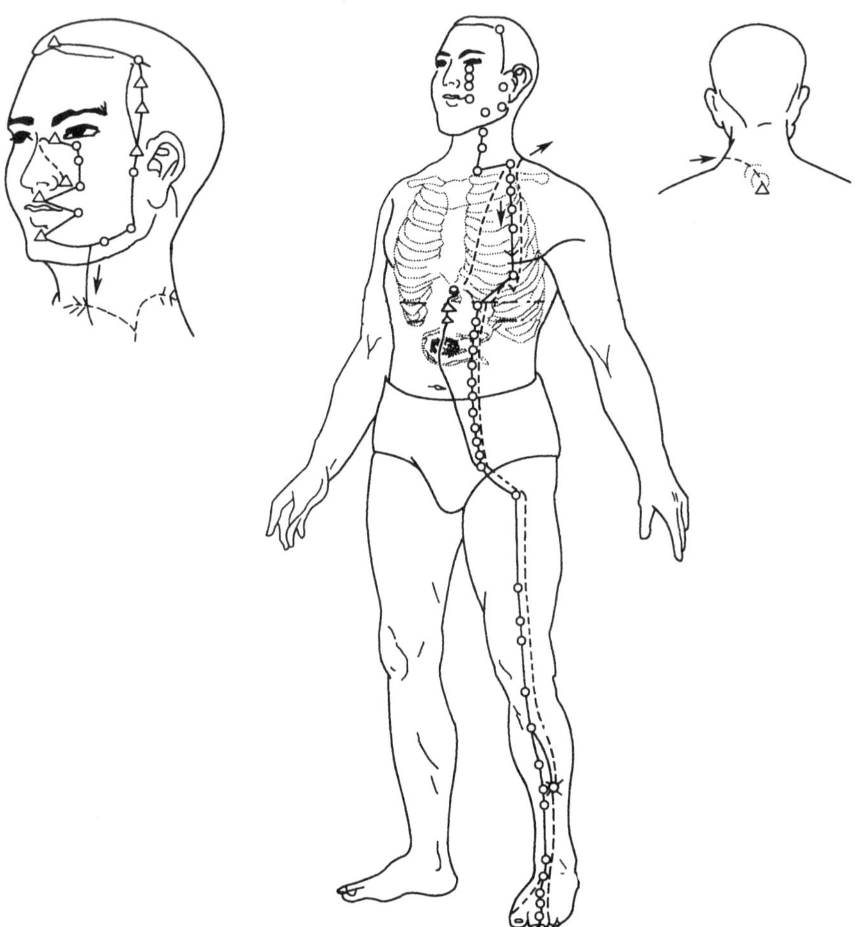

Fig.3-12　The distribution course of stomach meridian of foot-yangming

图 3-12　足阳明胃经循行示意图

2 Location of acupoints

The starting acupoint of the stomach meridian is Chengqi(ST 1) and the ending acupoint is Lidui (ST 45), totally 45 acupoints in each side. The location of acupoints is presented in Table 3 - 3 and Fig.3-13～3-19.

2 腧穴定位

本经首穴为承泣，末穴为厉兑，左右各 45 穴。腧穴定位见表 3 - 3、图 3 - 13～3-19。

Table 3-3 Location of acupoints of the stomach meridian of foot-yangming

Acupoint		Location	Specific feature
ST 1*	Chengqi	Between the eyeball and the infraorbital ridge, right below the pupils	Crossing acupoint of yang heel vessel, conception vessel and foot-yangming meridian
ST 2*	Sibai	In the depression at the infraorbital foramen	Crossing acupoint of yang heel vessel and foot-yangming meridian
ST 3	Juliao	Level with the lower border of the ala nasi and right below the pupil	
ST 4*	Dicang	0.4 cun lateral to the corner of the mouth	Crossing acupoint of yang heel vessel, hand and foot-yangming meridian
ST 5	Daying	Anterior to the angle of mandible, in the anterior depression of the attached part of masseter muscle, where facial artery can be felt	
ST 6*	Jiache	One finger-width anterior and superior to the lower angle of the mandible, at the prominence when teeth are clenched	
ST 7*	Xiaguan	In the depression between the zygomatic arch and mandibular notch	Crossing acupoint of the foot-yangming meridian and foot-shaoyang meridian
ST 8*	Touwei	0.5 cun above the forehead hairline, and 4.5 cun lateral to the anterior midline	Crossing acupoint of foot-shaoyang and foot-yangming meridian
ST 9*	Renying	Level with the Adam's apple, on the anterior border of the sternocleidomastoideus muscle, where the common carotid artery can be felt	
ST 10	Shuitu	Level with the thyroid cartilage, on the anterior border of the sternocleidomastoideus muscle	
ST 11	Qishe	On the superior border of the sternal extremity of the clavicle, in the depression between the sternal head and clavicular head of the sternocleidomastoideus muscle	
ST 12	Quepen	In the center of the supraclavicular fossa, 4 cun lateral to the anterior midline	

(continued)

Acupoint		Location	Specific feature
ST 13	Qihu	At the lower border of the clavicle, 4 cun lateral to the anterior midline	
ST 14	Kufang	In the first intercoastal space, 4 cun lateral to the anterior midline	
ST 15	Wuyi	In the second intercostal space, 4 cun lateral to the anterior midline	
ST 16	Yingchuang	In the third intercostal space, 4 cun lateral to the anterior midline	
ST 17	Ruzhong	In the center of the nipple	
ST 18	Rugen	In the fifth intercoastal space, 4 cun lateral to the anterior midline	
ST 19	Burong	6 cun above the navel and 2 cun lateral to the anterior midline	
ST 20	Chengman	5 cun above the navel and 2 cun lateral to the anterior midline	
ST 21*	Liangmen	4 cun above the navel and 2 cun lateral to the anterior midline	
ST 22	Guanmen	3 cun above the navel and 2 cun lateral to the anterior midline	
ST 23	Taiyi	2 cun above the navel and 2 cun lateral to the anterior midline	
ST 24	Huaroumen	1 cun above the navel and 2 cun lateral to the anterior midline	
ST 25*	Tianshu	Level with the navel and 2 cun lateral to the anterior midline	Front-Mu acupoint of the large intestine
ST 26	Wailing	1 cun below the navel and 2 cun lateral to the anterior midline	
ST 27	Daju	2 cun below the navel and 2 cun lateral to the anterior midline	
ST 28*	Shuidao	3 cun below the navel and 2 cun lateral to the anterior midline	
ST 29*	Guilai	4 cun below the navel and 2 cun lateral to the anterior midline	
ST 30*	Qichong	On the upper border of the pubic symphysis and 2 cun lateral to the anterior midline. Where the artery can be felt	

(continued)

Acupoint		Location	Specific feature
ST 31*	Biguan	In the depression between rectus femoris, sartorius and tensor fasciae latae	
ST 32*	Futu	6 cun superior to the laterosuperior border of the patella, on the line connecting the anterior iliac spine and the lateral border of the patella	
ST 33	Yinshi	3 cun superior to the laterosuperior border of the patella and the lateral border of the tendon of rectus femoris	
ST 34*	Liangqiu	2 cun superior to the laterosuperior border of the patella, between the tendons of vastus lateralis andrectus femoris	Xi-Cleft acupoint
ST 35*	Dubi	In the depression lateral to the patellar ligament	
ST 36*	Zusanli	3 cun below Dubi(ST 35), on the line between Dubi (ST 35) and Jiexi(ST 41)	He-Sea acupoint, Lower He-Sea acupoint of the stomach
ST 37*	Shangjuxu	6 cun below Dubi(ST 35), on the line between Dubi (ST 35) and Jiexi(ST 41)	Lower He-Sea acupoint of the large intestine
ST 38*	Tiaokou	8 cun below Dubi(ST 35), on the line between Dubi (ST 35) and Jiexi(ST 41)	
ST 39*	Xiajuxu	9 cun below Dubi(ST 35), on the line between Dubi (ST 35) and Jiexi(ST 41)	Lower He-Sea acupoint of the small intestine
ST 40*	Fenglong	8 cun above the tip of the external malleolus, on the lateral border of tibialis anterior	Luo-Connecting acupoint
ST 41*	Jiexi	In the depression in the front ankle and between the tendons of extensor digitorm longus muscle and hallucis longus	Jing-River acupoint
ST 42*	Chongyang	The joint between the base of the second metatarsal bones and cuneiform, where the dorsal artery can be felt	Yuan-Source acupoint
ST 43*	Xiangu	Between the second and third metatarsal bones, and in the depression near the second metatarsophalangeal joints	Shu-Stream acupoint
ST 44*	Neiting	Proximal to the web margin between the second and third toes	Ying-Spring acupoint
ST 45*	Lidui	On the lateral side of the second toe, 0.1 cun posterior to the corner of the nail	Jing-Well acupoint

表 3-3　足阳明胃经的腧穴定位

腧穴		定位	特定穴属性
承泣*	Chéngqì	眼球与眶下缘之间，瞳孔直下	阳蹻脉、任脉、足阳明经交会穴
四白*	Sìbái	眶下孔处	阳蹻脉、足阳明经交会穴
巨髎	Jùliáo	横平鼻翼下缘，瞳孔直下	
地仓*	Dìcāng	口角旁开 0.4 寸(指寸)	阳蹻脉、手足阳明经交会穴
大迎	Dàyíng	下颌角前方，咬肌附着部的前缘凹陷中，面动脉搏动处	
颊车*	Jiáchē	下颌角前上方约一横指，当咀嚼时咬肌隆起高点处	
下关*	Xiàguān	颧弓下缘中央与下颌切迹之间凹陷中	足阳明、少阳经交会穴
头维*	Tóuwéi	额角发际直上 0.5 寸，头正中线旁开 4.5 寸	足少阳、阳明经交会穴
人迎*	Rényíng	横平喉结，胸锁乳突肌前缘，颈总动脉搏动处	
水突	Shuǐtū	横平环状软骨，胸锁乳突肌前缘	
气舍	Qìshè	锁骨上小窝，锁骨胸骨端上缘，胸锁乳突肌胸骨头与锁骨头中间的凹陷中	
缺盆	Quēpén	锁骨上大窝，锁骨上缘凹陷中，前正中线旁开4 寸	
气户	Qìhù	锁骨下缘，前正中线旁开 4 寸	
库房	Kùfáng	第 1 肋间隙，前正中线旁开 4 寸	
屋翳	Wūyì	第 2 肋间隙，前正中线旁开 4 寸	
膺窗	Yīngchuāng	第 3 肋间隙，前正中线旁开 4 寸	
乳中	Rǔzhōng	乳头中央	
乳根	Rǔgēn	第 5 肋间隙，前正中线旁开 4 寸	
不容	Bùróng	脐中上 6 寸，前正中线旁开 2 寸	
承满	Chéngmǎn	脐中上 5 寸，前正中线旁开 2 寸	
梁门*	Liángmén	脐中上 4 寸，前正中线旁开 2 寸	
关门	Guānmén	脐中上 3 寸，前正中线旁开 2 寸	
太乙	Tàiyǐ	脐中上 2 寸，前正中线旁开 2 寸	
滑肉门	Huáròumén	脐中上 1 寸，前正中线旁开 2 寸	
天枢*	Tiānshū	横平脐中，前正中线旁开 2 寸	大肠募穴
外陵	Wàilíng	脐中下 1 寸，前正中线旁开 2 寸	
大巨	Dàjù	脐中下 2 寸，前正中线旁开 2 寸	
水道*	Shuǐdào	脐中下 3 寸，前正中线旁开 2 寸	

(续表)

腧穴		定位	特定穴属性
归来*	Guīlái	脐中下 4 寸,前正中线旁开 2 寸	
气冲*	Qìchōng	耻骨联合上缘,前正中线旁开 2 寸,动脉搏动处	
髀关*	Bìguān	股直肌近端、缝匠肌与阔筋膜张肌 3 条肌肉之间凹陷中	
伏兔*	Fútù	髌骨底上 6 寸,髂前上棘与髌骨底外侧端的连线上	
阴市	Yīnshì	髌骨底上 3 寸,股直肌肌腱外侧缘	
梁丘*	Liángqiū	髌骨底上 2 寸,股外侧肌与股直肌肌腱之间	郄穴
犊鼻*	Dúbí	髌韧带外侧凹陷中	
足三里*	Zúsānlǐ	犊鼻(ST35)下 3 寸,犊鼻(ST35)与解溪(ST41)连线上	合穴;胃下合穴
上巨虚*	Shàngjùxū	犊鼻(ST35)下 6 寸,犊鼻(ST35)与解溪(ST41)连线上	大肠下合穴
条口*	Tiáokǒu	犊鼻(ST35)下 8 寸,犊鼻(ST35)与解溪(ST41)连线上	
下巨虚*	Xiàjùxū	犊鼻(ST35)下 9 寸,犊鼻(ST35)与解溪(ST41)连线上	小肠下合穴
丰隆*	Fēnglóng	外踝尖上 8 寸,胫骨前肌的外缘	络穴
解溪*	Jiěxī	踝关节前面中央凹陷中,拇长伸肌腱与趾长伸肌腱之间	经穴
冲阳*	Chōngyáng	第 2 跖骨基底部与中间楔状骨关节处,可触及足背动脉	原穴
陷谷	Xiàngǔ	第 2、第 3 跖骨间,第 2 跖趾关节近端凹陷中	输穴
内庭*	Nèitíng	第 2、第 3 趾间,趾蹼缘后方赤白肉际处	荥穴
厉兑*	Lìduì	第 2 趾末节外侧,趾甲根角侧后方 0.1 寸(指寸)	井穴

3 Indications of acupoints

The acupoints of the stomach meridian are principally indicated for the diseases in the stomach and intestine, in the head, face and five sense organs, mental disorders, febrile diseases, and the conditions along the course of the stomach meridian. The diseases of the stomach and intestine are often treated by Tianshu (ST 25), Liangmen (ST

3 腧穴主治

本经腧穴主要用于治疗胃肠病、头面五官疾病、神志病、热病以及经脉所过部位的病证。治疗胃肠病常用天枢、梁门、足三里、上巨虚、下巨虚、梁丘和内庭;治疗头面五官疾病常用地仓、颊车、四

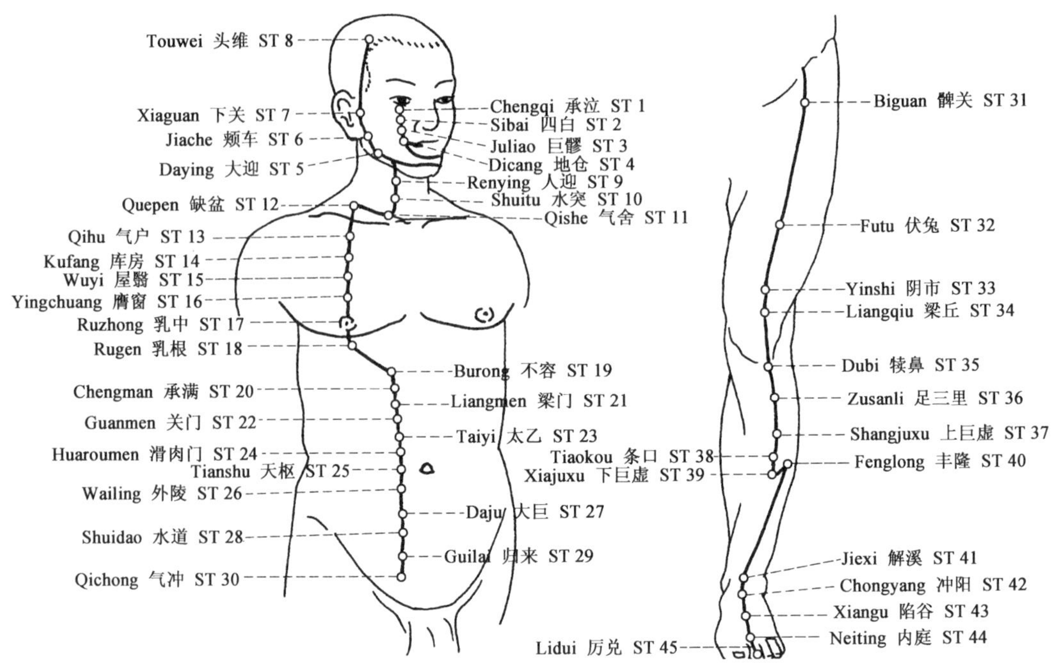

Fig.3-13　Acupoints of stomach meridian of foot-yangming

图 3-13　足阳明胃经腧穴总图

21), Zusanli(ST 36), Shangjuxu(ST 37), Xiajuxu (ST 39), Liangqiu(ST 34) and Neiting(ST 44); the diseases in the head, face and five sense organs are often treated by Dicang(ST 4), Jiache(ST 6), Sibai (ST 2), Touwei(ST 8), Xiaguan(ST 7), Neiting(ST 44) and Jiexi(ST 41); the mental disorders are often treated by Jiexi(ST 41), Lidui(ST 45) and Neiting (ST 44); Fenglong(ST 40) acts to remove phlegm; Shuidao(ST 28) functions to disinhibit water, and Zusanli (ST 36) serves to strengthen body and healthcare. The indications and needling manipulations are presented as follows.

白、头维、下关、内庭和解溪；治疗神志病常用解溪、厉兑和内庭；丰隆有祛痰的功能；水道有利水的功能；足三里有强身保健的功能。临床常用腧穴的主治及针刺操作如下。

3.1 Chengqi (ST 1) Crossing acupoint of yang heel vessel, conception vessel and foot-yangming

Indications: ① Redness, swelling and pain in the eyes, lacrimation, night blindness, blurred version; ② twitching eyelids, deviated mouth and eyes.

Needling: The patient is asked to close his eyes. Push the eyeball upwards with the left thumb and perpendicularly puncture 0.5～1.0 cun slowly along the infraorbital ridge; to avoid injuring blood vessels and causing hematoma, it is not advisable to lift and thrust the needle.

3.1 承泣 Chéngqì 阳蹻脉、任脉、足阳明经交会穴

主治：①目赤肿痛，迎风流泪，夜盲，视物不明；②眼睑瞤动，口眼㖞斜。

操作：让患者闭目，医者以左手拇指向上轻推眼球，紧靠眶缘缓慢直刺0.5～1.0寸，不宜提插，出针时按压针孔，以防出血。

3.2 Sibai (ST 2)

Indications: ① Redness, swelling and pain in the eyes, lacrimation, nebula, blurred vision; ② deviated mouth and eyes, twitching eyelids, facial pain, facial itching.

Needling: Puncture vertically or obliquely 0.3～0.5 cun.

3.2 四白 Sìbái

主治：①目赤肿痛，迎风流泪，目翳，视物不明；②口眼㖞斜，眼睑瞤动，面痛、面痒；③眩晕。

操作：直刺或斜刺0.3～0.5寸。

3.3 Dicang (ST 4) Crossing acupoint of yang heel vessel, hand and foot-yangming meridian

Indications: Deviated mouth and eyes, salivation, toothache, facial pain, and twitching face.

Needling: Puncture vertically 0.2 cun, obliquely or transversely 0.5～1.5 cun.

3.3 地仓 Dìcāng 阳蹻脉、手足阳明经交会穴

主治：口眼㖞斜，流涎，齿痛，面痛，面肌瞤动。

操作：直刺0.2寸，斜刺或平刺0.5～1.5寸。

3.4 Daying (ST 5)

Indications: Toothache, deviated mouth and eyes, swollen cheeck, facial pain, twitching face.

Needling: Puncture vertically 0.3～0.5 cun.

3.4 大迎 Dàyíng

主治：齿痛，口眼㖞斜，颊肿，面痛，面肌瞤动。

操作：直刺0.3～0.5寸。

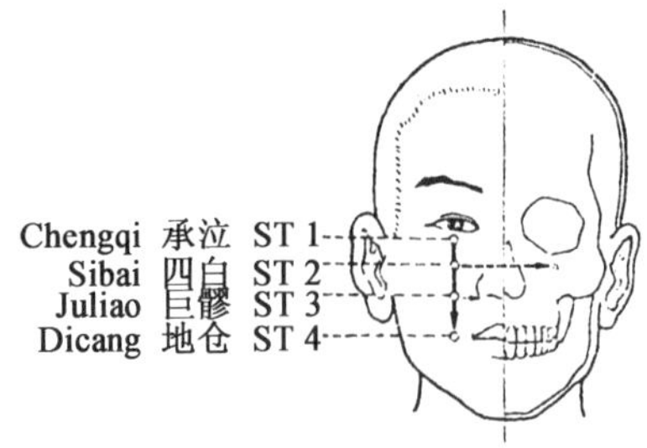

Fig.3-14　Head and face acupoints on the stomach meridian of foot-yangming

图 3-14　足阳明胃经头面部经穴图

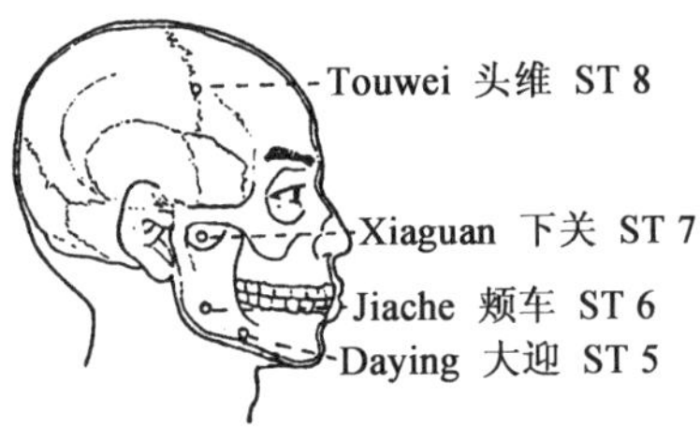

Fig.3-15　Head and face acupoints of the stomach meridian of foot-yangming

图 3-15　足阳明胃经头面部经穴图

3.5　Jiache (ST 6)

Indications: Deviated mouth and eyes, toothache, facial pain, twitching face, swollen cheeck.

Needling: Puncture vertically 0. 3～0. 5 cun, transversely 0.5～0.8 cun.

3.6　Xiaguan (ST 7)　Crossing acupoint of foot-yangming meridian and foot-shaoyang meridian

Indications: ① Pain in the lower mandible, lockjaw, deviated mouth and eyes, toothache, swollen cheeck, facial pain; ② deafness, tinnitus, and otorrhea.

Needling: Puncture vertically 0.3～0.5 cun.

3.7　Touwei (ST 8)　Crossing acupoint of foot-shaoyang meridian and foot-yangming meridian

Indications: ① Headache, vertigo; ② painful eyes, lacrimation; ③ twitching eyelids.

Needling: Puncture transversely 0.5～0.8 cun.

3.8　Liangmen (ST 21)

Indications: Stomachache, vomiting, poor appetite, abdominal distension.

Needling: Puncture vertically 0. 8～1. 2 cun. Needling is not indicated for those full stuffed or with enlarged liver.

3.5　颊车 Jiáchē

主治: 口眼㖞斜,齿痛,面痛,面肌瞤动,颊肿。

操作: 直刺 0.3～0.5 寸,平刺 0.5～0.8 寸。

3.6　下关 Xiàguān　足阳明、少阳经交会穴

主治: ①下颌疼痛,口噤,口眼㖞斜,齿痛,颊肿,面痛;②耳聋,耳鸣,聤耳。

操作: 直刺 0.3～0.5 寸。

3.7　头维 Tóuwéi　足少阳、阳明经交会穴

主治: ①头痛,眩晕;②目痛,迎风流泪;③眼睑瞤动。

操作: 平刺 0.5～0.8 寸。

3.8　梁门 Liángmén

主治: 胃痛,呕吐,食欲不振,腹胀。

操作: 直刺 0.8～1.2 寸。过饱或肝肿大者不宜针。

3.9 Tianshu (ST 25) Front-Mu acupoint of large intestine

Indications: ① Abdominal pain, abdominal distension, intestinal gurgling, diarrhea, dysentery, constipation, intestinal abscess; ② irregular menstruation and menstrual cramps; ③ edema.

Needling: Puncture vertically 0.8～1.2 cun.

3.9 天枢 Tiānshū 大肠募穴

主治：①腹痛，腹胀，肠鸣，泄泻，痢疾，便秘，肠痈；②月经不调，痛经；③水肿。

操作：直刺0.8～1.2寸。

3.10 Shuidao (ST 28)

Indications: ① Lower abdominal distension, difficulty urination; ② menstrual cramps; ③ hernia.

Needling: Puncture vertically 1.0～1.5 cun.

3.10 水道 Shuǐdào

主治：①小腹胀痛，小便不利；②痛经；③疝气。

操作：直刺1.0～1.5寸。

3.11 Guilai (ST 29)

Indications: ① Amenorrhea, proplased uterus, menstrual cramps, morbid leukorrhea, irregular menstruation; ② lower abdominal pain, hernia.

Needling: Puncture vertically 1.0～1.5 cun.

3.11 归来 Guīlái

主治：①经闭，阴挺，痛经，带下，月经不调；②小腹痛，疝气。

操作：直刺1.0～1.5寸。

3.12 Qichong (ST 30)

Indications: ① Abdominal pain, hernia; ② irregular menstruation, infertility, impotence, swelling of the external genitalia.

Needling: Puncture vertically 0.8～1.2 cun.

3.12 气冲 Qìchōng

主治：①腹痛，疝气；②月经不调，不孕，阳痿，阴肿痛。

操作：直刺0.8～1.2寸。

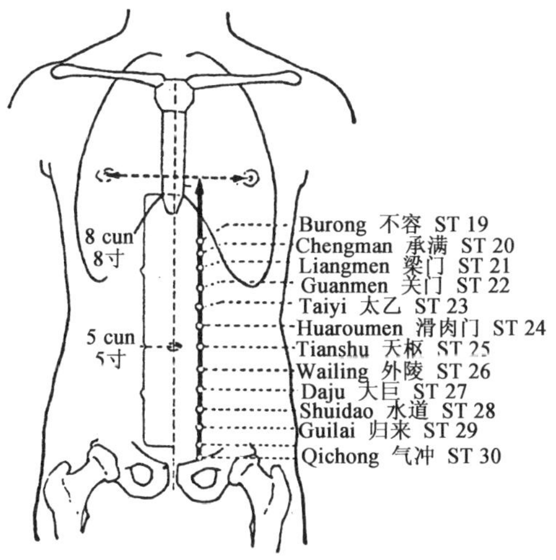

Fig.3-16 Abdomen acupoints on the stomach meridian of foot-yangming

图3-16 足阳明胃经腹部经穴图

3.13 Biguan (ST 31)

Indications: Muscular atrophy and motor impairment of the lower limbs, pain in the lower back and leg.

Needling: Puncture vertically 1.0～2.0 cun.

3.14 Futu (ST 32)

Indications: Muscular atrophy and motor impairment of the lower limbs, pain and coldness of the lower back and knees.

Needling: Puncture vertically 1.0～2.0 cun.

3.15 Liangqiu (ST 34) Xi-Cleft acupoint

Indications: ① Stomachache; ② knee pain, muscular atrophy and motor impairment of the lower limbs; ③ breast abscess.

Needling: Puncture vertically 1.0～1.5 cun.

3.13 髀关 Bìguān

主治：下肢痿痹不遂，腰腿疼痛。

操作：直刺1.0～2.0寸。

3.14 伏兔 Fútù

主治：下肢痿痹不遂，腰膝冷痛。

操作：直刺1.0～2.0寸。

3.15 梁丘 Liángqiū 郄穴

主治：①胃痛；②膝痛，下肢痿痹不遂；③乳痈。

操作：直刺1.0～1.5寸。

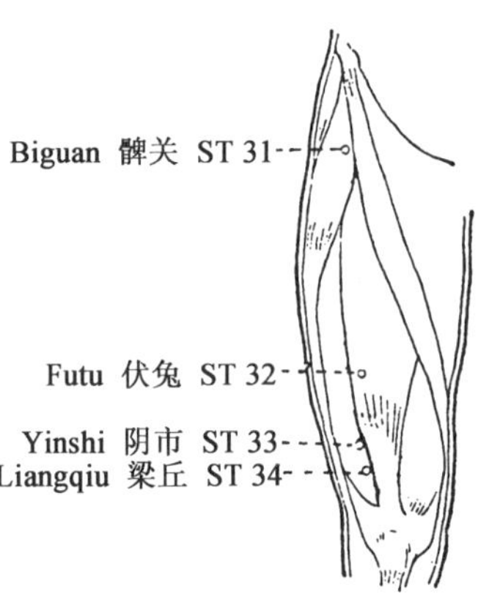

Fig.3-17 Lower limb acupoints on the stomach meridian of foot-yangming

图3-17 足阳明胃经下肢部经穴图

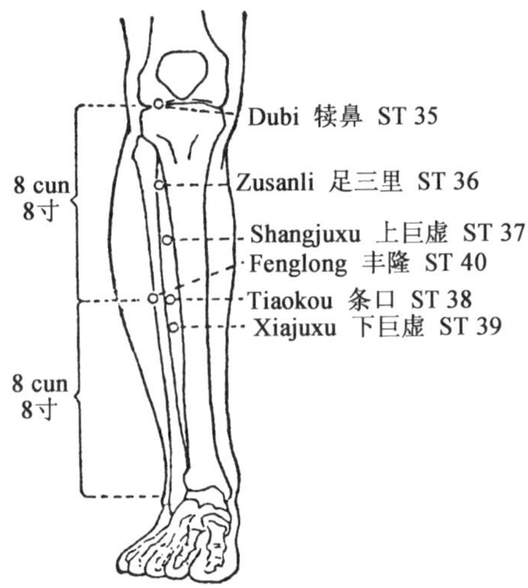

Fig.3-18 Lower limb acupoints on the stomach meridian of foot-yangming

图3-18 足阳明胃经下肢部经穴图

3.16 Dubi (ST 35)

Indications: Swelling and pain of the knees,

3.16 犊鼻 Dúbí

主治：膝肿痛、屈伸不

muscular atrophy and motor impairment of the lower limbs, and beriberi.

Needling: Puncture posteriorly-medially 0.8～1.5 cun.

利,脚气。

操作: 向后内斜刺0.8～1.5寸。

3.17 Zusanli (ST 36) He-Sea acupoint; Lower He-Sea acupoint of stomach

Indications: ① Stomachache, vomiting, abdominal pain, abdominal distension, diarrhea, dysentery, constipation, intestinal abscess; ② general emaciation and deficiency, palpitation and shortness of breath; ③ muscular atrophy and motor impairment of the lower limbs, beriberi, edema; ④ depressive and manic psychosis.

Needling: Puncture vertically 1.0～1.5 cun.

3.17 足三里 Zúsānlǐ 合穴;胃下合穴

主治: ①胃痛,呕吐,腹痛,腹胀,泄泻,痢疾,便秘,肠痈;②虚劳羸瘦,心悸气短;③下肢痿痹不遂,脚气,水肿;④癫狂痫。

操作: 直刺 1.0～1.5 寸。

3.18 Shangjuxu (ST 37) Lower He-Sea acupoint

Indications: ① Abdominal pain, diarrhea, dysentery, constipation, intestinal abscess; ② muscular atrophy and motor impairment of the lower limbs, beriberi.

Needling: Puncture vertically 1.0～1.5 cun.

3.18 上巨虚 Shàngjùxū 大肠下合穴

主治: ①腹痛,泄泻,痢疾,便秘,肠痈;②下肢痿痹不遂,脚气。

操作: 直刺 1.0～1.5 寸。

3.19 Tiaokou (ST 38)

Indications: ① Muscular atrophy and motor impairment of the lower limbs; ② abdominal pain; ③ pain in the arm and shoulder.

Needling: Puncture vertically 1.0～1.5 cun.

3.19 条口 Tiáokǒu

主治: ①下肢痿痹;②脘腹疼痛;③肩臂痛。

操作: 直刺 1.0～1.5 寸。

3.20 Xiajuxu (ST 39) Lower He-Sea acupoint of small intestine

Indications: ① Lower abdominal pain, intestinal gurgling, diarrhea; ② muscular atrophy and motor impairment of the lower limbs.

Needling: Puncture vertically 1.0～1.5 cun.

3.20 下巨虚 Xiàjùxū 小肠下合穴

主治: ①小腹痛,肠鸣,泄泻;②下肢痿痹不遂。

操作: 直刺 1.0～1.5 寸。

3.21 Fenglong (ST 40) Luo-Connecting acupoint

Indications: ① Cough with profuse sputum; ②

3.21 丰隆 Fēnglóng 络穴

主治: ①咳嗽痰多;②头

headache, vertigo, depressive and manic psychosis; ③ muscular atrophy and motor impairment of the lower limbs.

痛，眩晕，癫狂痫；③下肢痿痹。

Needling: Puncture vertically 1.0～1.5 cun.

操作: 直刺 1.0～1.5 寸。

3.22 Jiexi (ST 41) Jing-River acupoint

3.22 解溪 Jiěxī 经穴

Indications: ① Muscular atrophy and motor impairment of the lower limbs, ankle swelling; ② abdominal distension, constipation; ③ headache, vertigo, depressive and manic psychosis.

主治: ①下肢痿痹，足踝肿痛；②腹胀，便秘；③头痛，眩晕，癫狂痫。

Needling: Puncture vertically 0.5～1.0 cun.

操作: 直刺 0.5～1.0 寸。

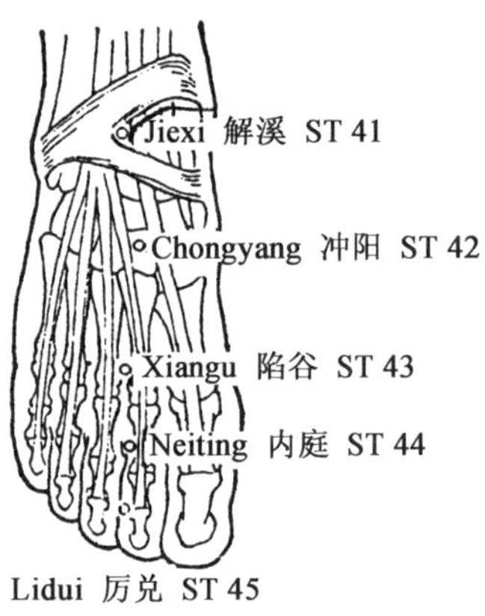

Fig.3-19 Foot dorsum acupoints on the stomach meridian of foot-yangming

图 3-19　足阳明胃经足背部经穴图

3.23 Chongyang (ST 42) Yuan-Source acupoint

3.23 冲阳 Chōngyáng 原穴

Indications: ① Stomachache, abdominal distension; ② deviated mouth, facial edema, toothache; ③ edema and pain in the dorsum of foot, paralysis and weakness of the foot.

主治: ①胃痛，腹胀；②口㖞，面肿，齿痛；③足背肿痛，足痿无力。

Needling: Avoid the artery and puncture vertically 0.3～0.5 cun.

操作: 避开动脉，直刺 0.3～0.5 寸。

3.24 Neiting (ST 44) Ying-Spring acupoint

3.24 内庭 Nèitíng 荥穴

Indications: ① Toothache, sore throat, nasal

主治: ①齿痛，咽喉肿

bleeding, deviated mouth; ② febrile diseases; ③ stomachache, sour regurgitation, diarrhea, dysentery, constipation; ④ paralysis and weakness of the foot.

Needling: Puncture vertically or obliquely 0.3～0.5 cun.

痛，鼻衄，口㖞；②热病；③胃痛，吐酸，泄泻，痢疾，便秘；④足背肿痛。

操作：直刺或斜刺0.3～0.5 寸。

3.25 Lidui (ST 45) Jing-Well acupoint

Indications: ① Toothahce, nasal beedling, sore throat; ② febrile diseases; ③ dreaminess, depressive and manic psychosis.

Needling: Puncture shallowly 0.1 cun.

3.25 厉兑 Lìduì 井穴

主治：①齿痛，鼻衄，咽喉肿痛；②热病；③多梦，梦魇，癫狂。

操作：浅刺 0.1 寸。

Section 4 Spleen Meridian of Foot-Taiyin and its Acupoints

第 4 节 足太阴脾经及其腧穴

1 Distribution course

The spleen meridian of foot-taiyin originates at the medial side of the big toe. It then runs along the medial aspect of the foot at the junction of the red and white skin, ascends in front of the medial malleolus up to the medial aspect of the leg. It follows the posterior border of the tibia, crosses and goes in front of the liver meridian of foot jueyin; passing through the anterior medial aspect of the knee and thigh to enter the abdominal cavity, it runs internally to the spleen, to which it pertains, and connects with the stomach(the external course of the meridian with acupoints is on the abdomen 4 cun lateral to the anterior midline). From there, the meridian continuously ascends to pass through the diaphragm (the external course of the meridian with acupoints is on the chest 6 cun lateral to the anterior midline)

1 经脉循行

足太阴脾经，起于大趾末端，沿大趾内侧赤白肉际，经第一跖趾关节后，从内踝前，上小腿内侧，沿胫骨后，在内踝上 8 寸处交出足厥阴肝经之前，上膝股内侧前缘，进入腹部，属于脾，络于胃（在腹部有穴位分布的外行经脉是旁开前正中线 4 寸），通过膈肌（在胸部有穴位分布的外行经脉是旁开前正中线 6 寸），挟食管旁，连舌根，散舌下。腹部支脉，从胃部分出，上经膈肌，流注心中，连接手少阴心经（图 3-20）。

and runs alongside the throat; then it reaches the root of the tongue, and spreads over the lower surface of the tongue. An internal branch from the stomach goes upwards through the diaphragm and flows into the heart, where it connects with the heart meridian of hand shaoyin(Fig.3-20).

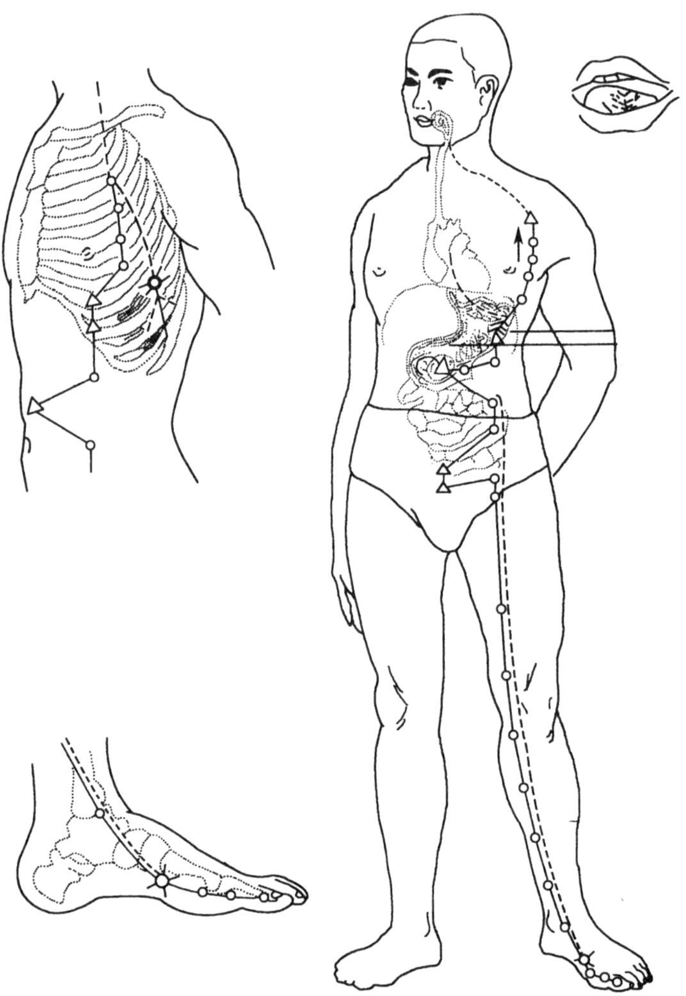

Fig.3-20　The distribution course of spleen meridian of foot-taiyin

图 3-20　足太阴脾经循行示意图

2 Location of acupoints

The starting acupoint of the spleen meridian is Yinbai(SP 1) and the ending acupoint is Dabao(SP 21), totally 21 acupoints in each side. The location of acupoints is presented in Table 3-4 and Fig. 3-21~3-26.

2 腧穴定位

本经首穴为隐白，末穴为大包，左右各 21 穴。腧穴定位见表 3-4、图 3-21～3-26。

Table 3-4 Location of acupoints of the spleen meridian of foot-taiyin

Acupoint		Location	Specific feature
SP 1*	Yinbai	At the medial side of the great toe, 0.1 cun posterior to the corner of the nail	Jing-Well acupoint
SP 2	Dadu	At the anterior border of the first metatarsodigital joint, at the junction of the red and white skin	Spring-Ying acupoint
SP 3*	Taibai	Just proximal to the first metatarsodigital joint, at the junction of the red and white skin	Shu-Stream acupoint, Yuan-Source acupoint
SP 4*	Gongsun	Anterior and inferior to the base of the first metatarsodigital joint, at the junction of the red and white skin	Luo-Connecting acupoint, Confluent acupoint communicating the thoroughfare vessel
SP 5	Shangqiu	In the depression anterior and inferior to the medial malleolus, midpoint between the tuberosity of the navicular bone and the tip of the medial malleolus	Jing-River acupoint
SP 6*	Sanyinjiao	3 cun above the tip of the medial malleolus, on the posterior border of the tibia	Crossing acupoint the three foot yin meridians
SP 7	Lougu	6 cun above the tip of the medial malleolus, on the posterior border of the tibia	
SP 8*	Diji	3 cun below Yinlingquan(SP 9), on the posterior border of the tibia	Xi-Cleft acupoint
SP 9*	Yinlingquan	On the lower border of the medial condyle of the tibia, in the depression on the medial border of the tibia	He-Sea acupoint
SP 10*	Xuehai	2 cun above the medial border of the petalla and on the bulge of medial side of quadriceps femoris muscle	
SP 11	Jimen	At the intersection of the upper one-third and lower two-thirds of the line between the medial border of the patella and Chongmen(SP 12), where the artery can be felt	
SP 12	Chongmen	In the inguinal groove, on the upper border of the pubic symphysis, on the lateral side of the femoral artery	Crossing acupoint of the spleen meridian and liver meridian
SP 13	Fushe	4.3 cun below the navel and 4 cun lateral to the anterior midline	Crossing acupoint of spleen meridian, liver meridian and yin link vessel

(continued)

Acupoint		Location	Specific feature
SP 14	Fujie	1.3 cun below the navel and 4 cun lateral to the anterior midline	
SP 15*	Daheng	4 cun lateral to the anterior midline	Crossing acupoint of the foot-taiyin meridian and yin link vessel
SP 16	Fuai	3 cun above the navel and 4 cun lateral to the anterior midline	Crossing acupoint of the spleen meridian and yin link vessel
SP 17	Shidou	In the fifth intercostal space, 6 cun lateral to the anterior midline	
SP 18	Tianxi	In the fourth intercostal space, 6 cun lateral to the anterior midline	
SP 19	Xiongxiang	In the third intercostal space, 6 cun lateral to the anterior midline	
SP 20	Zhourong	In the second intercostal space, 6 cun lateral to the anterior midline	
SP 21*	Dabao	In the sixth intercostal space, on the mid-axillary line	Major collateral of the spleen

表 3-4　足太阴脾经的腧穴定位

腧穴		定位	特定穴属性
隐白*	Yǐnbái	足大趾末节内侧，趾甲根角侧后方0.1寸(指寸)	井穴
大都	Dàdū	第1跖趾关节远端赤白肉际凹陷中	荥穴
太白*	Tàibái	第1跖趾关节近端赤白肉际凹陷中	输穴；原穴
公孙*	Gōngsūn	第1跖骨底的前下缘赤白肉际处	络穴；八脉交会穴(通冲脉)
商丘	Shāngqiū	内踝前下方，舟骨粗隆与内踝尖连线中点凹陷中	经穴
三阴交*	Sānyīnjiāo	内踝尖上3寸，胫骨内后缘	足三阴经交会穴
漏谷	Lòugǔ	内踝尖上6寸，胫骨内后缘	
地机*	Dìjī	阴陵泉下3寸，胫骨内后缘	郄穴
阴陵泉*	Yīnlíngquán	胫骨内侧髁下缘与胫骨内侧缘之间的凹陷中	合穴
血海*	Xuèhǎi	髌骨底内侧端上2寸，股内侧肌隆起处	
箕门	Jīmén	髌骨底内侧端与冲门的连线上1/3与下2/3交点，长收肌和缝匠肌交角的动脉搏动处	
冲门	Chōngmén	腹股沟斜纹中，平耻骨联合上缘，髂外动脉搏动处的外侧	足太阴、厥阴经交会穴
府舍	Fǔshě	脐中下4.3寸，前正中线旁开4寸	足太阴、厥阴经、阴维脉交会穴

（续表）

腧穴		定位	特定穴属性
腹结	Fùjié	脐中下 1.3 寸，前正中线旁开 4 寸	
大横*	Dàhéng	脐中旁开 4 寸	足太阴经、阴维脉交会穴
腹哀	Fùāi	脐中上 3 寸，前正中线旁开 4 寸	足太阴经、阴维脉交会穴
食窦	Shídòu	第 5 肋间隙，前正中线旁开 6 寸	
天溪	Tiānxī	第 4 肋间隙，前正中线旁开 6 寸	
胸乡	Xiōngxiāng	第 3 肋间隙，前正中线旁开 6 寸	
周荣	Zhōuróng	第 2 肋间隙，前正中线旁开 6 寸	
大包*	Dàbāo	第 6 肋间隙，在腋中线上	脾之大络

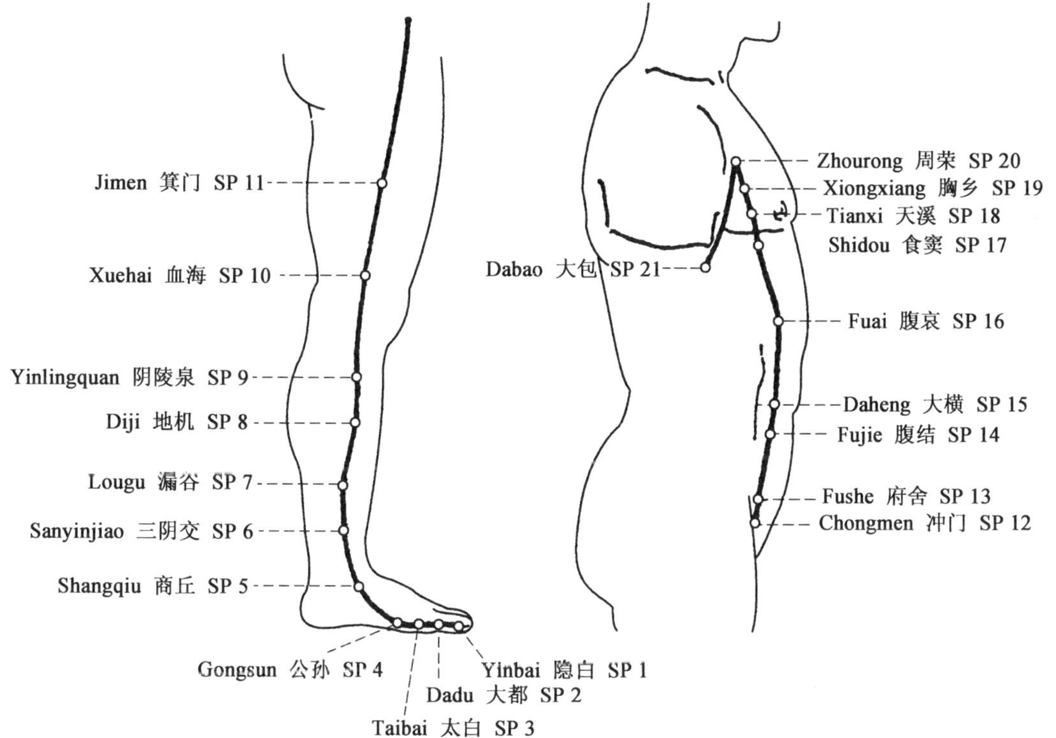

Fig.3-21 Acupoints of spleen meridian of foot-taiyin

图 3-21 足太阴脾经腧穴总图

3 Indications of acupoints

The acupoints of the spleen meridian are indicated for the diseases in the spleen and stomach, gynecology, external genital problems and conditions along the course of this meridian. The diseases of the spleen and stomach can be treated by Daheng (SP 15), Taibai(SP 3), Gongsun(SP 4), Yinbao(SP 1), Yinlingquan(SP 9) and Sanyinjiao(SP 6); the gynecological disorders can be treated by Yinbai(SP 1), Xuehai(SP 10), Gongsun(SP 4) and Sanyinjiao (SP 6); urinary difficulty can be treated by Yinlingquan(SP 6), Jimen(SP 11) and Sanyinjiao(SP 6). The indications and needling techniques of common acupoints are presented as follows.

3 腧穴主治

本经腧穴主要用于治疗脾胃病、妇科病、前阴病及经脉所过部位的病证。治疗脾胃病常用大横、太白、公孙、隐白、阴陵泉和三阴交；治疗妇科病常用隐白、血海、太白、公孙和三阴交；治疗小便不利常用阴陵泉、箕门和三阴交。临床常用腧穴的主治及针刺操作如下。

3.1 Yinbai (SP 1) Jing-Well acupoint

Indications: ① Menorrhagia, hematochezia, uterine bleeding, hematuria; ② abdominal distension; ③ depressive and manic psychosis, dreaminess, convulsion.

Needling: Puncture shallowly 0.1 cun; or moxibustion may be performed.

3.1 隐白 Yǐnbái 井穴

主治：①崩漏，月经过多，便血，尿血；②腹胀；③癫狂，多梦，惊风。

操作：浅刺 0.1 寸；或灸。

3.2 Taibai (SP 3) Shu-Stream acupoint, Yuan-Source acupoint

Indications: ① Stomachache, abdominal distension, diarrhea, dysentery, poor appetite; ② general heaviness and joint pain.

Needling: Puncture vertically 0.5～0.8 cun.

3.2 太白 Tàibái 输穴；原穴

主治：①胃痛，腹胀，腹痛，泄泻，痢疾，纳呆；②体重节痛。

操作：直刺 0.5～0.8 寸。

3.3 Gongsun (SP 4) Luo-Connecting acupoint; Confluent acupoint communicating with thoroughfare vessel

Indications: ① Stomachache, vomiting, abdominal distension, abdominal pain, diarrhea, dysentery; ② cardiac pain, chest fullness.

3.3 公孙 Gōngsūn 络穴；八脉交会穴（通冲脉）

主治：①胃痛，呕吐，腹胀，腹痛，泄泻，痢疾；②心痛，胸闷。

Needling: Puncture vertically 0.5～1.0 cun.

操作: 直刺 0.5～1.0 寸。

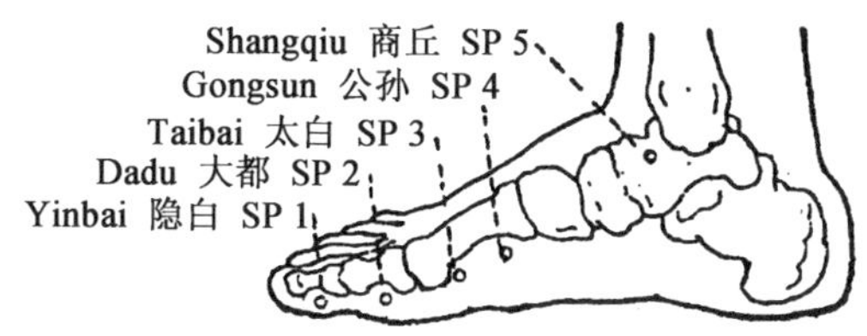

Fig.3-22 Foot acupoints on the spleen meridian of foot-taiyin

图 3-22 足太阴脾经足部经穴图

3.4 Sanyinjiao (SP 6) Crossing acupoint of foot-taiyin, foot-Jueyin and foot-Shaoyin meridians

Indications: ① Abdominal pain, abdominal distension, diarrhea; ② irregular menstruation, menstrual cramps, amenorrhea, morbid leucorrhea, prolapse of the uterine, delayed labor, infertility, sterility, impotence, seminal emission; ③ urinary difficulty, enuresis, edema; ④ insomnia, vertigo; ⑤ paralysis and motor impairment of the lower limbs, and beriberi.

Needling: Puncture vertically 1.0～1.5 cun; needling is contraindicated in the pregnant weomen.

3.4 三阴交 Sānyīnjiāo 足太阴、厥阴、少阴经交会穴

主治: ①腹痛,腹胀,肠鸣,泄泻;②月经不调,痛经,经闭,带下,阴挺,滞产,不孕,不育,阳萎,遗精;③小便不利,遗尿,水肿;④失眠,眩晕;⑤下肢痿痹,脚气。

操作: 直刺 1.0～1.5 寸;孕妇禁针。

3.5 Diji (SP 8) Xi-Cleft acupoint

Indications: ① Abdominal distension, abdominal pain, diarrhea; ② irregular menstruation, dysmenorrhea, uterine bleeding; ③ difficulty urination, edema; ④ paralysis and motor impairment of the lower limbs.

Needling: Puncture vertically 0.5～0.8 cun.

3.5 地机 Dìjī 郄穴

主治: ①腹胀,腹痛,泄泻;②月经不调,痛经,崩漏;③小便不利,水肿;④下肢痿痹。

操作: 直刺 0.5～0.8 寸。

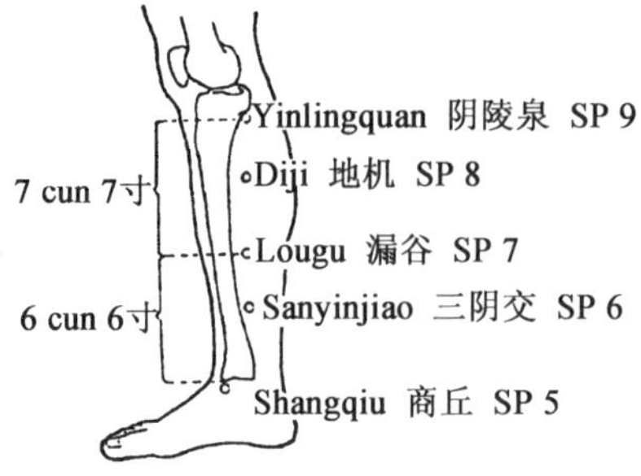

Fig.3-23 Lower limb acupoints on the spleen meridian of foot-taiyin

图 3-23 足太阴脾经下肢部经穴图

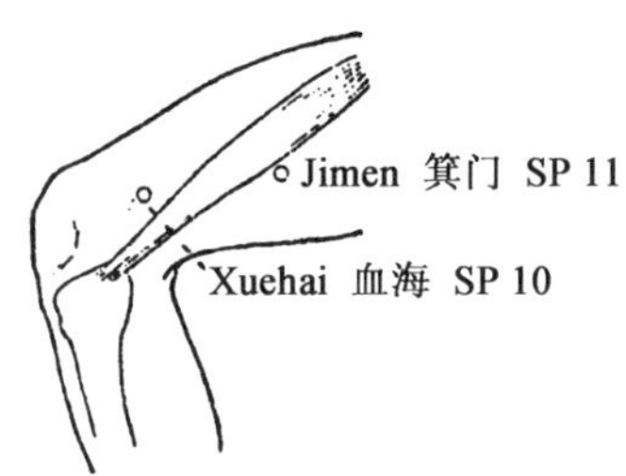

Fig.3-24 Lower limb acupoints on the spleen meridian of foot-taiyin

图 3-24 足太阴脾经下肢部经穴图

3.6 Yinlingquan (SP 9) He-Sea acupoint

Indications: ① Abdominal distension, diarrhea, jaundice; ② difficulty urination, edema; edema; ③ seminal emission, genital pain; ④ knee pain.

Needling: Puncture vertically 1.0～2.0 cun.

3.7 Xuehai (SP 10)

Indications: ① Irregular menstruation, uterine bleeding, amenorrhea; ② skin eruptions, eczema and erysipelas; ③ swelling and pain of the knee.

Needling: Puncture vertically 1.0～1.5 cun.

3.8 Daheng (SP 15) Crossing acupoint of foot-taiyin meridian and yin link vessel

Indications: Abdominal pain around the navel, diarrhea, and constipation.

Needling: Puncture vertically 1.0～1.5 cun.

3.9 Dabao (SP 21) Major collateral of the spleen

Indications: ① Cough and asthma; ② pain in the chest and flank; ③ general pain, and weakness of the limbs.

Needling: Puncture obliquely or transversely

3.6 阴陵泉 Yīnlíngquán 合穴

主治: ①腹胀,泄泻,黄疸;②小便不利,水肿;③遗精,阴痛;④膝痛。

操作: 直刺 1.0～2.0 寸。

3.7 血海 Xuèhǎi

主治: ①月经不调,崩漏,经闭;②瘾疹,湿疹,丹毒;③膝肿痛。

操作: 直刺 1.0～1.5 寸。

3.8 大横 Dàhéng 足太阴经、阴维脉交会穴

主治: 绕脐腹痛,泄泻,便秘。

操作: 直刺 1.0～1.5 寸。

3.9 大包 Dàbāo 脾之大络

主治: ①咳喘;②胸胁痛;③全身疼痛,四肢无力。

操作: 斜刺或平刺

0.5～0.8 cun; since lungs are lodged in the thoracic cavity, deep needling is not allowed.

0.5～0.8寸。穴位深部有肺脏，不宜深刺。

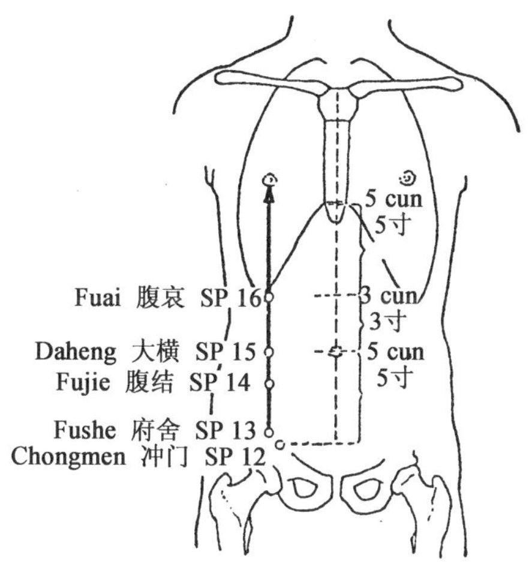

Fig.3-25 Abdomen acupoints on the spleen meridian of foot-taiyin

图3-25 足太阴脾经腹部经穴图

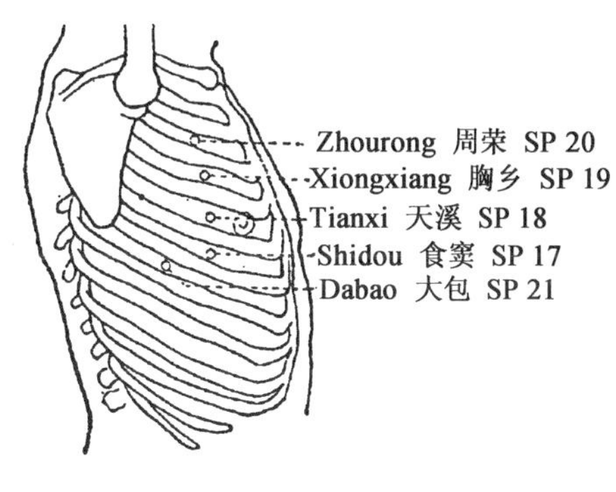

Fig.3-26 Chest acupoints on the spleen meridian of foot-taiyin

图3-26 足太阴脾经胸部经穴图

Section 5 Heart Meridian of Hand-Shaoyin and its Acupoints

第5节 手少阴心经及其腧穴

1 Distribution course

The heart meridian of hand-shaoyin starts from the heart. Emerging, it spreads over the heart system(i.e. the tissues connecting the heart with other zang-fu organs), and runs downwards through the diaphrgm to connect with the small intestine. A branch of thc mcridian from the heart system runs upwards alongside the throat to reach the eye system (i. e. the tissues connecting the eyes with the

1 经脉循行

手少阴心经，起于心中，出于心系（心与其他脏器相连的部位），向下通过横膈，联络小肠。心系支脉，从心系向上，沿咽喉至目系（眼后与脑相连的组织）。其直行主脉，从心系上行至肺，再向下浅出腋下，沿上臂内侧后

brain). The main branch of the meridian derives from the heart system and ascends to the lung; then it turns downwards and emerges in the underarm. It runs along the posterior border of the medial aspect of the upper arm down to the elbow; from there it descends along the posterior border of the medial aspect of the forearm to the pisiform region and enters the palm; then it follows the medial aspect of the little finger to its tip, where it connects with the small intestine meridian(Fig. 3-27).

缘到肘,沿前臂内侧后缘至掌后豌豆骨部,进入掌内,沿小指桡侧至末端,与手太阳小肠经相接(图 3-27)。

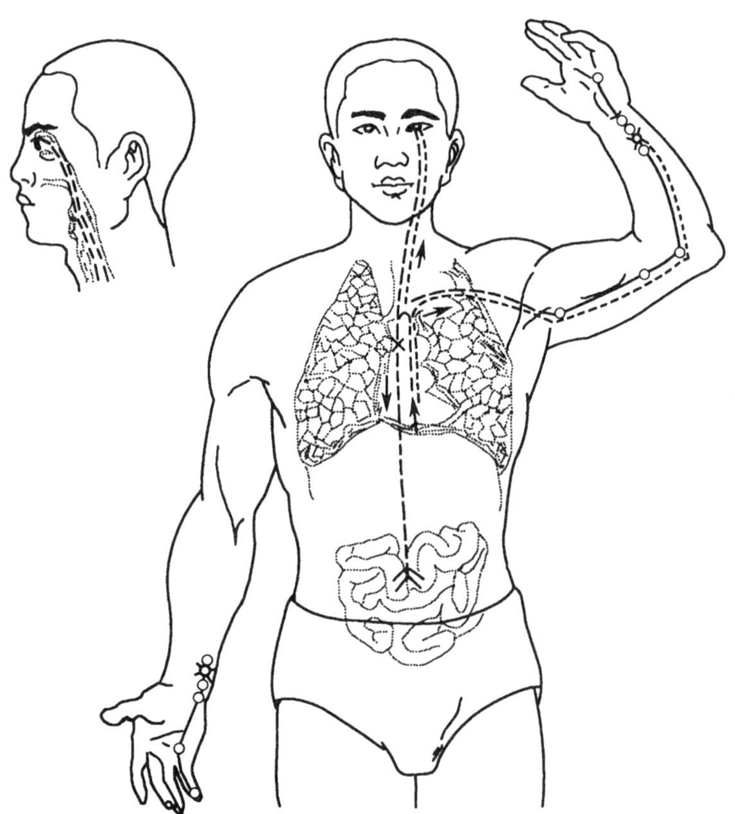

Fig.3-27 The distribution course of heart meridian of hand-shaoyin

图 3-27 手少阴心经循行示意图

2 Location of acupoints

The starting acupoint of the heart meridian is Jiquan(HT 1) and the ending acupoint is Shaochong (HT 9), totally 9 acupoints in each side. The location of acupoints is presented in Table 3-5 and Fig. 3-28～3-31.

2 腧穴定位

本经首穴为极泉，末穴为少冲，左右各 9 穴。腧穴定位见表 3-5、图 3-28～3-31。

Table 3-5 Location of acupoints of the heart meridian of hand-shaoyin

Acupoint		Location	Specific feature
HT 1*	Jiquan	In the center of the axilla, on the medial side of the axillary artery	
HT 2	Qingling	In the forearm, 3 cun above the cubital crease, in the groove medial to biceps brachii muscle	
HT 3*	Shaohai	In the cubital crease and the anterior border of the medial epicondyle	He-Sea acupoint
HT 4	Lingdao	In the forearm, 1.5 cun above the wrist crease, on the radial side of the tendon of the flexor carpi ulnaris muscle	Jing-River acupoint
HT 5*	Tongli	In the forearm, 1 cun above the wrist crease, on the radial side of the tendon of the flexor carpi ulnaris muscle	Luo-Connecting acupoint
HT 6*	Yinxi	In the forearm, 0.5 cun above the wrist crease, on the radial side of the tendon of the flexor carpi ulnaris muscle	Xi-Cleft acupoint
HT 7*	Shenmen	At the ulnar end of the wrist crease, on the radial side of the tendon of the flexor carpi ulnaris muscle	Shu-Stream acupoint; Yuan-Source acupoint
HT 8*	Shaofu	On the palm, at the level with the proximal end of the fifth metacarpophalangeal joint, between the fourth and fifth metacarpal bones	Ying-Spring acupoint
HT 9*	Shaochong	On the radial side of the little finger, 0.1 cun next to the corner of the nail	Jing-Well acupoint

表 3-5 手少阴心经的腧穴定位

腧穴		定位	特定穴属性
极泉*	Jíquán	在腋区，腋窝中央，腋动脉搏动处	
青灵	Qīnglíng	在臂前区，肘横纹上 3 寸，肱二头肌的内侧沟中	
少海*	Shàohǎi	在肘前区，横平肘横纹，肱骨内上髁前缘	合穴
灵道	Língdào	在前臂前区，腕掌侧远端横纹上 1.5 寸，尺侧腕屈肌腱的桡侧缘	经穴

(续表)

腧穴		定位	特定穴属性
通里*	Tōnglǐ	在前臂前区，腕掌侧远端横纹上1寸，尺侧腕屈肌腱的桡侧缘	络穴
阴郄*	Yīnxì	在前臂前区，腕掌侧远端横纹上0.5寸，尺侧腕屈肌腱的桡侧缘	郄穴
神门*	Shénmén	在腕前区，腕掌侧远端横纹尺侧端，尺侧腕屈肌腱的桡侧缘	输穴；原穴
少府*	Shàofǔ	在手掌，横平第5掌指关节近端，第4、5掌骨之间	荥穴
少冲*	Shàochōng	在手指，小指末节桡侧，指甲根角侧上方0.1寸(指寸)	井穴

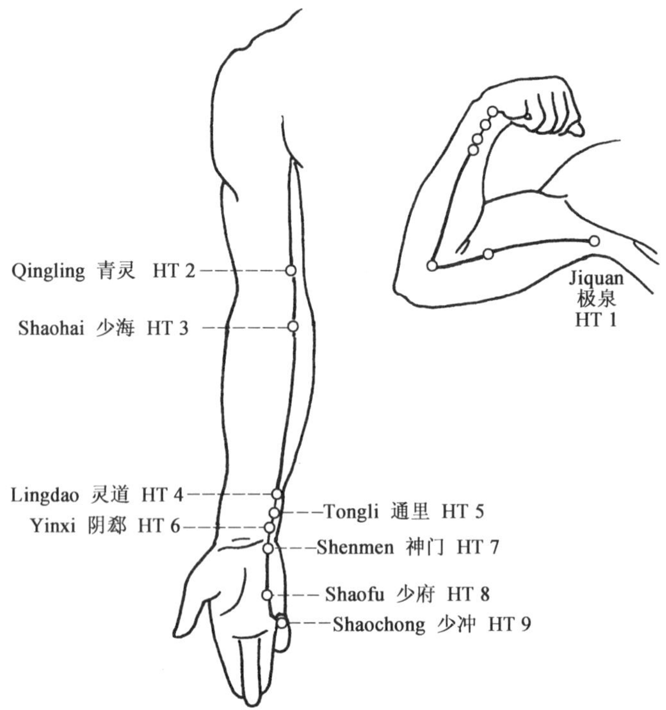

Fig.3-28　Acupoints of the heart meridian of hand-shaoyin

图3-28　手少阴心经腧穴总图

3　Indications of acupoints

The acupoints of the heart meridian are primarily indicated for the diseases of the heart and chest, mental disorders, and the conditions along the course of this meridian. Heart diseases are often

3　腧穴主治

本经腧穴主要用于治疗心、胸、神志病以及经脉所过部位的病证。治疗心脏病常用极泉、阴郄、神门；神志病

treated by Jiquan (HT 1), Yinxi (HT 6) and Shenmen (HT 7); mental disorders are treated by Shenmen (HT 7) and Shaochong (HT 9); pain and numbness along the the posterior border of the medial aspect of the upper limbs is treated by Jiquan (HT 1), Qingling (HT 2), Shaohai (HT 3) and Lingdao (HT 4); the diseases of the tongue and throat are treated by Tongli (HT 5) and Yinxi (HT 6). The indications and needling techniques are presented as follows.

常用神门、少冲;上肢内侧后缘疼痛、麻木用极泉、青灵、少海、灵道;舌咽病用通里、阴郄。临床常用腧穴的主治及针刺操作如下。

3.1 Jiquan (HT 1)

Indications: ① Cardiac pain, palpitation; ② flank pain; ③ pain in the shoulder and arm, paralysis of the upper limbs.

Needling: Avoid the axillary artery, puncture vertically 0.3～0.5 cun.

3.1 极泉 Jíquán

主治: ①心痛,心悸;②胁肋疼痛;③肩臂疼痛,上肢不遂。

操作: 避开腋动脉,直刺0.3～0.5寸。

3.2 Shaohai (HT 3) He-Sea acupoint

Indications: ① Cardiac pain; ② flank pain; ③ numbness and pain of the elbow and arm.

Needling: Puncture vertically 0.5～1.0 cun.

3.2 少海 Shàohǎi 合穴

主治: ①心痛;②腋胁痛;③肘臂麻痛。

操作: 直刺0.5～1.0寸。

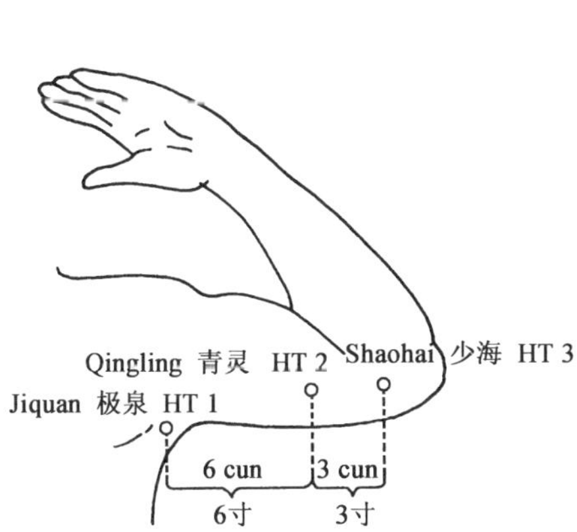

Fig.3-29 Upper arm acupoints on the heart meridian of hand-shaoyin

图3-29 手少阴心经上臂部经穴图

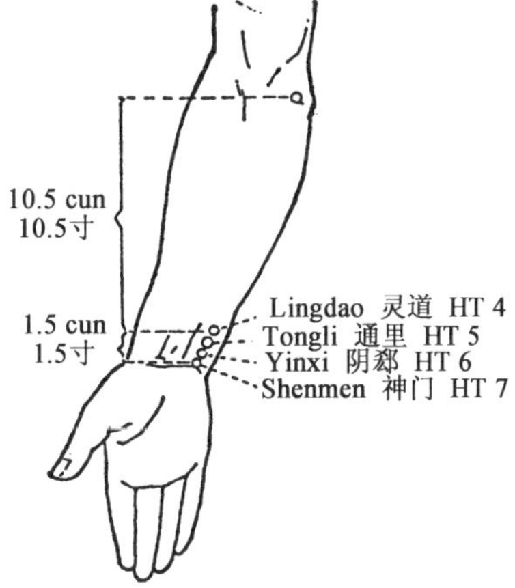

Fig.3-30 Forearm acupoints on the heart meridian of hand-shaoyin

图3-30 手少阴心经前臂部经穴图

3.3 Tongli (HT 5) Luo-Connecting acupoint

Indications: ① Sudden loss of voice, stiff tongue failing to speak; ② palpitation; ③ pain in the wrist and arm.

Needling: Puncture vertically 0.3～0.5 cun.

3.3 通里 Tōnglǐ 络穴

主治: ①暴喑,舌强不语;②心悸;③腕臂痛。

操作: 直刺0.3～0.5寸。

3.4 Yinxi (HT 6) Xi-Cleft acupoint

Indications: ① Cardiac pain, palpitation; ② hematemesis, epistaxis; ③ hectic tidal fever and night sweats; ④ sudden loss of voice.

Needling: Puncture vertically 0.3～0.5 cun.

3.4 阴郄 Yīnxì 郄穴

主治: ①心痛,惊悸;②吐血,衄血;③骨蒸盗汗;④暴喑。

操作: 直刺0.3～0.5寸。

3.5 Shenmen (HT 7) Shu-Stream acupoint; Yuan-Source acupoint

Indications: ① Insomnia, forgetfulness, dementia, depressive-manic psychosis; ② cardiac pain, palpitation.

Needling: Puncture vertically 0.3～0.5 cun.

3.5 神门 Shénmén 输穴;原穴

主治: ①失眠,健忘,呆痴,癫狂痫;②心痛,心悸。

操作: 直刺0.3～0.5寸。

3.6 Shaofu (HT 8) Ying-Spring acupoint

Indications: ① Palpitation, chest pain; ② itching and pain in the external genitalia; ③ convulsive pain of the little finger, palm fever.

Needling: Puncture vertically 0.3～0.5 cun.

3.6 少府 Shàofǔ 荥穴

主治: ①心悸,胸痛;②阴痒痛;③手小指挛痛,掌中热。

操作: 直刺0.3～0.5寸。

3.7 Shaochong (HT 9) Jing-Well acupoint

Indications: ① Cardiac pain, palpitation; ② depressive-manic psychosis, coma; ③ febrile disorders.

Needling: Puncture shallowly 0.1～0.2 cun; or prick to bleed.

3.7 少冲 Shàochōng 井穴

主治: ①心痛,心悸;②癫狂,昏迷;③热病。

操作: 浅刺0.1～0.2寸,或点刺出血。

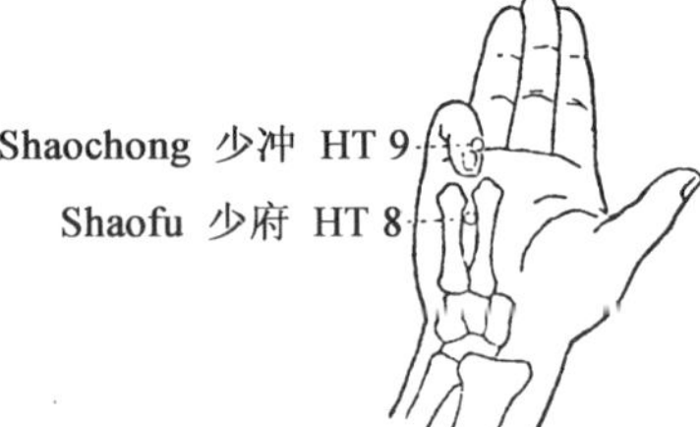

Fig.3-31 Hand acupoints on the heart meridian of hand-shaoyin

图3-31 手少阴心经手部经穴图

Section 6 Small Intestine Meridian of Hand-Taiyang and its Acupoints

第6节 手太阳小肠经及其腧穴

1 Distribution Course

The small intestine meridian of hand-taiyang originates from the ulnar side of the tip of the little finger, runs along the ulnar side of the dorsum of the hand to the wrist, where it emerges from the styloid process of the ulna; from there, the meridian goes upwards along the posterior aspect of the forearm, passes between the olecranon of the ulna and the medial epicondyle of the humerus, and continues upwards along the posterior border of the lateral aspect of the upper arm, circles behind the shoulder, and runs to the center of the uppermost part of the back. Then, the meridian turns down through the supraclavicular fossa to connect with the heart; from there it descends along the oesophagus, passes through the diaphragm, reaches the stomach and finally enters the small intestine to which it pertains. The branch from the supraclavicular fossa ascends along the neck, and further to the cheek; via the outer canthus, it enters the ear from its back. The branch leaves the meridian on the cheek, and runs upwards to the infraorbital region and further to the lateral aspect of the nose; then it reaches the inner canthus, where it connects with the bladder meridian(Fig.3-32).

1 经脉循行

手太阳小肠经,起于手小指外侧端,沿着手背尺侧至腕部,出于尺骨茎突,直上沿着前臂外侧后缘,经尺骨鹰嘴与肱骨内上髁之间,沿上臂外侧后缘,出于肩关节,绕行肩胛部,交会于肩上,向下进入缺盆(锁骨上窝),联络心脏,沿着食管,通过横膈,到达胃部,属于小肠。颈部支脉,从缺盆上行,沿着颈部,上经面颊至目外眦,弯曲向后进入耳中。面颊部支脉,从面颊部分出,上行颧骨抵于鼻旁,至目内眦,与足太阳膀胱经相接(图3-32)。

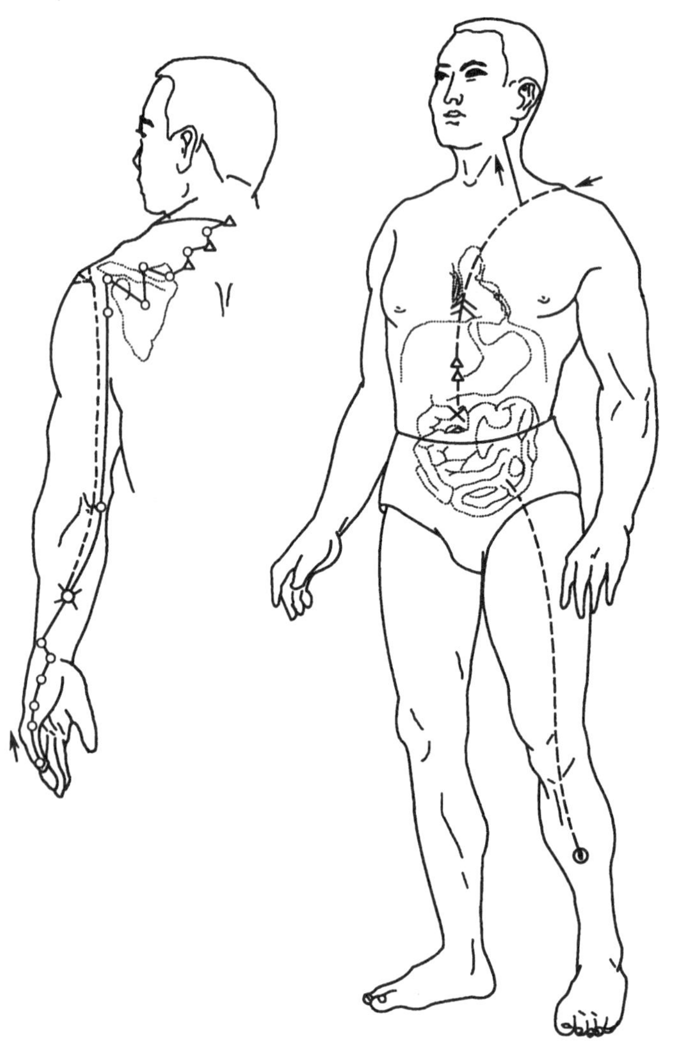
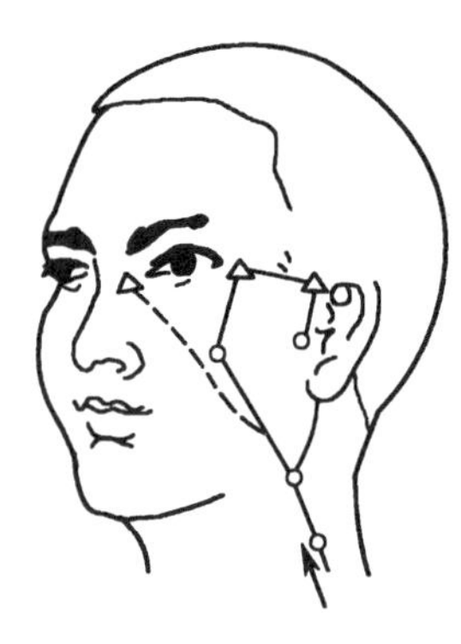

Fig.3-32　The distribution course of small intestine meridian of hand-taiyang

图 3-32　手太阳小肠经循行示意图

2　Location of acupoints

The starting acupoint of the small intestine meridian is Shaoze(SI 1) and the ending acupoint is Tinggong(SI 19), totally 19 acupoints in each side. The location of acupoints is presented in Table 3-6 and Figure 3-33～3-37.

2　腧穴定位

本经首穴为少泽，末穴为听宫，左右各 19 穴。腧穴定位见表 3-6、图 3-33～3-37。

Table 3-6 Location of acupoints of the small intestine meridian of hand-taiyang

Acupoint		Location	Specific feature
SI 1	Shaoze	On the ulnar side of the little finger, about 0.1 cun superior to the corner of the nail	Jing-Well acupoint
SI 2	Qiangu	On the ulnar side, distal to the fifth metacarpophalangeal joint, at the junction of the red and white skin	Ying-Spring acupoint
SI 3*	Houxi	On the ulnar side, proximal to the fifth metacarpophalangeal joint, at the junction of the red and white skin	Shu-Stream acupoint; Confluent acupoint connecting with the governor vessel
SI 4*	Wangu	On the ulnar aspect of the wrist crease, between the base of the fifth metacarpophalangeal joint and triquetral bone, at the junction of the red and white skin	Yuan-Source acupoint
SI 5	Yanggu	On the ulnar side of the wrist crease, in the depression between the styloid process of the ulna and the triquetral bone	Jing-Well acupoint
SI 6*	Yanglao	1 cun above the wrist crease, in the bony cleft on the radial side of the styloid process of the ulna	Xi-Cleft acupoint
SI 7*	Zhizheng	On the dorsolateral aspect of the forearm, 5 cun above the wrist crease, between the ulnar side of the ulna and the extensor carpiulnaris muscle	Luo-Connecting acupoint
SI 8*	Xiaohai	In the depression between the olecranon of the ulna and the medial epicondyle of the humerus	He-Sea acupoint
SI 9*	Jianzhen	Posterior and inferior to the shoulder joint, 1 cun above the end of the posterior axillary fold	
SI 10	Naoshu	Right above the end of the posterior axillary fold, in the depression inferior to the scapular spine	Crossing acupoint of the small intestine meridian, bladder meridian, yang link vessel and yang heel vessel
SI 11*	Tianzong	In the scapular region, in the center of the infraspinous fossa	
SI 12	Bingfeng	In the center of the suprascapular fossa	Crossing acupoint of the three yang meridians of the hand and foot shaoyang meridian
SI 13	Quyuan	In the scapular region, on the upper end of medial side of the suprascapular fossa	
SI 14	Jianwaishu	In the spinal area, 3 cun lateral to the lower border of the spinous process of the first thoracic vertebra	
SI 15	Jianzhongshu	In the spinal area, 2 cun lateral to the lower border of the spinous process of the seventh cervical vertebra	

(continued)

Acupoint		Location	Specific feature
SI 16	Tianchuang	On the posterior border of the sternocleidomastoideus muscle, at the level with the Adam's apple	
SI 17	Tianrong	Posterior to the angle of the mandible, in the depression anterior to the sternocleidomastoideus muscle	
SI 18*	Quanliao	In the depression on the lower border of the zygoma and directly below the outer canthus	Crossing acupoint of hand-shaoyang meridian and hand-taiyang meridian
SI 19*	Tinggong	In the depression between the tragus and the condyle of the mandible	Crossing acupoint of hand and foot-shaoyang meridian, hand-taiyang meridian

表 3-6　手太阳小肠经的腧穴定位

腧穴		定位	特定穴属性
少泽*	Shàozé	在手指，小指末节尺侧，指甲根角侧上方 0.1 寸(指寸)	井穴
前谷	Qiángǔ	在手指，第 5 掌指关节尺侧远端赤白肉际凹陷中	荥穴
后溪*	Hòuxī	在手内侧，第 5 掌指关节尺侧近端赤白肉际凹陷中	输穴；八脉交会穴(通督脉)
腕骨*	Wàngǔ	在腕区，第 5 掌骨底与三角骨之间的赤白肉际凹陷中	原穴
阳谷	Yánggǔ	在腕后区，尺骨茎突与三角骨之间的凹陷中	经穴
养老*	Yǎnglǎo	在前臂后区，腕背横纹上 1 寸，尺骨头桡侧凹陷中	郄穴
支正*	Zhīzhèng	在前臂后区，腕背侧远端横纹上 5 寸，尺骨尺侧与尺侧腕屈肌之间	络穴
小海*	Xiǎohǎi	在肘后区，尺骨鹰嘴与肱骨内上髁之间凹陷处	合穴
肩贞*	Jiānzhēn	在肩胛区，肩关节后下方，腋后纹头直上 1 寸	
臑俞	Nàoshū	在肩胛区，腋后纹头直上，肩胛冈下缘凹陷中	手足太阳经、阳维脉、阳蹻脉交会穴
天宗*	Tiānzōng	在肩胛区，肩胛冈中点与肩胛骨下角连线上 1/3 与下 2/3 交点凹陷中	
秉风	Bǐngfēng	在肩胛区，肩胛冈中点上方冈上窝中	手三阳经与足少阳经交会穴
曲垣	Qūyuán	在肩胛区，肩胛冈内侧端上缘凹陷中	
肩外俞	Jiānwàishū	在脊柱区，第 1 胸椎棘突下，后正中线旁开 3 寸	

(续表)

腧穴		定位	特定穴属性
肩中俞	Jiānzhōngshū	在脊柱区,第 7 颈椎棘突下,后正中线旁开 2 寸	
天窗	Tiānchuāng	在颈部,横平喉结,胸锁乳突肌的后缘	
天容	Tiānróng	在颈部,下颌角后方,胸锁乳突肌的前缘凹陷中	
颧髎*	Quánliáo	在面部,颧骨下缘,目外眦直下凹陷中	手少阳、太阳经交会穴
听宫*	Tīnggōng	在面部,耳屏正中与下颌骨髁突之间的凹陷中	手足少阳、手太阳经交会穴

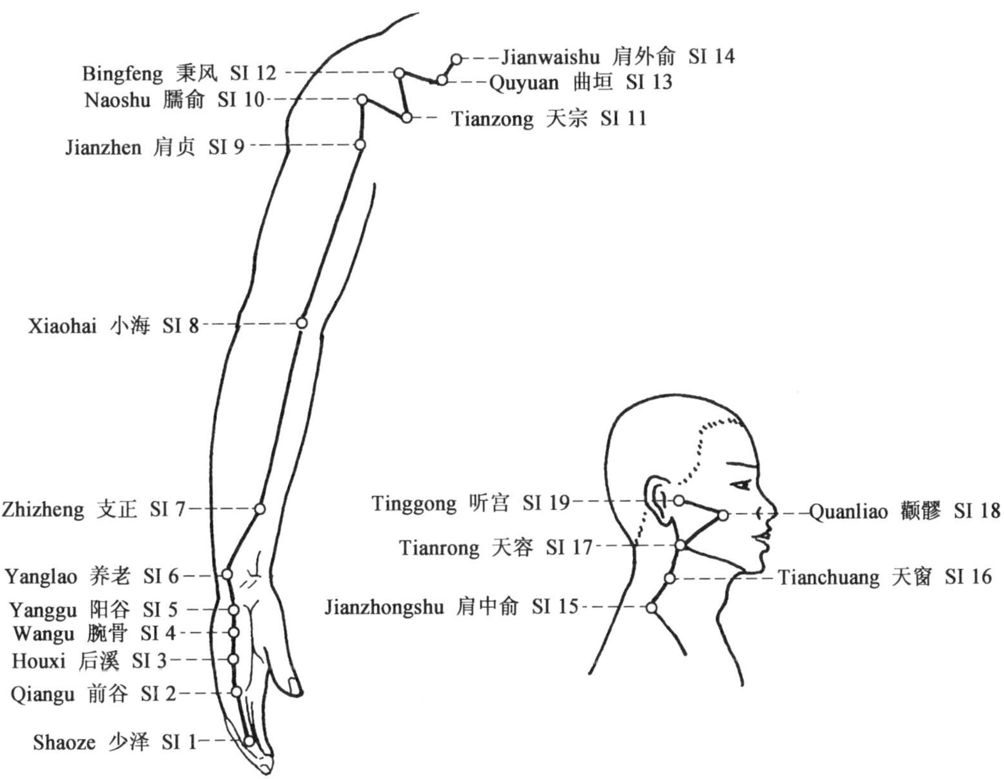

Fig.3-33 Acupoints of the small intestine meridian of hand-taiyang

图 3-33 手太阳小肠经腧穴总图

3 Indications of acupoints

The acupoints of the small intestine meridian are indicated for the diseases in the head, neck, ears, eyes and throat, febrile diseases, mental dis-

3 腧穴主治

本经腧穴主要用于治疗头、项、耳、目、咽喉病,热病,神志病以及经脉所过部位的

orders and the conditions along the meridian course. The disorders on the head and neck can be treated by Houxi(SI 3), Yanglao(SI 6), Zhizheng(SI 7), Tianchuang(SI 16) and Tianrong(SI 17); the ear diseases can be treated by Tinggong(SI 19), HouXi (SI 3) and Qiangu(SI 2); the eye diseases can be treated by Houxi(SI 3) and Yanglao(SI 6); teethache can be treated by Tinggong(SI 19) and Quanliao(SI 18); the throat diseases can be treated by Shaoze(SI 1), Qiangu(SI 2), Tianchuang(SI 16) and Tianrong(SI 17); breast diseases can be treated by Shaoze(SI 1) and Tianzong(SI 11); acute lumbago can be treated by Houxi(SI 3) and Yanglao(SI 6); pain in the shoulder and arm can be treated by Houxi(SI 3), Yanglao(SI 6), Zhizheng(SI 7), Jianzhen(SI 9), Naoshu(SI 10), Tianzong(SI 11), Bingfeng(SI 12), Quyuan(SI 13), Jianwaishu(SI 14) and Jianzhongshu(SI 15). The indications and needling techniques of the commonly used acupoints are presented as follows.

病证。治疗头项痛常用后溪、养老、支正、天窗、天容;治疗耳病常用听宫、后溪、前谷;治疗目疾常用后溪、养老;齿痛常用听宫、颧髎;咽喉痛可用少泽、前谷、天窗、天容;乳房病常用少泽、天宗;急性腰痛常用后溪、养老;肩臂背部疼痛常用后溪、养老、支正、肩贞、臑俞、天宗、秉风、曲垣、肩外俞、肩中俞等。临床常用腧穴的主治及针刺操作如下。

3.1 Shaoze (SI 1) Jing-Well acupoint

Indications: ① Headache, nebula, sore throat; ② breast abscess, insufficient lactation; ③ coma; ④ febrile disorders.

Needling: Puncture shallowly 0.1～0.2 cun, or prick to bleed.

3.1 少泽 Shàozé 井穴

主治: ①头痛,目翳,咽喉肿痛;②乳痈,乳汁少;③昏迷;④热病。

操作: 浅刺0.1～0.2寸,或点刺出血。

3.2 Houxi (SI 3) Shu-Stream acupoint; Confluent acupoint communicating with the governor vessel

Indications: ① Neck pain and stiffness, back pain; ② redness of the eye, deafness, sore throat; ③ night sweats, malaria; ④ depressive-manic syndrome, epilepsy; ⑤ convulsion of the fingers, elbow and arm.

3.2 后溪 Hòuxī 输穴;八脉交会穴(通督脉)

主治: ①头项强痛,腰背痛;②目赤,耳聋,咽喉肿痛;③盗汗,疟疾;④癫狂痫;⑤手指及肘臂挛急。

Needling: Puncture vertically 0.5～0.8 cun, or puncture with the needle tip towards Hegu(LI 4).

操作：直刺0.5～0.8寸，或向合谷方向透刺。

3.3 Wangu (SI 4) Yuan-Source acupoint

3.3 腕骨 Wàngǔ 原穴

Indications: ① Neck stiffness and pain, tinnitus, nebula; ② jaundice; ③ thirstiness, febrile diseases, malaria; ④ finger convulsion and wrist pain.

主治：①头项强痛，耳鸣，目翳；②黄疸；③消渴，热病，疟疾；④指挛腕痛。

Needling: Puncture vertically 0.3～0.5 cun.

操作：直刺0.3～0.5寸。

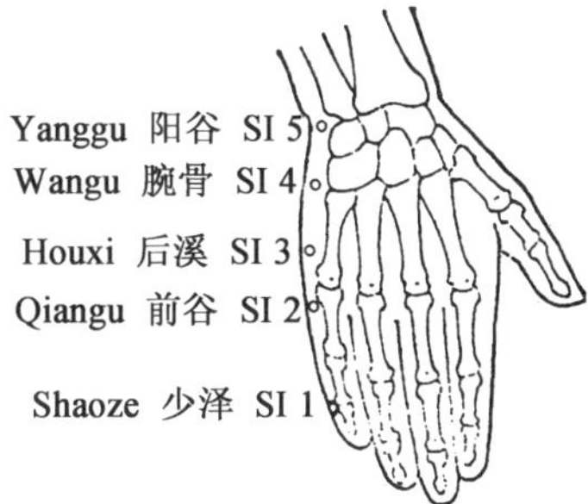

Fig.3-34 Hand acupoints on the small intestine meridian of hand-taiyang

图 3-34 手太阳小肠经手部经穴图

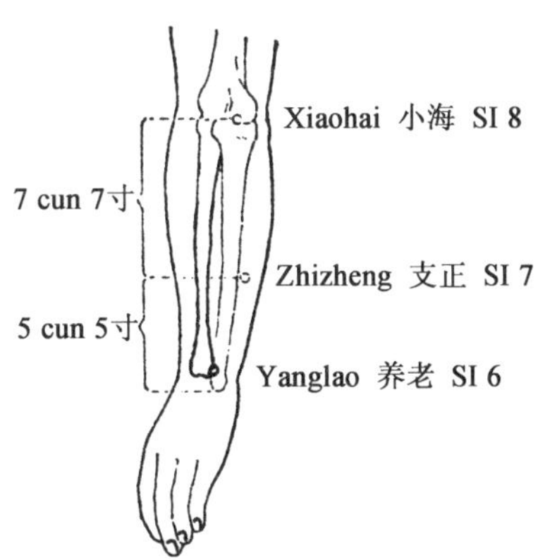

Fig.3-35 Forearm acupoints on the small intestine meridian of hand-taiyang

图 3-35 手太阳小肠经前臂部经穴图

3.4 Yanglao (SI 6) Xi-Cleft acupoint

3.4 养老 Yǎnglǎo 郄穴

Indications: ① Blurred vision; ② pain and numbness in the shoulder, back, elbow and arm, neck stiffness, acute lumbago.

主治：①目视不明；②肩背肘臂麻痛，项强，急性腰痛。

Needling: With the palm facing the chest, puncture 0.5～0.8 cun with the needle tip towards the elbow.

操作：掌心向胸，向肘方向斜刺0.5～0.8寸。

3.5 Zhizheng (SI 7) Luo-Connecting acupoint

3.5 支正 Zhīzhèng 络穴

Indications: ① Headache, neck stiffness; ② febrile diseases; ③ depressive-manic syndrome;

主治：①头痛，项强；②热病；③癫狂；④肘臂酸

④ aching pain in the elbow and arm.

Needling: Puncture vertically or obliquely 0.5～0.8 cun.

3.6 Xiaohai (SI 8)　He-Sea acupoint

Indicaitons: ① Pain in the elbow and arm; ② epilepsy.

Needling: Puncture vertically 0.3～0.5 cun.

3.7 Jianzhen (SI 9)

Indications: ① Numbness and pain in the shoulder and arm; ② tinnitus, deafness.

Needling: Puncture vertically 1.0～1.5 cun.

3.8 Tianzong (SI 11)

Indications: ① Scapular pain; ② breast abscess; ③ shortness of breath.

Needling: Puncture vertically or obliquely 0.5～1.0 cun.

痛。

操作： 直刺或斜刺0.5～0.8寸。

3.6 小海 Xiǎohǎi　合穴

主治： ①肘臂疼痛；②癫痫。

操作： 直刺 0.3～0.5 寸。

3.7 肩贞 Jiānzhēn

主治： ①肩臂麻痛；②耳鸣，耳聋。

操作： 直刺 1.0～1.5 寸。

3.8 天宗 Tiānzōng

主治： ①肩胛疼痛；②乳痈；③气喘。

操作： 直刺或斜刺0.5～1.0寸。

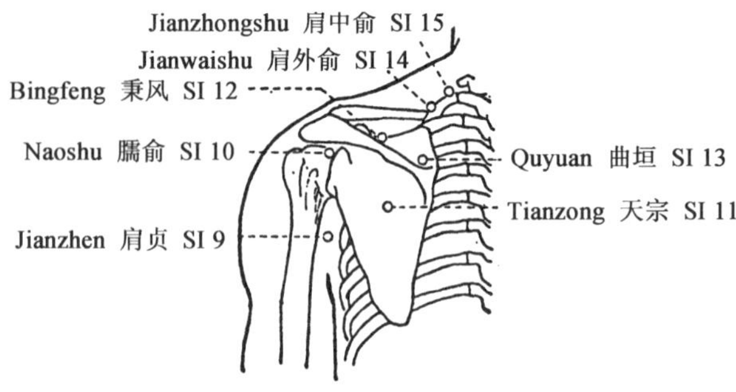

Fig.3-36　Shoulder and back acupoints on the small intestine meridian of hand-taiyang

图 3-36　手太阳小肠经肩背部经穴图

Tinggong 听宫 SI 19
Quanliao 颧髎 SI 18

Fig.3-37　Head and face acupoints on the small intestine meridian of hand-taiyang

图 3-37　手太阳小肠经头面部经穴图

3.9 Quanliao (SI 18)　Crossing acupoint of hand-shaoyang meridian and hand-taiyang meridian

Indications: Deviated mouth and eyes, twinkling eyelids, facial pain, toothache, cheeck swelling.

3.9 颧髎 Quánliáo　手少阳、太阳经交会穴

主治： 口眼㖞斜，眼睑瞤动，面痛，齿痛，颊肿。

Needling: Puncture vertically 0.3～0.5 cun, or obliquely 0.5～1.0 cun.

操作: 直刺 0.3～0.5 寸，或斜刺 0.5～1.0 寸。

3.10 Tinggong (SI 19) Crossing acupoint of hand and foot-shaoyang meridian, hand-taiyang meridian

3.10 听宫 Tīnggōng 手足少阳、手太阳经交会穴

Indications: ① Tinnitus, deafness, toothache; ② epilepsy.

主治: ①耳鸣，耳聋，齿痛；②癫痫。

Needling: With the mouth slightly opened, puncture vertically 0.5～1.0 cun.

操作: 微张口，直刺 0.5～1.0 寸。

Section 7 Bladder Meridian of Foot-Taiyang and its Acupoints

第 7 节 足太阳膀胱经及其腧穴

1 Distribution course

The bladder meridian of foot-taiyang starts from the inner canthus, and ascends across the forehead to the vertex of the head. From the vertex, a small branch arises and runs to the temple above the ear. A straight branch of this meridian enters the vertex and communicates with the brain; then it emerges and bifurcates to descend along the back of the head and neck. Running downwards alongside the medial aspect of the scapular area and parallel to the vertebral spine it reaches the lumbar region, where it enters the body cavity via the paravertebral muscles to connect with the kidneys and its pertaining organ, the bladder. The branch from the lumbar region descends through the gluteal region and ends in the popliteal fossa. The branch from the back of the neck goes straight downwards along the medial border of the scapula; passing through the gluteal region downwards along the lateral aspect of the thigh it meets the pre-

1 经脉循行

足太阳膀胱经，起于目内眦，上额交会于巅顶；头顶部的支脉，从头顶分出到耳上方。巅顶部直行的主脉，从头顶入里联络于脑，返回出项部而分开下行。一支沿着肩胛部内侧，挟着脊柱，到达腰部，从脊柱旁肌肉进入体腔，联络肾脏，属于膀胱；腰部的支脉，向下通过臀部，进入腘窝中。后项的另一支脉，通过肩胛骨内缘直下，经过臀部下行，沿着大腿后外侧，与腰部下来的支脉会合于腘窝。由此向下通过腓肠肌，出于外踝的后面，沿着第五跖骨粗隆，至小趾外侧端，与足少阴肾经相接(图 3-38)。

ceeding branch descending from the lumbar region in the popliteal fossa; from there it descends to the leg and further to the posterior aspect of the external malleolus; then running along the tuberosity of the fifth metatarsal bone, it reaches the lateral side of the tip of the little toe, where it connects with the kidney meridian of foot shaoyin(Fig. 3-38).

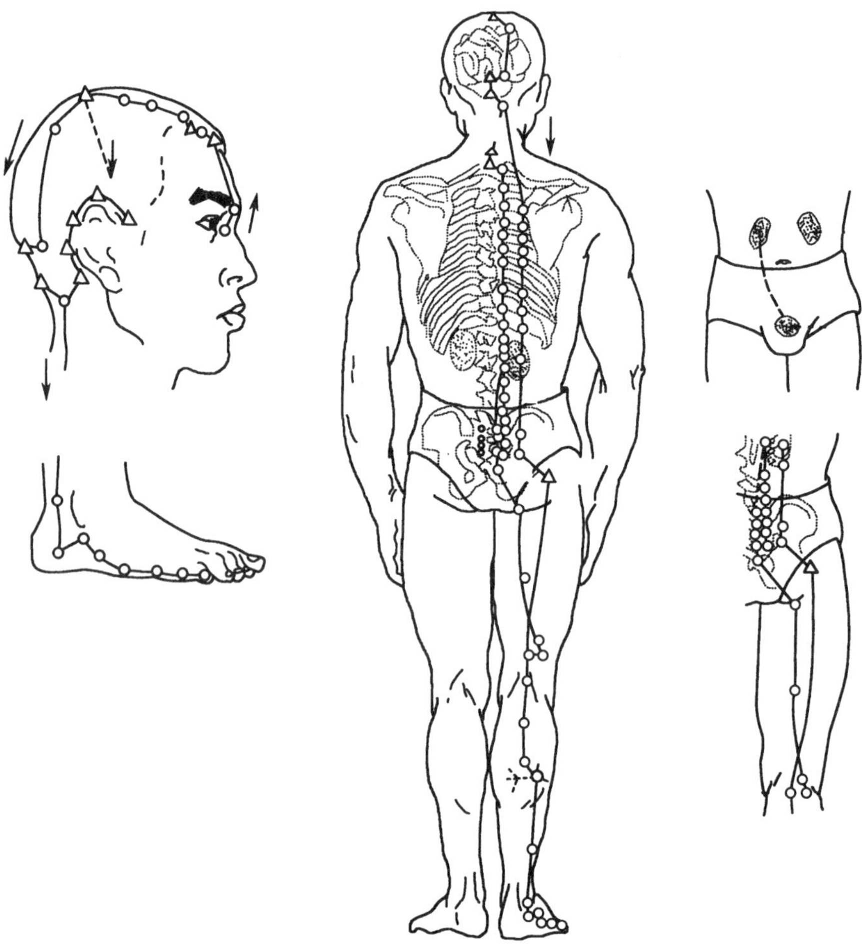

Fig.3-38　The distribution course of bladder meridian of foot-taiyang

图 3-38　足太阳膀胱经循行示意图

2 Location of acupoints

The starting acupoint of the bladder meridian is Jingming (BL 1) and the ending acupoint is Zhiyin (BL 67), totally 67 acupoints in each side. The location of acupoints is presented in Table 3-7 and Figure 3-39～3-46.

2 腧穴定位

本经首穴为睛明，末穴为至阴，左右各67穴。腧穴定位见表3-7、图3-39～3-46。

Table 3-7 Location of acupoints of the bladder meridian of foot-taiyang

Acupoint		Location	Specific feature
BL 1*	Jingming	In the depression superior to the inner canthus	Crossing acupoint of hand-taiyang meridian, foot-taiyang meridian, foot-yangming meridian, yin heel vessel and yang heel vessel
BL 2*	Cuanzhu	In the depression on the medial end of the eyebrow, on the supraorbital notch	
BL 3	Meichong	On the scalp, 0.5 cun right above the supraorbital notch	
BL 4	Qucha	On the scalp, 0.5 cun within anterior hairline, 1.5 cun lateral to front midline	
BL 5	Wuchu	On the scalp, 1.0 cun within anterior hairline, 1.5 cun lateral to front midline	
BL 6	Chengguang	On the scalp, 2.5 cun within anterior hairline, 1.5 cun lateral to front midline	
BL 7	Tongtian	On the scalp, 4.0 cun within anterior hairline, 1.5 cun lateral to front midline	
BL 8	Luoque	On the scalp, 5.5 cun within anterior hairline, 1.5 cun lateral to front midline	
BL 9	Yuzhen	On the scalp, at the level with the upper border of the external occipital protuberance, 1.3 cun lateral to the posterior hairline	
BL 10*	Tianzhu	On the nape, at the level with the upper border of the second cervical vertebra, in the depression on the lateral side of trapezius	
BL 11	Dazhu	Level with the lower border of the spinous process of the first thoracic vertebra, 1.5 cun lateral to posterior midline	Influential acupoint of bone; Crossing acupoint of bladder meridian and small intestine meridian
BL 12*	Fengmen	Level with the lower border of the spinous process of the second thoracic vertebra, 1.5 cun lateral to posterior midline	Crossing acupoint of foot-taiyang meridian and govenor vessel

(continued)

Acupoint		Location	Specific feature
BL 13*	Feishu	Level with the lower border of the spinous process of the third thoracic vertebra, 1.5 cun lateral to posterior midline	Back-Shu acupoint of the lung
BL 14	Jueyinshu	Level with the lower border of the spinous process of the fourth thoracic vertebra, 1.5 cun lateral to posterior midline	Back-Shu acupoint of the pericardium
BL 15*	Xinshu	Level with the lower border of the spinous process of the fifth thoracic vertebra, 1.5 cun lateral to posterior midline	Back-Shu acupoint of the heart
BL 16	Dushu	Level with the lower border of the spinous process of the sixth thoracic vertebra, 1.5 cun lateral to posterior midline	
BL 17*	Geshu	Level with the lower border of the spinous process of the seventh thoracic vertebra, 1.5 cun lateral to posterior midline	Influential acupoint of blood
BL 18*	Ganshu	Level with the lower border of the spinous process of the ninth thoracic vertebra, 1.5 cun lateral to posterior midline	Back-Shu acupoint of the liver
BL 19*	Danshu	Level with the lower border of the spinous process of the tenth thoracic vertebra, 1.5 cun lateral to posterior midline	Back-Shu acupoint of the gallbladder
BL 20*	Pishu	Level with the lower border of the spinous process of the eleventh thoracic vertebra, 1.5 cun lateral to posterior midline	Back-Shu acupoint of the spleen
BL 21*	Weishu	Level with the lower border of the spinous process of the twelth thoracic vertebra, 1.5 cun lateral to posterior midline	Back-Shu acupoint of the stomach
BL 22	Sanjiaoshu	Level with the lower border of the spinous process of the first lumbar vertebra, 1.5 cun lateral to posterior midline	Back-Shu acupoint of the triple energizer
BL 23*	Shenshu	Level with the lower border of the spinous process of the second lumbar vertebra, 1.5 cun lateral to posterior midline	Back-Shu acupoint of the kidney
BL 24	Qihaishu	Level with the lower border of the spinous process of the third lumbar vertebra, 1.5 cun lateral to posterior midline	
BL 25*	Dachangshu	Level with the lower border of the spinous process of the fourth lumbar vertebra, 1.5 cun lateral to posterior midline	Back-Shu acupoint of the large intestine
BL 26	Guanyuanshu	Level with the lower border of the spinous process of the fifth lumbar vertebra, 1.5 cun lateral to posterior midline	

(continued)

Acupoint		Location	Specific feature
BL 27	Xiaochang-shu	At the level of the first sacral foramen, 1.5 cun lateral to the posterior midline	Back-Shu acupoint of the small intestine
BL 28*	Pangguang-shu	At the level of the second sacral foramen, 1.5 cun lateral to the posterior midline	Back-Shu acupoint of the bladder
BL 29	Zhonglüshu	At the level of the third sacral foramen, 1.5 cun lateral to the posterior midline	
BL 30	Baihuanshu	At the level of the fourth sacral foramen, 1.5 cun lateral to the posterior midline	
BL 31	Shangliao	In the first posterior sacral foramen	
BL 32*	Ciliao	In the second posterior sacral foramen	
BL 33	Zhongliao	In the third posterior sacral foramen	
BL 34	Xialiao	In the fourth posterior sacral foramen	
BL 35	Huiyang	0.5 cun lateral to the tip of the coccyx	
BL 36*	Chengfu	In the middle of the transverse gluteal fold	
BL 37	Yinmen	On the posterior aspect of the thigh, 6 cun below the transverse gluteal fold and between the biceps femoris muscle and semitendinosus muscle	
BL 38	Fuxi	1 cun above the popliteal crease, on the medial side of the tendon of the biceps femoris	
BL 39*	Weiyang	On the transverse popliteal crease, on the medial side of the tendon of the biceps femoris	Lower He-Sea acupoint of the triple energizer
BL 40*	Weizhong	At the midpoint of the transverse popliteal crease	He-Sea acupoint; Lower He-Sea acupoint of the bladder
BL 41	Fufen	At the medial border of the scapula, 3 cun lateral to the posterior midline and at the level with the lower border of the second thoracic vertebra	Crossing acupoint of the hand and foot taiyang meridians
BL 42	Pohu	At the medial border of the scapula, 3 cun lateral to the posterior midline and at the level with the lower border of the third thoracic vertebra	
BL 43*	Gaohuang-shu	At the medial border of the scapula, 3 cun lateral to the posterior midline and at the level with the lower border of the fourth thoracic vertebra	
BL 44	Shentang	At the medial border of the scapula, 3 cun lateral to the posterior midline and at the level with the lower border of the fifth thoracic vertebra	
BL 45	Yixi	At the medial border of the scapula, 3 cun lateral to the posterior midline and at the level with the lower border of the sixth thoracic vertebra	

(continued)

Acupoint		Location	Specific feature
BL 46	Geguan	At the medial border of the scapula, 3 cun lateral to the posterior midline and at the level with the lower border of the seventh thoracic vertebra	
BL 47	Hunmen	At the medial border of the scapula, 3 cun lateral to the posterior midline and at the level with the lower border of the ninth thoracic vertebra	
BL 48	Yanggang	At the medial border of the scapula, 3 cun lateral to the posterior midline and at the level with the lower border of the tenth thoracic vertebra	
BL 49	Yishe	At the medial border of the scapula, 3 cun lateral to the posterior midline and at the level with the lower border of the eleventh thoracic vertebra	
BL 50	Weicang	At the medial border of the scapula, 3 cun lateral to the posterior midline and at the level with the lower border of the twelfth thoracic vertebra	
BL 51	Huangmen	On the lower back, 3 cun lateral to the posterior midline and at the level with the lower border of the first lumbar vertebra	
BL 52*	Zhishi	On the lower back, 3 cun lateral to the posterior midline and at the level with the lower border of the second lumbar vertebra	
BL 53	Baohuang	3 cun lateral to the median sacral crest and at the level with the second sacral posterior foremen	
BL 54*	Zhibian	3 cun lateral to the median sacral crest and at the level with the fourth sacral posterior foremen	
BL 55	Heyang	2 cun directly below popliteal crease and between the medial and lateral heads of muscle gastrocnemius	
BL 56	Chengjin	5 cun directly below popliteal crease and in the center of the belly of muscle gastrocnemius	
BL 57*	Chengshan	In the depression below the two bellies and tendons of the muscle gastrocnemius	
BL 58*	Feiyang	7 cun directly above Kunlun (BL 60) and between the lateral-inferior border of muscle gastrocnemius and heel tendon	Luo-Connecting acupoint
BL 59	Fuyang	3 cun directly above Kunlun (BL 60) and between the calf and heel tendon	Xi-Cleft acupoint of yang heel vessel
BL 60*	Kunlun	In the depression between the Achilles tendon and the lateral malleolus	Jing-River acupoint

(continued)

Acupoint		Location	Specific feature
BL 61	Pucan	Directly below Kunlun (BL 60), lateral to calcaneum, and at the junction of the red and white skin	
BL 62*	Shenmai	Directly below the lateral malleolus, and in the depression between the lower border of the lateral malleolus and heel tendon.	Influential acupoint communicating with yang heel vessel
BL 63	Jinmen	On the lateral side of the foot, directly below the anterior border of the external malleolus and below the border of femur	Xi-Cleft acupoint
BL 64*	Jinggu	Below the tuberosity of the fifth metatarsal bone and at the junction of the red and white skin	Yuan-Source acupoint
BL 65	Shugu	Posterior to the head of the fifth metatarsal bone and at the junction of the red and white skin	Shu-Stream acupoint
BL 66	Zutonggu	Anterior to the head of the fifth metatarsal bone and at the junction of the red and white skin	Ying-Spring acupoint
BL 67	Zhiyin	On the lateral side of the small toe, about 0.1 cun from the corner of the nail	Jing-Well acupoint

表 3-7 足太阳膀胱经的腧穴定位

腧穴		定位	特定穴属性
睛明*	Jīngmíng	在面部，目内眦内上方眶内侧壁凹陷中	手足太阳、足阳明经、阴蹻脉、阳蹻脉交会穴
攒竹*	Cuánzhú	在面部，眉头凹陷中，额切迹处	
眉冲	Méichōng	在头部，额切迹直上入发际 0.5 寸	
曲差	Qūchā	在头部，前发际正中直上 0.5 寸，旁开 1.5 寸	
五处	Wǔchù	在头部，前发际正中直上 1 寸，旁开 1.5 寸	
承光	Chéngguāng	在头部，前发际正中直上 2.5 寸，旁开 1.5 寸	
通天	Tōngtiān	在头部，前发际正中直上 4 寸，旁开 1.5 寸	
络却	Luòquè	在头部，前发际正中直上 5.5 寸，旁开 1.5 寸	
玉枕	Yùzhěn	在头部，横平枕外隆凸上缘，后发际正中旁开 1.3 寸	
天柱*	Tiānzhù	在颈后区，横平第 2 颈椎棘突上际，斜方肌外缘凹陷中	
大杼	Dàzhù	在脊柱区，第 1 胸椎棘突下，后正中线旁开 1.5 寸	八会穴(骨会)；手足太阳经交会穴
风门*	Fēngmén	在脊柱区，第 2 胸椎棘突下，后正中线旁开 1.5 寸	足太阳经、督脉交会穴

（续表）

腧穴		定位	特定穴属性
肺俞*	Fèishū	在脊柱区，第 3 胸椎棘突下，后正中线旁开 1.5 寸	肺之背俞穴
厥阴俞	Juéyīnshū	在脊柱区，第 4 胸椎棘突下，后正中线旁开 1.5 寸	心包之背俞穴
心俞*	Xīnshū	在脊柱区，第 5 胸椎棘突下，后正中线旁开 1.5 寸	心之背俞穴
督俞	Dūshū	在脊柱区，第 6 胸椎棘突下，后正中线旁开 1.5 寸	
膈俞*	Géshū	在脊柱区，第 7 胸椎棘突下，后正中线旁开 1.5 寸	八会穴（血会）
肝俞*	Gānshū	在脊柱区，第 9 胸椎棘突下，后正中线旁开 1.5 寸	肝之背俞穴
胆俞*	Dǎnshū	在脊柱区，第 10 胸椎棘突下，后正中线旁开 1.5 寸	胆之背俞穴
脾俞*	Píshū	在脊柱区，第 11 胸椎棘突下，后正中线旁开 1.5 寸	脾之背俞穴
胃俞*	Wèishū	在脊柱区，第 12 胸椎棘突下，后正中线旁开 1.5 寸	胃之背俞穴
三焦俞	Sānjiāoshū	在脊柱区，第 1 腰椎棘突下，后正中线旁开 1.5 寸	三焦之背俞穴
肾俞*	Shènshū	在脊柱区，第 2 腰椎棘突下，后正中线旁开 1.5 寸	肾之背俞穴
气海俞	Qìhǎishū	在脊柱区，第 3 腰椎棘突下，后正中线旁开 1.5 寸	
大肠俞*	Dàchángshū	在脊柱区，第 4 腰椎棘突下，后正中线旁开 1.5 寸	大肠之背俞穴
关元俞	Guānyuánshū	在脊柱区，第 5 腰椎棘突下，后正中线旁开 1.5 寸	
小肠俞	Xiǎochángshū	在骶区，横平第 1 骶后孔，骶正中嵴旁开 1.5 寸	小肠之背俞穴
膀胱俞*	Pángguāngshū	在骶区，横平第 2 骶后孔，骶正中嵴旁开 1.5 寸	膀胱之背俞穴
中膂俞	zhōnglǚshū	在骶区，横平第 3 骶后孔，骶正中嵴旁开 1.5 寸	
白环俞	Báihuánshū	在骶区，横平第 4 骶后孔，骶正中嵴旁开 1.5 寸	
上髎	Shàngliáo	在骶区，正对第 1 骶后孔中	
次髎*	Cìliáo	在骶区，正对第 2 骶后孔中	
中髎	Zhōngliáo	在骶区，正对第 3 骶后孔中	
下髎	Xiàliáo	在骶区，正对第 4 骶后孔中	
会阳	Huìyáng	在骶区，尾骨端旁开 0.5 寸	
承扶*	Chéngfú	在股后区，臀沟的中点	
殷门	Yīnmén	在股后区，臀沟下 6 寸，股二头肌与半腱肌之间	
浮郄	Fúxì	在膝后区，腘横纹上 1 寸，股二头肌腱的内侧缘	
委阳*	Wěiyáng	在膝部，腘横纹上，股二头肌腱的内侧缘	三焦下合穴

（续表）

腧穴		定位	特定穴属性
委中*	Wěizhōng	在膝后区，腘横纹中点	合穴；膀胱下合穴
附分	Fùfēn	在脊柱区，第 2 胸椎棘突下，后正中线旁开 3 寸	手、足太阳经交会穴
魄户	Pòhù	在脊柱区，第 3 胸椎棘突下，后正中线旁开 3 寸	
膏肓俞*	Gāohuāngshū	在脊柱区，第 4 胸椎棘突下，后正中线旁开 3 寸	
神堂	Shéntáng	在脊柱区，第 5 胸椎棘突下，后正中线旁开 3 寸	
譩譆	Yìxǐ	在脊柱区，第 6 胸椎棘突下，后正中线旁开 3 寸	
膈关	Géguān	在脊柱区，第 7 胸椎棘突下，后正中线旁开 3 寸	
魂门	Húnmén	在脊柱区，第 9 胸椎棘突下，后正中线旁开 3 寸	
阳纲	Yánggāng	在脊柱区，第 10 胸椎棘突下，后正中线旁开 3 寸	
意舍	Yìshè	在脊柱区，第 11 胸椎棘突下，后正中线旁开 3 寸	
胃仓	Wèicāng	在脊柱区，第 12 胸椎棘突下，后正中线旁开 3 寸	
肓门	Huāngmén	在腰区，第 1 腰椎棘突下，后正中线旁开 3 寸	
志室*	Zhìshì	在腰区，第 2 腰椎棘突下，后正中线旁开 3 寸	
胞肓	Bāohuāng	在骶区，横平第 2 骶后孔，骶正中嵴旁开 3 寸	
秩边*	Zhìbiān	在骶区，横平第 4 骶后孔，骶正中嵴旁开 3 寸	
合阳	Héyáng	在小腿后区，腘横纹下 2 寸，腓肠肌内外侧头之间	
承筋	Chéngjīn	在小腿后区，腘横纹下 5 寸，腓肠肌两肌腹之间	
承山*	Chéngshān	在小腿后区，腓肠肌两肌腹与肌腱交角处	
飞扬*	Fēiyáng	在小腿后区，昆仑直上 7 寸，腓肠肌外下缘与跟腱移行处	络穴
跗阳	Fūyáng	在小腿后区，昆仑直上 3 寸，腓骨与跟腱之间	阳蹻郄穴
昆仑*	Kūnlún	在踝区，外踝尖与跟腱之间的凹陷中	经穴
仆参	Púcān	在跟区，昆仑直下，跟骨外侧，赤白肉际处	
申脉*	Shēnmài	在踝区，外踝尖直下，外踝下缘与跟骨之间凹陷中	八脉交会穴（通阳蹻脉）
金门	Jīnmén	在足背，外踝前缘直下，第 5 跖骨粗隆后方，骰骨下缘凹陷中	郄穴
京骨*	Jīnggǔ	在跖区，第 5 跖骨关节粗隆前下方，赤白肉际处	原穴
束骨	Shùgǔ	在跖区，第 5 跖趾关节的近端，赤白肉际处	输穴
足通谷	Zútōnggǔ	在足趾，第 5 跖趾关节的远端，赤白肉际处	荥穴
至阴*	Zhìyīn	在足趾，小趾末节外侧，趾甲根角侧后方 0.1 寸（指寸）	井穴

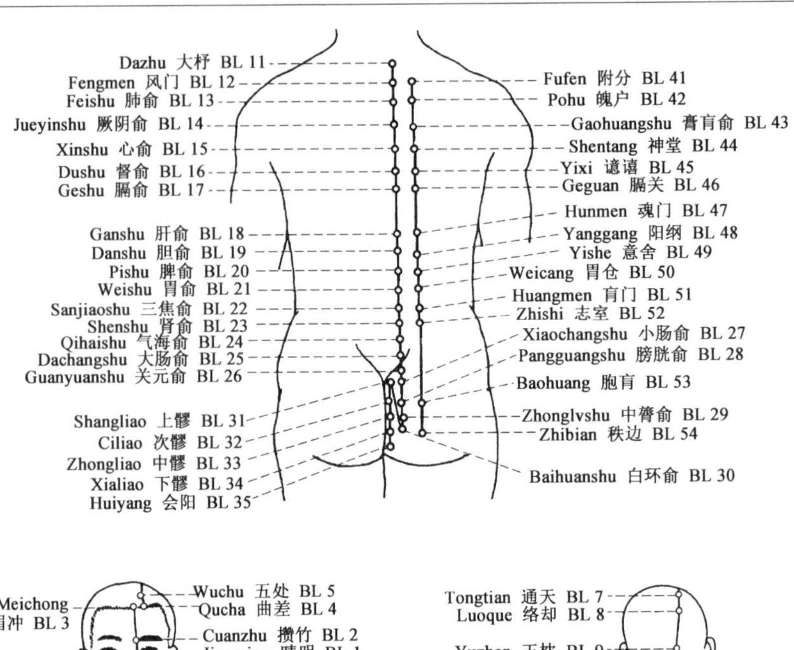

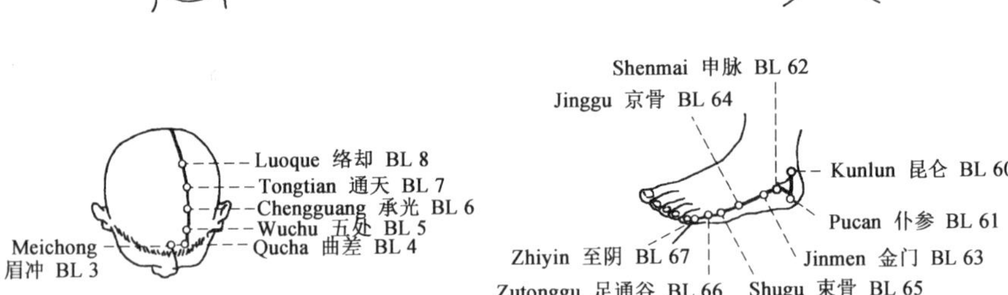

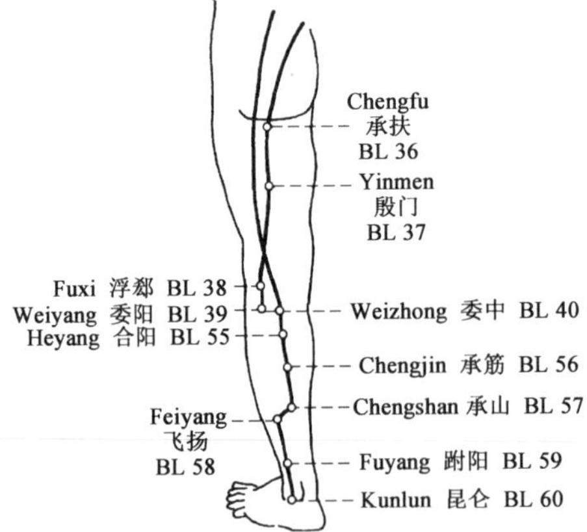

Fig.3-39　Acupoints of bladder meridian of Foot-taiyang

图 3-39　足太阳膀胱经腧穴总图

3 Indications of acupoints

The acupoints of the bladder meridian are indicated for the disorders of the head, eyes, neck, back, low back, lower limbs, and mental diseases; the Back-Shu acupoints on the first lateral line, and the acupoints on the second lateral line which are level with those Back-Shu acupoints on the first lateral line are indicated for the diseases of their related zang-fu organs and tissues. The acupoints from the first to the sixth thoracic vertebrae are indicated for the heart and lung diseases; the acupoints from the seventh to twelfth thoracic vertebrae are indicated for the diseases in the liver, gallbladder, spleen and stomach; the acupoints from the first lumbar vertebrae to the fifth sacral vertebrae are indicated for the diseases in the kidneys, bladder, large intestine, small intestine and uterus. The disorders on the head and face are usually treated by Jinggu(BL 64), Cuanzhu(BL 2) and Meichong(BL 3); lumbago is often treated by Weizhong(40) and Kunlun (BL 60). The indications and needling methods are presented as below.

3 腧穴主治

本经腧穴主要用于治疗头、目、项、背、腰、下肢部病证以及神志病；背部第一侧线的背俞穴及第二侧线相平的腧穴主治与其相关的脏腑及组织器官病证。第一至六胸椎之间两侧的腧穴治心肺疾病；第七至十二胸椎之间两侧的腧穴治肝、胆、脾、胃等疾病；第一腰椎至第五骶椎两侧腧穴治疗肾、膀胱、大小肠、子宫等疾病。头面部疾病常用京骨、攒竹、眉冲等；腰痛常用委中、昆仑。临床常用腧穴的主治及针刺操作如下。

3.1 Jingming (BL 1) Crossing acupoint of hand-taiyang meridian, foot-taiyang meridian, foot-yangming meridian, yin heel vessel and yang heel vessel

Indications: Reddened and swollen eyes, lacrimation, nearsightedness, blurred vision, vertigo, night blindness and color blindness.

Needling: Ask the patient to close the eyes when gently pushing the eyeball to the lateral side; then puncture slowly and vertically 0.5～1.0 cun close against the orbital wall. It is not advisable to rotate

3.1 睛明 Jīngmíng 手足太阳、足阳明经、阴蹻脉、阳蹻脉交会穴

主治：目赤肿痛，流泪，近视，视物不明，目眩，夜盲，色盲。

操作：患者闭目，医者押手轻推眼球向外侧固定，刺手持针，紧靠眶缘缓慢直刺0.5～1.0寸，不宜提插和大幅

or lift and thrust the needle. To avoid bleeding, press the punctured site for a while; moxibustion is contraindicated on this acupoint.

度捻转，出针按压，以防出血；禁灸。

3.2 Cuanzhu (BL 2)

Indications: ① Blurred vision, reddened and swollen eyes, lacrimation, twitching of the eyelids; ② headache, pain in the supraorbital region, facial paralysis; ③ hiccup.

Needling: Puncture downwards or laterally or obliquely 0.5～0.8 cun; moxibustion is contraindicated.

3.2 攒竹 Cuánzhú

主治：①目视不明，目赤肿痛，流泪，眼睑瞤动；②头痛，眉棱骨痛，面瘫；③呃逆。

操作：向下或向外平刺或斜刺0.5～0.8寸；禁灸。

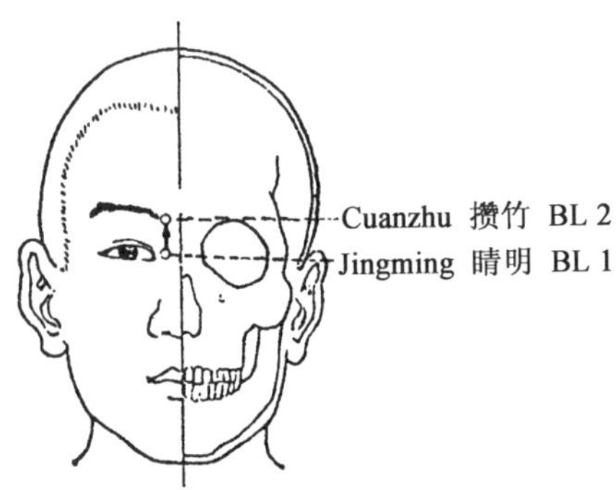

Fig.3-40 Head and face acupoints on the bladder meridian of foot-taiyang

图3-40 足太阳膀胱经头面部经穴图

Luoque 络却 BL 8
Yuzhen 玉枕 BL 9
Tianzhu 天柱 BL 10
4 cun
4寸
2.5 cun
2.5寸

Fig.3-41 Head and face acupoints on the bladder meridian of foot-taiyang

图3-41 足太阳膀胱经头部经穴图

3.3 Tianzhu (BL 10)

Indications: ① Headache, dizziness; ② blurred vision, nasal stuffiness; ③ stiff neck, painful shoulder and back.

Needling: Puncture vertically or obliquely 0.5～0.8 cun, puncturing in a medial or upward direction is forbidden to avoid injuring the medulla.

3.3 天柱 Tiānzhù

主治：①头痛，眩晕；②目视不明，鼻塞；③项强，肩背痛。

操作：直刺或斜刺0.5～0.8寸，不可向内上方深刺，以免伤及延髓。

3.4 Fengmen (BL 12) Crossing acupoint of the foot-taiyang meridian and governor vessel

Indications: ① Common cold, cough, fever,

3.4 风门 Fēngmén 足太阳经、督脉交会穴

主治：①感冒，咳嗽，发

headache; ② stiff neck, painful chest and back.

Needling: Puncture obliquely 0.5~0.8 cun.

3.5 Feishu (BL 13) Back-Shu acupoint of the lung

Indications: ① Cough, common cold, nasal stuffiness; ② hectic fever, night sweating; ③ itching skin, urticaria.

Needling: Puncture obliquely 0.5~0.8 cun.

3.6 Xinshu (BL 15) Back-Shu acupoint of the heart

Indications: ① Heart pain, palpitation, insomnia, forgetfulness, epilepsy; ② cough, vomiting of blood; ③ nocturnal emission, nigh sweating.

Needling: Puncture obliquely 0.5~0.8 cun.

3.7 Geshu (BL 17) Influential acupoint of blood

Indications: ① Stomachache, vomiting, hiccup; ② cough and asthma, vomiting of blood, hectic fever, night sweating; ③ urticaria.

Needling: Puncture obliquely 0.5~0.8 cun.

3.8 Ganshu (BL 18) Back-Shu acupoint of the liver

Indications: ① Jaundice, flank pain; ② reddened eyes, blurred vision, night blindness; ③ vomiting of blood, bleeding condition; ④ dizziness, depressive-manic psychosis and epilepsy.

Needling: Puncture obliquely 0.5~0.8 cun.

3.9 Danshu (BL 19) Back-Shu acupoint of the gallbladder

Indications: ① Jaundice, bitter taste in the mouth, flank pain; ② lung tuberculosis, hectic fever.

Needling: Puncture obliquely 0.5~0.8 cun.

热,头痛;②项强,胸背痛。

操作: 斜刺 0.5~0.8 寸。

3.5 肺俞 Fèishū 肺之背俞穴

主治: ①咳喘,感冒,鼻塞;②骨蒸潮热,盗汗;③皮肤瘙痒,瘾疹。

操作: 斜刺 0.5~0.8 寸。

3.6 心俞 Xīnshū 心之背俞穴

主治: ①心痛,心悸,失眠,健忘,癫痫;②咳嗽,吐血;③梦遗,盗汗。

操作: 斜刺 0.5~0.8 寸。

3.7 膈俞 Géshū 八会穴(血会)

主治: ①胃痛,呕吐,呃逆;②咳喘,吐血,潮热,盗汗;③瘾疹。

操作: 斜刺 0.5~0.8 寸。

3.8 肝俞 Gānshū 肝之背俞穴

主治: ①黄疸,胁痛;②目赤,目视不明,夜盲;③吐血,衄血;④眩晕,癫狂痫。

操作: 斜刺 0.5~0.8 寸。

3.9 胆俞 Dǎnshū 胆之背俞穴

主治: ①黄疸,口苦,胁痛;②肺痨,潮热。

操作: 斜刺 0.5~0.8 寸。

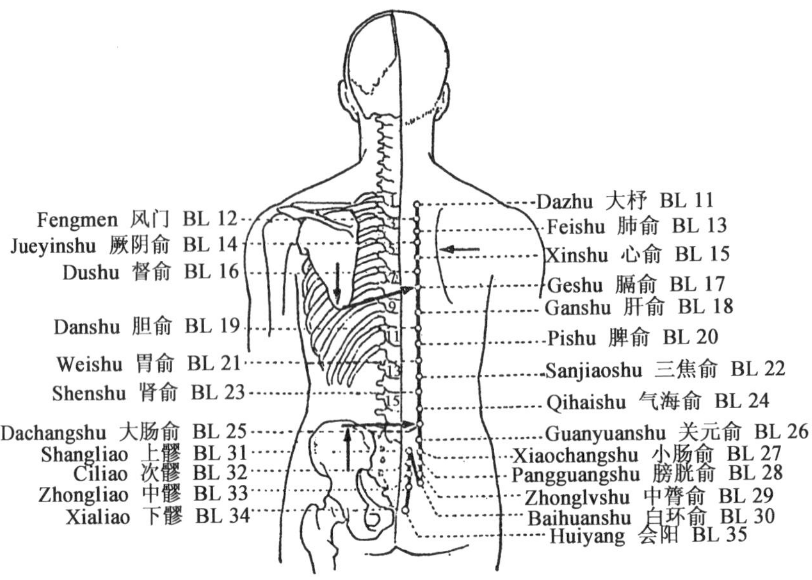

Fig.42 Back acupoints on the bladder meridian of foot-taiyang

图 3-42 足太阳膀胱经背腰部经穴图

3.10 Pishu (BL 20) Back-Shu acupoint of the spleen

Indications: ① Abdominal distension, diarrhea, dysentery, bloody stools, poor appetite; ② edema, jaundice.

Needling: Puncture obliquely 0.5～0.8 cun.

3.10 脾俞 Píshū 脾之背俞穴

主治: ①腹胀,泄泻,痢疾,便血,纳呆;②水肿,黄疸。

操作: 斜刺 0.5～0.8 寸。

3.11 Weishu (BL 21) Back-Shu acupoint of the stomach

Indications: ① Stomachache, vomiting, abdominal distension, intestinal gurgling; ② chest and flank pain.

Needling: Puncture obliquely 0.5～0.8 cun.

3.11 胃俞 Wèishū 胃之背俞穴

主治: ①胃脘痛,呕吐,腹胀,肠鸣;②胸胁痛。

操作: 斜刺 0.5～0.8 寸。

3.12 Shenshu (BL 23) Back-Shu acupoint of the kidneys

Indications: ① Tinnitus, deafness; ② seminal emission, impotence, irregular menstruation, mor-

3.12 肾俞 Shènshū 肾之背俞穴

主治: ①耳鸣,耳聋;②遗精,阳痿,月经不调,带

bid leukorrhea, enuresis, difficulty in urination, edema; ③ lumbago; ④ cough and shortness of breath.

下,遗尿,小便不利,水肿;③腰痛;④咳喘少气。

Needling: Puncture vertically 0.5～1.0 cun.

操作: 直刺 0.5～1.0 寸。

3.13 Dachangshu (BL 25) Back-Shu acupoint of the large intestine

3.13 大肠俞 Dàchángshū 大肠之背俞穴

Indications: ① Pain in the loin and legs; ② abdominal pain, diarrhea, constipation, dysentery, and hemorrhoids.

主治: ①腰腿痛;②腹痛,泄泻,便秘,痢疾,痔疾。

Needling: Puncture vertically 0.8～1.2 cun.

操作: 直刺0.8～1.2 寸。

3.14 Pangguangshu (BL 28) Back-Shu acupoint of the bladder

3.14 膀胱俞 Pángguāngshū 膀胱之背俞穴

Indications: ① Difficulty in urination, frequent urination, enuresis; ② diarrhea, constipation; ③ spinal stiffness and pain.

主治: ①小便不利,尿频,遗尿;②泄泻,便秘;③腰脊强痛。

Needling: Puncture vertically or obliquely 0.8～1.2 cun.

操作: 直刺或斜刺0.8～1.2 寸。

3.15 Ciliao (BL 32)

3.15 次髎 Cìliáo

Indications: ① Irregular menstruation, menstrual cramp, morbid leucorrhea, seminal emission, impotence, difficulty in urination, enuresis; ② sacral pain, paralysis of the lower limbs.

主治: ①月经不调,痛经,带下,遗精,阳痿,小便不利,遗尿;②腰骶痛,下肢痿痹。

Needling: Puncture vertically 1.0～1.5 cun.

操作: 直刺 1.0～1.5 寸。

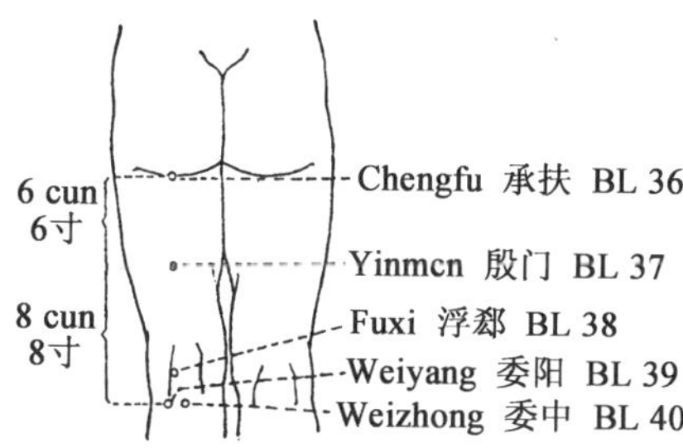

Fig.3-43 Lower limb acupoints on the bladder meridian of foot-taiyang

图 3-43 足太阳膀胱经下肢部经穴图

3.16 Chengfu (BL 36)

Indications: ① Pain in the loin and legs, paralysis of the lower limbs; ② hemorrhoids.

Needling: Puncture vertically 1.5～2.0 cun.

3.17 Weiyang (BL 39) Lower He-Sea acupoint of the triple energizer

Indications: ① Abdominal floating, urinary difficulty; ② spinal stiffness and pain, convulsion and pain in the legs.

Needling: Puncture vertically 1.0～1.5 cun.

3.18 Weizhong (BL 40) He-Sea acupoint; Lower He-Sea acupoint of the bladder

Indications: ① Lumbago, spasms of the legs, paralysis of the lower limbs; ② difficulty in urination, enuresis; ③ erysipelas, urticaria, carbuncle.

Needling: Puncture vertically 1.0～1.5 cun; or prick to bleed with a three-edged needle.

3.19 Gaohuangshu(BL 43)

Indications: ① Cough and asthma, lung tuberculosis; ② forgetfullness, seminal emission, night sweating, deficiency condition; ③ pain in the shoulder and back.

Needling: Puncture obliquely 0.5～0.8 cun.

3.20 Zhishi (BL 52)

Indications: ① Seminal emission, impotence; ② difficulty in urination, edema; ③ spinal stiffness and pain.

Needling: Puncture obliquely 0.5～0.8 cun.

3.21 Zhibian (BL 54)

Indications: ① Pain in the loin and legs, paralysis of the lower limbs; ② hemorrhoids, constipation, and difficulty in urination.

Needling: Puncture vertically 1.5～2.0 cun.

3.16 承扶 Chéngfú

主治: ①腰腿痛,下肢痿痹;②痔疾。

操作: 直刺1.5～2.0寸。

3.17 委阳 Wěiyáng 三焦下合穴

主治: ①腹满,水肿,小便不利;②腰脊强痛,腿足挛痛。

操作: 直刺1.0～1.5寸。

3.18 委中 Wěizhōng 合穴;膀胱下合穴

主治: ①腰痛,腘筋挛急,下肢痿痹;②小便不利,遗尿;③丹毒,瘾疹,疔疮。

操作: 直刺1.0～1.5寸,或三棱针点刺出血。

3.19 膏肓俞 Gāohuāngshū

主治: ①咳喘,肺痨;②健忘,遗精,盗汗,虚劳;③肩胛背痛。

操作: 斜刺0.5～0.8寸。

3.20 志室 Zhìshì

主治: ①遗精,阳痿;②小便不利,水肿;③腰脊强痛。

操作: 斜刺0.5～0.8寸。

3.21 秩边 Zhìbiān

主治: ①腰腿痛,下肢痿痹;②痔疾,便秘,小便不利。

操作: 直刺1.5～2.0寸。

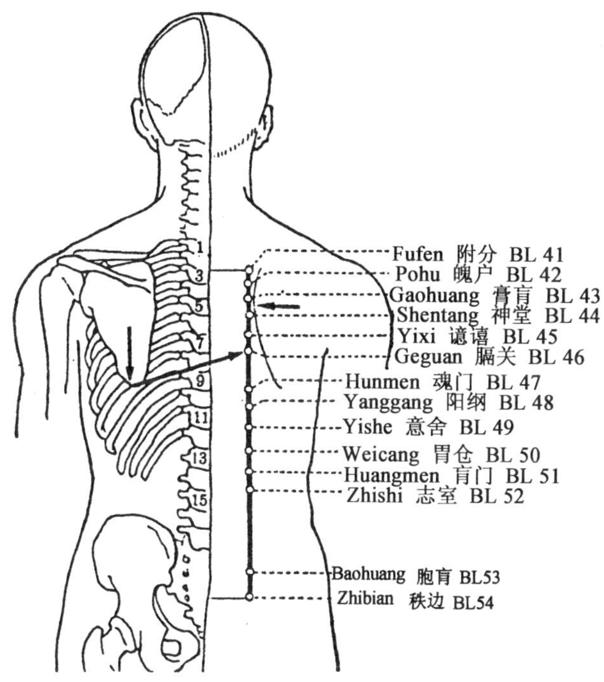

Fig.3-44 Back acupoints on the bladder meridian of foot-taiyang

图 3-44 足太阳膀胱经背腰部经穴图

3.22 Chengshan (BL 57)

Indications: ① Convulsive pain in the loin and legs; ② hemorrhoids, and constipation.

Needling: Puncture vertically 1.0～2.0 cun.

3.23 Fciyang (BL 58) Luo-Connecting acupoint

Indications: ① Pain in the loin and legs; ② headache, dizziness, and nasal bleeding; ③ hemorrhoids.

Needling: Puncture vertically 1.0～1.5 cun.

3.24 Kunlun (BL 60) Jing-River acupoint

Indications: ① Headache and stiff neck; ② lumbago and heel pain; ③ delayed labor; ④ epilepsy.

3.22 承山 Chéngshān

主治: ①腰腿拘急疼痛;②痔疾,便秘。

操作: 直刺 1.0～2 寸。

3.23 飞扬 Fēiyáng 络穴

主治: ①腰腿疼痛;②头痛,目眩,鼻衄;③痔疾。

操作: 直刺 1.0～1.5 寸。

3.24 昆仑 Kūnlún 经穴

主治: ①头痛,项强;②腰痛,足跟痛;③滞产;④癫痫。

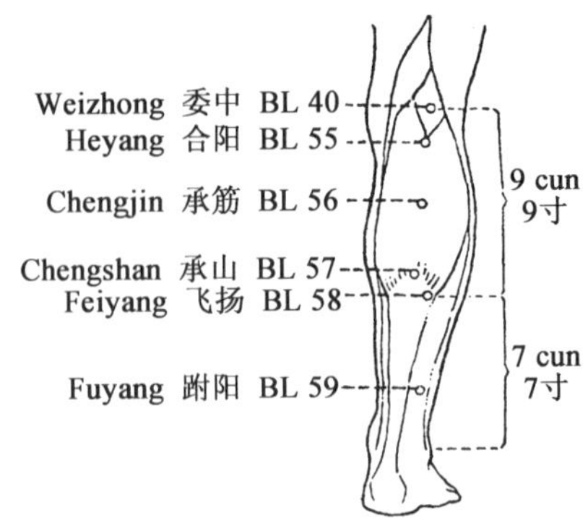

Fig.3-45 Lower limb acupoints on the bladder meridian of foot-taiyang

图 3-45 足太阳膀胱经下肢部经穴图

Needling: Puncture vertically 0.5～0.8 cun. Puncturing at this acupoint is forbidden in the pregnant women.

操作: 直刺0.5～0.8寸。孕妇禁用。

3.25 Shenmai (BL 62) Confluent acupoint communicating with the yang heel vessel

Indications: ① Insomnia, epilepsy; ② headache, stiff neck, and pain in the loin and legs; ③ dropping eyelids and sleepiness.

Needling: Puncture vertically 0.3～0.5 cun.

3.25 申脉 Shēnmài 八脉交会穴(通阳蹻脉)

主治: ①失眠,癫狂痫;②头痛,项强,腰腿痛;③眼睑下垂,嗜睡。

操作: 直刺0.3～0.5寸。

3.26 Jinggu (BL 64) Yuan-Source acupoint

Indications: ① Headache, stiff neck and nebula; ② pain in the loin and legs; ③ epilepsy.

Needling: Puncture vertically 0.3～0.5 cun.

3.26 京骨 Jīnggǔ 原穴

主治: ①头痛,项强,目翳;②腰腿痛;③癫痫。

操作: 直刺0.3～0.5寸。

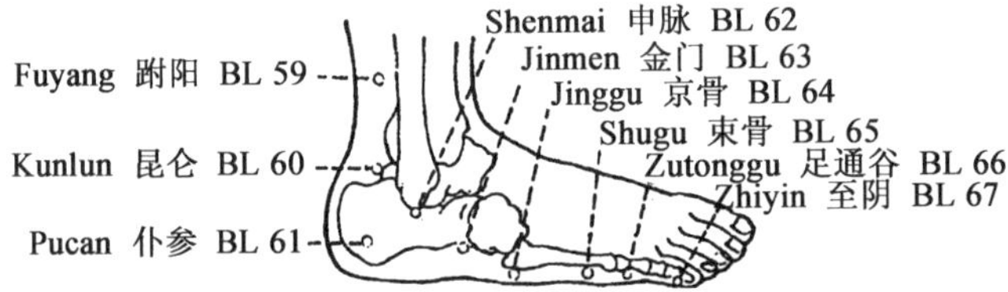

Fig.3-46 Foot acupoints on the bladder meridian of foot-taiyang

图 3-46 足太阳膀胱经足部经穴图

3.27 Zhiyin (BL 67) Jing-Well acupoint

Indications: ① Malposition of the fetus, delayed labor; ② headache, painful eyes, nasal stuffiness and bleeding.

Needling: Puncture shallowly 0.1 cun; for malposition of the fetus, moxibustion is applied.

3.27 至阴 Zhìyīn 井穴

主治: ①胎位不正,滞产;②头痛,目痛,鼻塞,鼻衄。

操作: 浅刺 0.1 寸;胎位不正用灸法。

Section 8 Kidney Meridian of Foot-Shaoyin and its Acupoints

第 8 节 足少阴肾经及其腧穴

1 Distribution course

The kidney meridian of foot-shaoyin starts from the inferior aspect of the small toe, and runs obliquely across the sole of the foot; emerging from the lower aspect of the tuberosity of the navicular bone and running behind the inner ankle, it enters the heel. It then ascends along the medial side of the lower leg to the medial side of the popliteal crease, climbs upwards along the innermost aspect of the thigh towards the vertebral column, where it enters the kidney, its pertaining organ, and connects with the bladder(returning to the surface of the abdomen above the pubic bone and running upwards over the abdomen and chest to the inferior border of the clavicle). The main portion of the meridian reemerges from the kidney, ascends through the liver and diaphragm, and enters the lung. A branch emerges from the lungs, continues along the throat and terminates at the root of the tongue. Another branch leaves the lung, joins the heart, and flows into the chest to connect with the

1 经脉循行

足少阴肾经,起于足小趾之下,斜走足心,出于舟骨粗隆下,沿内踝后,进入足跟,再向上行于小腿内侧,出腘窝内侧,向上行大腿内后缘,通向脊柱,属于肾脏,联络膀胱(腧穴通路:浅出腹前,上行经腹胸部,终止于锁骨下缘)。肾脏直行的主脉,从肾向上,通过肝和横膈,进入肺中,沿喉咙挟舌根;肺部支脉,从肺部出来,联络心脏,流注于胸中,与手厥阴心包经相接(图 3-47)。

pericardium meridian(Fig. 3-47).

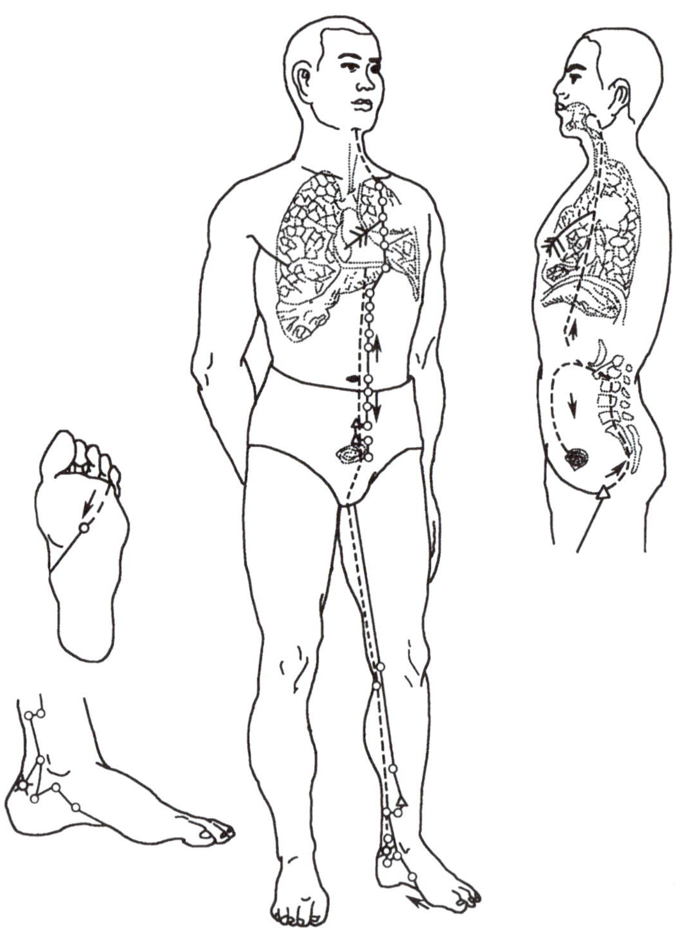

Fig.3-47 The distribution course of kidney meridian of foot-shaoyin

图 3-47 足少阴肾经循行示意图

2 Location of acupoints

The starting acupoint of the kidney meridian is Yongquan (KI 1), and the ending acupoint is Shufu (KI 27), totally 27 acupoints in each side. The location of acupoints is presented in Table 3-8 and Fig. 3-48～3-52.

2 腧穴定位

本经首穴为涌泉，末穴为俞府，左右各 27 穴。腧穴定位见表 3-8、图 3-48～3-52。

Table 3-8 Location of acupoints of the kidney meridian of foot-shaoyin

Acupoint		Location	Specific features
KI 1*	Yongquan	On the sole, in the depression when the foot is in plantar flexion	Jing-Well acupoint
KI 2*	Rangu	In the depression below the lower border of the tuberosity of the navicular bone, at the junction of the red and white skin	Ying-Spring acupoint
KI 3*	Taixi	In the depression between the tip of the medial malleolus and the heel tendon	Shu-Stream acupoint; Yuan-Source acupoint
KI 4*	Dazhong	Posterior and inferior to the medial malleolus, in the depression anterior to the medial side of the attachment of Achilles' tendon	Luo-Connecting acupoint
KI 5	Shuiquan	1 cun directly below Taixi (KI 3), in the depression of the medial side of the tuberisity of the calcaneum	Xi-Cleft acupoint
KI 6*	Zhaohai	1 cun below the tip of the medial malleolus, in the depression below the lower border of the medial malleolus	Confluent acupoint communicating with yin heel vessel
KI 7*	Fuliu	2 cun directly above the tip of the medial malleolus, on the anterior border of Achilles' tendon	Jing-River acupoint
KI 8	Jiaoxin	2 cun above the tip of the medial malleolus, in the depression posterior to the medial border of tibia	Xi-Cleft acupoint of yin heel vessel
KI 9	Zhubin	5 cun directly above Taixi (KI 3), between soleus muscle and Achilles' tendon	Xi-Cleft acupoint of yin link vessel
KI 10	Yingu	On the medial side of the popliteal crease, between the tendons of muscle semitendinosus and semimembranosus	He-Sea acupoint
KI 11	Henggu	On the lower abdomen, 5 cun below the navel, and 0.5 cun lateral to the anterior midline	Crossing acupoint of the foot-shaoyin and thoroughfare vessel
KI 12*	Dahe	On the lower abdomen, 4 cun below the navel, and 0.5 cun lateral to the anterior midline	Crossing acupoint of the foot-shaoyin and thoroughfare vessel
KI 13	Qixue	On the lower abdomen, 3 cun below the navel, and 0.5 cun lateral to the anterior midline	Crossing acupoint of the foot-shaoyin and thoroughfare vessel
KI 14	Siman	On the lower abdomen, 2 cun below the navel, and 0.5 cun lateral to the anterior midline	Crossing acupoint of the foot-shaoyin and thoroughfare vessel
KI 15	Zhongzhu	On the lower abdomen, 1 cun below the navel, and 0.5 cun lateral to the anterior midline	Crossing acupoint of the foot-shaoyin and thoroughfare vessel
KI 16	Huangshu	On the abdomen, 0.5 cun lateral to the navel	Crossing acupoint of the foot-shaoyin and thoroughfare vessel
KI 17	Shangqu	On the upper abdomen, 2 cun above the navel, and 0.5 cun lateral to the anterior midline	Crossing acupoint of the foot-shaoyin and thoroughfare vessel

(continued)

Acupoint		Location	Specific features
KI 18	Shiguan	On the upper abdomen, 3 cun above the navel, and 0. 5 cun lateral to the anterior midline	Crossing acupoint of the foot-shaoyin and thoroughfare vessel
KI 19	Yindu	On the upper abdomen, 4 cun above the navel, and 0. 5 cun lateral to the anterior midline	Crossing acupoint of the foot-shaoyin and thoroughfare vessel
KI 20	Futonggu	On the upper abdomen, 5 cun above the navel, and 0. 5 cun lateral to the anterior midline	Crossing acupoint of the foot-shaoyin and thoroughfare vessel
KI 21	Youmen	On the upper abdomen, 6 cun above the navel, and 0. 5 cun lateral to the anterior midline	Crossing acupoint of the foot-shaoyin and thoroughfare vessel
KI 22	Bulang	On the chest, in the fifth intercostal space, 2 cun lateral to the anterior midline	
KI 23	Shenfeng	On the chest, in the fourth intercostal space, 2 cun lateral to the anterior midline	
KI 24	Lingxu	On the chest, in the third intercostal space, 2 cun lateral to the anterior midline	
KI 25	Shencang	On the chest, in the second intercostal space, 2 cun lateral to the anterior midline	
KI 26	Yuzhong	On the chest, in the first intercostal space, 2 cun lateral to the anterior midline	
KI 27	Shufu	On the chest, at the lower border of the clavicle, 2 cun lateral to the anterior midline	

表 3-8　足少阴肾经的腧穴定位

腧穴		定位	特定穴属性
涌泉*	Yǒngquán	在足底，屈足蜷趾时足心最凹陷中	井穴
然谷*	Rángǔ	在足内侧，足舟骨粗隆下方，赤白肉际处	荥穴
太溪*	Tàixī	在踝区，内踝尖与跟腱之间的凹陷中	输穴；原穴
大钟*	Dàzhōng	在跟区，内踝后下方，跟骨上缘，跟腱附着部前缘凹陷中	络穴
水泉	Shuǐquán	在跟区，太溪直下 1 寸，跟骨结节内侧凹陷中	郄穴
照海*	Zhàohǎi	在踝区，内踝尖下 1 寸，内踝下缘边际凹陷中	八脉交会穴(通阴蹻脉)
复溜*	Fùliū	在小腿内侧，内踝尖上 2 寸，跟腱的前缘	经穴
交信	Jiāoxìn	在小腿内侧，内踝尖上 2 寸，胫骨内侧缘后际凹陷中	阴蹻郄穴
筑宾	Zhùbīn	在小腿内侧，太溪直上 5 寸，比目鱼肌与跟腱之间	阴维郄穴
阴谷	Yīngǔ	在膝后区，腘横纹上，半腱肌肌腱外侧缘	合穴
横骨	Hénggǔ	在下腹部，脐中下 5 寸，前正中线旁开 0.5 寸	足少阴经、冲脉交会穴
大赫*	Dàhè	在下腹部，脐中下 4 寸，前正中线旁开 0.5 寸	足少阴经、冲脉交会穴
气穴	Qìxué	在下腹部，脐中下 3 寸，前正中线旁开 0.5 寸	足少阴经、冲脉交会穴

（续表）

腧穴		定位	特定穴属性
四满	Sìmǎn	在下腹部，脐中下 2 寸，前正中线旁开 0.5 寸	足少阴经、冲脉交会穴
中注	Zhōngzhù	在下腹部，脐中下 1 寸，前正中线旁开 0.5 寸	足少阴经、冲脉交会穴
肓俞	Huāngshū	在腹部，脐中旁开 0.5 寸	足少阴经、冲脉交会穴
商曲	Shāngqū	在上腹部，脐中上 2 寸，前正中线旁开 0.5 寸	足少阴经、冲脉交会穴
石关	Shíguān	在上腹部，脐中上 3 寸，前正中线旁开 0.5 寸	足少阴经、冲脉交会穴
阴都	Yīndū	在上腹部，脐中上 4 寸，前正中线旁开 0.5 寸	足少阴经、冲脉交会穴
腹通谷	Fùtōnggǔ	在上腹部，脐中上 5 寸，前正中线旁开 0.5 寸	足少阴经、冲脉交会穴
幽门	Yōumén	在上腹部，脐中上 6 寸，前正中线旁开 0.5 寸	足少阴经、冲脉交会穴
步廊	Bùláng	在胸部，第 5 肋间隙，前正中线旁开 2 寸	
神封	Shénfēng	在胸部，第 4 肋间隙，前正中线旁开 2 寸	
灵墟	Língxū	在胸部，第 3 肋间隙，前正中线旁开 2 寸	
神藏	Shéncáng	在胸部，第 2 肋间隙，前正中线旁开 2 寸	
彧中	Yùzhōng	在胸部，第 1 肋间隙，前正中线旁开 2 寸	
俞府	Shūfǔ	在胸部，锁骨下缘，前正中线旁开 2 寸	

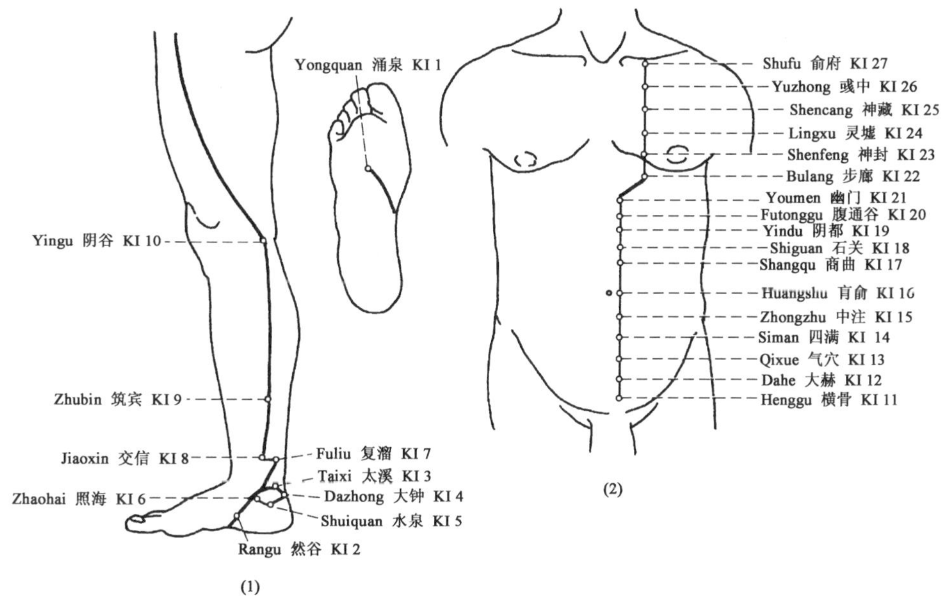

Fig.3-48 Acupoints of kidney meridian of Foot-shaoyin

图 3-48 足少阴肾经腧穴总图

3 Indications of acupoints

The acupoints of this meridian are indicated for the diseases of gynecology, external genitalia, kidney, lung and throat, and other diseases at the areas it supplies. For seminal emission, impotence and urinary difficulty, Dahe (KI 12), Shuiquan (KI 5), Yingu (KI 10) and Fuliu (KI 7) are often used; for irregular menstruation, Siman (KI 14), Taixi (KI 3), Rangu (KI 2), Fuliu (KI 7) and Zhaohai (KI 6) are usually used. The indications and needling methods of the commonly used acupoints are presented as follows.

3 腧穴主治

本经腧穴主要用于治疗妇科病，前阴病，肾、肺、咽喉病以及经脉所过部位的病证。治疗遗精、阳痿、小便不利常用大赫、水泉、阴谷和复溜；治疗月经不调常用四满、太溪、然谷、复溜、照海。临床常用腧穴的主治及针刺操作如下。

3.1 Yongquan (KI 1) Jing-Well acupoint

Indications: ① Pain in the vertex of the head, vertigo and dizziness; ② sore throat, sudden loss of voice; ③ insomnia, depressive-manic psychosis, infantile convulsions; ④ feverish in the soles; ⑤ constipation and urinary difficulty.

Needling: Puncture vertically 0.5～0.8 cun.

3.1 涌泉 Yǒngquán 井穴

主治： ①顶心头痛，头晕，目眩；②咽喉痛，失音；③失眠，癫狂，小儿惊风；④足心热；⑤便秘，小便不利。

操作： 直刺0.5～0.8寸。

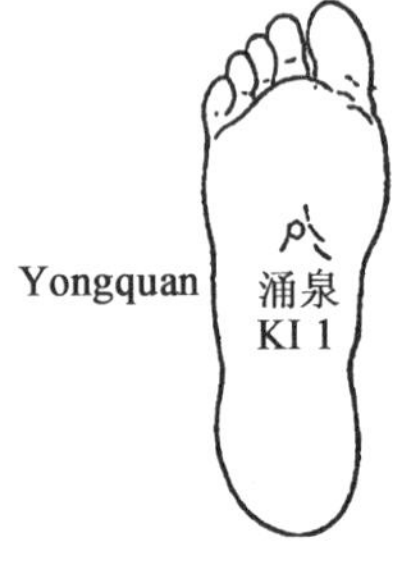

Fig.3-49 Sole acupoints on the kidney meridian of foot-shaoyin

图3-49 足少阴肾经足底部经穴图

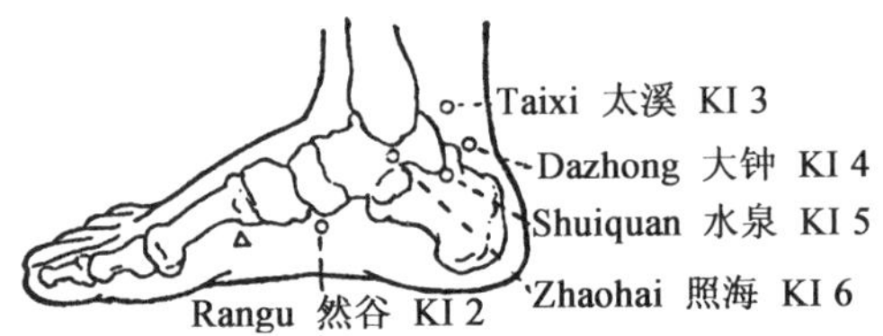

Fig.3-50 Foot acupoints on the kidney meridian of foot-shaoyin

图3-50 足少阴肾经足部经穴图

3.2 Rangu (KI 2) Ying-Spring acupoint

Indications: ① Irregular menstruation, prolapse

3.2 然谷 Rángǔ 荥穴

主治： ①月经不调，阴

of uterus, pruritus vuluae, morbid leucorrhea, seminal emission and urinary difficulty; ② diarrhea; ③ diabetes; ④ infantile omphalitis and trismus; ⑤ congested and sore throat, and coughing blood.

Needling: Puncture vertically 0.5～0.8 cun.

挺，阴痒，带下，遗精，小便不利；②泄泻；③消渴；④小儿脐风，口噤；⑤咽喉肿痛，咳血。

操作： 直刺 0.5～0.8 寸。

3.3 Taixi (KI 3) Shu-Stream acupoint; Yuan-Source acupoint

Indications: ① Headache, vertigo, insomnia and forgetfulness; ② congested and sore throat, toothache, tinnitus and deafness; ③ cough and shortness of breath; ④ lumbago; ⑤ irregular menstruation, seminal emission, impotence and frequent urination; ⑥ diabetes.

Needling: Puncture vertically 0.5～1.0 cun.

3.3 太溪 Tàixī 输穴；原穴

主治： ①头痛，眩晕，失眠，健忘；②咽喉肿痛，齿痛，耳鸣，耳聋；③咳嗽，气喘；④腰痛，⑤月经不调，遗精，阳痿，小便频数；⑥消渴。

操作： 直刺 0.5～1.0 寸。

3.4 Dazhong (KI 4) Luo-Connecting acupoint

Indications: ① Heel pain, lumbago; ② dementia, sleepiness; ③ retention of urine, enuresis and constipation.

Needling: Puncture vertically 0.3～0.5 cun.

3.4 大钟 Dàzhōng 络穴

主治： ①足跟痛，腰痛；②呆痴，嗜睡；③癃闭，遗尿，便秘。

操作： 直刺 0.3～0.5 寸。

3.5 Zhaohai (KI 6) Confluent acupoint communicating with yin heel vessel

Indications: ① Irregular menstruation, menstrual cramps, morbid leucorrhea, prolapse of uterus; ② frequent urination, retention of urine, constipation; ③ sore and dry throat; ④ insomnia and epilepsy.

Needling: Puncture vertically 0.5～0.8 cun.

3.5 照海 Zhàohǎi 八脉交会穴(通阴跷脉)

主治： ①月经不调，痛经，带下，阴挺；②小便频数，癃闭，便秘；③咽喉干痛；④失眠，癫痫。

操作： 直刺 0.5～0.8 寸。

3.6 Fuliu (KI 7) Jing-River acupoint

Indications: ① Edema, abdominal distension, diarrhea; ② night sweating, absence of sweating, or copious sweating; ③ paralysis of the lower limbs.

Needling: Puncture vertically 0.8～1.0 cun.

3.6 复溜 Fùliū 经穴

主治： ①水肿，腹胀，泄泻；②盗汗，无汗，多汗；③下肢痿痹。

操作： 直刺 0.8～1.0 寸。

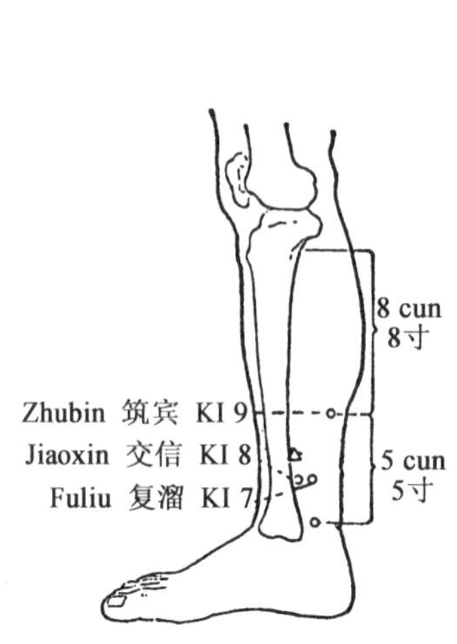

Fig.3-51　Lower limb acupoints on the kidney meridian of foot-shaoyin

图 3-51　足少阴肾经下肢部经穴图

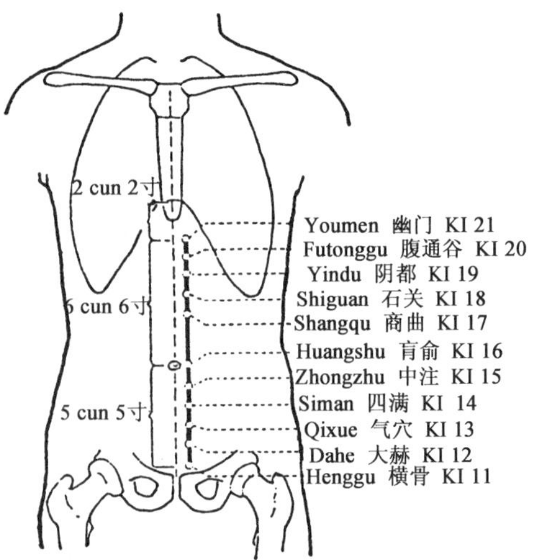

Fig.3-52　Abdomen acupoints on the kidney meridian of foot-shaoyin

图 3-52　足少阴肾经腹部经穴图

3.7 Dahe (KI 12)　Crossing acupoint of foot-shaoyin meridian and thoroughfare vessel

Indications: ① Seminal emission and impotence; ② prolapse of uterus and morbid leucorrhea.

Needling: Puncture vertically 1.0～1.5 cun.

3.7 大赫 Dàhè　足少阴经、冲脉交会穴

主治: ①遗精，阳痿；②阴挺，带下。

操作: 直刺 1.0～1.5 寸。

Section 9　Pericardium Meridian of Hand-Jueyin and its acupoints

第 9 节　手厥阴心包经及其腧穴

1　Distribution course

The pericardium meridian of hand-jueyin originates from the chest and the pericardium, its pertaining organ, and descends through the diaphragm to link the upper, middle and lower portions of the triple energizer. A branch of the meridian arises from the chest, goes out to the surface at the flank regions and

1　经脉循行

手厥阴心包经起于胸中，出属心包络，向下通过横膈，从胸至腹依次联络上、中、下三焦。胸部支脉沿着胸中，出于胁部，至腋下 3 寸处，上行抵腋窝中，沿上臂内

emerges from the costal area at a point 3 cun below the anterior axillary fold. The meridian then ascends to the armpit and follows along the medial aspect of the upper arm between the hand-taiyin meridian and hand-shaoyin meridian to the elbow crease. It runs further along the forearm between the two tendons to the palm, ending at the tip of the middle finger. A short branch splits off from the palm at Laogong (PC 8), goes along the ring finger to its tip, and then connects with the triple energizer meridian of hand shaoyang(Fig. 3-53).

侧,行于手太阴和手少阴经之间,进入肘窝,向下行于前臂两筋的中间,进入掌中,沿着中指到指端。掌中支脉从劳宫穴分出,沿无名指到指端, 接 手 少 阳 三 焦 经(图 3-53)。

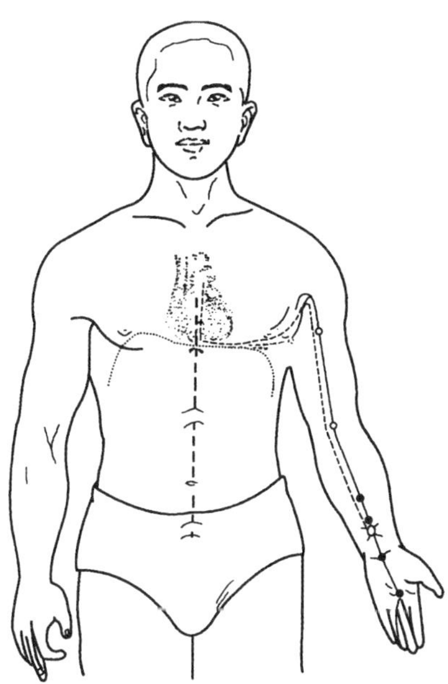

Fig.3-53 The distribution course of pericardium meridian of hand-jueyin

图 3-53 手厥阴心包经循行示意图

2 Location of acupoints

The starting acupoint of with pericardium meridian is Tianchi (PC 1), and the ending acupoint is Zhongchong (PC 9), totally 9 acupoints in each side. The location of acupoints is presented in Table 3-9 and Fig. 3-54~3-58.

2 腧穴定位

本经腧穴首穴为天池,末穴为中冲,左右各 9 穴。腧穴定位见表 3-9、图3-54~3-58。

Table 3-9　Location of acupoints of the pericardium meridian of hand-jueyin

Acupoint		Location	Specific feature
PC 1*	Tianchi	On the chest, at the fourth intercostal space, 5 cun lateral to the anterior midline	
PC 2	Tianquan	On the palmar side of the upper arm, 2 cun below the anterior axillary fold, between the two heads of the muscle bicepsbrachii	
PC 3*	Quze	On the transverse cubital crease, in the depression lateral to the tendon of the muscle biceps brachii	He-Sea acupoint
PC 4*	Ximen	5 cun above the transverse crease of the wrist, between the tendons of the muscle palmaris lungus and muscle flexor carpi radialis	Xi-Cleft acupoint
PC 5*	Jianshi	3 cun above the transverse crease of the wrist, between the tendons of the muscle palmaris lungus and muscle flexor carpi radialis	Jing-River acupoint
PC 6*	Neiguan	2 cun above the transverse crease of the wrist, between the tendons of the muscle palmaris lungus and muscle flexor carpi radialis	Luo-Connecting acupoint; Confluent acupoint communicating with yin link vessel
PC 7*	Daling	In the middle of the transverse crease of the wrist, between the tendons of the muscle palmaris lungus and muscle flexor carpi radialis	Shu-Stream acupoint; Yuan-Source acupoint
PC 8*	Laogong	On the palm, at the proximal end of the third metacarpophalangeal joint, between the second and third metacarpal bones	Ying-Spring acupoint
PC 9*	Zhongchong	In the center of the tip of the middle finger	Jing-Well acupoint

表 3-9　手厥阴心包经的腧穴定位

腧穴		定位	特定穴属性
天池*	Tiānchí	在胸部，第4肋间隙，前正中线旁开5寸	
天泉	Tiānquán	在臂前区，腋前纹头下2寸，肱二头肌的长短头之间	
曲泽*	Qūzé	在肘前区，肘横纹上，肱二头肌腱的尺侧缘凹陷中	合穴
郄门*	Xìmén	在前臂前区，腕掌侧远端横纹上5寸，掌长肌腱与桡侧腕屈肌腱之间	郄穴
间使*	Jiānshǐ	在前臂前区，腕掌侧远端横纹上3寸，掌长肌腱与桡侧腕屈肌腱之间	经穴
内关*	Nèiguān	在前臂前区，腕掌侧远端横纹上2寸，掌长肌腱与桡侧腕屈肌腱之间	络穴；八脉交会穴(通阴维脉)
大陵*	Dàlíng	在腕前区，腕掌侧远端横纹中，掌长肌腱与桡侧腕屈肌腱之间	输穴；原穴
劳宫*	Láogōng	在掌区，横平第3掌指关节近端，第2、3掌骨之间偏于第3掌骨	荥穴
中冲*	Zhōngchōng	在手指，中指末端最高点	井穴

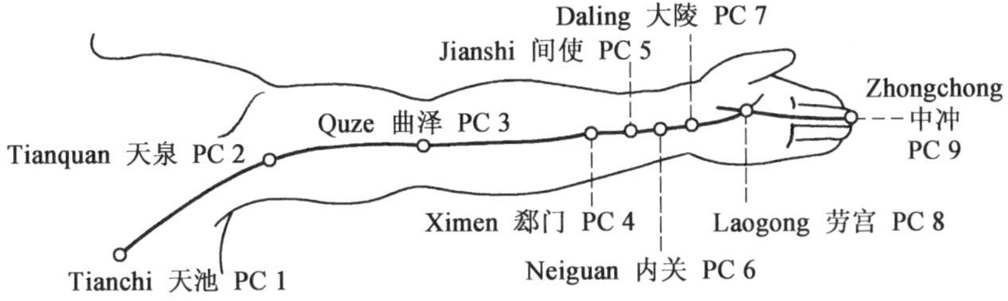

Fig.3-54 Acupoints of pericardium meridian of hand-jueyin

图 3-54 手厥阴心包经腧穴总图

3 Indications of acupoints

The acupoints of the pericardium meridian are indicated for the diseases of the heart, chest and stomach, and mental disorders, and other diseases of the areas this meridian supplies. For disorders in the heart, chest and stomach, Quze (PC 3), Ximen(PC 4), Jianshi (PC 5), Neiguan (PC 6) and Daling(PC 7) are usually used; for mental disorders, Jianshi(PC 5), Laogong (PC 8) and Zhongchong (PC 9) are often used. The indications and needling methods of common acupoints are presented as follows.

3 腧穴主治

本经腧穴主要用于治疗心、胸、胃病，神志病以及经脉循行部位的病证。治疗心、胸、胃病常用曲泽、郄门、间使、内关和大陵；治疗神志病常用间使、劳宫、中冲；临床常用腧穴的主治及针刺操作如下。

3.1 Tianchi (PC 1)

Indications: ① Breast abscess, insufficient lactation; ② cough and shortness of breath; ③ cardiac pain.

Needling: Puncture obliquely or transversely 0.5～0.8 cun; deep needling is contraindicated so as not to injure the lungs.

3.1 天池 Tiānchí

主治：①乳痈，乳少；②咳嗽，气喘；③心胸疼痛。

操作：斜刺或平刺0.5～0.8 寸，不可深刺，以免伤及肺脏。

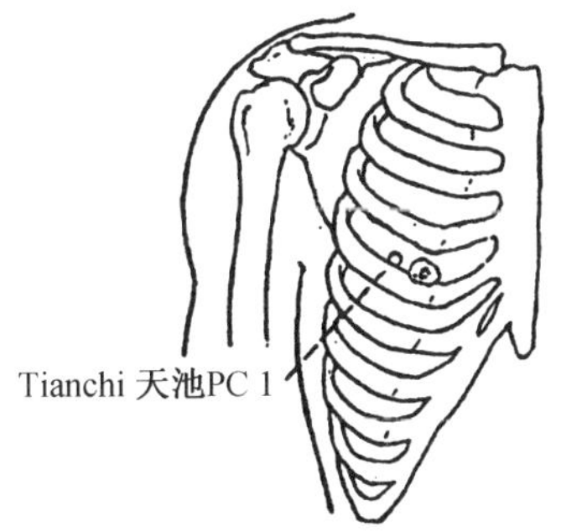

Fig.3-55 Chest acupoints on the pericardium meridian of hand-jueyin

图 3-55 手厥阴心包经胸部经穴图

3.2 Quze (PC 3) He-Sea acupoint

Indications: ① Cardiac pain, palpitation; ② stomachache, vomiting, diarrhea; ③ summer-heat disorder.

Needling: Puncture 0.8～1.0 cun; or prick to bleed with a three-edged needle.

3.3 Ximen (PC 4) Xi-Cleft acupoint

Indications: ① Cardiac pain, palpitation; ② vomiting blood, coughing blood; ③ epilepsy.

Needling: Puncture vertically 0.5～1.0 cun.

3.4 Jianshi (PC 5) Jing-River acupoint

Indications: ① Cardiac pain, palpitation, and depressive-manic psychosis; ② stomachache, vomiting; ③ fever disorders and malaria.

Needling: Puncture vertically 0.5～1.0 cun; the median nerve should not be punctured.

3.5 Neiguan (PC 6) Luo-Connecting acupoint; Confluent acupoint communicating with the yin link vessel

Indications: ① Cardiac pain, palpitation, chest stuffiness; ② vomiting, hiccup and stomachache; ③ dizziness, insomnia, epilepsy and depression; ④ convulsive pain in the elbow and arms.

Needling: Puncture vertically 0.5～1.0 cun; the median nerve should not be punctured.

3.6 Daling (PC 7) Shu-Stream acupoint; Yuan-Source acupoint

Indications: ① Cardiac pain and palpitation; ② depressive-manic psychosis; ③ pain in the wrist and arms; ④ stomachache and vomiting.

Needling: Puncture vertically 0.3～0.5 cun.

3.7 Laogong (PC 8) Ying-Spring acupoint

Indications: ① Cardiac pain and palpitation; ② apoplectic coma, heatstroke; ③ vomiting, canker

3.2 曲泽 Qūzé　合穴

主治: ①心痛,心悸;②胃痛,呕吐,泄泻;③暑热病。

操作: 直刺0.8～1.0寸;或用三棱针点刺出血。

3.3 郄门 Xìmén　郄穴

主治: ①心痛,心悸;②呕血,咳血;③癫痫。

操作: 直刺0.5～1.0寸。

3.4 间使 Jiānshǐ　经穴

主治: ①心痛,心悸,癫狂痫;②胃痛,呕吐;③热病,疟疾。

操作: 直刺0.5～1.0寸,注意避开正中神经。

3.5 内关 Nèiguān　络穴;八脉交会穴(通阴维脉)

主治: ①心痛,心悸,胸闷;②呕吐,呃逆,胃痛;③眩晕,失眠,癫痫,郁证;④肘臂挛痛。

操作: 直刺0.5～1.0寸,注意避开正中神经。

3.6 大陵 Dàlíng　输穴;原穴

主治: ①心痛,心悸;②癫狂;③腕臂痛;④胃痛,呕吐。

操作: 直刺0.3～0.5寸。

3.7 劳宫 Láogōng　荥穴

主治: ①心痛,心悸;②中风昏迷,中暑;③呕吐,口

sore and bad breath in the mouth.

Needling: Puncture vertically 0.3～0.5 cun.

3.8 Zhongchong (PC 9) Jing-Well acupoint

Indications: ① Apoplectic coma, heat-stroke, coma, and feverish conditions; ② cardiac pain; ③ infantile convulsion.

Needling: Puncture shallowly 0.1 cun; or prick to bleed with a three-edged needle.

疮，口臭。

操作： 直刺 0.3～0.5 寸。

3.8 中冲 Zhōngchōng 井穴

主治： ① 中风昏迷，中暑，昏厥，热病；②心痛；③小儿惊风。

操作： 浅刺 0.1 寸，或用三棱针点刺出血。

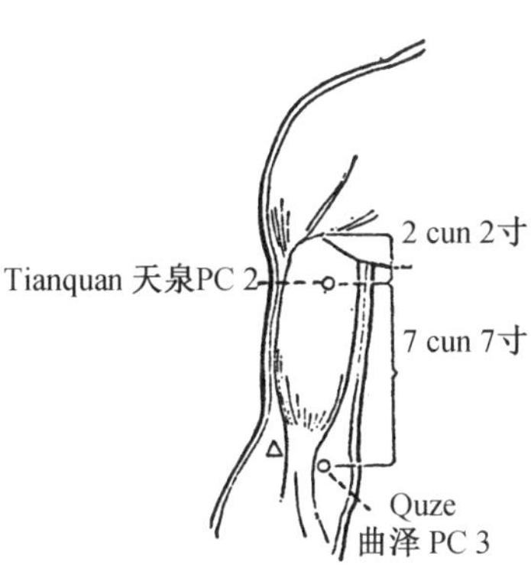

Fig.3-56 Upper arm acupoints on the pericardium meridian of hand-jueyin

图 3-56 手厥阴心包经上臂部经穴图

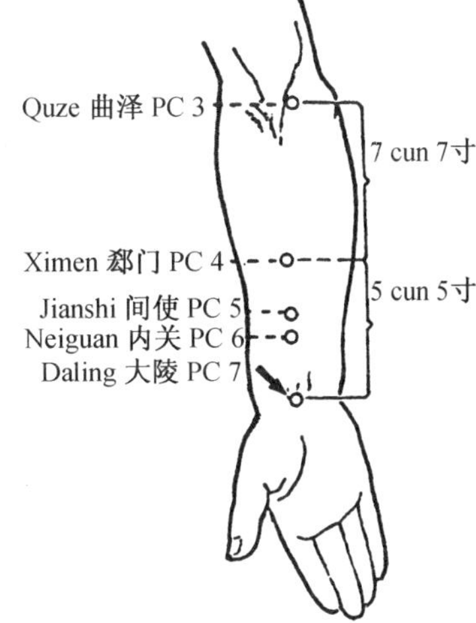

Fig.3-57 Forearm acupoints on the pericardium meridian of hand-jueyin

图 3-57 手厥阴心包经前臂部经穴图

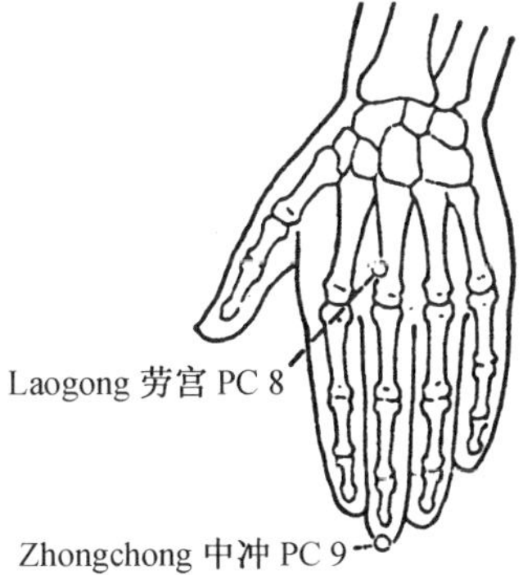

Fig.3-58 Hand acupoints on the pericardium meridian of hand-jueyin

图 3-58 手厥阴心包经手部经穴图

Section 10 Triple Energizer Meridian of Hand-Shaoyang and its acupoints

1 Distribution course

The triple energizer meridian of hand-shaoyang starts from the outside tip of the ring finger, proceeds over between the fourth and fifth metacarpal bones, along the back of the hand and wrist to the lateral aspect of the forearm between the radius and ulna; passing through the olecranon and along the lateral aspect of the upper arm, it reaches the posterior shoulder region, where it runs across and passes behind the gallbladder meridian of foot shaoyang; winding over to the supraclavicular fossa, it spreads in the chest to connect with the pericardium; then it descends through the diaphragm down to the abdomen, and connects with the upper, middle and lower energizers. A branch starts from the chest; running upwards it emerges from the supraclavicular fossa; from there it ascends to the neck, running along the posterior border of the ear, and further to the corner of the anterior hairline; then it turns downwards to the cheek and terminates in the infraorbital region. The auricular branch originates behind the ear, enters the ear, and then emerges in front of the ear to reach the outer canthus to connect with the gallbladder meridian of foot shaoyang(Fig. 3-59).

2 Location of acupoints

The starting acupoint of the triple energizer meridian is Guanchong(TE 1), and the ending acu-

第10节 手少阳三焦经及其腧穴

1 经脉循行

手少阳三焦经起于无名指末端，向上行于小指与无名指之间，沿着手背，出于前臂外侧桡骨和尺骨之间，向上通过肘尖，沿上臂外侧，上达肩部，交出足少阳胆经的后面，向上进入缺盆部，分布于胸中，散络于心包，向下通过横膈，从胸至腹，属上、中、下三焦。胸中支脉，从胸向上，出于缺盆部，上走颈旁，连系耳后，沿耳后直上，出于耳部上行额角，再屈而下行至面颊部，到达眼下部。耳部支脉，从耳后进入耳中，出耳前，与前脉交叉于面颊部，到达目外眦，接足少阳胆经(图3-59)。

2 腧穴定位

本经腧穴首穴为关冲，末穴为丝竹空，左右各23

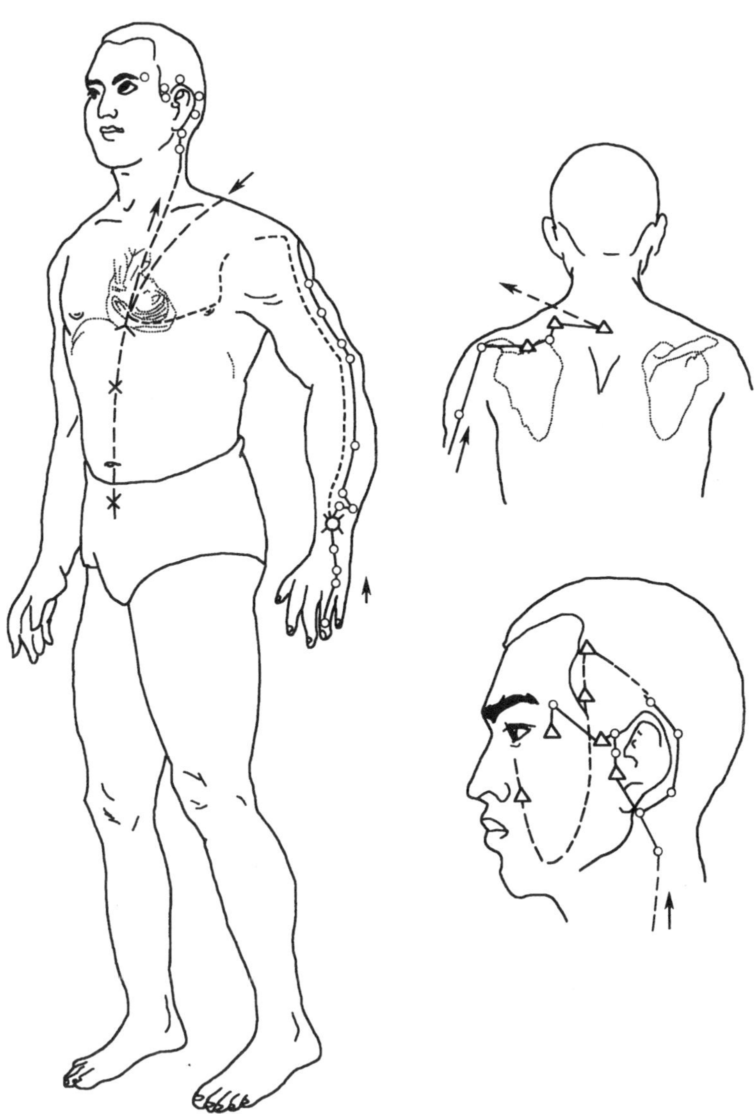

Fig.3-59 The distribution course of triple energizer meridian of hand-shaoyang

图 3-59 手少阳三焦经循行示意图

point is Sizhukong(TE 23), totally 23 acupoints in each side. The location of the acupoints is presented in Table 3-10 and Fig. 3-60～3-64.

穴。腧穴定位见表 3-10、图 3-60～3-64。

Table 3-10　Location of acupoints of the triple energizer meridian of hand-shaoyang

Acupoint		Location	Specific feature
TE 1*	Guanchong	On the ulnar side of the ring finger, about 0.1 cun posterior to the corner of the nail	Jing-Well acupoint
TE 2	Yemen	Between the ring and small fingers, in the depression proximal to the margin of the web, at the junction of the red and white skin	Ying-Spring acupoint
TE 3*	Zhongzhu	On the back of the hand between the fourth and fifth metacarpal bones, in the depression proximal to the metacarpophalangral joint	Shu-Stream acupoint
TE 4*	Yangchi	On the transverse crease of the dorsum of wrist, in the depression on the ulnar side of the tendon of the muscle extensor digitorum communis	Yuan-Source acupoint
TE 5*	Waiguan	2 cun above the transverse crease of the dorsum of wrist, between the radius and ulna	Luo-Connecting acupoint; Confluent acupoint communicating with yang link vessel
TE 6*	Zhigou	3 cun above the transverse crease of the dorsum of wrist, between the radius and ulna	Jing-River acupoint
TE 7	Huizong	3 cun above the transverse crease of the dorsum of wrist, on the radial side of the ulna	Xi-Cleft acupoint
TE 8	Sanyangluo	4 cun above the transverse crease of the dorsum of wrist, between the radius and ulna	
TE 9	Sidu	5 cun below the olecranon of the ulna, between the radius and ulna	
TE 10	Tianjing	In the depression 1 cun above the olecranon of the ulna	He-Sea acupoint
TE 11	Qinglengyuan	On the line connecting the olecranon of the ulna and acromial angle, 2 cun above the olecranon	
TE 12	Xiaoluo	On the line connecting the olecranon of the ulna and acromial angle, 5 cun above the olecranon	
TE 13	Naohui	3 cun below the olecranon, on the posterior-inferior border of the muscle deltoideus	
TE 14*	Jianliao	Posterior to Jianyu(LI 15), in the depression posterior to the acromion when the arm is abducted	
TE 15	Tianliao	In the depression on the superior angle of the scapula	
TE 16	Tianyou	At the level with mandibular angle, in the depression of the posterior border of the muscle sternocleidomastoideus	
TE 17*	Yifeng	Behind the ear lobe, in the depression anterior to lower end of the mastoid process	

(continued)

Acupoint		Location	Specific feature
TE 18	Chimai	In the center of the mastoid process, at the junction of the lower one-third and upper two-thirds of the curved line connecting Jiaosun(TE 20) and Yifeng(TE 17)	
TE 19	Luxi	At the junction of the upper one-third and lower two-thirds of the curved line connecting Jiaosun(TE 20) and Yifeng(TE 17)	
TE 20*	Jiaosun	On the hairline directly above the ear apex	
TE 21*	Ermen	In the depression between the supratragic notch and the condylar process of the mandible	
TE 22	Erheliao	On the posterior border of the hairline where the superficial temporal artery passes, at the level with the root of the auricle	
TE 23*	Sizhukong	In the depression at the lateral depression of the eyebrow	

表 3-10 手少阳三焦经的腧穴定位

腧穴		定位	特定穴属性
关冲*	Guānchōng	在手指,第 4 指末节尺侧,指甲根角侧上方 0.1 寸(指寸)	井穴
液门	Yèmén	在手背,第 4、5 指间,指蹼缘上方赤白肉际凹陷中	荥穴
中渚*	Zhōngzhǔ	在手背,第 4、5 掌骨间,第 4 掌指关节近端凹陷中	输穴
阳池*	Yángchí	在腕后区,腕背侧远端横纹上,指伸肌腱的尺侧缘凹陷中	原穴
外关*	Wàiguān	在前臂后区,腕背侧远端横纹上 2 寸,尺骨与桡骨间隙中点	络穴;八脉交会穴(通阳维脉)
支沟*	Zhīgōu	在前臂后区,腕背侧远端横纹上 3 寸,尺骨与桡骨间隙中点	经穴
会宗	Huìzōng	在前臂后区,腕背侧远端横纹上 3 寸,尺骨的桡侧缘	郄穴
三阳络	Sānyángluò	在前臂后区,腕背侧远端横纹上 4 寸,尺骨与桡骨间隙中点	
四渎	Sìdú	在前臂后区,肘尖下 5 寸,尺骨与桡骨间隙中点	
天井	Tiānjǐng	在肘后区,肘尖上 1 寸凹陷中	合穴
清冷渊	Qīnglěngyuān	在臂后区,肘尖与肩峰角连线上,肘尖上 2 寸	
消泺	Xiāoluò	在臂后区,肘尖与肩峰角连线上,肘尖上 5 寸	
臑会	Nàohuì	在臂后区,肩峰角下 3 寸,三角肌的后下缘	
肩髎*	Jiānliáo	在肩部,肩髃后方,当臂外展时,于肩峰后下方呈现凹陷处	
天髎	Tiānliáo	在肩胛区,肩胛骨上角骨际凹陷中	
天牖	Tiānyǒu	在颈部,横平下颌角,胸锁乳突肌的后缘凹陷中	
翳风*	Yìfēng	在颈部,耳垂后方,乳突下端前方凹陷中	
瘈脉	Chìmài	在头部,乳突中央,角孙与翳风沿耳轮弧形连线的上 2/3 与下 1/3 的交点处	
颅息	Lúxī	在头部,角孙与翳风沿耳轮弧形连线的上 1/3 与下 2/3 的交点处	

(续表)

腧穴		定位	特定穴属性
角孙*	Jiǎosūn	在头部,耳尖正对发际处	
耳门*	Ermén	在耳区,耳屏上切迹与下颌骨髁突之间的凹陷中	
耳和髎	Erhéliáo	在头部,鬓发后缘,耳郭根的前方,颞浅动脉的后缘	
丝竹空*	Sīzhúkōng	在面部,眉梢凹陷中	

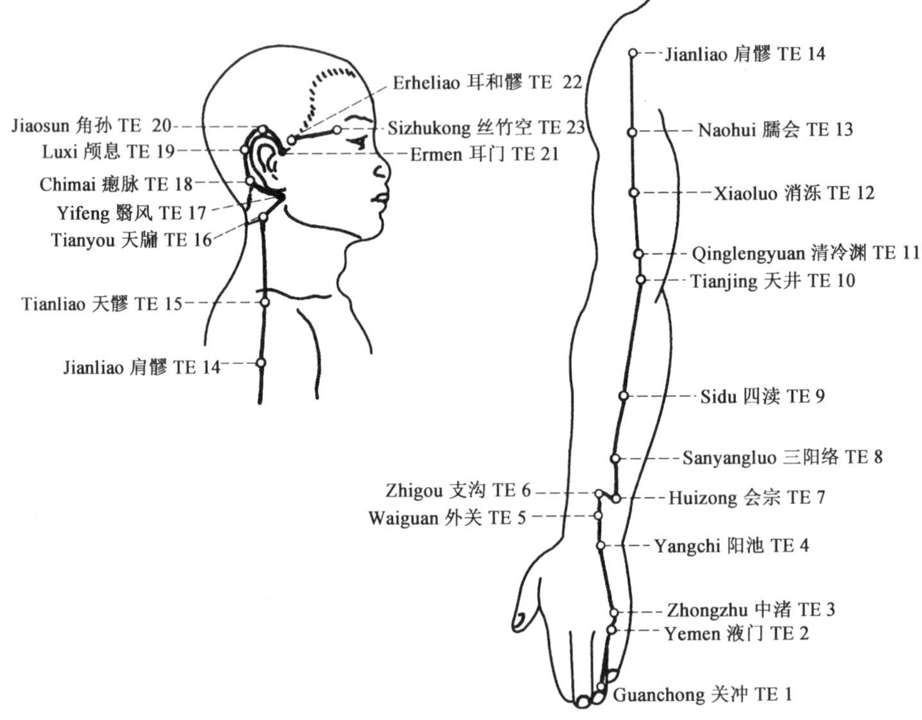

Fig.3-60　Acupoints of triple energizer meridian of hand-shaoyang

图 3-60　手少阳三焦经腧穴总图

3　Indications of acupoints

The acupoints of the triple energizer meridian are indicated for the diseases of the lateral aspect of the head, of the throat, ear and flanks; febrile diseases and other diseases of the areas this meridian supplies. For migraine headache, Sizhukong (TE 23), Jiaosun(TE 20), Waiguan(TE 5) and Tianjing (TE 10) are often used; for eye disorders,

3　腧穴主治

本经腧穴主要用于治疗侧头部、咽喉、耳部病,胸胁病,热病以及经脉所过部位的病证。治疗偏头痛常用丝竹空、角孙、外关、天井;治疗目疾常用丝竹空、液门、关冲;治疗咽喉病常用关冲、液

Sizhukong(TE 23), Yemen(TE 2) and Guanchong (TE 1) are often used; for throat diseases, Guanchong(TE 1), Yemen(TE 2) and Yangchi(TE 4) are often used; for ear diseases, Ermen(TE 21), Yifeng(TE 17), Zhongzhu(TE 3), Waiguan(TE 5) and Yemen(TE 2) are often used; for fever diseases, Guanchong(TE 1), Zhongzhu(TE 3), Waiguan (TE 5) and Zhigou(TE 6) are often used. The indications and needling methods of common acupoints are presented as follows.

门、阳池；治疗耳疾常用耳门、翳风、中渚、外关、液门；治疗热病常用关冲、中渚、外关、支沟。临床常用腧穴的主治及针刺操作如下。

3.1 Guanchong (TE 1) Jing-Well acupoint

Indications: ① Fever disease, coma; ② headache, reddened eyes, deafness, sore throat.

Needling: Puncture shallowly 0.1 cun; or prick to bleed with a three-edged needle.

3.1 关冲 Guānchōng 井穴

主治： ①热病，昏厥；②头痛，目赤，耳聋，咽喉肿痛。

操作： 浅刺 0.1 寸；或用三棱针点刺出血。

3.2 Zhongzhu (TE 3) Shu-Stream acupoint

Indications: ① Tinnitus, deafness, headache, reddened eyes, throat obstruction; ② pain and numbness in the arms; ③ febrile diseases.

Needling: Puncture vertically 0.3~0.5 cun.

3.2 中渚 Zhōngzhǔ 输穴

主治： ①耳鸣，耳聋，头痛，目赤，喉痹；②手臂痛麻；③热病。

操作： 直刺 0.3~0.5 寸。

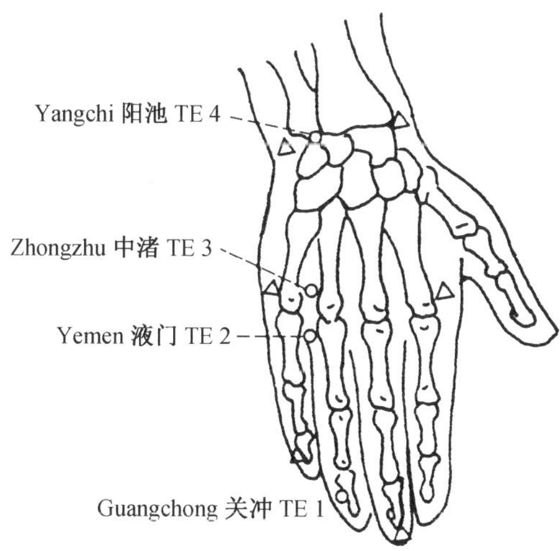

Fig.3-61 Hand acupoints on the triple energizer meridian of hand-shaoyang

图 3-61 手少阳三焦经手部经穴图

3.3 Yangchi (TE 4) Yuan-Source acupoint

Indications: ① Pain in the wrist and arms; ② headache, reddened and swollen eyes, deafness, and throat obstruction; ③ malaria; ④ diabetes.

Needling: Puncture vertically 0.3～0.5 cun.

3.4 Waiguan (TE 5) Luo-Connecting acupoint; Confluent acupoint communicating with yang link vessel

Indications: ① Headache, cheek pain, reddened and swollen eyes, tinnitus and deafness; ② flank pain; ③ febrile diseases.

Needling: Puncture vertically 0.5～1.0 cun.

3.5 Zhigou (TE 6) Jing-River acupoint

Indications: ① Constipation; ② flank pain; ③ tinnitus and deafness; ④ febrile diseases.

Needling: Puncture vertically 0.5～1.0 cun.

3.3 阳池 Yángchí　原穴

主治：①腕臂痛；②头痛，目赤肿痛，耳聋，喉痹；③疟疾；④消渴。

操作：直刺0.3～0.5寸。

3.4 外关 Wàiguān　络穴；八脉交会穴（通阳维脉）

主治：①头痛，颊痛，目赤肿痛，耳鸣，耳聋；②胁肋痛；③热病。

操作：直刺0.5～1.0寸。

3.5 支沟 Zhīgōu　经穴

主治：①便秘；②胁痛；③耳鸣，耳聋；④热病。

操作：直刺0.5～1.0寸。

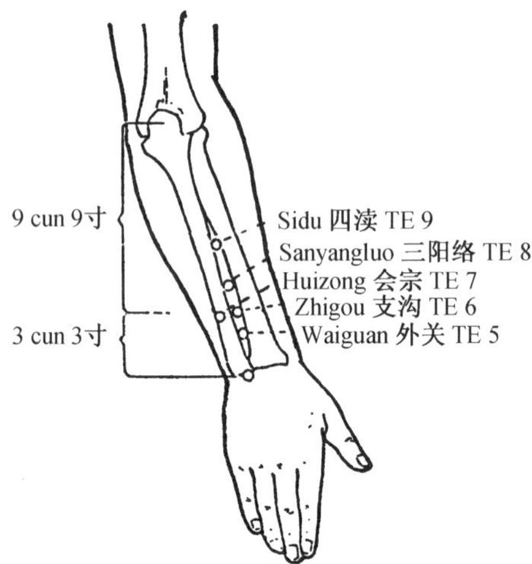

Fig.3-62　Forearm acupoints on the triple energizer meridian of hand-shaoyang

图3-62　手少阳三焦经前臂部经穴图

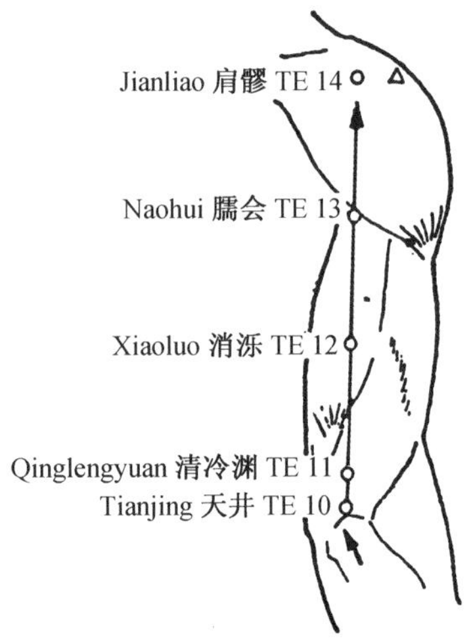

Fig.3-63　Upper arm acupoints on the triple energizer meridian of hand-shaoyang

图3-63　手少阳三焦经上臂部经穴图

3.6 Jianliao (TE 14)

Indications: ① Pain in the shoulder and arms and inability to raise objects; ② flank pain.

Needling: Puncture vertically 1.0～1.5 cun towards the shoulder joint.

3.7 Yifeng (TE 17)

Indications: ① Tinnitus and deafness; ② deviated mouth and eyes, lockjaw, and toothache.

Needling: Puncture vertically 0.5～1.0 cun.

3.8 Jiaosun (TE 20)

Indications: ① Migraine headache, stiff neck; ② swollen cheek, nebula and toothache.

Needling: Puncture transversely 0.3～0.5 cun.

3.9 Ermen (TE 21)

Indications: ① Tinnitus and deafness; ② toothache.

Needling: With mouth open, puncture vertiucally 0.5～1.0 cun.

3.10 Sizhukong (TE 23)

Indications: ① Reddened and swollen eyes, twitching of eyelids; ② migraine headache; ③ depressive-manic psychosis and epilepsy.

Needling: Puncture transversely 0.3～0.5 cun.

3.6 肩髎 Jiānliáo

主治：①肩臂痛，肩重不能举；②胁肋疼痛。

操作：向肩关节直刺1.0～1.5寸。

3.7 翳风 Yìfēng

主治：①耳鸣，耳聋；②口眼㖞斜，牙关紧闭，齿痛。

操作：直刺0.5～1.0寸。

3.8 角孙 Jiǎosūn

主治：①偏头痛，项强；②颊肿，目翳，齿痛。

操作：平刺0.3～0.5寸。

3.9 耳门 Ermén

主治：①耳鸣，耳聋；②齿痛。

操作：张口，直刺0.5～1寸。

3.10 丝竹空 Sīzhúkōng

主治：①目赤肿痛，眼睑瞤动；②偏头痛；③癫狂痫。

操作：平刺0.3～0.5寸。

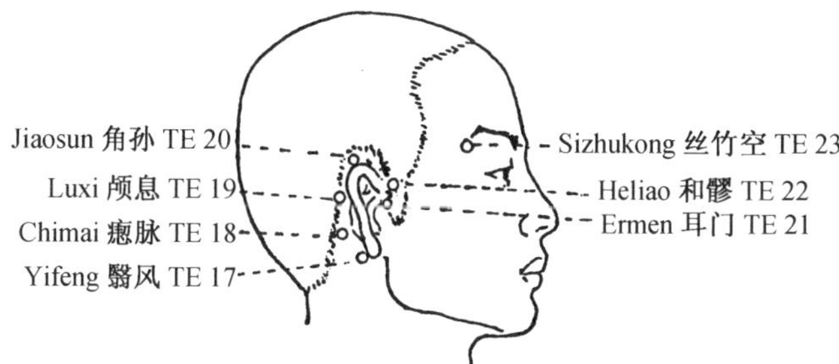

Fig.3-64 Head and face acupoints on the triple energizer meridian of hand-shaoyang

图3-64 手少阳三焦经头面部经穴图

Section 11 Gallbladder Meridian of Foot-Shaoyang and its Acupoints

1 Distribution course

The gallbladder meridian of foot-shaoyang begins at the outer canthus, ascends to the corner of the forehead, then curves downwards to the retroauricular region and goes along the side of the neck to the shoulder and then down to the supraclavicular fossa. A branch arises from the retroauricular region and enters the ear, then it comes out and passes the preauricular region to the posterior aspect of the outer canthus. A branch arising from the outer canthus runs downwards to Daying(ST 5) and meets triple energizer in the infraorbital region; then passing through Jiache(ST 6), it descends to the neck and enters the supraclavicular fossa; from there it further descends into the chest, passes through the diaphragm to link with the liver and enter the gallbladder, the organ it pertains to; then it runs along the flank regions and descends to the inguinal region near the femoral artery; from there it goes along the margin of the pubic hair and goes transversely into the hip region. The straight portion of the meridian goes downwards from the supraclavicular fossa, passes in front of the axilla along the lateral aspect of the chest and through the free ends of the floating ribs to the hip region where it meets the previous branch; then it descends along the lateral aspect of the thigh and the knee; going further

第 11 节 足少阳胆经及其腧穴

1 经脉循行

足少阳胆经起于目外眦，上行额角部，下行至耳后，沿颈项部至肩上，下入缺盆。耳部支脉，从耳后入耳中，经耳前，到目外眦后方；目外眦支脉，从目外眦下走大迎，再向上到达目眶下，下行经颊车，至颈部会合前脉于缺盆，内行进入胸中，通过横膈，联络肝，属于胆，沿胁肋内，下达腹股沟动脉部，经过外阴部毛际，横入髋关节部。直行主脉从缺盆下经腋部、侧胸、胁肋部，下合前脉于髋关节部，再向下沿着大腿外侧、膝外缘、腓骨之前，达外踝之前，循足背部，止于足第四趾外侧端。足背部支脉，从足背上分出，沿第一、二跖骨之间，止于大趾端，接足厥阴肝经（图 3-65）。

downwards along the anterior aspect of the fibula to its lower end, it reaches the anterior aspect of the external malleolus; it then follows the back of the foot to the lateral side of the tip of the fourth toe. A branch leaves the meridian from the back of foot, goes between the first and second metatarsal bones to the great toe, where it connects with the liver meridian of foot jueyin(Fig. 3-65).

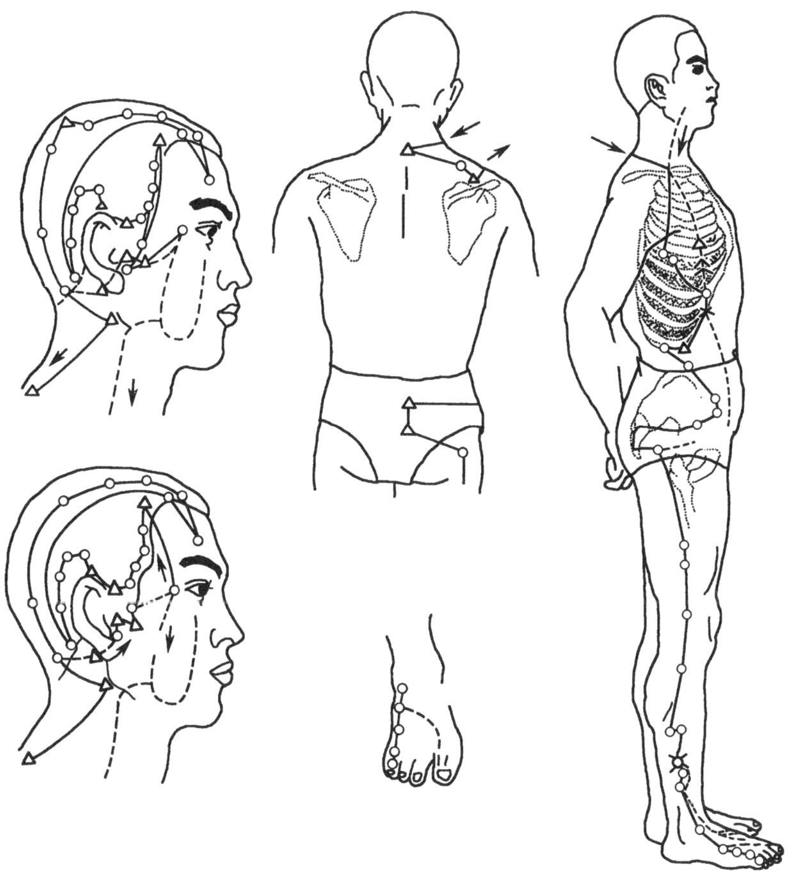

Fig.3-65 The distribution course of gallbladder meridian of foot-jueyin

图 3-65 足少阳胆经循行示意图

2 Location of acupoints

The starting acupoint of the gallbladder meridian is Tongziliao (GB 1), and the ending acupoint is Zuqiaoyin (GB 44), totally 44 acupoints in each side. The location of acupoints is presented in Table 3-11 and Figure 3-66～3-75.

2 腧穴定位

本经腧穴首穴为瞳子髎，末穴为足窍阴，左右各44穴。腧穴定位见表3-11、图3-66～3-75。

Table 3-11 Location of acupoints of the gaubladder meridian of foot-shaoyang

Acupoint		Location	Specific feature
GB 1*	Tongziliao	In the depression 0.5 cun lateral to the outer canthus	Crossing acupoint of hand-taiyang meridian, hand and foot-shaoyang meridians
GB 2*	Tinghui	In the depression between the intertragic notch and the condylar process of the mandible	
GB 3	Shangguan	In the depression at the midpoint of the upper border of the zygomatic arch	Crossing acupoint of hand and foot-shaoyang meridians, foot-yangming meridian
GB 4	Hanyan	At the junction of the upper one-fourth and the lower three-fourths of the curved line linking Touwei(ST 8) and Qubin(ST 7)	Crossing acupoint of hand and foot- shaoyang meridians, foot-yangming meridian
GB 5	Xuanlu	At the midpoint of the curved line linking Touwei (ST 8) and Qubin(ST 7)	
GB 6	Xuanli	At the junction of the upper three-fourths and the lower one-fourth of the curved line linking Touwei (ST 8) and Qubin(ST 7)	Crossing acupoint of hand and foot- shaoyang meridians, foot-yangming meridian
GB 7*	Qubin	The crossing point between the posterior border of the pre-auricular hairline and the line at the level with the apex of the ear	
GB 8*	Shuaigu	Directly above the ear apex, 1.5 cun within the hairline	Crossing acupoint of foot-shaoyang meridian and foot-taiyang meridian
GB 9	Tianchong	Above the posterior border of the root of the auricle, 2 cun within the hairline	Crossing acupoint of foot-shaoyang and foot-taiyang meridians
GB 10	Fubai	Posterior and superior to the mastoid process, at the junction of the upper one-third and lower two-thirds of the curved line linking Tianchong (GB 9) and Wangu (GB 12)	Crossing acupoint of foot-shaoyang meridian and foot-tai-yang meridian
GB 11	Touqiaoyin	Posterior and superior to the mastoid process, at the junction of the upper two-thirds and lower one-third of the curved line linking Tianchong (GB 9) and Wangu (GB 12)	Crossing acupoint of foot- shaoyang meridian and foot-tai-yang meridian

(continued)

Acupoint		Location	Specific feature
GB 12*	Wangu	In the depression posterior and inferior to the mastoid process	Crossing acupoint of foot-shao yang meridian and foot-tai-yang meridian
GB 13*	Benshen	0.5 cun above the anterior hairline, 3 cun lateral to the anterior head midline	Crossing acupoint of foot-shaoyang meridian and yang link vessel
GB 14*	Yangbai	1 cun above the eyebrow, directly above the pupils	Crossing acupoint of foot-shaoyang meridian and yang link vessel
GB 15*	Toulinqi	0.5 cun above the anterior hairline, directly above the pupils	Crossing acupoint of foot-shaoyang meridian, foot-taiyang meridian and yang link vessel
GB 16	Muchuang	1.5 cun above the anterior hairline, directly above the pupils	Crossing acupoint of foot-shaoyang meridian and yang link vessel
GB 17	Zhengying	2.5 cun above the anterior hairline, directly above the pupils	Crossing acupoint of foot-shaoyang meridian and yang link vessel
GB 18	Chengling	4 cun above the anterior hairline, directly above the pupils	Crossing acupoint of foot-shaoyang meridian and yang link vessel
GB 19	Naokong	At the level with the upper border of the external occipital protuberance, directly above Fengchi (GB 20)	Crossing acupoint of foot-shaoyang meridian and yang link vessel
GB 20*	Fengchi	Below the occipital bone, in the depression between the upper ends of the muscle sternocleidomastoideus and muscle trapezius	Crossing acupoint of foot-shaoyang meridian and yang link vessel
GB 21*	Jianjing	At the midpoint of the line linking the spinous process of the seventh cervical vertebra and the acromion	Crossing acupoint of hand and foot-shaoyang meridians, foot yangming meridian and yang link vessel
GB 22	Yuanye	On the mid axillary line, at the fourth intercostal space	
GB 23	Zhejin	At the fourth intercostal space, 1 cun anterior to the mid-axillary line	
GB 24*	Riyue	At the seventh intercostal space, 4 cun lateral to the anterior midline	Front-Mu acupoint of the gallbladder; Crossing acupoint of the foot-shaoyang meridian and foot-taiyin meridian

(continued)

Acupoint		Location	Specific feature
GB 25*	Jingmen	On the free end of the twelfth rib	Front-Mu acupoint the kidney
GB 26*	Daimai	Directly below the free end of the eleventh rid, level with the navel	Crossing acupoint of foot-shaoyang meridian and belt vessel
GB 27	Wushu	3 cun below the level of the navel, anterior to the superior iliac spine	Crossing acupoint of foot-shaoyang meridian and belt vessel
GB 28	Weidao	0.5 cun anterior and inferior to the superior iliac spine	Crossing acupoint of foot-shaoyang meridian and belt vessel
GB 29	Juliao	At the midpoint of the line linking the anterio-superior iliac spine and the highest point of the great trochanter	Crossing acupoint of foot-shaoyang meridian and belt vessel
GB 30*	Huantiao	At the junction of the lateral one-third and the medial two-thirds of the line linking the highest point of the great trochanter and the hiatus of the sacrum	Crossing acupoint of foot-shaoyang meridian and foot-tai-yang meridian
GB 31*	Fengshi	7 cun above the transverse popliteal crease, between the musculus vastus lateralis and biceps femoris; when the patient is standing erect with hands hanging down, the acupoint is at the tip of the middle finger touching	
GB 32	Zhongdu	On the lateral aspect of the thigh, 5 cun above the transverse popliteal crease, on the posterior border of iliotibial band	
GB 33	Xiyangguan	On the posterior-superior border of external epicondyle of femur, in the depression between the bicep femoris and iliotibial band	
GB 34*	Yanglingquan	In the depression anterior and inferior to the small head of the fibula	He-Sea acupoint; Lower He-Sea acupoint of the gallbladder; Influential acupoint of the tendons
GB 35	Yangjiao	On the lateral aspect of the leg, 7 cun above the tip of the external malleolus, at the posterior border of the fibula	Xi-Cleft acupoint of yang link vessel
GB 36	Waiqiu	On the lateral aspect of the leg, 7 cun above the tip of the external malleolus, at the anterior border of the fibula	Xi-Cleft acupoint
GB 37*	Guangming	On the lateral aspect of the leg, 5 cun above the tip of the external malleolus, at the anterior border of the fibula	Luo-Connecting acupoint
GB 38	Yangfu	On the lateral aspect of the leg, 4 cun above the tip of the external malleolus, at the anterior border of the fibula	Jing-Spring acupoint

(continued)

Acupoint		Location	Specific feature
GB 39	Xuanzhong	On the lateral aspect of the leg, 3 cun above the tip of the external malleolus, at the anterior border of the fibula	Confluent acupoint of marrow
GB 40	Qiuxu	Anterior and inferior to the external malleolus, in the depression lateral to the tendon of the muscle extensor digitorum longus	Yuan-Source acupoint
GB 41	Zulinqi	In the depression distal to the junction of the fourth and fifth metatarsal bones, on the lateral side of the tendon of the muscle extensor digiti minimi of the foot	Shu-Stream acupoint; Confluent acupoint communicating with the belt vessel
GB 42	Diwuhui	Between the fourth and fifth metatarsal bones, in the depression proximal to the fourth metatarsophalangeal joint	
GB 43	Xiaxi	Between the fourth and fifth metatarsal bones, proximal to the margin of the web and at the junction of the red and white skin	Ying-Spring acupoint
GB 44	Zuqiaoyin	On the lateral side of the fourth toe, about 0.1 cun posterior to the corner of the nail	Jing-Well acupoint

表 3-11 足少阳胆经的腧穴定位

腧穴		定位	特定穴属性
瞳子髎*	Tóngzǐliáo	在面部，目外眦外侧 0.5 寸凹陷中	手太阳、手足少阳经交会穴
听会*	Tīnghuì	在面部，耳屏间切迹与下颌骨髁突之间的凹陷中	
上关	Shàngguān	在面部，颧弓上缘中央凹陷中	手足少阳、足阳明经交会穴
颔厌	Hànyàn	在头部，从头维至曲鬓的弧形连线(其弧度与鬓发弧度相应)的上 1/4 与下 3/4 的交点处	手足少阳、足阳明经交会穴
悬颅	Xuánlú	在头部，从头维至曲鬓的弧形连线(其弧度与鬓发弧度相应)的中点处	
悬厘	Xuánlí	在头部，从头维至曲鬓的弧形连线(其弧度与鬓发弧度相应)的上 3/4 与下 1/4 的交点处	手足少阳、足阳明经交会穴
曲鬓*	Qūbìn	在头部，耳前鬓角发际后缘与耳尖水平线的交点处	
率谷*	Shuàigǔ	在头部，耳尖直上入发际 1.5 寸	足少阳、足太阳经交会穴
天冲	Tiānchōng	在头部，耳根后缘直上，入发际 2 寸	足少阳、足太阳经交会穴
浮白	Fúbái	在头部，耳后乳突的后上方，从天冲至完骨的弧形连线(其弧度与耳郭弧度相应)的上 1/3 与下 2/3 交点处	足少阳、足太阳经交会穴

（续表）

腧穴		定位	特定穴属性
头窍阴	Tóuqiàoyīn	在头部，耳后乳突的后上方，从天冲到完骨的弧形连线(其弧度与耳郭弧度相应)的上 2/3 与下 1/3 交点处	足少阳、足太阳经交会穴
完骨*	Wángǔ	在头部，耳后乳突的后下方凹陷中	足少阳、足太阳经交会穴
本神*	Běnshén	在头部，前发际上 0.5 寸，头正中线旁开 3 寸	足少阳经、阳维脉交会穴
阳白*	Yángbái	在头部，眉上 1 寸，瞳孔直上	足少阳经、阳维脉交会穴
头临泣*	Tóulínqì	在头部，前发际上 0.5 寸，瞳孔直上	足少阳、太阳经、阳维脉交会穴
目窗	Mùchuāng	在头部，前发际上 1.5 寸，瞳孔直上	足少阳经、阳维脉交会穴
正营	Zhèngyíng	在头部，前发际上 2.5 寸，瞳孔直上	足少阳经、阳维脉交会穴
承灵	Chénglíng	在头部，前发际上 4 寸，瞳孔直上	足少阳经、阳维脉交会穴
脑空	Nǎokōng	在头部，横平枕外隆凸的上缘，风池直上	足少阳经、阳维脉交会穴
风池*	Fēngchí	在颈后区，枕骨之下，胸锁乳突肌上端与斜方肌上端之间的凹陷中	足少阳经、阳维脉交会穴
肩井*	Jiānjǐng	在肩胛区，第 7 颈椎棘突与肩峰最外侧点连线的中点	手足少阳、足阳明经、阳维脉交会穴
渊腋	Yuānyè	在胸外侧区，第 4 肋间隙中，在腋中线上	
辄筋	Zhèjīn	在胸外侧区，第 4 肋间隙中，在腋中线前 1 寸	
日月*	Rìyuè	在胸部，第 7 肋间隙中，前正中线旁开 4 寸	胆募穴；足少阳、足太阴经交会穴
京门*	Jīngmén	在上腹部，第 12 肋骨游离端的下际	肾募穴
带脉*	Dàimài	在侧腹部，第 11 肋骨游离端垂线与脐水平线的交点上	足少阳经、带脉交会穴
五枢	Wǔshū	在下腹部，横平脐下 3 寸，髂前上棘内侧	足少阳经、带脉交会穴
维道	Wéidào	在下腹部，髂前上棘内下 0.5 寸	足少阳经、带脉交会穴
居髎	Jūliáo	在臀区，髂前上棘与股骨大转子最凸点连线的中点处	足少阳经、带脉交会穴
环跳*	Huántiào	在臀区，股骨大转子最凸点与骶管裂孔连线的外 1/3 与内 2/3 交点处	足少阳、足太阳经交会穴
风市*	Fēngshì	在股部，腘横纹上 7 寸，股外侧肌与股二头肌之间直立垂手，掌心贴于大腿时，中指尖所指凹陷中	
中渎	Zhōngdú	在股部，腘横纹上 5 寸，髂胫束后缘	
膝阳关	Xīyángguān	在膝部，股骨外上髁后上缘，股二头肌腱与髂胫束之间的凹陷中	

（续表）

腧穴		定位	特定穴属性
阳陵泉*	Yánglíngquán	在小腿外侧，腓骨头前下方凹陷中	合穴；胆下合穴；八会穴（筋会）
阳交	Yángjiāo	在小腿外侧，外踝尖上7寸，腓骨后缘	阳维脉之郄穴
外丘	Wàiqiū	在小腿外侧，外踝尖上7寸，腓骨前缘	郄穴
光明*	Guāngmíng	在小腿外侧，外踝尖上5寸，腓骨前缘	络穴
阳辅	Yángfǔ	在小腿外侧，外踝尖上4寸，腓骨前缘	经穴
悬钟*	Xuánzhōng	在小腿外侧，外踝尖上3寸，腓骨前缘	八会穴（髓会）
丘墟*	Qiūxū	在踝区，外踝的前下方，趾长伸肌腱的外侧凹陷中	原穴
足临泣*	Zúlínqì	在足背，第4、第5跖骨底结合部的前方，第5趾长伸肌腱外侧凹陷中	输穴；八脉交会穴（通带脉）
地五会	Dìwǔhuì	在足背，第4、第5跖骨间，第4跖趾关节近端凹陷中	
侠溪*	Xiáxī	在足背，第4、第5趾间，趾蹼缘后方赤白肉际处	荥穴
足窍阴	Zúqiàoyīn	在足趾，第4趾末节外侧，趾甲根角侧后方0.1寸（指寸）	井穴

3 Indications of acupoints

The acupoints of the gallbladder meridian are indicated for the diseases of the lateral head, eyes, ears and throat, mental diseases, febrile disorders, and the diseases of the areas the meridian supplies. For migraine headache, Xuanlu(GB 5), Xuanli(GB 6), Qiuxu(GB 40) and Zulinqi(GB 41) are primarily used; for eye diseases, Tongziliao(GB 1), Muchuang(GB 16), Toulinqi(GB 15), Fengchi(GB 20) and Zulinqi(GB 41) are often used; for ear diseases, Tinghui(GB 2), Qiuxu(GB 40) and Zulinqi(GB 41) are often used; for breast diseases, Riyue(GB 24), Jianjing(GB 21) and Guangming(GB 37) are often used; for chest and flank pain, Riyue(GB 24), Yanglingquan(GB 34), Waiqiu(GB 36) and Xuanzhong(GB 39) are often used. The indications and needling methods of some common acupoints are presented as follows.

3 腧穴主治

本经腧穴主要用于治疗侧头、目、耳、咽喉病，神志病，热病及经脉循行部位的病证。治疗偏头痛常用悬颅、悬厘、丘墟和足临泣；治疗目疾常用瞳子髎、目窗、头临泣、风池和足临泣；治疗耳疾常用听会、丘墟和足临泣；治疗乳房疾患常用日月、肩井和光明；治疗胸胁疼痛常用日月、阳陵泉、外丘和悬钟。临床常用腧穴的主治及针刺操作如下。

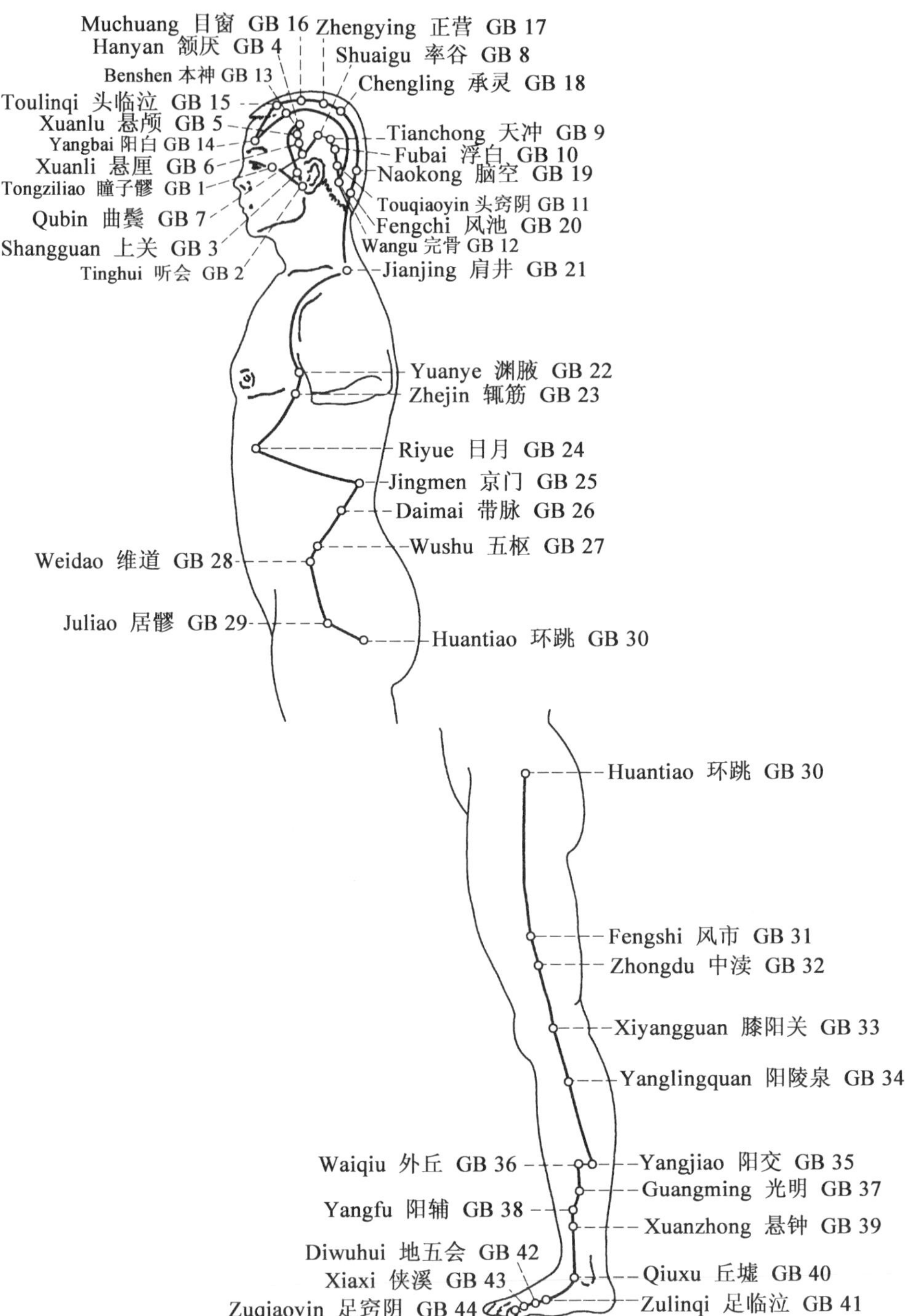

Fig.3-66　Acupoints of the gallbladder meridian of foot-shaoyang

图3-66　足少阳胆经腧穴总图

3.1 Tongziliao (GB 1) Crossing acupoint of the hand-taiyang meridian, hand and foot-shaoyang meridians

Indications: ① Painful eyes, reddened eyes and nebula; ② migraine headache, deviated mouth and eyes.

Needling: Puncture transversely 0.3～0.5 cun; or prick to bleed with a three-edged needle.

3.2 Tinghui (GB 2)

Indications: ① Tinnitus and deafness; ② deviated mouth and eyes, toothache, and facial pain.

Needling: Puncture vertically 0.5～1.0 cun.

3.3 Qubin (GB 7)

Indications: ① Migraine headache, vertigo, toothache, tinnitus, and reddened and swollen eyes.

Needling: Puncture transversely and backwards 0.5～0.8 cun.

3.4 Shuaigu (GB 8) Crossing acupoint of foot-shaoyang meridian and foot-taiyang meridian

Indications: ① Migraine headache, vertigo, tinnitus and deafness; ② infantile convulsion.

Needling: Puncture transversely 0.5～1.0 cun.

3.5 Wangu (GB 12) Crossing acupoint of foot-shaoyang and foot-taiyang meridian

Indications: ① Migraine headache, tinnitus, and deviated mouth and eyes; ② neck stiffness and pain; ③ epilepsy.

Needling: Punctre obliquely 0.5～0.8 cun.

3.6 Benshen (GB 13) Crossing acupoint of foot-shaoyang meridian and yang link vessel

Indications: ① Headache, dizziness, insomnia and epilepsy; ② infantile convulsion.

Needling: Puncture transversely 0.5～0.8 cun.

3.1 瞳子髎 Tóngzǐliáo 手太阳、手足少阳经交会穴

主治: ①目痛,目赤,目翳;②偏头痛,口眼㖞斜。

操作: 平刺0.3～0.5寸;或三棱针点刺出血。

3.2 听会 Tīnghuì

主治: ①耳鸣,耳聋;②口眼㖞斜,齿痛,面痛。

操作: 直刺0.5～1.0寸。

3.3 曲鬓 Qūbìn

主治: ①偏头痛,眩晕,齿痛,耳鸣,目赤肿痛。

操作: 向后平刺0.5～0.8寸。

3.4 率谷 Shuàigǔ 足少阳、足太阳经交会穴

主治: ①偏头痛,眩晕,耳鸣,耳聋;②小儿惊风。

操作: 平刺0.5～1.0寸。

3.5 完骨 Wángǔ 足少阳、足太阳经交会穴

主治: ①偏头痛,耳鸣,口眼㖞斜;②颈项强痛;③癫痫。

操作: 斜刺0.5～0.8寸。

3.6 本神 Běnshén 足少阳经、阳维脉交会穴

主治: ①头痛,眩晕,不寐,癫痫;②小儿惊风。

操作: 平刺0.5～0.8寸。

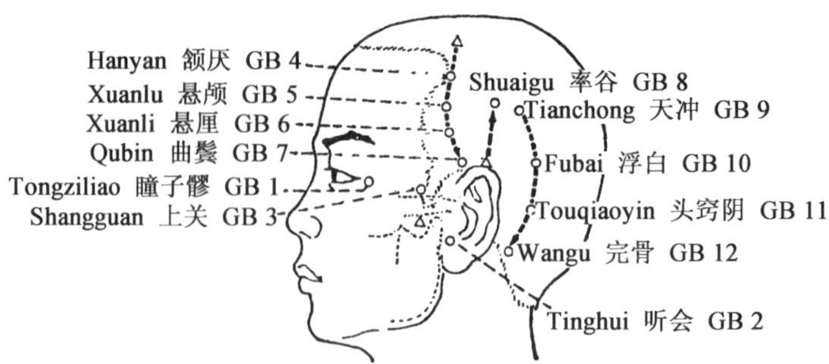

Fig.3-67　Head acupoints on the gallbladder meridian of foot-shaoyang

图 3-67　足少阳胆经头部经穴图

3.7　Yangbai (GB 14)　Crossing acupoint of foot-shaoyang meridian and yang link vessel

Indications: ① Forehead pain, reddened and swollen eyes, dropping eyelids, and deviated mouth and eyes.

Needling: Puncture transversely 0.3～0.5 cun.

3.7　阳白 Yángbái　足少阳经、阳维脉交会穴

主治: ①前头痛，目赤肿痛，眼睑下垂，口眼㖞斜。

操作: 平刺 0.3～0.5 寸。

3.8　Toulinqi (GB 15)　Crossing acupoint of foot-shaoyang meridian, foot taiyang meridian and yang link vessel

Indications: ① Headache, eye pain, lacrimation, and nasal sinusitis; ② infantile convulsion and epilepsy.

Needling: Puncture transversely 0.3～0.5 cun.

3.8　头临泣 Tóulínqì　足少阳、太阳经、阳维脉交会穴

主治: ①头痛，目痛，流泪，鼻渊；②小儿惊痫，癫痫。

操作: 平刺 0.3～0.5 寸。

3.9　Fengchi (GB 20)　Crossing acupoint of foot-shaoyang meridian and yang link vessel

Indications: ① Headache, dizziness, reddened and swollen eyes, nasal stuffiness, nasal sinusitis and tinnitus; ② insomnia, stroke and epilepsy; ③ neck stiffness and pain; ④ common cold and febrile condition.

Needling: With the needle tip slightly downwards, puncture obliquely 0.8～1.2 cun towards the tip of the nose; or puncture transversely towards

3.9　风池 Fēngchí　足少阳经、阳维脉交会穴

主治: ①头痛，眩晕，目赤肿痛，鼻塞，鼻渊，耳鸣；②失眠，中风，癫痫；③颈项强痛；④感冒，热病。

操作: 针尖微下，向鼻尖方向斜刺 0.8～1.2 寸；或平刺透风府穴。不可向内上方

Fengfu(GV 16). The needle should not be deep inserted upwards and inwards to avoid injuring the medulla.

深刺,以免伤及延髓。

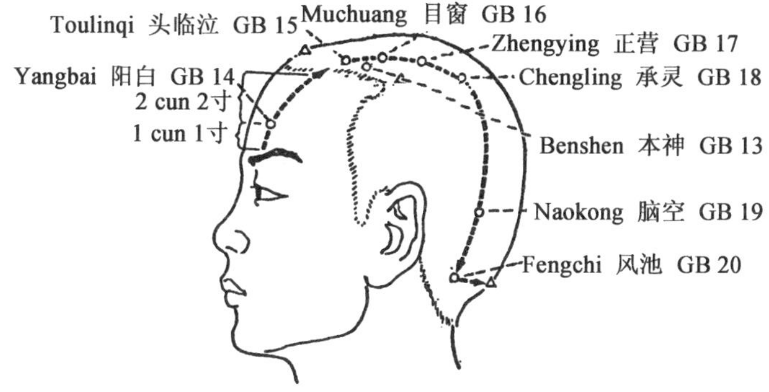

Fig.3-68 Head acupoints on the gallbladder meridian of foot-shaoyang

图3-68 足少阳胆经头部经穴图

3.10 Jianjing (GB 21) Crossing acupoint of hand and foot-shaoyang meridian, foot-yangming meridian and yang link vessel

Indications: ① Pain in the shoulder and back, stiffness and pain in the neck; ② breast abscess, insufficient lactation; ③ delayed labor; ④ scrofula.

Needling: Puncture vertically 0.3~0.5 cun; underneath is the apex of the lung and deep needling is forbidden. Contraindicated for pregnant women.

3.10 肩井 Jiānjǐng 手足少阳、足阳明经、阳维脉交会穴

主治: ①肩背痹痛,颈项强痛;②乳痈,乳汁不下;③滞产;④瘰疬。

操作: 直刺0.3~0.5寸,深部正当肺尖,不可深刺;孕妇禁针。

3.11 Riyue (GB 24) Front-Mu acupoint of the gallbladder; crossing acupoint of foot-shaoyang meridian and foot-taiyin meridian

Indications: ① Flank pain; ② stomachache, vomiting, hiccup; ③ jaundice.

Needling: Puncture obliquely 0.5~0.8 cun.

3.11 日月 Rìyuè 胆募穴;足少阳、足太阴经交会穴

主治: ①胁肋疼痛;②胃脘痛,呕吐,呃逆;③黄疸。

操作: 斜刺0.5~0.8寸。

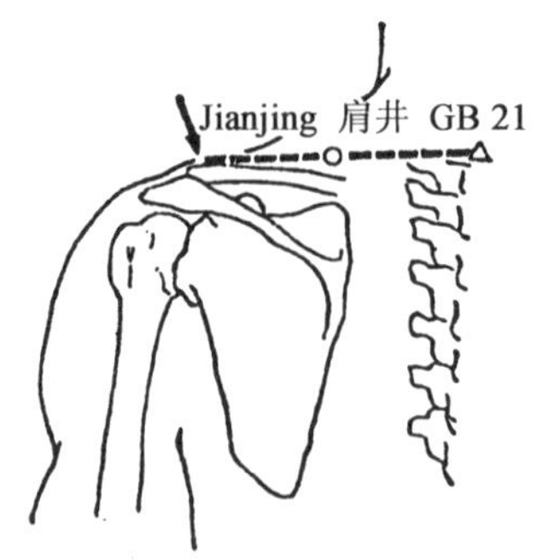

Fig.3-69　Shoulder acupoints on the gallbladder meridian of foot-shaoyang

图3-69　足少阳胆经肩部经穴图

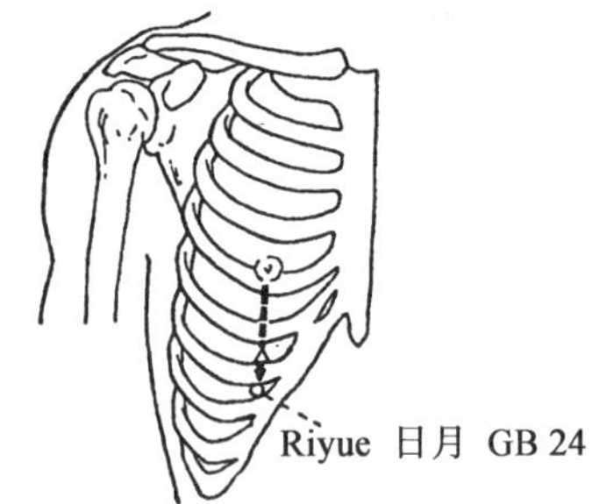

Fig.3-70　Chest acupoints on the gallbladder meridian of foot-shaoyang

图3-70　足少阳胆经胸部经穴

3.12 Jingmen (GB 25) Front-Mu acupoint of the kidney

Indications: ① Urinary difficulty and edema; ② flank pain and lumbago; ③ abdominal distention, diarrhea and intestinal gurgling.

Needling: Puncture obliquely 0.5～1.0 cun.

3.12 京门 Jīngmén　肾募穴

主治: ①小便不利,水肿;②胁痛,腰痛;③腹胀,泄泻,肠鸣。

操作: 斜刺0.5～1.0寸。

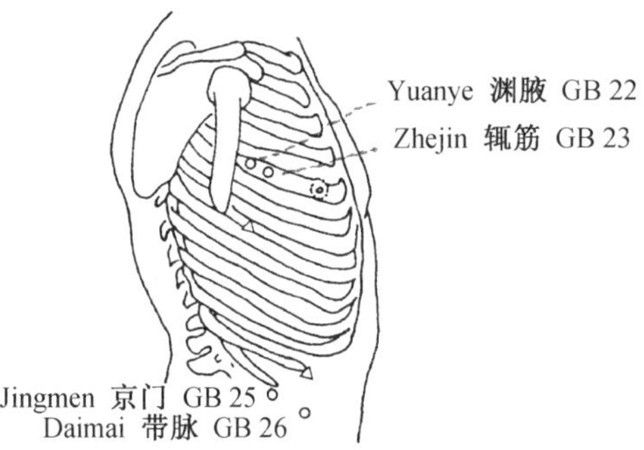

Fig.3-71　Chest and rib-side acupoints on the gallbladder meridian of foot-shaoyang

图3-71　足少阳胆经胸胁部经穴图

3.13 Daimai (GB 26) Crossing acupoint of foot-shaoyang meridian and belt vessel

Indications: ① Irregular menstruation, morbid leucorrhea, absence of menstruation, and lower abdominal pain; ② lumbago.

Needling: Puncture obliquely 0.8～1.0 cun.

3.13 带脉 Dàimài　足少阳经、带脉交会穴

主治: ①月经不调,带下,经闭,小腹痛;②腰痛。

操作: 斜刺0.8～1.0寸。

3.14 Huantiao (GB 30) Crossing acupoint of foot-shaoyang meridian and foot taiyang meridian

Indications: ① Pain in the loin and legs, flaccidity of the lower limbs, and half-side paralysis.

Needling: Puncture vertically 2.0～3.0 cun.

3.14 环跳 Huántiào 足少阳、足太阳经交会穴

主治: 腰腿痛，下肢痿痹，半身不遂。

操作: 直刺 2.0～3.0 寸。

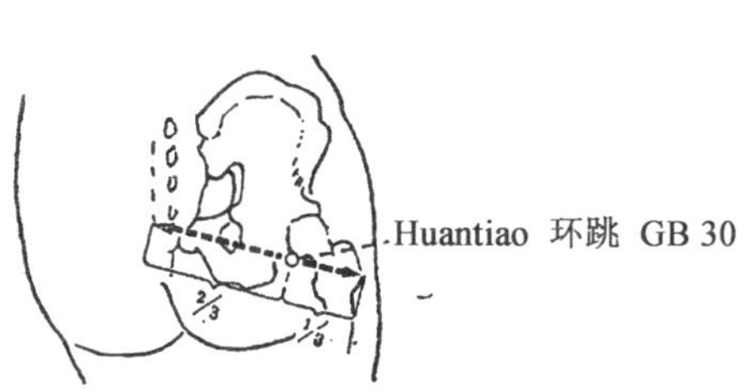

Fig.3-72 Hip acupoints on the gallbladder meridian of foot-shaoyang

图 3-72 足少阳胆经髋部经穴图

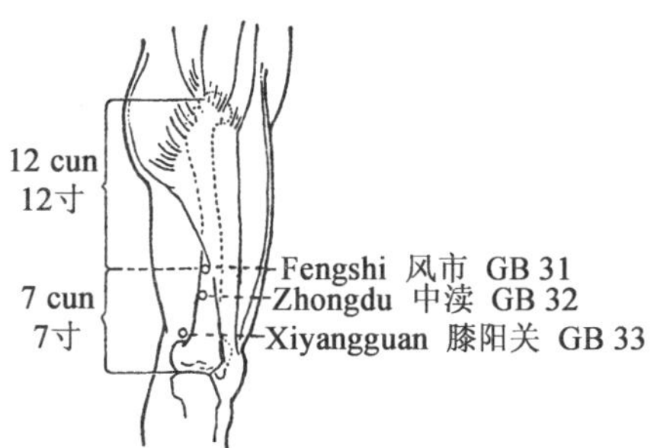

Fig.3-73 Lower limb acupoints on the gallbladder meridian of foot-shaoyang

图 3-73 足少阳胆经下肢部经穴图

3.15 Fengshi (GB 31)

Indications: ① Paralysis of lower limbs and beriberi; ② itchiness throughout the body.

Needling: Puncture vertically 1.0～1.5 cun.

3.15 风市 Fēngshì

主治: ①下肢痿痹，脚气；②遍身瘙痒。

操作: 直刺 1.0～1.5 寸。

3.16 Yanglingquan (GB 34) He-Sea acupoint; Lower He-Sea acupoint; Influential acupoint of the tendons

Indications: ① Jaundice, bitter taste in the mouth, hiccup and vomiting; ② flank pain; ③ swollen and painful knees and paralysis of the lower limbs.

Needling: Puncture vertically 1.0～1.5 cun.

3.16 阳陵泉 Yánglíngquán 合穴;胆下合穴;八会穴(筋会)

主治: ①黄疸，口苦，呃逆，呕吐；②胁肋疼痛；③膝膑肿痛，下肢痿痹。

操作: 直刺 1.0～1.5 寸。

3.17 Guangming (GB 37)

Indications: ① Eye pain, night blindness, and blurred vision; ② breast distention and insufficient lactation; ③ paralysis of lower limbs.

Needling: Puncture vertically 1.0～1.5 cun.

3.17 光明 Guangmíng 络穴

主治: ①目痛，夜盲，目视不明；②乳房胀痛，乳少；③下肢痿痹。

操作: 直刺 1.0～1.5 寸。

3.18 Xuanzhong (GB 39) Influential acupoint of the marrow

Indications: ① Neck stiffness nad pain, and distending pain in the flank; ② dementia and stroke; ③ paralysis of the lower limbs.

Needling: Puncture vertically 1.0～1.5 cun.

3.18 悬钟 Xuánzhōng 八会穴(髓会)

(绝骨 Juégǔ)

主治: ①颈项强痛,胸胁胀痛;②痴呆,中风;③下肢痿痹。

操作: 直刺 1.0～1.5 寸。

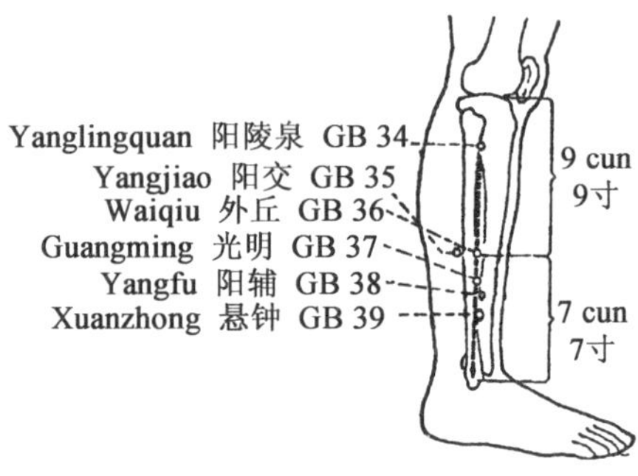

Fig.3-74 Lower limb acupoints on the gallbladder meridian of foot-shaoyang

图 3-74 足少阳胆经下肢部经穴图

3.19 Qiuxu (GB 40) Yuan-Source acupoint

Indications: ① Blurred vision; ② distending pain in the flank; ③ malaria; ④ paralysis of the lower limbs and beriberi.

Needling: Puncture vertically 0.5～0.8 cun.

3.19 丘墟 Qiūxū 原穴

主治: ①目视不明;②胸胁胀痛;③疟疾;④下肢痿痹,脚气。

操作: 直刺 0.5～0.8 寸。

3.20 Zulinqi (GB 41) Shu-Stream acupoint; Confluent acupoint communicating with the belt vessel

Indications: ① Migraine headache, dizziness, and eye pain; ② breast abscess and irregular menstruation; ③ flank pain, swelling and pain in the dorsum of foot.

Needling: Puncture vertically 0.3～0.5 cun.

3.20 足临泣 Zúlínqì 输穴;八脉交会穴(通带脉)

主治: ①偏头痛,眩晕,目痛;②乳痈,月经不调;③胁痛,足跗肿痛。

操作: 直刺 0.3～0.5 寸。

3.21 Xiaxi (GB 43) Ying-Spring acupoint

Indications: ① Headache, tinnitus, deafness, eyepain, dizziness; ② febrile condition; ③ distending

3.21 侠溪 Xiáxī 荥穴

主治: ①头痛,耳鸣,耳聋,目痛,眩晕;②热病;③胸

pain in the flank, swelling and pain in the dorsum of the foot.

胁胀痛，足跗肿痛。

Needling: Puncture perpendicularly 0.3～0.5 cun.

操作：直刺 0.3～0.5 寸。

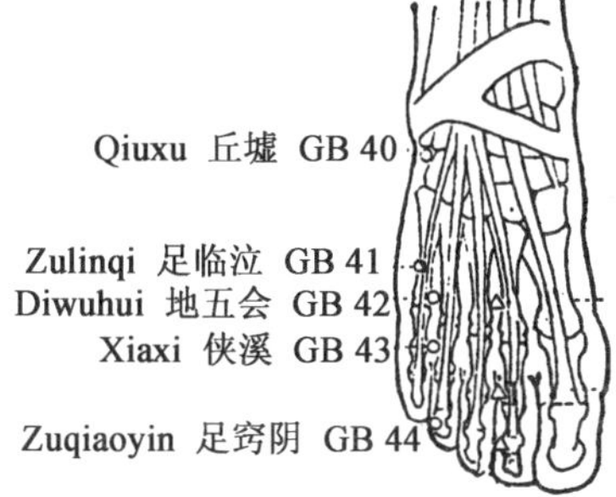

Fig.3-75 Foot acupoints on the gallbladder meridian of foot-shaoyang

图 3-75 足少阳胆经足部经穴图

Section 12 Liver Meridian of Foot-Jueyin and its Acupoints

第 12 节 足厥阴肝经及其腧穴

1 Distribution course

The liver meridian of foot-jueyin begins from the dorsal hairy region of the great toe; ascending along the back of the foot and passing through the front of the medial malleolus and along the medial aspect of the lower leg, it ascends to the area 8 cun above the medial malleolus, where it goes across and behind the spleen meridian of foot-taiyin. Then it runs continuously upwards to the medial aspect of knee and along the medial aspect of thigh to the pubic region, where it encircles the external genitalia before entering the lower abdomen. It ascends internally and curves the stomach to connect with its pertaining organ, the liver, and with the gallblad-

1 经脉循行

起于足大趾背上丛毛部，上沿足跗到内踝前，至内踝上 8 寸处交到足太阴经之后，上经膝股内侧，入阴毛中，环绕阴器，达小腹，挟胃，属于肝，联络胆，上过横膈，分布于胁肋，经喉咙的后面，上入鼻咽部，连目系，上出额部，与督脉会于巅顶。目系支脉，从目系下循颊里，环绕唇内。肝部支脉，从肝分出，通过横膈，行于肺，与手太阴肺经相接(图 3-76)。

der. From there it continues to ascend, passing through the diaphragm and spreading over the costal and hypochondriac regions. It goes up along the posterior aspect of the throat to the nasopharynx and connects with the eye system; running further upwards, it emerges from the forehead and meets the governor vessel at the vertex. A branch arising from the eye system goes downwards to the cheek and curves around the lips. Another branch arises from the liver, passing through the diaphragm, and runs upwards into the lung, where it links with the lung meridian of hand-taiyin(Fig. 3-76).

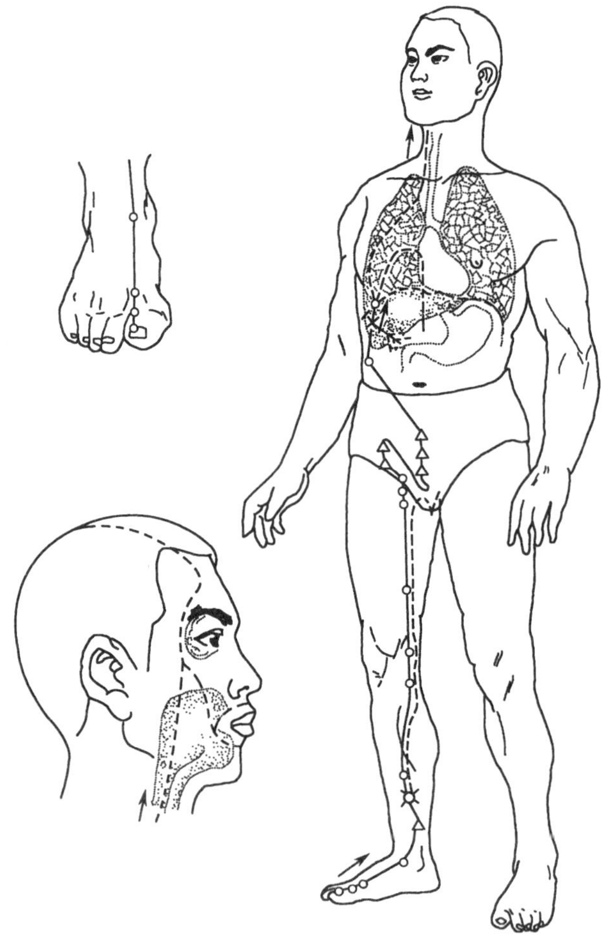

Fig.3-76　The distribution course of liver meridian of foot-jueyin

图 3-76　足厥阴肝经循行示意图

2 Location of acupoints

The starting acupoint of the liver meridian is Dadun(LR 1), and the ending acupoint is Qimen (LR 14), totally 14 acupoints in each side. The location of acupoints is presented in Table 3-12 and Figure 3-77～3-81.

2 腧穴定位

本经腧穴首穴为大敦，末穴为期门，左右各 14 穴。腧穴定位见表 3 - 12、图 3-77～3-81。

Table 3-12 Location of acupoints of the Liver meridian of foot-jueyin

Acupoint		Location	Specific feature
LR1*	Dadun	On the lateral side of the great toe, about 0.1 cun posterior to the corner of the nail	Jing-Well acupoint
LR2*	Xingjian	On the dorsum of the foot between the first and second toes, proximal to the margin of the web	Ying-Spring acupoint
LR3*	Taichong	On the dorsum of the foot, in the depression distal to the junction of the first and second metatarsal bones; artery pulsation may be felt	Shu-Stream acupoint; Yuan-Source acupoint
LR4	Zhongfeng	Before the medial malleolus, in the depression on the medial border of the tendon of the muscle tibialis anterior	Jing-River acupoint
LR5*	Ligou	5 cun above the tip of the medial malleolus, at the middle of the medial aspect of the tibia	Luo-Connecting acupoint
LR6	Zhongdu	7 cun above the tip of the medial malleolus, at the middle of the medial aspect of the tibia	Xi-Cleft acupoint
LR7	Xiguan	Inferior to the medial condyle of the tibia, 1 cun posterior to Yinlingquan(SP 9)	
LR8*	Ququan	At the medial end of the transverse popliteal crease, in the depression on the medial border of the tendon of the muscle semitendinosus	He-Sea acupoint
LR9	Yinbao	4 cun above the medial epicondyle of the femur, between the gracilis and sartorius muscles	
LR10	Zuwuli	3 cun directly below Qichong(ST 30), where the femoral artery may be felt	
LR11	Yinlian	2 cun directly below Qichong(ST 30)	
LR12	Jimai	In the inguinal groove, at the level with the upper border of the symphysis pubica and 2.5 cun lateral to the anterior midline	
LR13*	Zhangmen	At the free end of the eleventh floating rib	Front-Mu acupoint of the spleen; Influential acupoint of the zang-organs; Crossing acupoint of foot-jueyin and shaoyang meridians
LR14*	Qimen	At the sixth intercostal space, 4 cun lateral to the anterior midline	Front-Mu acupoint; Crossing acupoint of foot-jueyin meridian, foot-taiyang meridian and yin link vessel

表 3-12　足厥阴肝经的腧穴定位

腧穴		定位	特定穴属性
大敦*	Dàdūn	在足趾，大趾末节外侧，趾甲根角侧后方 0.1 寸（指寸）	井穴
行间*	Xíngjiān	在足背，第 1、2 趾之间，趾蹼缘后方赤白肉际处	荥穴
太冲*	Tàichōng	在足背，第 1、2 跖骨间，跖骨底结合部前方凹陷中，或触及动脉搏动	输穴；原穴
中封	Zhōngfēng	在踝区，内踝前，胫骨前肌肌腱的内侧缘凹陷中	经穴
蠡沟*	Lígōu	在小腿内侧，内踝尖上 5 寸，胫骨内侧面的中央	络穴
中都	Zhōngdū	在小腿内侧，内踝尖上 7 寸，胫骨内侧面的中央	郄穴
膝关	Xīguān	在膝部，胫骨内侧髁的下方，阴陵泉后 1 寸	
曲泉*	Qūquán	在膝部，腘横纹内侧端，半腱肌肌腱内缘凹陷中	合穴
阴包	Yīnbāo	在股前区，髌骨底上 4 寸，股薄肌与缝匠肌之间	
足五里	Zúwǔlǐ	在股前区，气冲直下 3 寸，动脉搏动处	
阴廉	Yīnlián	在股前区，气冲直下 2 寸	
急脉	Jímài	在腹股沟区，横平耻骨联合上缘，前正中线旁开 2.5 寸	
章门*	Zhāngmén	在侧腹部，在第 11 肋游离端的下际	脾募穴；八会穴（脏会）；足厥阴、足少阳经交会穴
期门*	Qīmén	在胸部，第 6 肋间隙，前正中线旁开 4 寸	肝募穴；足厥阴、太阳经、阴维脉交会穴

3　Indications of acupoints

The acupoints of the liver meridian are indicated for the diseases of the liver and gallbladder, gynecology, and external genitals, and diseases at the areas the meridian supplies. For the distending pain in the flank due to the liver and gallbladder disorders and emotional depression, Taichong(LR 3) and Qimen(LR 14) are used; for hernia, reproductive disorders and lower abdominal pain, Taichong(LR 3) and Dadun(LR 1) are often used; for genital urticaria, Ligou(LR 5) and Zhongdu(LR 6) are often used; for dizziness and eye disorders, Xingjian(LR 3) and Taichong(LR 3) are used. The indications and needling methods of common acupoints are presented as follows.

3　腧穴主治

本经腧穴主要用于治疗肝胆病、妇科病、前阴病及经脉循行部位的病证。治疗肝胆病之胸胁胀满疼痛、情志抑郁常用太冲、期门；治疗疝气、生殖系统疾病、小腹疼痛常用太冲、大敦；治疗阴部湿疹常用蠡沟、中都；治疗眩晕、目疾，常用行间、太冲。临床常用腧穴的主治及针刺操作如下。

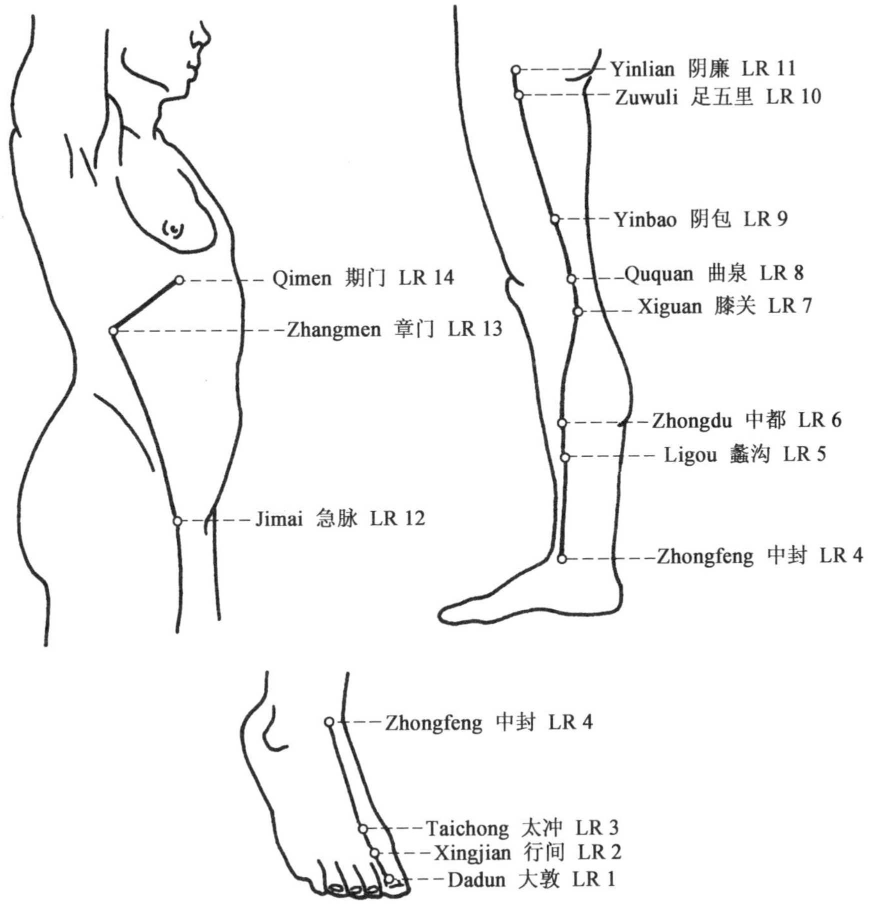

Fig.3-77 Acupoints of liver meridian of foot-jueyin

图 3-77 足厥阴肝经腧穴总图

3.1 Dadun (LR l) Jing-Well acupoint

Indications: ① Hernia, menstrual blockage, uterine bleeding, prolapse of uterus, enuresis and urinary difficulty; ② epilepsy.

Needling: Puncture shallowly 0.1～0.2 cun; or prick to bleed with a three-edged needle.

3.2 Xingjian (LR 2) Ying-Spring acupoint

Indications: ① Headache, vertigo, reddened

3.1 大敦 Dàdūn) 井穴

主治: ①疝气，经闭，崩漏，阴挺，遗尿，小便不利；②癫痫。

操作: 浅刺 0.1～0.2 寸；或三棱针点刺出血。

3.2 行间 Xíngjiān 荥穴

主治: ①头痛，目眩，目

and swollen eyes, blindness and deviated mouth; ② stroke and epilepsy; ③ irregular menstruation, menstrual cramps, uterine bleeding, morbid leucorrhea, enuresis and urinal obstruction; ④ distending pain in the chest and flank.

赤肿痛,青盲,口祸;②中风,癫痫;③月经不调,痛经,崩漏,带下,遗尿,癃闭;④胸胁胀痛。

Needling: Puncture vertically 0.5～0.8 cun.

操作: 直刺0.5～0.8寸。

3.3 Taichong (LR 3) Shu-Stream acupoint; Yuan-Source acupoint

3.3 太冲 Tàichōng 输穴;原穴

Indications: ① Headache, dizziness, reddened and swollen eyes, blindness and deviated mouth; ② epilepsy, depression, irritability, infantile convulsion and stroke; ③ jaundice, flank pain; ④ irregular menstruation, menstrual cramps, absence of menstruation, morbid leucorrhea, enuresis and urinal obstruction; ⑤ paralysis of lower limbs.

主治: ①头痛,眩晕,目赤肿痛,青盲,口祸;②癫痫,抑郁,易怒,小儿惊风,中风;③黄疸,胁痛;④月经不调,痛经,经闭,带下,遗尿,癃闭;⑤下肢痿痹。

Needling: Puncture vertically 0.5～1.0 cun.

操作: 直刺0.5～1.0寸。

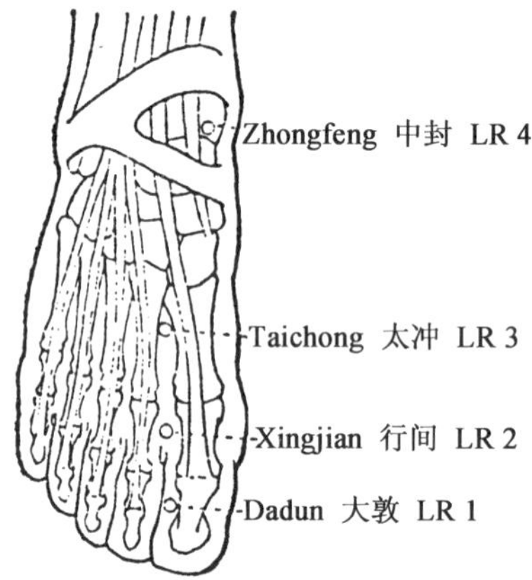

Fig.3-78 Foot acupoints on the liver meridian of foot-jueyin

图3-78 足厥阴肝经足部经穴图

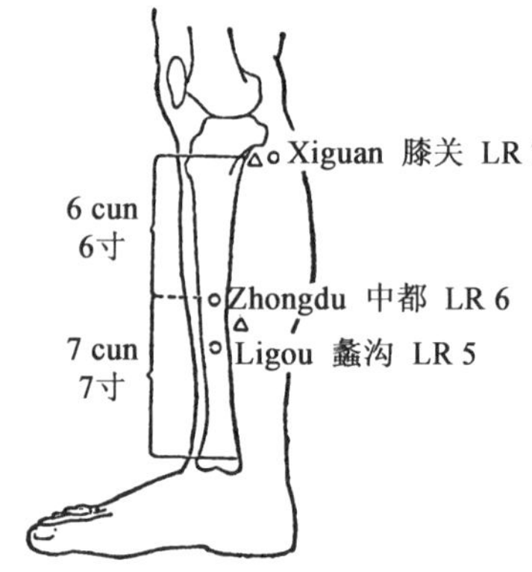

Fig.3-79 Lower limb acupoints on the liver meridian of foot-jueyin

图3-79 足厥阴肝经下肢部经穴图

3.4 Ligou (LR 5) Luo-Connecting acupoint

Indications: ① Irregular menstruation, morbid leucorrhea, priapism, painful and swollen testis, urinary difficulty and hernia; ② tibial pain.

Needling: Puncture transversely 0.5～0.8 cun.

3.5 Ququan (LR 8) He-Sea acupoint

Indications: ① Urinary difficulty, painful and obstructed urination, impotence, seminal emission, irregular menstruation, menstrual cramps, morbid leucorrhea and prolapse of uterine; ② swollen and painful knee, and paralysis of the lower limbs.

Needling: Puncture vertically 1.0～1.5 cun.

3.4 蠡沟 Lígōu 络穴

主治: ①月经不调,带下,阳强,睾丸肿痛,小便不利,疝气;②足胫疼痛。

操作: 平刺 0.5～0.8 寸。

3.5 曲泉 Qūquán 合穴

主治: ①小便不利,尿频涩痛,阳痿,遗精,月经不调,痛经,白带,阴挺;②膝膑肿痛,下肢痿痹。

操作: 直刺 1.0～1.5 寸。

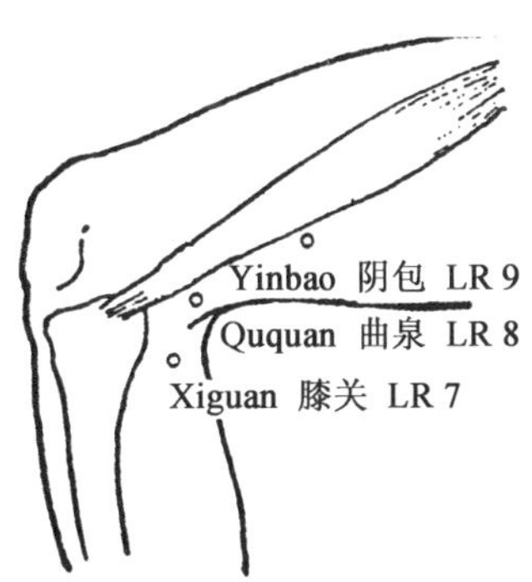

Fig.3-80 Medial knee acupoints on the liver meridian of foot-jueyin

图 3-80 足厥阴肝经膝内侧经穴图

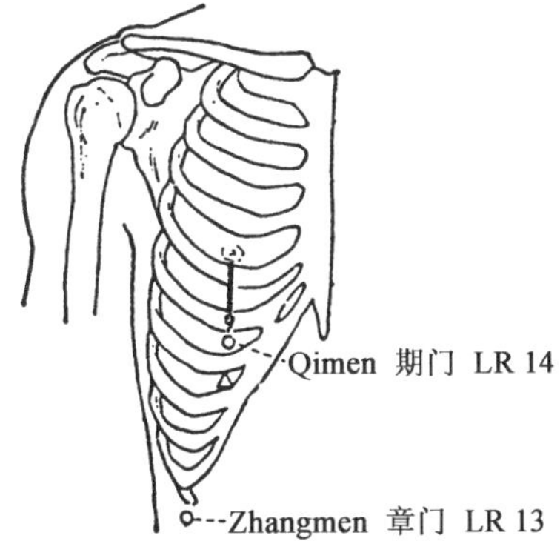

Fig.3-81 Hypochondrium and rib-side acupoints on the liver meridian of foot-jueyin

图 3-81 足厥阴肝经胁肋部经穴图

3.6 Zhangmen (LR 13) Front-Mu acupoint of the spleen; Influential acupoint of zang-organs; Crossing acupoint of foot-jueyin and foot-shaoyang meridian

Indications: ① Flank pain, jaundice; ② abdominal distention, diarrhea and vomiting; ③ ab-

3.6 章门 Zhāngmén 脾募穴;八会穴(脏会);足厥阴、足少阳经交会穴

主治: ①胁痛,黄疸;②腹胀,泄泻,呕吐;③痞块。

dominal lumps.

Needling: Puncture obliquely 0.5～0.8 cun.

操作：斜刺0.5～0.8寸。

3.7 Qimen (LR 14) Front-Mu acupoint of the liver; Crossing acupoint of the foot-jueyin meridian, foot-taiyang meridian and yin link vessel

3.7 期门 Qīmén 肝募穴；足厥阴、太阳经、阴维脉交会穴

Indications: ① Distending pain in the chest and flank, mental depression; ② breast abscess; ③ abdominal distention, hiccup and acid regurgitation.

Needling: Puncture vertically 0.5～0.8 cun.

主治： ①胸胁胀痛，抑郁；②乳痈；③腹胀，呃逆，泛酸。

操作： 斜刺0.5～0.8寸。

Section 13 Extraordinary Vessels and Their Acupoints

第13节 奇经八脉及其腧穴

1 Governor vessel and its acupoints

1.1 Distribution course

The governor vessel begins from the lower abdomen and emerges from the perineum. Then it runs backwards and goes up inside the spinal column to Fengfu(GV 16) at the nape, where it enters the brain. It further ascends to the vertex and descends across the forehead to the columnella of the nose(Fig. 3-82).

1.2 Location of acupoints

The starting acupoint of the governor vessel is Changqiang(GV 1), and the ending acupoint is Yinjiao(GV 28), totally 28 acupoints. The location of acupoint is presented in Table 3-13 and Fig. 3-83～3-85.

1 督脉及其腧穴

1.1 经脉循行

起于小腹内，下出于会阴部，向后行于脊柱的内部，向上到达项后风府，进入脑内，上行巅顶，沿前额下行鼻柱(图3-82)。

1.2 腧穴定位

本经首穴为长强，末穴为龈交，一名一穴，共28穴。腧穴定位见表3-13、图3-83～3-85。

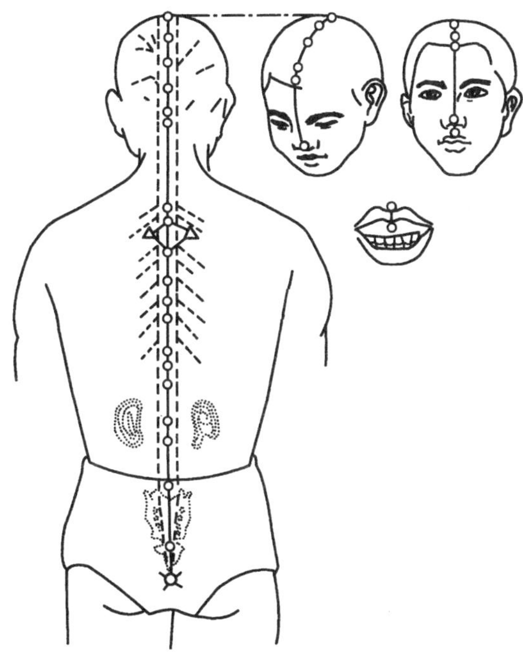

Fig.3-81 Distribution course of governor vessel

图 3-81 督脉循行示意图

Table 3-13 Location of acupoints of the Governor Vessel

Acupoint		Location	Specific feature
GV1*	Changqiang	Below the coccyx, at the midpoint of the line linking the tip of the coccyx and the anus	Luo-Connecting acupoint; Crossing acupoint of governor vessel, foot-shaoyang meridian and foot-shaoyin meridian
GV2	Yaoshu	In the hiatus of the sacrum and on the posterior midline	
GV3*	Yaoyangguan	Below the spinous process of the fourth lumbar vertebra, and on the posterior midline	
GV4*	Mingmen	Below the spinous process of the second lumbar vertebra, and on the posterior midline	
GV5	Xuanshu	Below the spinous process of the first lumbar vertebra, and on the posterior midline	
GV6	Jizhong	Below the spinous process of the eleventh thoracic vertebra, and on the posterior midline	
GV7	Zhongshu	Below the spinous process of the tenth thoracic vertebra, and on the posterior midline	
GV8*	Jinsuo	Below the spinous process of the nineth thoracic vertebra, and on the posterior midline	

(continued)

Acupoint		Location	Specific feature
GV9*	Zhiyang	Below the spinous process of the seventh thoracic vertebra, and on the posterior midline	
GV10	Lingtai	Below the spinous process of the sixth thoracic vertebra, and on the posterior midline	
GV11	Shendao	Below the spinous process of the fifth thoracic vertebra, and on the posterior midline	
GV12*	Shenzhu	Below the spinous process of the third thoracic vertebra, and on the posterior midline	
GV13	Taodao	Below the spinous process of the first thoracic vertebra, and on the posterior midline	Crossing acupoint of governor vessel and foot-taiyang meridian
GV14*	Dazhui	Below the spinous process of the seventh vertical vertebra, and on the posterior midline	Crossing acupoint of governor vessel and hand-foot yang meridians
GV15*	Yamen	Below the spinous process of the second cervical vertebra, and on the posterior midline	Crossing acupoint of governor vessel and yang link vessel
GV16*	Fengfu	Directly below the external occipital protuberance, in the depression between bilateral trapezius muscles	Crossing acupoint of governor vessel and yang link vessel
GV17	Naohu	In the depression superior to the external occipital protuberance, on the posterior midline	Crossing acupoint of governor vessel and foot-taiyang meridian
GV18	Qiangjian	4 cun directly above the posterior hairline and on the posterior midline	
GV19	Houding	5.5 cun directly above the posterior hairline and on the posterior midline	
GV20*	Baihui	5 cun directly above the anterior hairline and on the anterior midline	Crossing acupoint of governor vessel, hand and foot-shaoyang meridians, foot-taiyang and foot-jueyin meridians
GV21	Qianding	3.5 cun directly above the anterior hairline and on the anterior midline	
GV22	Xinhui	2 cun directly above the anterior hairline and on the anterior midline	
GV23*	Shangxing	1 cun directly above the anterior hairline and on the anterior midline	
GV24*	Shenting	0.5 cun directly above the anterior hairline and on the anterior midline	Crossing acupoint of governor vessel, foot-taiyang and foot-yangming meridians
GV25	Suliao	On the tip of the nose	
GV26*	Shuigou	At the junction of the upper one-third and lower two-thirds of the philtrum	Crossing acupoint of governor vessel, hand and foot-yangming meridians
GV27	Duiduan	At the midpoint of the labial tubercle of the upper lip	
GV28	Yinjiao	At the junction of the gum and the frenulum of the upper lip	

表 3-13 督脉的腧穴定位

腧穴		定位	特定穴属性
长强*	Chángqiáng	在会阴区，尾骨下方，尾骨端与肛门连线的中点处	络穴；督脉、足少阳、足少阴经交会穴
腰俞	Yāoshū	在骶区，正对骶管裂孔，后正中线上	
腰阳关*	Yāoyángguān	在脊柱区，第 4 腰椎棘突下凹陷中，后正中线上	
命门*	Mìngmén	在脊柱区，第 2 腰椎棘突下凹陷中，后正中线上	
悬枢	Xuánshū	在脊柱区，第 1 腰椎棘突下凹陷中，后正中线上	
脊中	Jǐzhōng	在脊柱区，第 11 胸椎棘突下凹陷中，后正中线上	
中枢	Zhōngshū	在脊柱区，第 10 胸椎棘突下凹陷中，后正中线上	
筋缩*	Jīnsuō	在脊柱区，第 9 胸椎棘突下凹陷中，后正中线上	
至阳*	Zhìyáng	在脊柱区，第 7 胸椎棘突下凹陷中，后正中线上	
灵台	Língtái	在脊柱区，第 6 胸椎棘突下凹陷中，后正中线上	
神道	Shéndào	在脊柱区，第 5 胸椎棘突下凹陷中，后正中线上	
身柱*	Shēnzhù	在脊柱区，第 3 胸椎棘突下凹陷中，后正中线上	
陶道	Táodào	在脊柱区，第 1 胸椎棘突下凹陷中，后正中线上	督脉、足太阳经交会穴
大椎*	Dàzhuī	在脊柱区，第 7 颈椎棘突下凹陷中，后正中线上	督脉、手足三阳经交会穴
哑门*	Yǎmén	在颈后区，第 2 颈椎棘突上际凹陷中，后正中线上	督脉、阳维脉交会穴
风府*	Fēngfǔ	在颈后区，枕外隆凸直下，两侧斜方肌之间凹陷中	督脉、阳维脉交会穴
脑户	Nǎohù	在头部，枕外隆凸的上缘凹陷中	督脉、足太阳经交会穴
强间	Qiángjiān	在头部，后发际正中直上 4 寸	
后顶	Hòudǐng	在头部，后发际正中直上 5.5 寸	
百会*	Bǎihuì	在头部，前发际正中直上 5 寸	督脉、手足少阳、足太阳、足厥阴经交会穴
前顶	Qiándǐng	在头部，前发际正中直上 3.5 寸	
囟会	Xìnhuì	在头部，前发际正中直上 2 寸	
上星*	Shàngxīng	在头部，前发际正中直上 1 寸	
神庭*	Shéntíng	在头部，前发际正中直上 0.5 寸	督脉、足太阳、足阳明经交会穴
素髎	Sùliáo	在面部，鼻尖的正中央	
水沟*	Shuǐgōu	在面部，人中沟的上 1/3 与中 1/3 交点处	督脉、手足阳明经交会穴
兑端	Duìduān	在面部，上唇结节的中点	
龈交	Yínjiāo	在上唇内，上唇系带与上牙龈的交点	

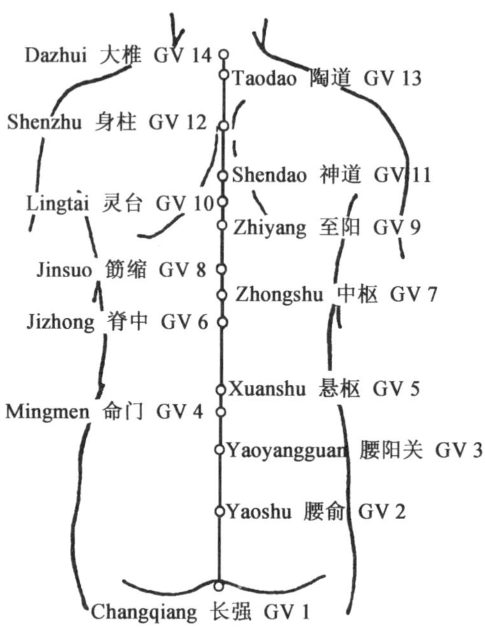

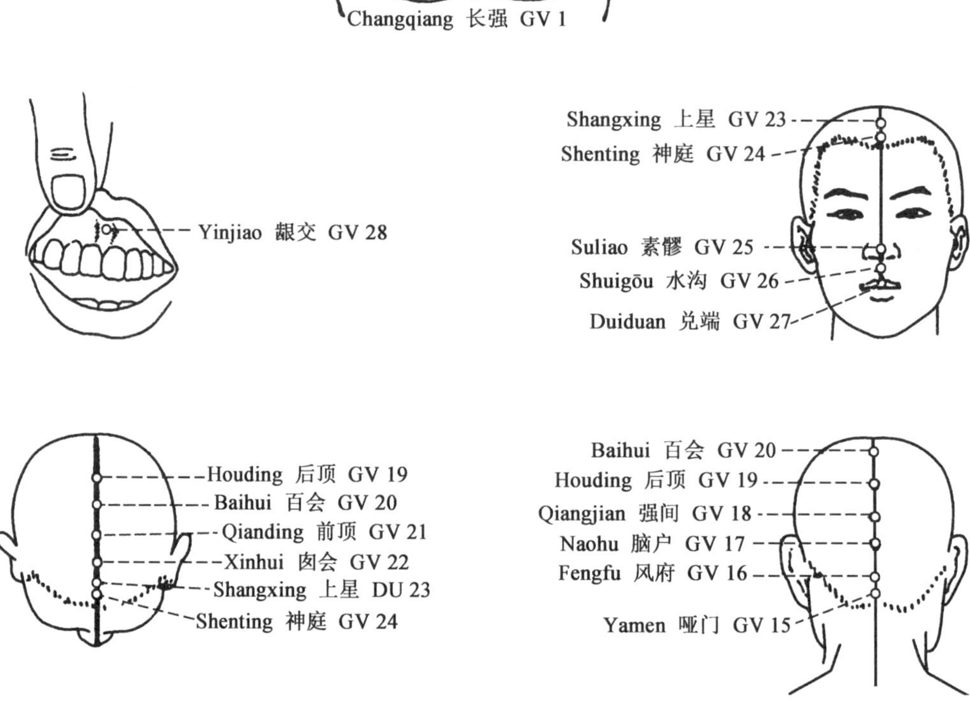

Fig.3-83　The acupoints of the governor vessel

图 3-83　督脉腧穴总图

1.3 Indications of acupoints

The acupoints of the governor vessel are indicated for mental disorders, febrile diseases, and diseases pf the loin, sacrum and head, and the disorders of associated zang-fu organs. For emergency conditions, Shuigou(GV 26), Suliao(GV 25) and Baihui (GV 20) are used; for depressive-manic psychosis and epilepsy, Changqiang(GV 1), Shendao(GV 11), Yamen(GV 15), Fengfu(GV 16), Baihui(GV 20) and Shenting(GV 24) are often used; for febrile diseases, Dazhui(GV 14), Taodao(GV 13) and Shenzhu(GV 12) are often used; for hemorrhoids and bloody stools, Changqiang(GV 1) and Yaoshu (GV 2) are used; for prolapse of rectum, Baihui (GV 20) and Changqiang(GV 1) are used; for pain in the lumbar spine and sacrum, Changqiang(GV 1), Yaoshu(GV 2), Yaoyangguan(GV 3) and Mingmen(GV 4) are used; for headache, Fengfu (GV 16), Baihui(GV 20), Qianding(GV 21) and Shangxing(23) are often used. The indications and needling methods of the common acupoints are presented as follows.

1.3 腧穴主治

本经腧穴主治神志病、热病,腰骶、项背、头部病证及相应的内脏疾病。急救常用水沟、素髎、百会;治疗癫痫、癫狂常用长强、神道、哑门、风府、百会、神庭;热病常用大椎、陶道、身柱;痔疾、便血常用长强、腰俞;脱肛常用百会、长强;腰脊、尾骶疼痛常用长强、腰俞、腰阳关、命门等;头痛常用风府、百会、前顶、上星等。临床常用腧穴的主治及针刺操作如下。

1.3.1 Changqiang (GV 1) Luo-Connecting acupoint; Crossing acupoint of governor vessel, foot-shaoyang meridian and foot-shaoyin meridian

Indications: ① Hemorrhoids, prolapse of rectum, bloody stools, diarrhea and constipation; ② depressive-manic psychosis and epilepsy; ③ lumbago and sacral pain.

Needling: Puncture obliquely close to the front of the coccyx 0.8～1.0 cun; vertical puncture is not allowed to prevent injuring the rectum.

1.3.1 长 强 Chángqiáng 络穴;督脉、足少阳、足少阴经交会穴

主治: ①痔疾,脱肛,便血,腹泻,便秘;②癫狂痫;③腰痛,尾骶痛。

操作: 紧靠尾骨前向上斜刺0.8～1.0寸;不宜直刺,以防刺伤直肠。

1.3.2　Yaoyangguan (GV 3)

Indications: ① Lumbago, paralysis of the lower limbs; ② irregular menstruation, mobid leucorrhea, seminal emission and impotence.

Needling: Puncture upwards and obliquely 0.5～1.0 cun; moxibustion is usually applied.

1.3.3　Mingmen (GV 4)

Indications: ① Seminal emission, impotence, irregular menstruation and morbid leucorrhea; ② lumbago, paralysis of lower limbs; ③ diarrhea.

Needling: Puncture upwards 0.5～1.0 cun; moxibustion is usually applied.

1.3.4　Jinsuo (GV 8)

Indications: ① Epilepsy; ② spinal stiffness, rigidity and convulsion of the limbs; ③ stomachache.

Needling: Puncture upwards 0.5～1.0 cun.

1.3.2　腰阳关 Yāoyángguān

主治： ①腰痛，下肢痿痹；②月经不调，带下，遗精，阳痿。

操作： 向上斜刺0.5～1.0寸；多用灸法。

1.3.3　命门 Mìngmén

主治： ①遗精，阳痿，月经不调，带下；②腰痛，下肢痿痹；③泄泻。

操作： 向上斜刺0.5～1.0寸；多用灸法。

1.3.4　筋缩 Jīnsuō

主治： ①癫痫；②脊强，四肢不收，筋挛拘急；③胃痛。

操作： 向上斜刺0.5～1.0寸。

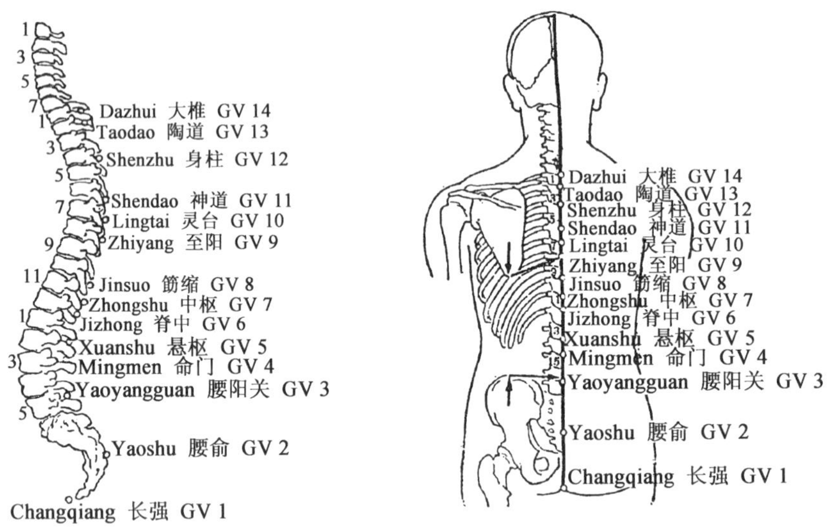

Fig.3-84　Back acupoints on the governor vessel

图3-84　督脉背腰部经穴图

1.3.5 Zhiyang (GV 9)

Indications: ① Jaundice, distention in the chest and flank; ② cough and shortness of breath; ③ spinal stiffness and backache.

Needling: Puncture upwards 0.5～1.0 cun.

1.3.5 至阳 Zhìyáng

主治: ①黄疸,胸胁胀满;②咳嗽,气喘;③脊强,背痛。

操作: 向上斜刺 0.5～1.0 寸。

1.3.6 Shenzhu (GV 12)

Indications: ① Cough and shortness of breath; ② bodily fever; ③ headache, spinal stiffness and pain; ④ carbuncle in the back; ⑤ epilepsy.

Needling: Puncture upwards 0.5～1.0 cun.

1.3.6 身柱 Shēnzhù

主治: ①咳嗽,气喘;②身热;③头痛,脊背强痛;④疔疮发背;⑤癫痫。

操作: 向上斜刺 0.5～1.0 寸。

1.3.7 Dazhui (GV 14) Crossing acupoint of governor vessel and hand-foot three yang meridians

Indications: ① Febrile conditions, tidal fever, night sweating, and malaria; ② cough; ③ depressive-manic psychosis and epilepsy, infantile convulsion; ④ wind wheals and acne.

Needling: Puncture upwards 0.5～1.0 cun; or prick to bleed with a three edged needle.

1.3.7 大椎 Dàzhuī 督脉、手足三阳经交会穴

主治: ①热病,骨蒸盗汗,疟疾;②咳喘;③癫狂痫,小儿惊风; ④风疹,痤疮。

操作: 向上斜刺 0.5～1.0 寸;或三棱针点刺出血。

1.3.8 Yamen (GV 15) Crossing acupoint of governor vessel and yang link vessel

Indications: ① Sudden loss of voice, stiff tongue and inability to speak; ② depressive-manic psychosis and epilepsy; ③ headache and stiff neck.

Needling: With upright sitting position and the head slightly bent, nape relaxed; puncture 0.5～1.0 cun towards the mandible, upward deep puncture is forbidden to avoid injuring the medullary bulb.

1.3.8 哑门 Yǎmén 督脉、阳维脉交会穴

主治: ①暴喑,舌强不语;②癫狂痫;③头痛,项强。

操作: 伏案正坐位,头微前倾,项部放松,向下颌方向缓慢刺入 0.5～1.0 寸。不可向上深刺,以防刺伤延髓。

1.3.9 Fengfu (GV 16) Crossing acupoint of governor vessel and yang link vessel

Indications: ① Stroke, depressive-manic psychosis and epilepsy; ② headache, stiff neck, dizzi-

1.3.9 风府 Fēngfǔ 督脉、阳维脉交会穴

主治: ①中风,癫狂痫;②头痛,项强,眩晕;③咽喉

ness; ③ sore throat and loss of voice.

Needling: With upright sitting position and the head slightly bent, nape relaxed; puncture 0.5～1.0 cun towards the mandible, upward deep puncture is forbidden to avoid injuring the medullary bulb.

1.3.10 Baihui (GV 20) Crossing acupoint of governor vessel, hand-foot shaoyang meridians, foot-taiyang meridian and foot-jueyin meridian

Indications: ① Headache, dizziness, insomnia, forgetfulness, stroke, depressive-manic psychosis and epilepsy; ② prolapse of rectum and uterus, gastroptosis, and long-term diarrhea.

Needling: Puncture transversely 0.5～0.8 cun; to lift yang and arrest collapse, moxibustion is frequently applied.

1.3.11 Shangxing (GV 23)

Indications: ① Nasal sinusitis, nasal bleeding, painful eyes; ② headache, dizziness, depressive-manic psychosis; ③ febrile condition and malaria.

Needling: Puncture transversely 0.5～0.8 cun.

1.3.12 Shenting (GV 24) Crossing acupoint of governor vessel, foot-taiyang meridian and foot-yangming meridian

Indications: ① Headache, dizziness, nasal sinusitis, nasal bleeding, reddened eyes, nebula; ② insomnia; ③ depressive-manic psychosis.

Needling: Puncture transversely 0.5～0.8 cun.

1.3.13 Shuigou (GV 26) Crossing acupoint of governor vessel and hand-foot yangming meridian

Indications: ① Coma, fainting, depressive-manic psychosis and epilepsy, stroke, heat-stroke, and shock; ② deviated mouth, nasal stuffiness, nasal

肿痛，失音。

操作：伏案正坐位，头微前倾，项部放松，向下颌方向缓慢刺入0.5～1.0寸，不可向上深刺，以防刺伤延髓。

1.3.10 百会 Bǎihuì 督脉、手足少阳、足太阳、足厥阴经交会穴

主治：①头痛，眩晕，失眠，健忘，中风，癫狂痫；②脱肛，子宫下垂，胃下垂，久泻。

操作：平刺0.5～0.8寸；升阳举陷时多用灸法。

1.3.11 上星 Shàngxīng

主治：①鼻渊，鼻衄，目痛；②头痛，眩晕，癫狂；③热病，疟疾。

操作：平刺0.5～0.8寸。

1.3.12 神庭 Shéntíng 督脉、足太阳、足阳明经交会穴

主治：①头痛，眩晕，鼻渊，鼻衄，目赤，目翳；②失眠；③癫狂。

操作：平刺0.5～0.8寸。

1.3.13 水沟 Shuǐgōu 督脉、手足阳明经交会穴

主治：①昏迷，晕厥，癫狂痫，中风，中暑，休克；②口㖞，鼻塞，鼻衄，牙关紧闭；

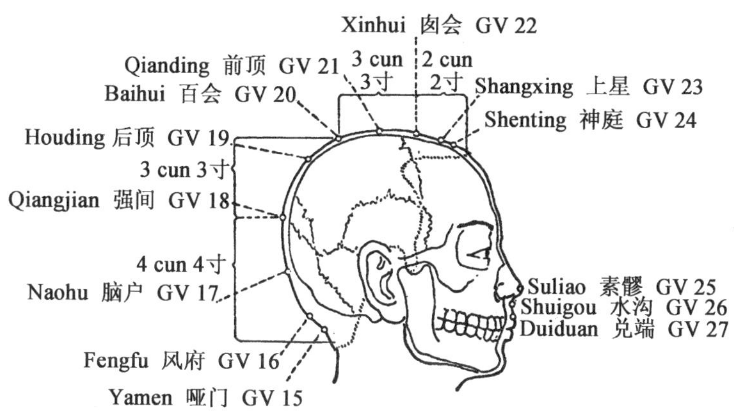

Fig.3-85 Head and neck acupoints on the governor vessel

图 3-85 督脉头颈部经穴图

bleeding, and lockjaw; ③ lumbago by sprain and contusion.

Needling: Puncture upwards 0.3～0.5 cun; or press the acupoint with nails.

2 Conception vessel and its acupoints

2.1 Distribution course

The conception vessel begins from the lower abdomen and emerges from the perineum. It goes forwards to the pubic region and ascends along the midline of the abdomen, chest, and throat; ascending further, it encircles around the lips, passes through the cheek and reaches the infraorbital region(Fig.3-86).

2.2 Location of acupoints

The starting acupoint of the conception vessel is Huiyin(CV 1), and the ending acupoint is Chengjiang (CV 24), totally 24 acupoints. The location of acupoints is presented in Table 3-14 and Fig.3-87～3-90.

③闪挫腰痛。

操作：向上斜刺0.3～0.5寸;或指甲掐按。

2 任脉及其腧穴

2.1 经脉循行

起于小腹内,下出于会阴部,向前行于阴毛部,在腹内沿前正中线上行,到达咽喉部,再上行环绕口唇,经过面部,进入目眶下(图3-86)。

2.2 腧穴定位

本经首穴为会阴,末穴为承浆,一名一穴,共24穴。腧穴定位见表3-14、图3-87～3-90。

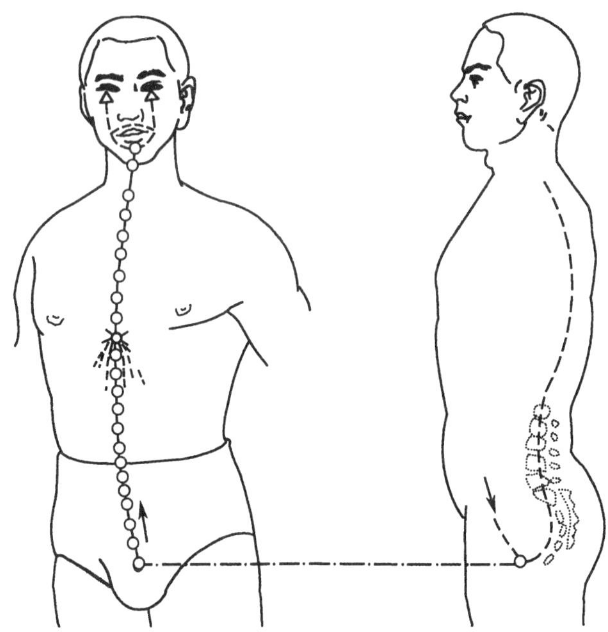

Fig.3-86　Distribution course of conception vessel

图 3-86　任脉循行示意图

Table 3-14　Location of acupoints of the conception vessel

Acupoint		Location	Specific feature
CV1	Huiyin	At the midpoint between the anus and the root of the scrotum in males and between the anus and the posterior labial commissure in females	Crossing acupoint of conception vessel, governor vessel and thoroughfare vessel
CV2	Qugu	At the level with the upper border of the symphysis pubis, on the anterior midline	Crossing acupoint of conception vessel and foot-jueyin meridian
CV3*	Zhongji	4 cun below the navel, on the anterior midline	Front-Mu acupoint the bladder; Crossing acupoint of conception vessel and three foot-yin meridians
CV4*	Guanyuan	3 cun below the navel, on the anterior midline	Front-Mu acupoint the small intestine; Crossing acupoint of conception vessel and three foot-yin meridians
CV5	Shimen	2 cun below the navel, on the anterior midline	Front-Mu acupoint of triple energizer
CV6*	Qihai	1.5 cun below the navel, on the anterior midline	

(continued)

Acupoint		Location	Specific feature
CV7	Yinjiao	1 cun below the navel, on the anterior midline	Crossing acupoint of conception and thoroughfare vessels
CV8*	Shenque	In the center of the navel	
CV9*	Shuifen	1 cun above the navel, on the anterior midline	
CV10*	Xiawan	2 cun above the navel, on the anterior midline	Crossing acupoint of conception vessel and foot taiyin meridian
CV11*	Jianli	3 cun above the navel, on the anterior midline	
CV12*	Zhongwan	4 cun above the navel, on the anterior midline	Front-Mu acupoint of stomach; Influential acupoint of fu-organs; Crossing acupoint of conception vessel, hand-taiyin and foot yangming meridians
CV13	Shangwan	5 cun above the navel, on the anterior midline	Crossing acupoint of Conception Vessel, hand-taiyang and foot yangming meridians
CV14*	Juque	6 cun above the navel, on the anterior midline	Front-Mu acupoint of heart
CV15*	Jiuwei	1 cun below the xiphosternal synchondrosis, on the anterior midline	Luo-Connecting acupoint
CV16	Zhongting	At the midpoint of the junction of sternum and xiphoid, on the anterior midline	
CV17*	Danzhong	At the level with the fourth intercostal space, on the anterior midline	Front-Mu acupoint of pericardium; Influential acupoint of qi
CV18	Yutang	At the level with the third intercostal space, on the anterior midline	
CV19	Zigong	At the level with the second intercostal space, on the anterior midline	
CV20	Huagai	At the level with the first intercostal space, on the anterior midline	
CV21	Xuanji	1 cun below the suprasternal fossa, on the anterior midline	
CV22*	Tiantu	In the center of the suprasternal fossa, on the anterior midline	Crossing acupoint of conception vessel and yin link vessel
CV23*	Lianquan	Above the Adam's apple, in the depression of the upper border of the hyoid bone, on the anterior midline	Crossing acupoint of conception vessel and yin link vessel
CV24*	Chengjiang	In the depression in the center of the mentolabial groove	Crossing acupoint of conception vessel and foot-yangming meridian

表 3-14　任脉的腧穴定位

腧穴		定位	特定穴属性
会阴	Huìyīn	在会阴区，男性在阴囊根部与肛门连线的中点，女性在大阴唇后联合与肛门连线的中点	任脉、督脉、冲脉交会穴
曲骨	Qūgǔ	在下腹部，耻骨联合上缘，前正中线上	任脉、足厥阴经交会穴
中极*	Zhōngjí	在下腹部，脐中下 4 寸，前正中线上	膀胱募穴；任脉、足三阴经交会穴
关元*	Guānyuán	在下腹部，脐中下 3 寸，前正中线上	小肠募穴；任脉、足三阴经交会穴
石门	Shímén	在下腹部，脐中下 2 寸，前正中线上	三焦募穴
气海*	Qìhǎi	在下腹部，脐中下 1.5 寸，前正中线上	
阴交	Yīnjiāo	在下腹部，脐中下 1 寸，前正中线上	任脉、冲脉交会穴
神阙*	Shénquè	在脐区，脐中央	
水分*	Shuǐfēn	在上腹部，脐中上 1 寸，前正中线上	
下脘*	Xiàwǎn	在上腹部，脐中上 2 寸，前正中线上	任脉、足太阴经交会穴
建里*	Jiànlǐ	在上腹部，脐中上 3 寸，前正中线上	
中脘*	Zhōngwǎn	在上腹部，脐中上 4 寸，前正中线上	胃募穴；八会穴（腑会）；任脉、手太阳、足阳明经交会穴
上脘	Shàngwǎn	在上腹部，脐中上 5 寸，前正中线上	任脉、手太阳、足阳明经交会穴
巨阙*	Jùquè	在上腹部，脐中上 6 寸，前正中线上	心募穴
鸠尾*	Jiūwěi	在上腹部，剑胸结合下 1 寸，前正中线上	络穴
中庭	Zhōngtíng	在胸部，剑胸结合中点处，前正中线上	
膻中*	Dànzhōng	在胸部，横平第 4 肋间隙，前正中线上	心包募穴；八会穴（气会）
玉堂	Yùtáng	在胸部，横平第 3 肋间隙，前正中线上	
紫宫	Zǐgōng	在上腹部，横平第 2 肋间隙，前正中线上	
华盖	Huágài	在胸部，横平第 1 肋间隙，前正中线上	
璇玑	Xuánjī	在胸部，胸骨上窝下 1 寸，前正中线上	
天突*	Tiāntū	在颈前区，胸骨上窝中央，前正中线上	任脉、阴维脉交会穴
廉泉*	Liánquán	在颈前区，喉结上方，舌骨上缘凹陷中，前正中线上	任脉、阴维脉交会穴
承浆*	Chéngjiāng	在面部，颏唇沟的正中凹陷处	任脉、足阳明经交会穴

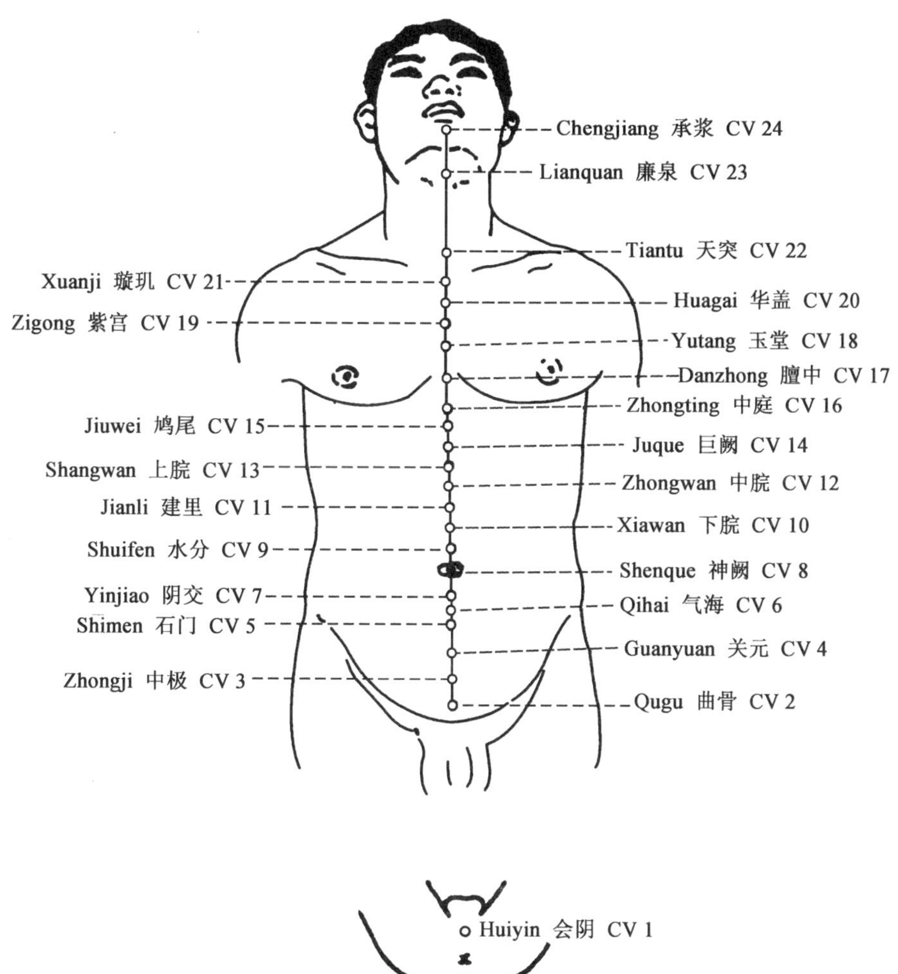

Fig.3-87 The acupoints of the conception vessel

图 3-87 任脉腧穴总图

2.3 Indications of acupoints

The acupoints of the conception vessel are indicated for the diseases in the abdomen, chest, neck, head and face, and disorders of their related zang-fu organs; many acupoints have tonic functions and a few acupoints act to treat mental disorders. For the diseases of gynecology and andrology, Guanyuan (GV 4), Zhongji(CV 3) and Qihai(CV 6) are often

2.3 腧穴主治

本经腧穴主要治疗腹、胸、颈、头面的局部病证及相应的内脏器官病证，部分腧穴有保健作用，少数腧穴可治疗神志病。治疗妇科、男科病证，常用关元、中极、气海等；治疗癃闭、遗尿，常用

used; for urinary retention and incontinence, Zhongji(CV 3), Qugu(GV 2), Guanyuan(CV 4) and Shimen(CV 5) are often used; for di-seases of stomach and intestine, Zhongwan(CV 12), Shenque(CV 8) and Jianli(CV 11) are often used; for cough and asthma, Danzhong(CV 17), Tiantu(CV 22) and Huagai(CV 20) are often used; for post-stroke aphasia, Lianquan(CV 23) is usually used; for deviated mouth and drooling, Chengjiang(CV 24) is often used; for drowning, Huiyin(CV 1) is used; for epilepsy, Jiuwei(CV 15) is used; Qihai (CV 6) and Guanyuan(CV 4) have tonic effects; Guanyuan(CV 4) and Shenque(CV 8) function to return yang and rectify adversity. The indications and needling methods are prsented as follows.

中极、曲骨、关元、石门等；治疗胃肠病常用中脘、神阙、下脘、建里等；治疗咳嗽、气喘常用膻中、天突、华盖等；中风失语常取廉泉；口喎流涎常取承浆；会阴主溺水急救；鸠尾主治癫痫；气海、关元有强身保健作用；关元、神阙有回阳救逆功效。临床常用腧穴的主治及针刺操作如下。

2.3.1 Zhongji (CV 3) Front-Mu acupoint; Crossing acupoint of conception vessel and three foot yin meridians

Indications: Urinary difficulty, enuresis, seminal emission, impotence, irregular menstruation, uterine bleeding, morbid leucorrhea, and infertility.

Needling: Puncture vertically 1.0～1.5 cun after the bladder is emptied; this acupoint is contraindicated for pregnant women.

2.3.1 中极 Zhōngjí 膀胱募穴；任脉、足三阴经交会穴

主治： 小便不利，遗尿，遗精，阳痿，月经不调，崩漏，带下，不育，不孕。

操作： 直刺1.0～1.5寸，需在排尿后针刺；孕妇禁用。

2.3.2 Guanyuan (CV 4) Front-Mu acupoint; Crossing acupoint of conception vessel and three foot yin meridians

Indications: ① Deficiency conditions, collapse syndrome of wind-stroke, and prolapse of rectum; ② seminal emission, impotence, irregular menstruation, morbid leucorrhea, infertility, urinary difficulty and enuresis;③ abdominal pain and diarrhea.

Needling: Puncture vertically 1.0～1.5 cun after the bladder is emptied; moxibustion is mostly

2.3.2 关元 Guānyuán 小肠募穴；任脉、足三阴经交会穴

主治： ①虚劳，中风脱证，脱肛；②遗精，阳痿，月经不调，痛经，崩漏，带下，不育，不孕，小便不利，遗尿；③腹痛，腹泻。

操作： 直刺1.0～1.5寸，需在排尿后针刺；多用灸法；

applied; this acupoint is contraindicated for pregnant women.

孕妇禁用。

2.3.3 Qihai (CV 6)

2.3.3 气海 Qìhǎi

Indications: ①Deficiency conditions; ② abdominal pain, diarrhea, constipation, dysentery; ③ irregular menstruation, menstrual cramps, seminal emission and impotence.

主治: ①虚脱;②腹痛,腹泻,便秘,痢疾;③月经不调,痛经,遗精,阳痿。

Needling: Puncture vertically 1.0～1.5 cun after the bladder is emptied; moxibustion is mostly applied; this acupoint is contraindicated for pregnant women.

操作: 直刺1.0～1.5寸;多用灸法;孕妇禁用。

2.3.4 Shenque (CV 8)

2.3.4 神阙 Shénquè

Indications: ① Prostration or shock, collapse stroke in wind-stroke; ② abdominal pain, abdominal distention, constipation and diarrhea; ③ edema and urinary difficulty.

主治: ①虚脱,中风脱证;②腹痛,腹胀,便秘,泄泻;③水肿,小便不利。

Needling: Generally needling is not applied; moxibustion with moxa stick or cones over a layer of salt is applicable.

操作: 一般不针,多用艾条灸或艾炷隔盐灸法。

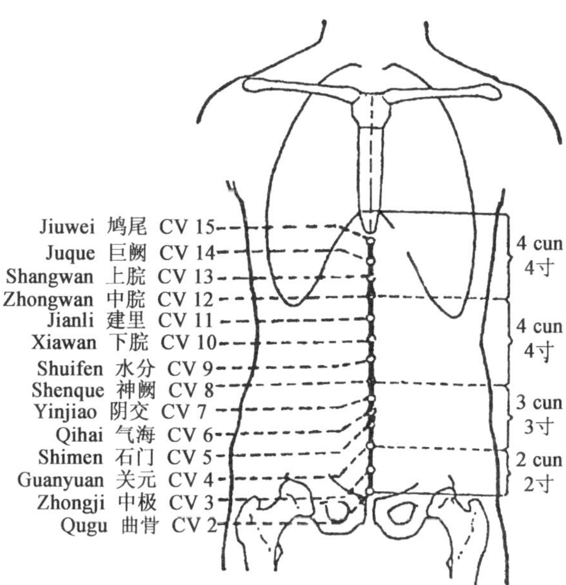

Fig.3-88 Abdomen acupoints on the conception vessel

图 3-88 任脉腹部经穴图

2.3.5 Shuifen (CV 9)

Indications: ① Edema, urinary difficulty; ② abdominal pain, abdominal distention, diarrhea, and vomiting.

Needling: Puncture vertically 1.0～1.5 cun; moxibustion is mostly applied.

2.3.6 Xiawan (CV 10) Crossing acupoint of conception vessel and foot-taiyin meridian

Indication: ① Abdominal pain, abdominal distention, diarrhea, and vomiting with undigested foods; ② abdominal lumps.

Needling: Puncture vertically 1.0～1.5 cun.

2.3.7 Jianli (CV 11)

Indications: ① Stomachache, abdominal distention, vomiting and poor appetite; ② edema.

Needling: Puncture vertically 1.0～1.5 cun.

2.3.8 Zhongwan (CV 12) Front-Mu acupoint of stomach; Influential acupoint of fu-organs; Crossing acupoint of conception vessel, hand-taiyang and foot-yangming meridians

Indications: ① Abdominal distention, diarrhea, stomachache, vomiting, acid regurgitation, hiccup and poor appetite; ② jaundice; ③ depressive-manic psychosis.

Needling: Puncture vertically 1.0～1.5 cun.

2.3.9 Juque (CV 14) Front-Mu acupoint of heart

Indications: ① Cardiac pain and palpitation; ② depressive-manic psychosis and epilepsy; ③ stomachache, vomiting and acid regurgitation.

Needling: Puncture downward obliquely 0.5～1.0 cun; deep needling is forbidden to avoid injuring the liver.

2.3.5 水分 Shuǐfēn

主治：①水肿，小便不利；②腹痛，腹胀，泄泻，反胃吐食。

操作：直刺1.0～1.5寸；多用灸法。

2.3.6 下脘 Xiàwǎn 任脉、足太阴经交会穴

主治：①腹痛，腹胀，泄泻，呕吐，食谷不化；②痞块。

操作：直刺1.0～1.5寸。

2.3.7 建里 Jiànlǐ

主治：①胃痛，腹胀，呕吐，食欲不振；②水肿。

操作：直刺1.0～1.5寸。

2.3.8 中脘 Zhōngwǎn 胃募穴；八会穴（腑会）；任脉、手太阳、足阳明经交会穴

主治：①腹胀，泄泻，胃痛，呕吐，吞酸，呃逆，食欲不振；②黄疸；③癫狂痫。

操作：直刺1.0～1.5寸。

2.3.9 巨阙 Jùquè 心募穴

主治：①胸痛，心悸；②癫狂痫；③胃痛，呕吐，吞酸。

操作：向下斜刺0.5～1.0寸；不可深刺，以防刺伤肝脏。

2.3.10 Jiuwei (CV 15) Luo-Connecting acupoint

Indications: ① Chest distress, chest pain and palpitation; ② depressive-manic psychosis and epilepsy; ③ abdominal distention, hiccup, and vomiting.

Needling: Puncture downwards obliquely 0.5～1.0 cun.

2.3.11 Danzhong (CV 17) Front-Mu acupoint; Influential acupoint of qi

Indications: ① Chest distress, shortness of breath, chest pain, and palpitation; ② cough and asthma; ③ vomiting and dysphagia; ④ insufficient lactation.

Needling: Puncture transversely 0.3～0.5 cun.

2.3.12 Tiantu (CV 22) Crossing acupoint of conception vessel and yin link vessel

Indications: ① Cough, asthma and chest pain; ② sore throat, sudden loss of voice, dysphagia and blobus hystericus; ③ goiter.

Needling: Puncture vertically 0.2～0.3 cun first, then insert the needle downwards along the posterior aspect of the stern 1.0～1.5 cun; correct angle and depth of needling should be stressed so as not to injure the lung and related arteries.

2.3.10 鸠尾 Jiūwěi 络穴

主治：①胸闷，胸痛，心悸；②癫狂痫；③腹胀，呃逆，呕吐。

操作：向下斜刺0.5～1.0寸。

2.3.11 膻中 Dànzhōng 心包募穴；八会穴(气会)

主治：①胸闷，气短，胸痛，心悸；②咳嗽，气喘；③呕吐，噎膈；④乳少。

操作：平刺0.3～0.5寸。

2.3.12 天突 Tiāntū 任脉、阴维脉交会穴

主治：①咳嗽，气喘，胸痛；②咽喉肿痛，暴喑，噎膈，梅核气；③瘿气。

操作：先直刺0.2～0.3寸，然后将针尖向下，紧靠胸骨柄后方刺入1.0～1.5寸；注意针刺的角度和深度，以防刺伤肺脏和血管。

Xuanji 璇玑 CV 21
Huagai 华盖 CV 20
Zigong 紫宫 CV 19
Yutang 玉堂 CV 18
Danzhong 膻中 CV 17
Zhongting 中庭 CV 16

Fig.3-89 Chest acupoints on the conception vessel

图 3-89 任脉胸部经穴图

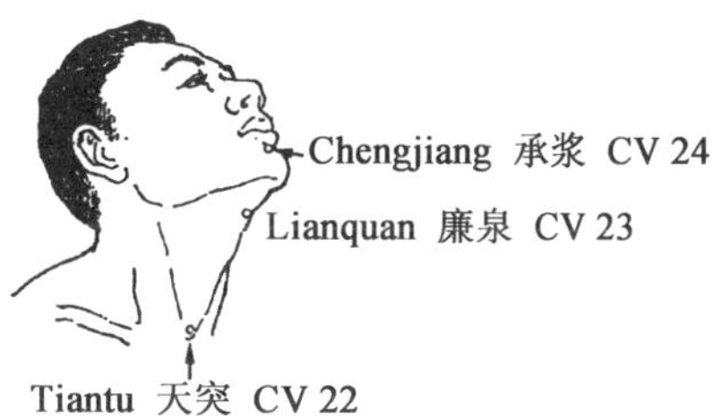

Fig.3-90 Neck acupoints on the conception

图 3-90 任脉颈颏部经穴图

2.3.13 Lianquan (CV 23) Crossing acupoint of conception vessel and yin link vessel

Indications: Stiff tongue failing to speak, painful and swollen tongue, drooling, swallowing difficulty, sudden loss of voice and dusphagia.

Needling: Puncture obliquely towards the root of the tongue 0.5～0.8 cun.

2.3.14 Chengjiang (CV 24) Crossing acupoint of conception vessel and foot-yangming meridian

Indications: ① Deviated mouth, drooling, tongue sores, painful and swollen gums, and sudden loss of voice; ② depressive-manic psychosis .

Needling: Puncture obliquely 0.3～0.5 cun.

3 Thoroughfare vessel

The thoroughfare vessel originates from the inside of the lower abdomen, emerges downwards at the perineum; and then goes up inside the spinal column. Its superficial branch passes through the region of Qichong(ST 30) to meet the kidney meridian of foot-shaoyin. Running along both sides of the abdomen, it ascends to the chest and scatters; a branch goes up to the throat and encircle the lips (Fig.3-91).

4 Belt vessel

The belt vessel originates below the hypochondriac regions and goes obliquely downwards through Daimai(GB 26), Wushu(GB 27) and Weidao(GB 28); it encircles the waist like a belt(Fig.3-92).

2.3.13 廉泉 Liánquán 任脉、阴维脉交会穴

主治: 舌强不语，舌下肿痛，流涎，吞咽困难，暴喑，喉痹。

操作: 向舌根斜刺0.5～0.8寸。

2.3.14 承浆 Chéngjiāng 任脉、足阳明经交会穴

主治: ①口㖞，流涎，口舌生疮，齿龈肿痛，暴喑；②癫狂。

操作: 斜刺0.3～0.5寸。

3 冲脉

起于小腹内，下出于会阴部，向上行于脊柱之内。其外行者经气冲与足少阴经交会，沿着腹部两侧，上行至胸中而散，其分支上达咽喉，环绕口唇(图3-91)。

4 带脉

起于季胁部的下面，斜向下行到带脉、五枢、维道穴，横行绕身一周(图3-92)。

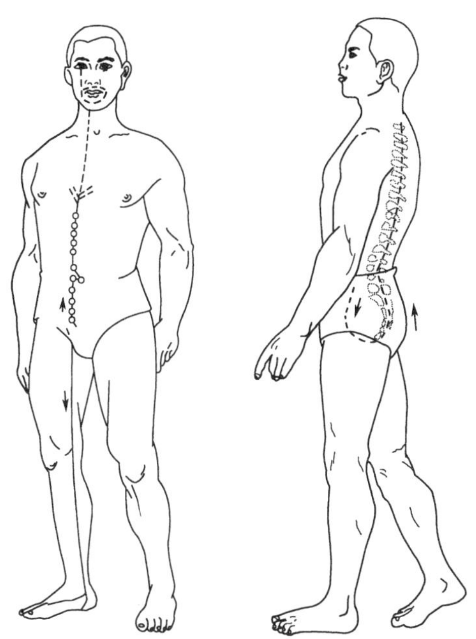

Fig.3-91 Flowing route of the thoroughfare vessel

图 3-91 冲脉循行示意图

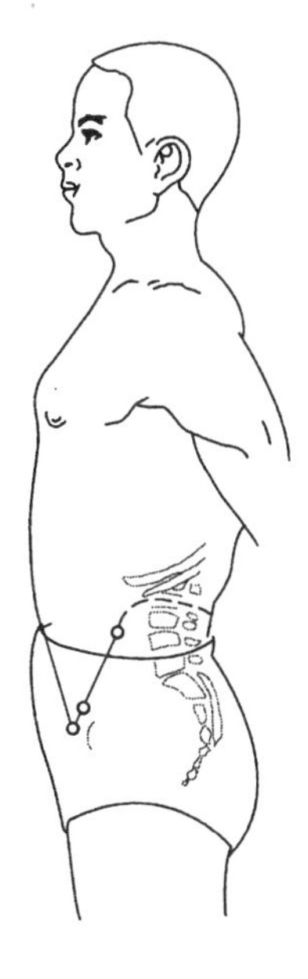

Fig.3-92 Flowing route of the belt vessel

图 3-92 带脉循行示意图

5 Yin link vessel

The Yin link vessel originates from the medial aspect of the lower leg, and goes up along the medial aspect of the thigh to the abdomen to meet the spleen meridian of foot-taiyin; it then reaches the chest and meets the conception vessel at the neck (Fig. 3-93).

5 阴维脉

起于小腿内侧，沿大腿内侧上行到腹部，与足太阴经相合，过胸部，与任脉会于颈部(图 3-93)。

6 Yang link vessel

Yang link vessel originates from the lateral aspect of the heel and emerges from the external malleolus; ascending along the foot-shaoyang meridian, it reaches the hip region; then it goes further upwards along the posterior aspect of hypochondriac and costal regions, and arrives through the posterior axilla at the shoulder and forehead; then it turns

6 阳维脉

起于足跟外侧，向上经过外踝，沿足少阳经上行至髋关节部，经胁肋后侧，从腋后上肩，至前额，再到项后，合于督脉(图 3-94)。

backwards to the back of the neck to meet the governor vessel(Fig. 3-94).

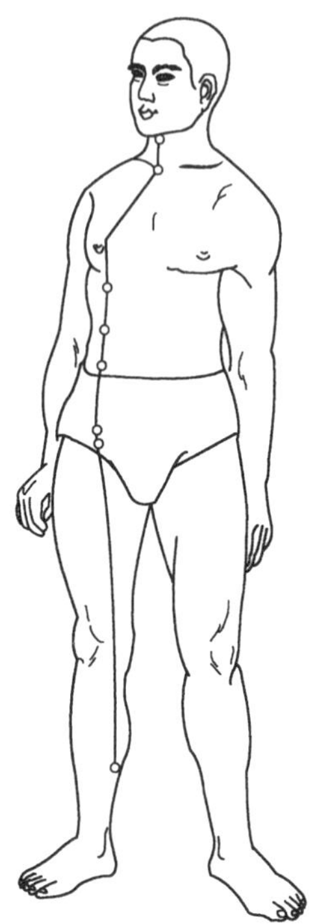

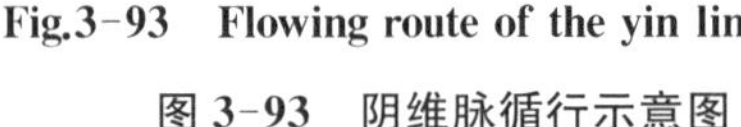

Fig.3-93　Flowing route of the yin link vessel

图 3-93　阴维脉循行示意图

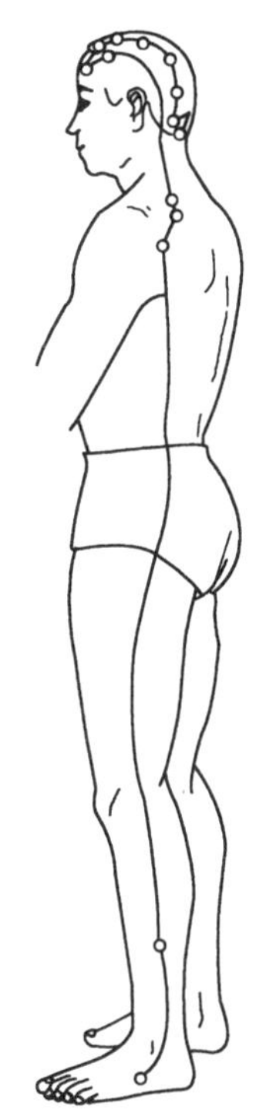

Fig.3-94　Flowing route of the yang link vessel

图 3-94　阳维脉循行示意图

7　Yin heel vessel

Yin heel vessel originates from the posterior aspect of the navicular bone; ascending to the upper portion of the medial malleolus, it goes straight upwards along the medial aspect of the lower leg and thigh to the external genitalia; then it goes upwards along the medial aspect of the chest to enter the supraclavicular fossa, and passes through the front of Renying(ST 7) and cheeks to reach the inner canthus, where it meets the yang heel vessel and the bladder meridian of foot-taiyang(Fig. 3-95).

7　阴蹻脉

起于足舟骨的后方，上行内踝的上面，沿小腿、大腿的内侧直上，经过阴部，向上沿胸部内侧，进入锁骨上窝，上经人迎的前面，过颧部，到目内眦，与足太阳膀胱经和阳蹻脉相会合(图 3-95)。

8 Yang heel vessel

Yang heel vessel originates from the lateral aspect of the heel and runs upwards along the external malleolus and the posterior border of the fibula; then it goes onwards along the lateral side of the thigh and the posterior side of the flank to the shoulder; from there it passes through the neck to the corner of the mouth and enters the inner canthus, where it meets the yin heel vessel; then it runs up along the bladder meridian of foot-taiyang to the forehead and converges at Fengchi (GB 20) with the foot-shaoyang meridian(Fig. 3-96).

8 阳蹻脉

起于足跟外侧，经外踝上行腓骨后缘，沿股外侧和胁后上肩，过颈部上挟口角，进入目内眦，与阴蹻脉会合，再沿足太阳膀胱经上额，与足少阳经合于风池（图 3-96）。

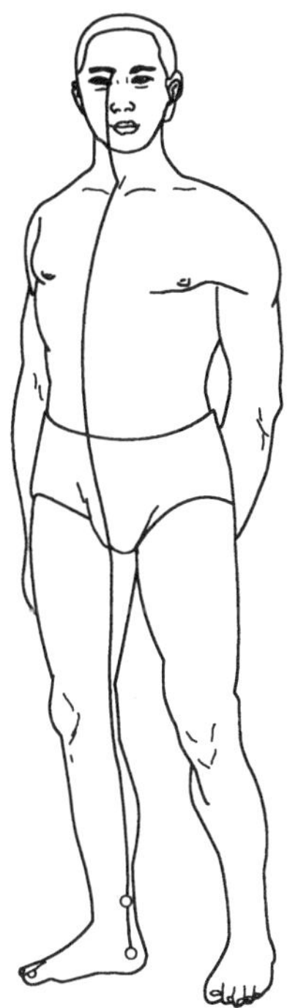

Fig.3-95 Flowing route of the yin heel vessel

图 3-95 阴蹻脉循行示意图

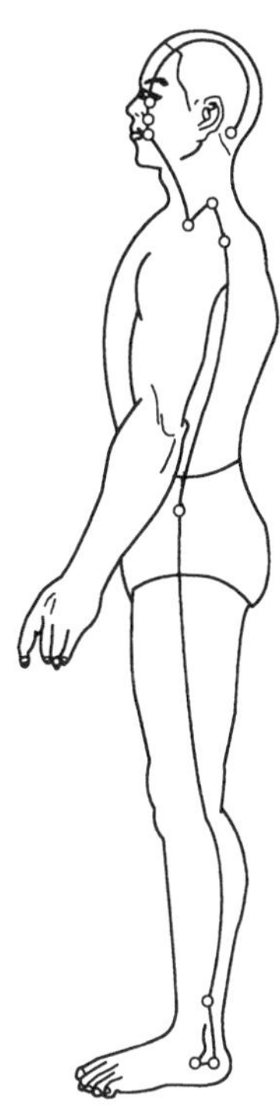

Fig.3-96 Flowing route of the yang heel vessel

图 3-96 阳蹻脉循行示意图

Section 14 Extraordinary Acupoints

1 On head and neck

1.1 Sishencong (EX-HN 1)

Location: On the head, 1 cun respectively anterior, posterior and bilateral to Baihui(GV 20), four acupoints in all(Fig.3-97).

Indications: ① Headache and dizziness; ② insomnia, forgetfulness; ③ epilepsy.

Needling: Puncture transversely 0.5～0.8 cun; moxibustion may be applied.

1.2 Yintang (EX-HN 3)

Location: On the head, in the depression at the midpoint between the medial ends of the eyebrows (Fig.3-98).

Indications: ① Headache, dizziness; ② insomnia, forgetfulness; ③ epilepsy, infantile convulsion; ④ nasal bleeding and sinusitis.

Needling: Puncture transversely 0.3～0.5 cun; or prick to bleed with a three-edged needle.

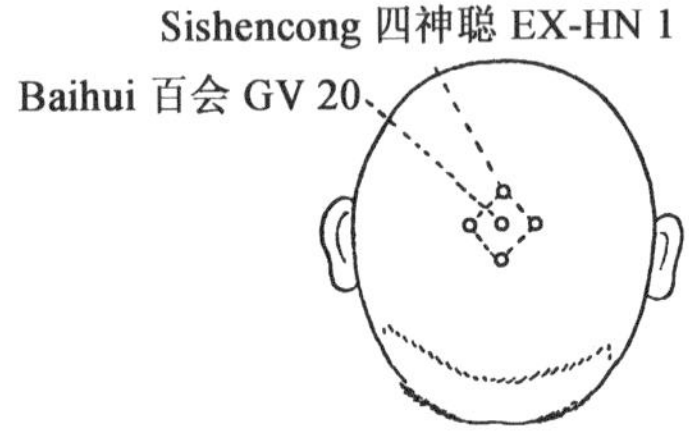

Fig.3-97 Extraordiary acupoints on the head

图 3-97 头顶部奇穴图

1.3 Yuyao (EX-HN 4)

Location: On the head, directly above the pu-

第14节 经外奇穴

1 头颈部穴

1.1 四神聪 Sìshéncōng

定位: 在头部,百会前后左右各旁开1寸,共4穴(图3-97)。

主治: ①头痛,眩晕;②失眠,健忘;③癫痫。

操作: 平刺0.5～0.8寸;可灸。

1.2 印堂 Yìntáng

定位: 在头部,两眉毛内侧端中间的凹陷中(图3-98)。

主治: ①头痛,眩晕;②失眠,健忘;③癫痫,小儿惊风;④鼻衄,鼻渊。

操作: 平刺0.3～0.5寸;或三棱针点刺出血。

Dangyang 当阳 EX-HN 2
Yintang 印堂 EX-HN 3
Yuyao 鱼腰 EX-HN 4
Qiuhou 球后 EX-HN 7
Shangyingxiang 上迎香 EX-HN 8

Fig.3-98 Extraordinary acupoints on the head and face

图 3-98 头面部奇穴图

1.3 鱼腰 Yúyāo

定位: 在头部,瞳孔直

pils, at the midpoint of the eyebrows(Fig.3-98).

Indications: Pain in the supraorbital region, twitching of eyelids, ptosis of eyelids, reddened and swollen eyes, nebula, and deviated mouth and eyes.

Needling: Puncture transversely 0.3～0.5 cun.

上，眉毛中(图 3-98)。

主治： 眉棱骨痛，眼睑瞤动，眼睑下垂，目赤肿痛，目翳，口眼㖞斜。

操作： 平刺 0.3～0.5 寸。

1.4 Taiyang (EX-HN 5)

Location: On the head, in the depression 1 cun posterior to the midpoint between the lateral end of the eyebrow and the outer canthus(Fig.3-99).

Indications: ① Headache, dizziness and insomnia; ② eye disorders and facial paralysis.

Needling: Puncture vertically or obliquely 0.3～0.5 cun; or prick to bleed with a three-edged needle.

1.4 太阳 Tàiyáng

定位： 在头部，眉梢与目外眦之间，向后约一横指的凹陷中(图 3-99)。

主治： ①头痛，眩晕，失眠；②目疾，面瘫。

操作： 直刺或斜刺0.3～0.5 寸；或三棱针点刺出血。

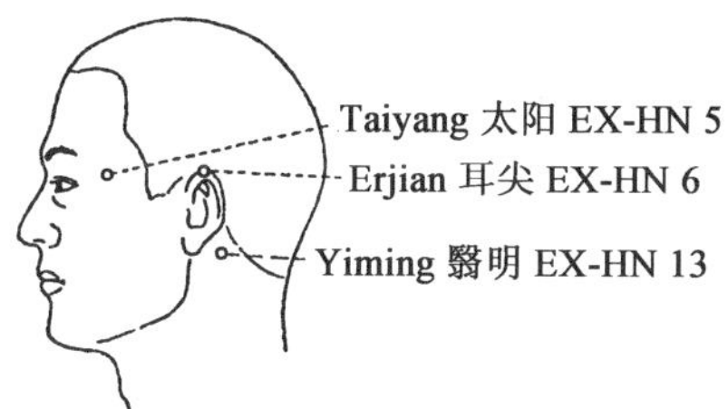

Fig.3-99 Extraordinary acupoints on the head and neck

图 3-99 头颈部奇穴图

1.5 Erjian (EX-HN 6)

Location: On the ear, at the apex of the auricle (Fig.3-99).

Indication: ① Reddened and swollen eyes, stye; ② sore throat; ③ headache and dizziness.

Needling: Puncture vertically 0.1～0.2 cun; or prick to bleed with a three-edged needle.

1.5 耳尖 Ěrjiān

定位： 在耳区，在外耳轮的最高点(图 3-99)。

主治： ①目赤肿痛，麦粒肿；②咽喉肿痛；③头痛，眩晕。

操作： 直刺 0.1～0.2 寸；或三棱针点刺出血。

1.6 Qiuhou (EX-HN 7)

Location: On the face, at the junction of the lateral one-fourth and the medial three-fourths of the infraorbital margin(Fig.3-98).

Indications: Eye disorders.

1.6 球后 Qíuhòu

定位： 在面部，眶下缘外 1/4 与内 3/4 交界处(图 3-98)。

主治： 目疾。

Needling: Gently push the eyeball downwards, puncture 0.5～1.5 cun vertically and slowly along the orbital margin, without lifting and thrusting manipulation.

操作：轻压眼球向下，向眶缘缓慢直刺 0.5～1.5 寸，不提插。

1.7 Shangyingxiang (EX-HN 8)

1.7 上迎香 Shàngyíng xiāng

Location: On the face, at the junction of alar cartilages and turbinate, close to the upper end of nasolabial sulcus(Fig. 3-98).

定位：在面部，鼻翼软骨与鼻甲的交界处，近鼻翼沟上端处(图 3-98)。

Indications: Nasal stuffiness, nasal sinusitis, nasal carbuncles.

主治：鼻塞，鼻渊，鼻部疮疖。

Needling: Puncture 0.3～0.5 cun transversely inwards and upwards.

操作：向内上方平刺 0.3～0.5 寸。

1.8 Neiyingxiang (EX-HN 9)

1.8 内迎香 Nèiyíngxiāng

Location: Inside the nostrils, at the membrane between alar cartilages and turbinate(Fig. 3-100).

定位：在鼻孔内，鼻翼软骨与鼻甲交界的黏膜处(图 3-100)。

Indications: ① Nasal disorders, throat blockage, reddened and swollen eyes; ② febrile conditions, heat-stroke; ③ dizziness and vertigo.

主治：①鼻疾，喉痹，目赤肿痛；②热病，中暑；③眩晕。

Needling: Prick to bleed with a long filiform needle; but this method is not allowed in patients with susceptibility to bleed.

操作：用较长的毫针点刺出血；有出血倾向者忌用。

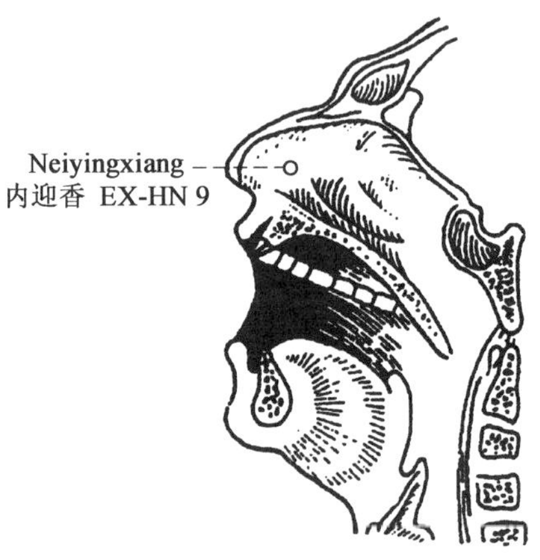

Fig.3-100　Neiyingxiang EX-HN 9

图 3-100　内迎香

1.9 Jinjin and Yuye (EX-HN 12, EX-HN 13)

Location: Inside the oral cavity, on the veins on both sides of the frenulum of the tongue, Jinjin on the left and Yuye on the right(Fig. 3-101).

Indications: ① Canker sore, stiff tongue failing to speak, and swollen tongue; ② vomiting; ③ diabetes.

Needling: Prick to bleed.

1.9 金津、玉液 Jīnjīn, Yùyè

定位: 在口腔内,舌下系带两侧的静脉上,左为金津、右为玉液(图 3-101)。

主治: ① 口疮,舌强不语,舌肿;②呕吐;③消渴。

操作: 点刺出血。

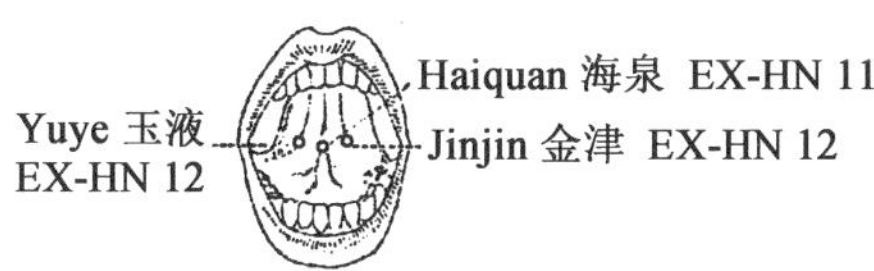

Fig.3-101 Extraordinary acupoints below the tongue

图 3-101 舌底部奇穴图

1.10 Yiming (EX-HN 14)

Location: On the neck, 1 cun posterior to Yifeng(TE 17) (Fig. 3-99).

Indications: Headache, dizziness, insomnia and tinnitus.

Needling: Puncture vertically 0.5～1.0 cun.

1.10 翳明 Yìmíng

定位: 在颈部,翳风后 1 寸(图 3-99)。

主治: 头痛,眩晕,失眠,耳鸣。

操作: 直刺 0.5～1.0 寸。

2 On trunk

2 躯干部穴

2.1 Zigong (EX-CA 1)

Location: On lower abdomen, 4 cun below the navel and 3 cun lateral to the anterior midline(Fig. 3-102).

Indications: Prolapse of the uterus, irregular menstruation, menstrual cramps, uterine bleeding and infertility.

Needling: Puncture vertically 0.8～1.2 cun.

2.1 子宫 Zǐgōng

定位: 在下腹部,脐中下 4 寸,前正中线旁开 3 寸(图 3-102)。

主治: 子宫脱垂,月经不调,痛经,崩漏,不孕。

操作: 直刺 0.8～1.2 寸。

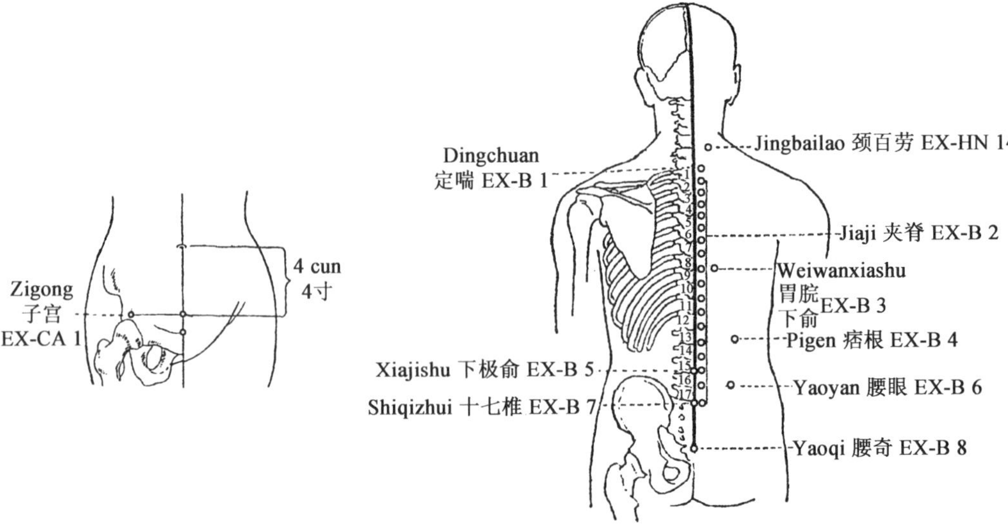

Fig.3-102 Extraordinary acupoints on the abdomen

图 3-102 腹部奇穴图

Fig.3-103 Extraordinary acupoints on the back

图 3-103 背腰部奇穴图

2.2 Dingchuan (EX-B 1)

Location: On the upper back, at the level with the lower spinous process of the seventh cervical vertebra, 0.5 cun bilateral to the posterior midline (Fig.3-103).

Indications: ① Asthma and cough; ② stiff neck and pain in the shoulder and back.

Needling: Puncture vertically 0.5～0.8 cun.

2.3 Jiaji (EX-B 2)

Location: On the upper back, 0.5 cun bilateral to the lower border of the spinous processes from the first thoracic vertebra to the fifth lumbar vertebra, 17 acupoints in each side(Fig.3-103).

Indications: ① Jiaji from the first to fifth thoracic vertebrae: disorders of the heart, lung, chest and upper limbs; ② Jiaji from the sixth to twelfth

2.2 定喘 Dìngchuǎn

定位：在脊柱区，横平第7颈椎棘突下，后正中线旁开0.5寸(图3-103)。

主治：①哮喘，咳嗽；②落枕，肩背痛。

操作：直刺0.5～0.8寸。

2.3 夹脊 Jiájǐ

定位：在脊柱区，第1胸椎至第5腰椎棘突下两侧，后正中线旁开0.5寸，一侧17穴(图3-103)。

主治：主治范围较广泛，其中①胸1～5夹脊：心肺、胸部及上肢疾病；②胸6～12

thoracic vertebrae: disorders of the stomach, intestine, liver, spleen and gallbladder; ③ Jiaji from the first to fifth lumbar vertebrae: disorders of the lower limbs, waist, sacrum and lower abdomen.

夹脊：胃肠、肝、脾、胆疾病；③腰1～5夹脊：下肢疼痛，腰、骶、小腹部疾病。

Needling: Puncture obliquely 0.5～1.0 cun; correct needling angle and depth should be stressed so as to avoid injuring the internal organs or cause pneumothoax; plum-blossom needles may be applied to tap these acupoints.

操作： 斜刺0.5～1.0寸。注意进针的角度和深度，以防刺伤内脏或引起气胸；也可用梅花针叩刺。

2.4 Weiwanxiashu (EX-B 3)

2.4 胃脘下俞 Wèiwǎnxiàshū

Location: On the back, at the level with the lower border of the spinous process of the eighth thoracic vertebra and 1.5 cun bilateral to the posterior midline(Fig.3-103).

定位： 在脊柱区，横平第8胸椎棘突下，后正中线旁开1.5寸(图3-103)。

Indications: ① Stomachache, abdominal pain and flank pain; ② diabetes.

主治： ①胃痛，腹痛，胸胁痛；②消渴。

Needling: Puncture obliquely 0.3～0.5 cun.

操作： 斜刺0.3～0.5寸。

2.5 Yaoyan (EX-B 6)

2.5 腰眼 Yāoyǎn

Location: On the low back, at the level with the lower border of the spinous process of fourth lumbar vertebra and 3.5 cun bilateral to the posterior midline(Fig.3-103).

定位： 在腰区，横平第4腰椎棘突下，后正中线旁开约3.5寸凹陷中(图3-103)。

Indications: ① Lumbago; ② irregular menstruation and morbid leucorrhea.

主治： ①腰痛；②月经不调，带下。

Needling: Puncture vertically 1.0～1.5 cun.

操作： 直刺1.0～1.5寸。

2.6 Shiqizhui (EX-B 7)

2.6 十七椎 Shíqīzhuī

Location: On the lower back, in the depression below the spinous process of the fifth lumbar vertebra(Fig.3-103).

定位： 在腰区，第5腰椎棘突下凹陷中(图3-103)。

Indications: ① Irregular menstruation, menstrual cramps, uterine bleeding; ② pain in the loin and legs, and paralysis of the lower limbs.

主治： ①月经不调，痛经，崩漏；②腰腿痛，下肢瘫痪。

Needling: Puncture vertically 0.5～1.0 cun.

操作： 直刺0.5～1.0寸。

2.7 Yaoqi (EX-B 8)

Location: On the sacrum, 2 cun directly above the tip of the coccyx, in the depression between sacral horns(Fig.3-103).

Indications: ① Epilepsy, headache and insomnia; ② constipation.

Needling: Puncture transversely upwards 1.0～1.5 cun.

2.7 腰奇 Yāoqí

定位: 在骶区,尾骨端直上2寸,骶角之间凹陷中(图3-103)。

主治: ①癫痫,头痛,失眠;②便秘。

操作: 向上平刺1.0～1.5寸。

3 On limbs

3.1 Zhoujian (EX-UE 1)

Location: On the tip of the ulnar olecranon when the elbow is flexed(Fig.3-104).

Indication: Carbuncle.

Needling: 7～15 maxa cones with moxibustion.

3 四肢部穴

3.1 肘尖 Zhǒujiān

定位: 在肘后区,尺骨鹰嘴的尖端(图3-104)。

主治: 痈疽。

操作: 艾炷灸7～15壮。

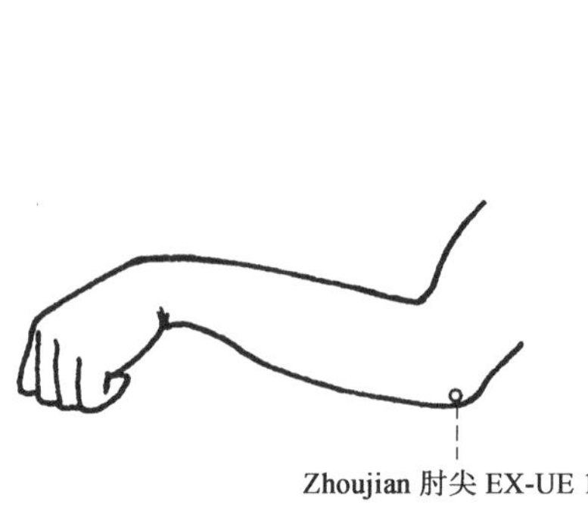

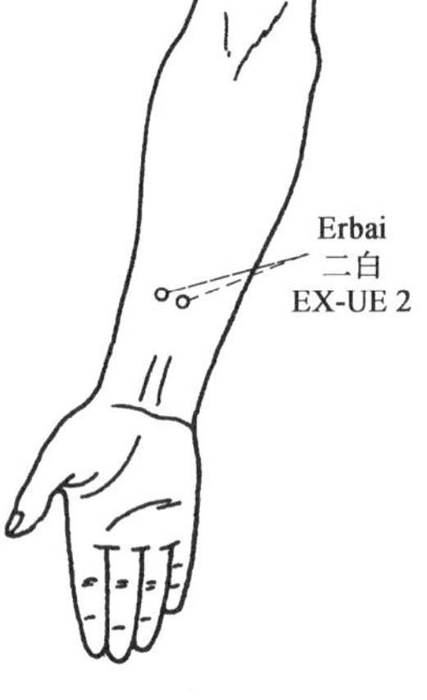

Fig.3-104　Extraordinary acupoints on the upper limb

图3-104　上肢奇穴图

3.2 Erbai (EX-UE 2)

Location: On the forearm, 4 cun above the transverse crease of the wrist, on both sides of the tendon of the muscle flexor carpi radialis, two acupoints in each side (Fig.3-104).

Indications: ① Hemorrhoids and prolapse of

3.2 二白 Èrbái (EX-UE 2)

定位: 在前臂前区,腕掌侧远端横纹上4寸,桡侧腕屈肌腱的两侧,一肢2穴(图3-104)。

主治: ①痔疾,脱肛;

rectum; ② pain in the chest and flank.

Needling: Puncture vertically 0.5～0.8 cun.

3.3 Zhongkui (EX-UE 4)

Location: On the midpoint of the proximal interphalangeal joint of the middle finger at the dorsal aspect(Fig.3-105).

Indications: Dysphagia, vomiting, hiccup and poor appetite.

Needling: Puncture vertically 0.2～0.3 cun; 5～7 moxa cones with moxibustion.

3.4 Yaotongdian (EX-UE 7)

Location: On the dorsum of the hand, midpoint between the transverse wrist crease and metacarpophalangeal joint, between the second and third metacarpal bones, and between the fourth and fifth metacarpal bones, 2 acupoints in each hand(Fig.3-106).

Indications: Acute lumbar sprain.

Needling: Puncture obliquely 0.5～0.8 cun toward the center of the palm.

3.5 Wailaogong (EX-UE 8)

Location: On the dorsum of hand, between the second and third metacarpal bones, and in the depression 0.5 cun below metacarpophalangeal joints(Fig.3-106).

Indications: ① Stiff neck; ② swelling and pain in the arms.

Needling: Puncture vertically 0.5～0.8 cun.

3.6 Baxie (EX-UE 9)

Location: On the dorsum of the hand, at the junction of the red and white skin of the hand webs, 8 acupoints in all(Fig.3-105).

Indications: ① Swelling and pain in the dorsum of hand, and numbness of fingers; ② vexation feverish; ③ painful eyes; poisonous snake bites.

②胸胁痛。

操作：直刺0.5～0.8寸。

3.3 中魁 Zhōngkuí

定位：在手指，中指背面，近侧指间关节的中点处(图3-105)。

主治：噎膈，呕吐，呃逆，食欲不振。

操作：直刺0.2～0.3寸；或艾炷灸5～7壮。

3.4 腰痛点 Yāotòngdiǎn

定位：在手背，第2、3掌骨间及第4、5掌骨间，腕背侧远端横纹与掌指关节的中点处，一手2穴(图3-106)。

主治：急性腰扭伤。

操作：由两侧向掌中斜刺0.5～0.8寸。

3.5 外劳宫 Wàiláogōng

定位：在手背，第2、3掌骨间，掌指关节后0.5寸(指寸)凹陷中(图3-106)。

主治：①落枕；②手臂肿痛。

操作：直刺0.5～0.8寸。

3.6 八邪 Bāxié

定位：在手背，第1～5指间，指蹼缘后方赤白肉际处，左右共8穴(图3-105)。

主治：①手背肿痛，手指麻木；②烦热；③目痛；④毒蛇咬伤。

Needling: Puncture obliquely 0.5～0.8 cun; or prick to bleed.

操作：斜刺0.5～0.8寸；或点刺出血。

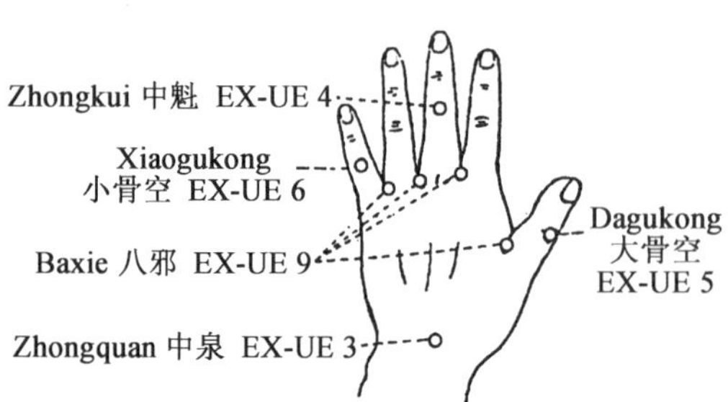

Fig.3-105 Extraordinary acupoints on the dorsum of hand

图3-105 手背部奇穴图

Wailaogong 外劳宫 EX-UE 8
Yaotongdian 腰痛点 EX-UE 7

Fig.3-106 Extraordinary acupoints on the dorsum of hand

图3-106 手背部奇穴图

3.7 Sifeng (EX-UE 10)

Location: On the palmar surface, in the midpoint of the transverse crease of the proximal interphalangeal joints of the second to fifth fingers, 4 acupoints in each hand (Fig.3-107).

Indications: ①Infantile malnutrition; ② whooping cough.

Needling: Prick to cause bleeding, or squeeze out some yellowish-whitish viscous fluid.

3.7 四缝 Sìfèng

定位：在手指，第2～5指掌面的近侧指间关节横纹的中央，一手4穴（图3-107）。

主治：①小儿疳积；②百日咳。

操作：点刺出血或挤出少许黄白色透明黏液。

3.8 Shixuan (EX-UE 11)

Location: On the tips of the ten fingers, about 0.1 cun distal to the nails, 10 acupoints in each hand (Fig.3-107).

Indications: ① Coma and high fever; ② sore throat; ③ epilepsy; ④ finger numbness.

Needling: Puncture shallowly 0.1～0.2 cun; or prick to bleed with a three-edged needle.

3.8 十宣 Shíxuān

定位：在手指，十指尖端，距指甲游离缘0.1寸（指寸），左右共10穴（图3-107）。

主治：①昏迷，高热；②咽喉肿痛；③癫痫；④手指麻木。

操作：浅刺0.1～0.2寸；或三棱针点刺出血。

3.9 Heding (EX-LE 2)

Location: In the depression at the midpoint of the upper border of the petella(Fig.3-108).

Indications: Knee pain, weakness of legs and paralysis.

Needling: Puncture vertically 0.8～1.0 cun.

3.9 鹤顶 Hèdǐng

定位：在膝前区，髌骨底中点的上方凹陷中（图3-108）。

主治：膝痛，腿足无力，瘫痪。

操作：直刺0.8～1.0寸。

3.10 Baichongwo (EX-LE 3)

Location: On the front thigh, 3 cun above the median-upper border of the petella(Fig.3-108).

Indications: ① Itching skin, ulcers in the lower body, wind wheals and urticaria; ② parasitic diseases.

Needling: Puncture vertically 1.5～2.0 cun.

3.10 百虫窝 Bǎichóngwō

定位：在股前区，髌骨底内侧端上3寸(图3-108)。

主治：①皮肤瘙痒，下部生疮，风疹，湿疹；②虫积。

操作：直刺1.5～2.0寸。

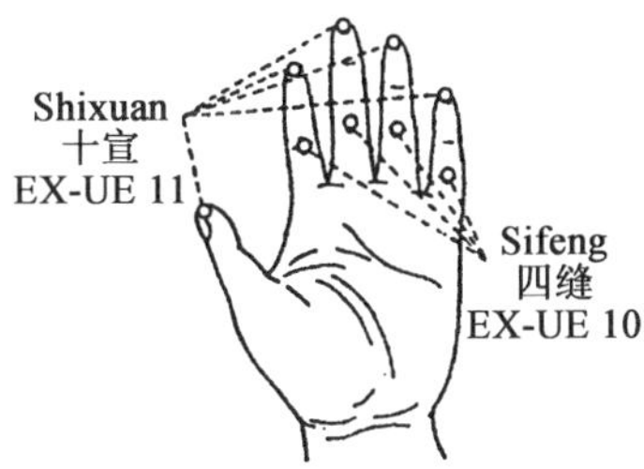

Fig.3-107 Extraordinary acupoints on the palm

图3-107 手掌部奇穴图

3.11 Neixiyan (EX-LE 5)

Location: In the depression medial to the patellar ligament(Fig.3-108).

Indications: Knee pain and paralysis of the lower limbs.

Needling: Puncture 0.5～1.0 cun outwards at the angle of 45°.

3.11 内膝眼 Nèixīyǎn

定位：在膝部，髌韧带内侧凹陷处的中央(图3-108)。

主治：膝痛，下肢痿痹。

操作：从前内向后外与额状面成45°角斜刺0.5～1.0寸。

3.12 Dannang (EX-LE 6)

Location: On the lateral aspect of lower leg, 2 cun directly below the capitulum fibulae(Fig.3-108).

3.12 胆囊 Dǎnnáng

定位：在小腿外侧，腓骨小头直下2寸(图3-108)。

Indications: ① Acute and chronic cholecystitis, cholelithiasis, biliary ascariasis and colic; ② paralysis of the lower limbs.

Needling: Puncture vertically 1.0～2.0 cun.

主治: ①急慢性胆囊炎，胆石症，胆绞痛，胆道蛔虫症；②下肢痿痹。

操作: 直刺 1.0～2.0 寸。

3.13 Lanwei (EX-LE 7)

Location: On the lateral side of the lower leg, 5 cun below the depression lateral to the the patellar ligament and one-finger breadth lateral to the anterior crest of tibia(Fig.3-108).

Indications: ① Acute and chronic appendicitis; ② indigestion; ③ paralysis of the lower limbs.

Needling: Puncture vertically 1.5～2.0 cun.

3.13 阑尾 Lánwěi

定位: 在小腿外侧，髌韧带外侧凹陷下 5 寸，胫骨前嵴外一横指（中指）（图 3-108）。

主治: ①急慢性阑尾炎；②消化不良；③下肢痿痹。

操作: 直刺 1.5～2.0 寸。

3.14 Neihuaijian (EX-LE 8)

Location: At the tip of medial malleolus (Fig.3-108).

Indications: ① Toothache and sore throat; ② inability to speech in children; ③ cramps.

Needling: Puncture is not allowed, and moxibustion is often applied.

3.14 内踝尖 Nèihuáijiān (EX-LE 8)

定位: 在踝区，内踝的最凸起处(图 3-108)。

主治: ① 牙痛，咽喉肿痛；②小儿不语；③转筋。

操作: 禁刺；常用灸法。

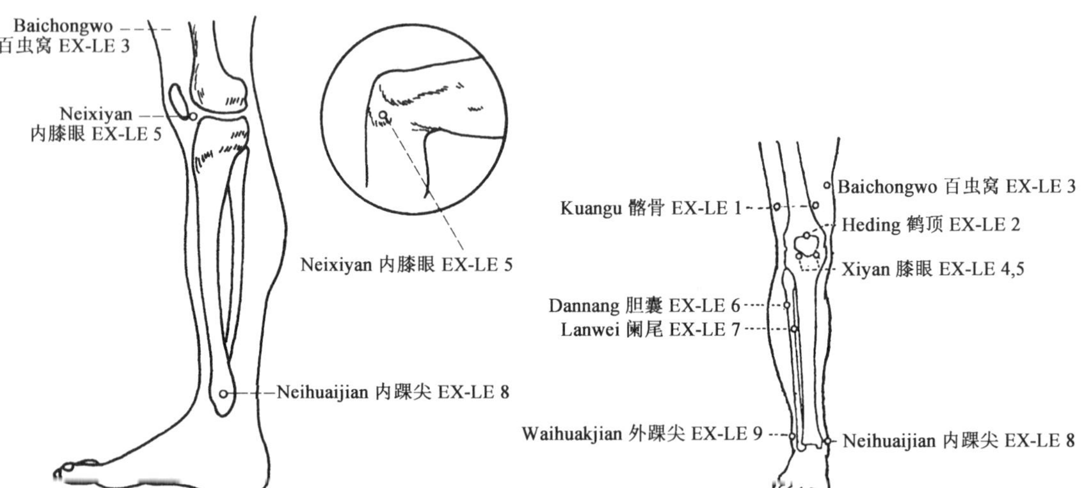

Fig.3-108 Extraordinary acupoints on the lower limb

图 3-108 下肢部奇穴图

3.15 Waihuaijian (EX-LE 9)

Location: At the tip of external malleolus (Fig.3-108).

Indications: ① Toe convulsion, and leg cramps; ② beriberi; ③ toothache.

Needling: Puncture is not allowed, and moxibustion is often applied.

3.15 外踝尖 Wàihuáijiān

定位: 在踝区,外踝的最凸起处(图 3-108)。

主治: ①足趾拘急,足外廉转筋;②脚气;③牙痛。

操作: 禁刺;常用灸法。

3.16 Bafeng (EX-LE 10)

Location: On the dorsum of the foot, at the junction of the red and white skin of the foot webs, 8 acupoints in all(Fig.3-109).

Indications: ① Swelling and pain in the dorsum of the foot, and toe pain; ② poisonous snakebites; ③ beriberi.

Needling: Puncture obliquely 0.5～0.8 cun; or prick to bleed.

3.16 八风 Bāfēng

定位: 在足背,第 1～5 趾间,趾蹼缘后方赤白肉际处,左右共 8 穴(图 3-109)。

主治: ① 足跗肿痛,趾痛;②毒蛇咬伤;③脚气。

操作: 斜刺 0.5～0.8 寸;或点刺出血。

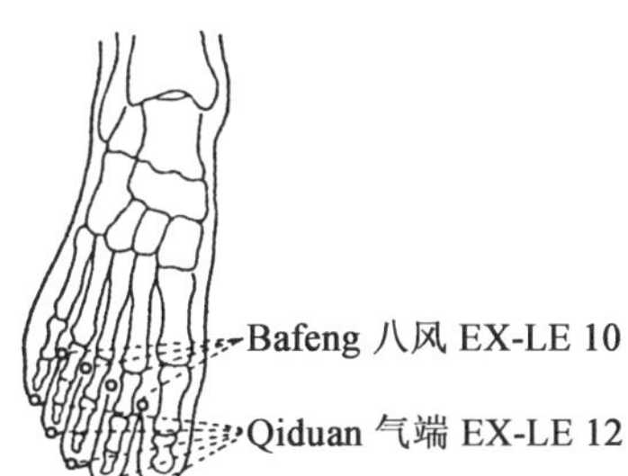

Fig.3-109 Extraordinary acupoints on the foot

图 3-109 足部奇穴图

3.17 Qiduan (EX-LE 12)

Location: At the tips of the ten toes, 0.1 cun anterior to the nails, 10 acupoints in all (Fig. 3-109).

Indications: ① Toe numbness, and swelling and pain in the dorsum of the foot; ② stroke.

Needling: Puncture vertically 0.1～0.2 cun.

3.17 气端 Qìduān

定位: 在足趾,十趾端的中央,距趾甲游离缘 0.1 寸(指寸),左右共 10 穴(图 3-109)。

主治: ①足趾麻木,足背红肿疼痛;②卒中。

操作: 直刺 0.1～0.2 寸。

Chapter 4 Filiform Needling Techniques

第4章 毫针刺法

Section 1 Structure and Specification of Filiform Needles

第1节 毫针的材料、结构和规格

1 Structure of a filiform needle

In ancient times, a filiform needle is made of stone, and thereafter of bone, bamboo, gold, silver, copper, steel, etc. In modern times, a filiform needle is primarily made of stainless steel, since the stainless steel is of good elasticity, toughness and strength.

In structure, a filifirm needle is divided into five parts: needle tip, needle shaft, needle root, needle handle and needle tail(Fig. 4-1).

1 毫针的材料和构造

古代最早的针具由砭石制成，其后有骨针、竹针及金、银、铜、铁等金属针。现代临床所用的毫针多由不锈钢制成，因不锈钢毫针具有较好的弹性、韧性和强度。

毫针的结构可分为5个部分，即针尖、针身、针根、针柄、针尾(图4-1)。

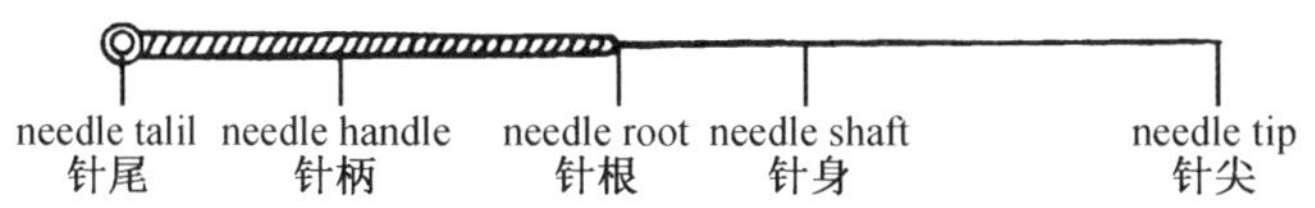

Fig.4-1 Structure of a filiform needle

图 4-1 毫针的结构

2 Specification of a filiform needle

The specification of a needle refers to the length of the needle body and its diameter. The

2 毫针的规格

毫针的规格主要指针身的长短和粗细，以毫米为计量

length and diameter are listed as follows(Tables 4-1, 4-2). The commonly used needle is of 40 mm and 75 mm in length and 0.30 mm and 0.25 mm in diameter.

单位。现将其长短、粗细规格分别列表如下(表 4-1，4-2)。其中临床较为常用的长度是 40 毫米和 75 毫米，粗细是直径 0.30 毫米和 0.25 毫米。

Table 4-1 The length of filiform needles
表 4-1 毫针的长度规格

Length(mm) 长度(毫米)	13	25	40	50	60	75	100	115	125

Table 4-2 The diameter of filiform needles
表 4-2 毫针的粗细规格

Diameter(mm) 直径(毫米)	0.45	0.40	0.35	0.30	0.25	0.22	0.20	0.18	0.16

Section 2 Filiform Needling Practice

第 2 节 毫针刺法的训练

Filiform needling practice refers to practising the needling manipulations of filiform needles, which is essential to skillful needle insertion and manipulation, and improvement of clinical efficacy. The practice comprises of practising finger force and manipulation techniques.

毫针刺法的训练是指毫针操作基本功的训练，它是熟练进针、行针和提高疗效的基本保证。主要包括指力和手法的训练。

1 Practising finger force

The finger force can be practised on packet of papers. Fold some soft tissue paper into a small packet about 8 cm in length, 5 cm in breadth and 3 cm in thickness, surround it with gauze and then bind it with

1 指力训练

指力的训练需在纸垫上进行。可用松软的纸张，折叠做成长 8 厘米、宽 5 厘米、厚约 3 厘米的纸垫，再用线如“井”字形扎紧。练针时，左手平执纸垫，右手持针使针垂直抵于纸

thread into the shape of the Chinese character "井". In practising needling, hold the packet horizontally in the left hand, and place the needle right on the packet and then rotate the handle with the right thumb, index and middle fingers clockwise and counter-clockwise with increasing pressure till the needle penetrates through the packet. Repeat the same practice at another place, again and again(Fig. 4-2).

垫，然后拇、食、中指来回捻转针柄，并渐加压力，待针刺透纸垫后，再换一处如前锻炼指力(图 4-2)。

2　Practising manipulation techniques

2.1　Practising with a cotton ball

Wrap some cotton into a cushion about 7 cm in diameter and surround it with gauze. The cotton cushion is soft and suitable for practising many manipulation techniques (Fig. 4-3).

2　手法训练

2.1　棉团练针

取棉絮一团，外包棉布一层，缝制成直径约 7 厘米的棉球。棉团柔软，可以用来练习各种进针、行针等毫针操作手法(图 4-3)。

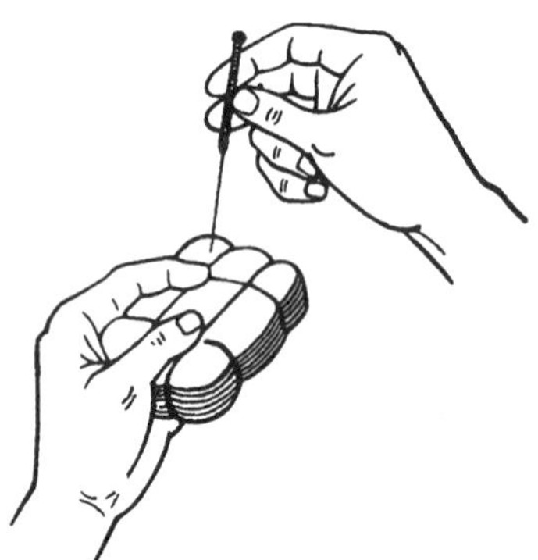

Fig. 4-2　Needling practice with paper packet

图 4-2　纸垫练针

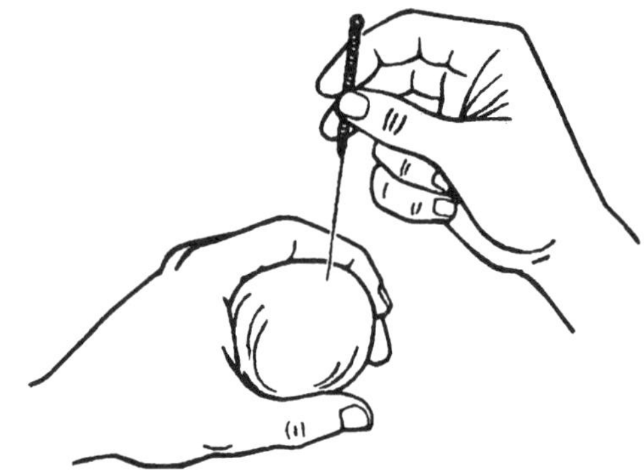

Fig. 4-3　Needling practice with cotton cushion

图 4-3　棉团练针

2.2　Practising on human body

After needling practice on paper packet and cotton cushion, it is necessary to practise needling on human body as clinical practice. The practice may be performed on one's own body and/or other body,

2.2　人体练针

在纸垫和棉团练针的基础上，模拟临床实际进行人体实训操作。自身练针和相互练针可交替进行，以先四

first on the limbs, then on the head and face, and finally on the trunk to gain experience in controlling insertion methods, needling depth, needling angle, needling direction and differing techniques of promoting qi, moving qi and reinforcing-reducing techniques.

肢、后头面、再躯干穴位的方式循序渐进，掌握不同穴位的进针手法、针刺深度、角度和方向，以及催气、行气、补泻等各种操作手法。

Section 3 Preparations Before Acupuncture

第3节 针刺前的准备

1 Explanation prior to acupuncture

At the first-visit acupuncture, some patients may experience fear or nervous, or worry about puncturing the acupoints on the head, face, chest and abdomen, so the acupuncturists should make necessary explanation, especially for the possible pain and needling sensation, so as to eliminate their nervous tension and fear. Only the patients are relaxed can acupuncture treatment be given.

1 针前解释

初次接受针刺治疗的患者会对针刺有惧怕或紧张心理，或对头面、胸腹等部位的穴位针刺存在顾虑，医生应该作适当的解释工作，尤其需要对进针时可能出现的微痛或针刺过程中产生的得气感应进行解释，消除患者的紧张情绪和恐惧心理，在机体放松的情况下再给予针刺治疗。

2 Choice of a needle

Nowadays the most commonly used needles are made of stainless steel. The needle tip is required as sharp but smooth and pointed like a pine needle; the needle body should be smooth, straight, flexible and well-proportioned. Furthermore, needles of differing length and diameter are chosen on the basis of the patient's constitution, age, build and treatment areas. Generally speaking, a relatively thick and long needle is suitable for a person who is well built or insensitive to needling, or for acupoints on thick muscles; a thin and short needle is suitable

2 针具选择

目前临床多采用不锈钢的针具，针尖要求尖中带圆，圆而不钝，形如松针，针身要求挺直滑利，圆正匀称。此外，应根据患者的体质、年龄、胖瘦及针刺部位等因素，来选择使用不同规格的针具。一般而言，体壮形胖，皮肉丰厚处的穴位，或针感较迟钝的患者，可选较粗、较长的毫针；体弱形瘦，皮肉浅薄处的穴位，

for a person who is thin or children or sensitive to needling, or for the acupoints on thin muscles.

幼儿，或针感较敏感的患者，可选较细、较短的毫针。

3　Choice of posture

An appropriate posture for the patient is important for the correct location of acupoints, insertion and manipulation of needles, and also in preventing acupuncture accidents. In principle, the best posture facilitates the acupuncturists to correctly locate acupoints and perform needling, and enable patients to feel comfortable and maintain for a long time. Also, the patient is advised not to move his/her body during acupuncture treatment to avoid bending or even breaking a needle. The lying position is usualy to be preferred, especially for those patients who have never been treated by acupuncture before, or who are elderly, deficient or nervous to prevent acupuncture fainting. There are five commonly used postures adopted in clinical practice.

3　体位选择

针刺时患者体位的选择是否适当，对正确取穴和针刺施术及避免针刺意外都有影响。体位的选择，应以便于医者能正确取穴、针刺施术，患者感到舒适自然，并能持久为原则。并应叮嘱患者在针刺和留针过程中切不可移动体位，以免弯针、断针等意外发生。凡年老、体弱、精神过度紧张和初次接受针刺的患者，应考虑卧位，以防晕针。临床常用的体位有五种。

Supine posture　Suitable for acupoints on the head, face, neck, chest and abdomen, and some acupoints on the four limbs(Fig. 4-4).

仰卧位：适用于取头、面、颈、胸、腹部和部分四肢部的腧穴（图 4-4）。

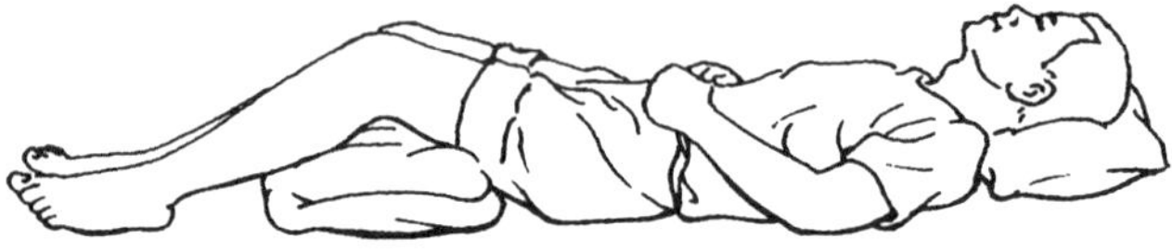

Fig.4-4　Supine posture

图 4-4　仰卧位

Lateral recumbent　Suitable for acupoints on the lateral side of the head, chest and abdomen, and some acupoints on the lateral side of limbs(Fig. 4-5).

侧卧位：适用于取侧头、侧胸、侧腹和部分四肢部的腧穴（图 4-5）。

Prone posture　Suitable for acupoints on the head, neck, back, lumbosacral and hip regions, and some acupoints on the four limbs(Fig. 4-6).

俯卧位：适用于取头、项、背、腰骶、臀和部分四肢部的腧穴（图 4-6）。

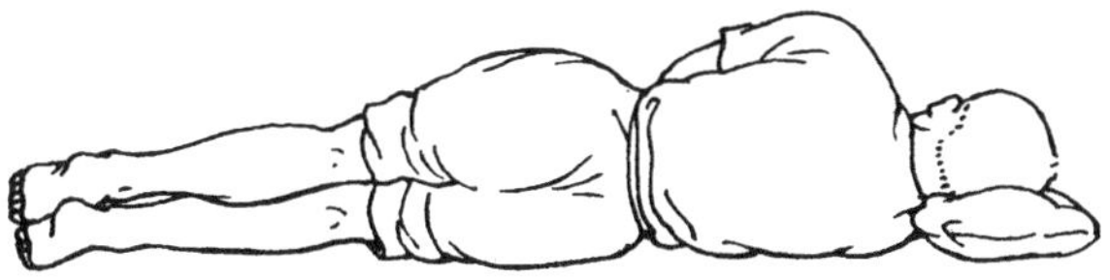

Fig.4-5 Lateral recumbent

图 4-5 侧卧位

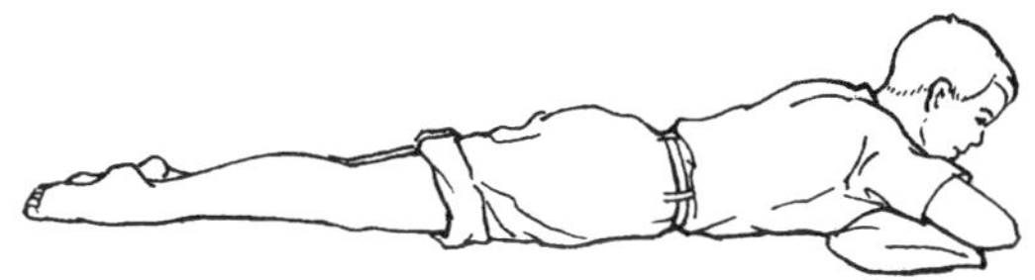

Fig.4-6 Prone posture

图 4-6 俯卧位

Sitting-reclining Suitable for acupoints on the anterior head, lateral head, face, neck and upper chest, and some acupoints on the four limbs(Fig. 4-7).

Sitting in flexion Suitable for acupoints on the posterior head, nape, shoulder and upper back, and some acupoints on the four limbs(Fig. 4-8).

仰靠坐位:适用于取前头、侧头、面、颈、上胸部和部分四肢部的腧穴(图 4-7)。

俯伏坐位:适用于取后头、项、肩、上背部和部分四肢部的腧穴(图 4-8)。

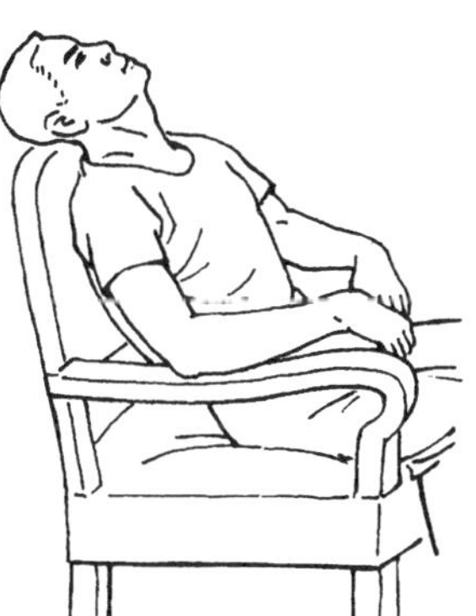

Fig.4-7 Sitting-reclining

图 4-7 仰靠坐位

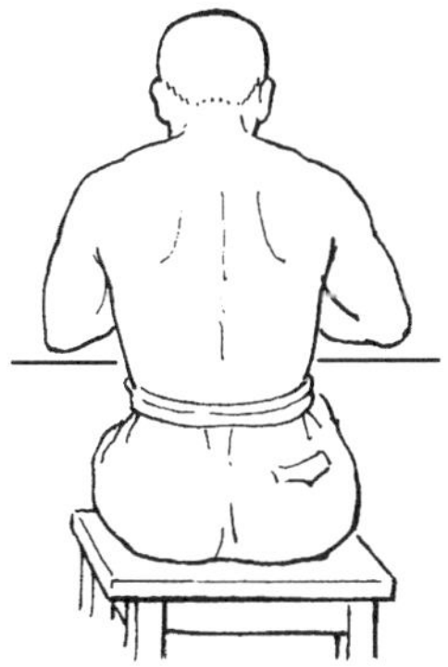

Fig.4-8 Sitting in flexion

图 4-8 俯伏坐位

4 Sterilization

Before the needles are inserted into the acupoints, sterilization must be applied. This includes

4 消毒

针刺治疗必须严格做好消毒工作,包括针具器械、医

the sterilization of the needles, the practitioner's fingers, the area around the acupoints and the therapeutic room.

者手指、施术部位及治疗室的消毒。

4.1 Needle sterilization

According to acupuncture rules, the aseptic disposable needles are adopted.

4.1 针具器械消毒

按规定使用一次性无菌针具。

4.2 Sterilization of practitioner's fingers

Before acupuncture, the practitioner should wash his/her hands with soap and rub the hands with 75% alcohol-soaked cotton balls.

4.2 医者手指消毒

医者在针刺前，须先用肥皂水将手洗净，待干后再用75%乙醇棉球涂擦，然后才可持针施术。

4.3 Sterilization of area around acupoint

The area on the body surface selected for needling should be sterilized by scraping the skin with 75% alcohol-soaked cotton balls in a circular manner from the center of the acupoint to the outside. Keep the sterilized area clean from dirt and contamination.

4.3 施术部位消毒

在患者需要针刺的部位，用75%的乙醇棉球，从中心点向外绕圈拭擦即可。消毒之处须避免接触污物，以防重新污染。

4.4 Sterilization of therapeutic room

The sheet and pillow towel on the therapeutic bed should be replaced in time if they are not disposable. The discarded medical objects like needles and cotton ball should be disposed differently from household garbage. After one-day treatments, the therapeutic room ought to be disinfected and its air circulated.

4.4 治疗室消毒

治疗床上的床单、枕巾等物品如非采用一次性的，要按时更换。使用过的针具、棉球等医用弃置物品要和生活垃圾分开处置。一天治疗结束后要对治疗室进行消毒，并保持空气流通。

Section 4 Needling Methods

第4节 针刺方法

1 Insertion

Insertion means piercing the skin with needle into the acupoint, and insertion of the needle should be swift. The right hand holding the needle is

1 进针法

进针法是指将针刺入皮肤的方法。其操作要点如古人所言：针入贵速。我们将

known as "puncturing hand", while the left hand pressing firmly on the area close to the acupoint with the finger nail and help to support the needle body, is known as "pressing hand". The correct method is to hold the handle of the needle with the thumb and index fingers, and the middle and ring fingers against the lower end of the needle body, with exposure to 2 mm of needle tip(Fig. 4-9). The commonly used needle-inserting methods are listed below.

持针操作的手称为"刺手"，而爪切按压所刺部位，或辅助针身，协助刺手进针的手称为"押手"。持针时，一般以右手拇、食二指指腹相对夹持针柄，中指和无名指抵住针身下端，针尖露出约2毫米(图4-9)。常用的的进针方法有单手进针和双手进针。

1.1 Inserting needle with one hand

In this method, the needle is held by one hand to insert into the skin. Hold the needle handle with the thumb and index fingers, and the lower needle body with the middle and ring fingers pressing on the acupoint. The needle can then be inserted quickly into the skin by exerting the force from the thumb and the index fingers. This method is suitable for the insertion of short needle(Fig. 4-10).

1.1 单手进针法

即单用刺手将针刺入穴位的方法。操作时以右手拇、食指夹持针柄，中指和无名指抵住针身下端，无名指指端靠近穴位，针尖轻抵穴位皮肤，然后通过拇、食指持针快速下插，使针尖刺透皮肤。适用于短针的进针(图4-10)。

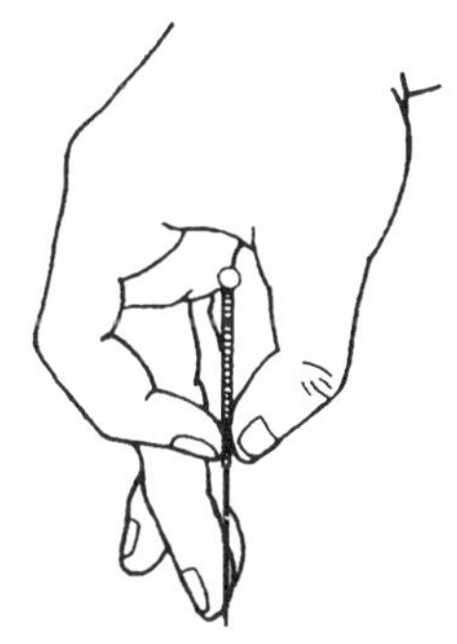

Fig.4-9 Holding the needle

图4-9 持针姿势

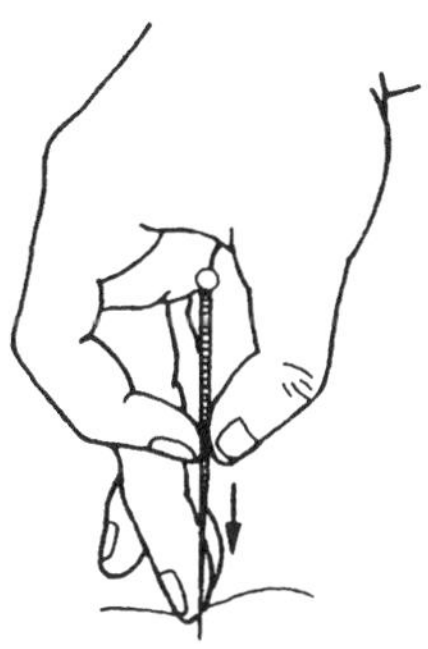

Fig.4-10 Inserting needle with one hand

图4-10 单手进针法

1.2 Inserting needle with both hands

1.2.1 Inserting the needle aided by pressing with the finger-nail Press the skin beside the acupoint with the nails of the thumb or index fingers of the left

1.2 双手进针法

1.2.1 指切进针法 以左手拇指或食指的指甲切按在穴位旁，右手持针，紧靠左手

hand. Hold the needle with the right hand and keep the needle-tip against the nail, and then insert the needle quickly into the skin. This method is suitable for insertion of the short needles(Fig.4-11).

切按手指的指甲，针尖轻抵穴位皮肤，然后通过持针之手快速下插，使针尖刺透皮肤。适用于短针的进针（图4-11）。

1.2.2 Inserting the needle with the help of both hands Hold and expose 2 mm of the needle-tip with the thumb and index fingers of the left hand, and point the needle-tip to the body surface of the acupoint. Hold the needle body and keep it upright with the right hand, then insert the needle into the acupoint with the help of both hands. This method is suitable for insertion of short and long needles (Fig.4-12).

1.2.2 夹持进针法 以左手拇、食二指夹住针身下端，露出针尖约2毫米，将针尖固定于穴位的皮肤表面，右手持针，使针身垂直，然后两手同时快速下插，协同将针刺入皮肤。适用于短针和长针的进针（图4-12）。

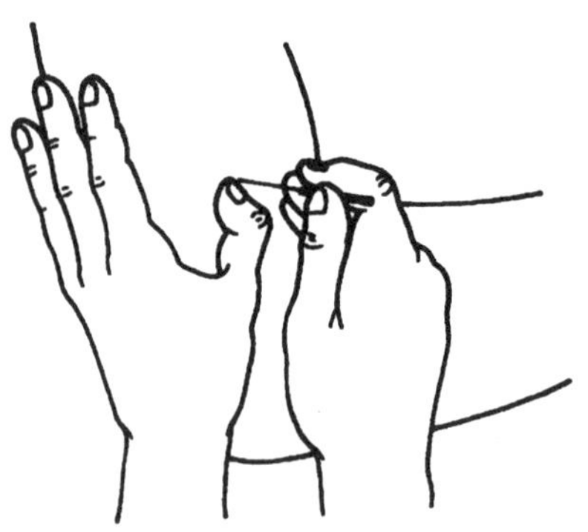

Fig.4-11 Inserting the needle aided by pressing with the finger-nail

图4-11 指切进针法

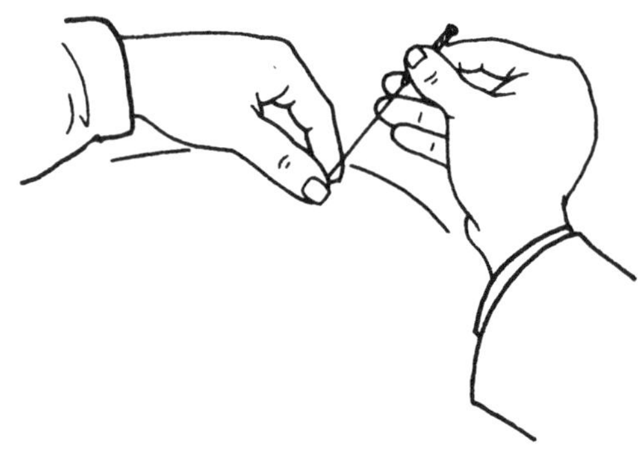

Fig.4-12 Inserting the needle with the help of both hands

图4-12 夹持进针法

1.2.3 Inserting the needle by pinching the skin Pinch the skin up around the acupoint with the thumb and index fingers of the left hand. Hold the needle with the right hand and insert the needle into the upper portion of the skin. This method is suitable for inserting needles into acupoints where the muscles and skin are thin(Fig.4-13).

1.2.3 提捏进针法 以左手拇、食指将针刺部位的皮肤捏起，右手持针从捏起部的上端快速将针刺入皮肤。适用于皮肉浅薄处穴位的进针（图4-13）。

1.2.4 Inserting the needle by stretching the skin

Stretch the skin where the acupoint is located with the thumb and index fingers of the left hand. Hold the needle with the right hand and then insert the needle into the space between the two fingers. This method is suitable for inserting the needle into the acupoints on areas where the skin is loose(Fig. 4-14).

1.2.4 舒张进针法 用左手拇、食二指将所刺腧穴部位的皮肤向两侧撑开绷紧，右手持针使针从左手拇、食二指的中间刺入。适用于皮肤松弛处穴位的进针(图 4-14)。

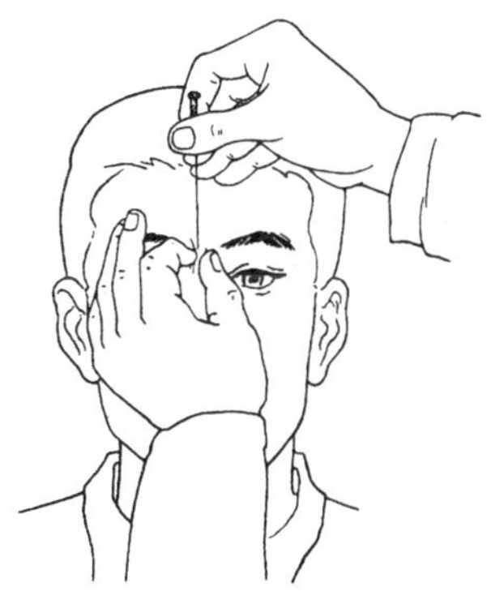

Fig.4-13 Inserting the needle by pinching the skin

图 4-13 提捏进针法

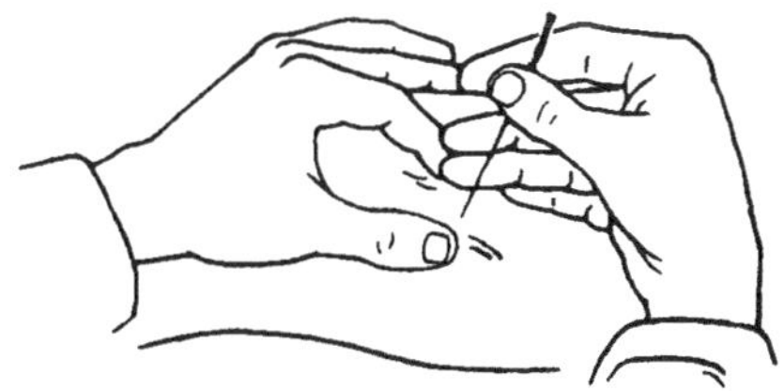

Fig.4-14 Inserting the needle by stretching the skin

图 4-14 舒张进针法

1.2.5 Inserting the needle with the help of guide tube

Hold the tube with the left hand and position the needle-tip directly on the selected acupoint. Tap the needle tail with the index finger of the right hand to insert the needle into the skin, and then remove the tube(Fig. 4-15).

1.2.5 管针进针法 左手夹持针管，将针尖所在的一端置于穴位皮肤上，右手食指快速叩打另一端针管上露出的针尾，使针尖刺入穴位皮肤，然后再退出针管(图 4-15)。

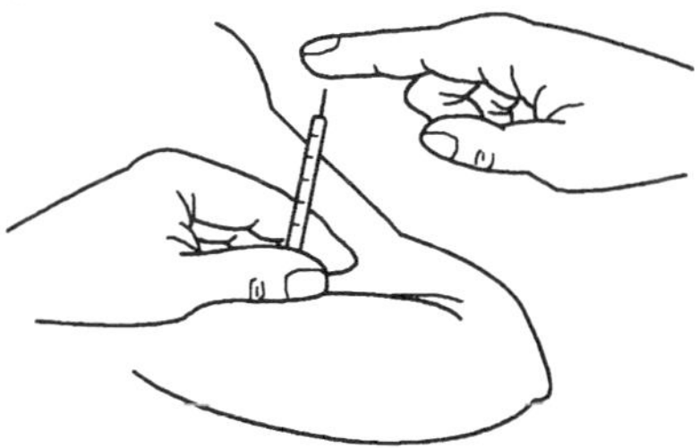

Fig.4-15 Inserting the needle with the help of guide tube

图 4-15 针管进针法

2 Direction, angle and depth of insertion

In the process of acupuncture, correct direction, angle and depth of needle insertion are of special importance in inducing needling sensation, enhancing therapeutic outcomes and avoiding accidents. Different acupoints are needled by varying needling direction, angle and depth. For the same acupoint, different needling direction, angle and depth may cause obviously different needling sensation and therapeutic effects.

2.1 Needling direction

Needling direction refers to the way in which the needle tip faces. The needling direction depends upon the meridian course, the area of acupoints and the therapeutic purposes.

2.1.1 According to meridian course To obtain therapeutic purpose of reinforcing or reducing, the needling direction should follow or head against the meridian course. Generally speaking, for reinforcing effects, the needle is inserted with the needle-tip along the meridian course; while for reducing effects, the needle is inserted with the needle-tip against the meridian course. For example, in puncturing Neiguan (PC 6), when the needle is inserted downwards, reinforcing effects are achieved; when the needle is inserted upwards, reducing effects are achieved.

2.1.2 According to anatomic structure The needling direction is sometimes determined by the anatomical structures near the acupounts, so some acupoints must be needled with the needle-tip toward a certain direction. For example, in needling Yamen

2 针刺的方向、角度和深度

正确的针刺方向、角度和深度，是加强针感、提高疗效、防止意外事故发生的重要环节。不仅不同的穴位需要不同的针刺方向、角度和深度，而且同一腧穴，如果方向、角度和深度不同，则针刺感应和治疗效果也会产生显著的差异。

2.1 针刺的方向

针刺的方向是指针刺时针尖的朝向。一般依经脉循行的方向、腧穴的部位特点和治疗的需要而定。

2.1.1 依经脉循行定方向 即针刺的方向结合经脉的循行走向，以达到“迎随补泻”的目的。当行迎随补法时，针尖所向与经脉循行的方向一致；当行迎随泻法时，针尖所向与经脉循行的方向则相反。如内关行补法时针尖朝下，行泻法时则针尖朝上。

2.1.2 依腧穴解剖定方向 即针刺的方向根据针刺腧穴所在部位的特点而定。某些穴位所在部位的解剖特点决定了针刺时必须朝向某一特

(GV 15) and Fengfu(GB 16), the needle tip should face downwards, not upwards to prevent the needle from entering great occipital foramen and injuring the marrow.

定的方向。如针刺哑门、风府穴时，针尖应向下而不可向上斜刺，以免刺入枕骨大孔伤及延髓。

2. 1. 3 According to diseased area In order to induce the needling sensation to the diseased area, the needle is usually inserted with the needle-tip towards the foci. For Lieque(LU 7), it is needled with the needle-tip upwards in the treatment of common cold, while it is needled with the needle-tip downwards in the treatment of tendovaginitis.

2. 1. 3 依病变位置定方向

为使针刺的感应达到病变所在的部位，所谓“气至病所”，在针刺时则要根据病位，采用针尖朝向病所的方法。如列缺治疗感冒时针尖向上，治疗腱鞘炎时则针尖向下。

2. 2 Needling angle

2. 2 针刺的角度

Needling angle refers to the angel formed by the needle and the skin surface. It depends on the anatomical structure and therapeutic purpose. Generally there are three types of angle: perpendicular, oblique and horizontal(Fig. 4-16).

针刺的角度是指进针时针身与所刺部位皮肤表面所形成的夹角，主要依腧穴所在部位的解剖特点而定。一般分为直刺、斜刺和横刺（图 4-16）。

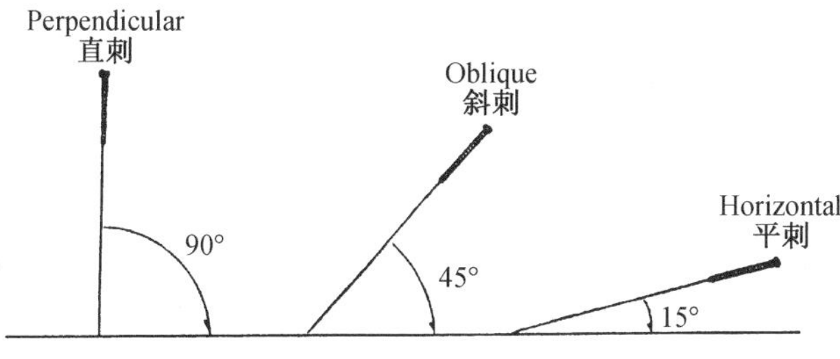

Fig.4-16 Needling angle

图 4-16 针刺的角度

2. 2. 1 Perpendicular The needle is inserted perpendicularly, forming a 90 degree angle with the skin surface. This method is suitable for most acupoints, especially for those on the thick muscles, such as the acupoints on the limbs, abdomen and low back.

2. 2. 1 直刺 针身与皮肤呈 90°角左右垂直刺入。适用于人体大部分腧穴尤其是肌肉丰厚部位的腧穴，如四肢、腹部、腰部的穴位。

2. 2. 2 Oblique The needle is inserted obliquely to form an angle of about 45 degree with the skin surface. This method is suitable for those acupoints

2. 2. 2 斜刺 针身与皮肤呈 45°角左右倾斜刺入。适用于骨骼边缘部位或内有重

close to the bones or vital viscera, such as the acupoints on the chest and upper back.

要脏器不宜深刺部位的腧穴,如胸背部的穴位。

2.2.3 Horizontal This is also known as transverse insertion or subcutaneous insertion. The needle is inserted horizontally at the angle of 15 degrees with the skin surface. This method is applicable to the areas where the muscles are thin, such as the acupoints on the head.

2.2.3 横刺 又称平刺,或称沿皮刺,针身与皮肤呈15°角左右横向刺入。适用于皮肉浅薄处的腧穴,如头部的穴位。

2.3 Needling depth

Needling depth means the length of a needle which is inserted into the body. Each acupoint has its own due needling depth. In principle, the needle is inserted into the body till "De Qi"(needling sensation comes) and the vital organs are nor injured. In addition, following conditions may be considered.

2.3 针刺的深度

针刺的深度是指针身刺入人体内的深浅度。虽然每个腧穴都有常规的针刺深度,但临床上多遵循在不损伤脏腑器官的前提下,以得气为度这样一个原则。在具体操作上还应综合考虑下列因素。

2.3.1 Age For the elderly whose constitution is weak or delicate, or in the case of infants, superficial insertion is applicable; for the young and middle-aged, and those with strong constitution, deep insertion is advisable.

2.3.1 年龄 年老体弱和小儿娇嫩之体,宜浅刺;中青年身强体壮者,宜深刺。

2.3.2 Constitution For strong constitution and fleshy body, deep insertion is advisable; for weak constitution and thin body, superficial insertion is adopted.

2.3.2 体质 体强形胖者宜深刺;体弱形瘦者应浅刺。

2.3.3 Condition of disease For exterior and yang syndrome and new illnesses, superficial insertion is advisable; for interior and yin syndrome and chronic illnesses, deep insertion is used.

2.3.3 病情 表证、阳证、新病,宜浅刺;里证、阴证、久病,宜深刺。

2.3.4 Location of acupoints For acupoints on the face and head, chest and upper back where the skin and muscles are thin, superficial insertion is adopted; for acupoints on the limbs, hip, and abdomen where the muscles are thick, deep insertion is advisable.

2.3.4 部位 头面和胸背等皮薄肉少处的腧穴,宜浅刺;四肢、臀、腹等肌肉丰厚处的腧穴,宜深刺。

2.3.5 Season In spring and summer, superficial

2.3.5 季节 春夏季节宜

insertion is used; while in autumn and winter, deep insertion is advisable.

浅刺;秋冬季节宜深刺。

Section 5 Needle Manipulations

第5节 行针手法

Needle manipulation refers to particular kinds of hand techniques, which are performed after inserting the needle in order to gain "De Qi", regulate needling sensation and achieve reinforcing or reducing purposes. It is divided into fundamental manipulation and auxiliary manipulation.

行针又名运针,是指将针刺入腧穴一定深度后,为得气、调节针感和进行补泻而施行的各种针刺操作手法。行针的手法可分为基本手法和辅助手法。

1 Fundamental manipulation

1 基本手法

1.1 Lifting-thrusting

1.1 提插法

After the needle-tip reaches a certain depth, the needle body is perpendicularly lifted and thrusted(Fig. 4-17). The needle penetrating in from the superficial region to the deep region is known as thrusting manipulation, while withdrawal of the needle from the deep region to the superficial region is known as lifting manipulation. In manipulation, the needle body should be kept upright, with the middle finger or ring finger against the acupoint, to avoid dragging pain induced by the skin movement with the needle. The amplitude and velocity of lifting and thrusting manipulation must be uniform, usually at an amplitude of about 0.3 ～ 0.5 cun and a frequency of about 60～90 times per minute.

将针刺入腧穴一定深度后,拇、食指持针柄施以上提下插的操作手法(图 4-17)。针由浅层向下刺入深层谓之插,从深层向上退至浅层谓之提。操作时应保持针身垂直,中指或无名指指端抵于穴旁,避免皮肤随针体的上下而牵拉疼痛。同时提和插的幅度、速度要保持一致。一般以幅度 0.3～0.5 寸、频率每分钟 60～90 次为宜。

1.2 Rotating

1.2 捻转法

After the needle-tip reaches a certain depth, the needle body is rotated, backwards and forwards, by the thumb and index-middle fingers of the right hand(Fig. 4-18). Rotating the needle with

将针刺入一定深度后,拇指与食、中指夹持针柄作一前一后来回转动的操作手法(图 4-18)。拇指向前转动

the thumb forwards is called left rotation, whereas rotating the needle with the thumb backwards is called right rotation. In manipulation, the needle should be rotated backwards and forwards, and not rotated in on-way direction to prevent the muscle fibers from stucking the needle. The amplitude and velocity of rotating the needle backwards and forwards should be uniform, generally at the angle of 90°～360° and frequency of 120～160 times per minute.

谓之左转，拇指向后转动谓之右转。操作时应前后来回转动，不可单向捻针，以免肌纤维缠绕针身而导致滞针。同时拇指向前和向后转动的角度、速度要保持一致。一般以角度 90°～360°、频率每分钟 120～160 次为宜。

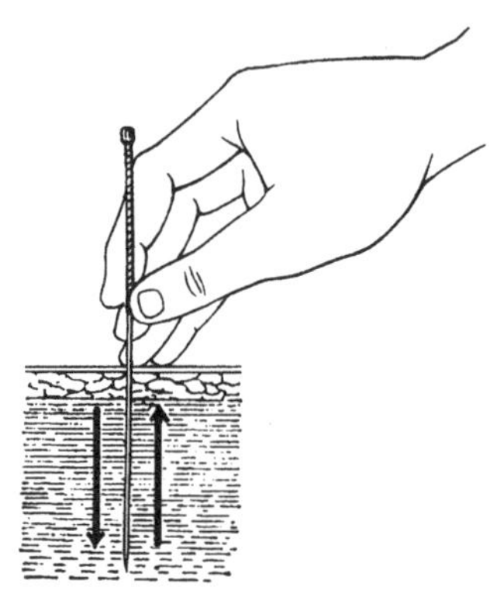

Fig.4-17 Lifting-thrusting manipulation

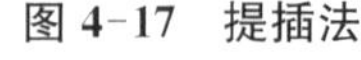

图 4-17 提插法

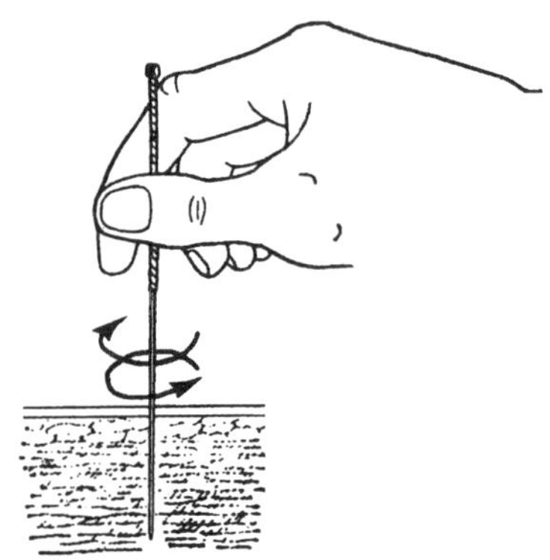

Fig.4-18 Rotating manipulation

图 4-18 捻转法

In clinical practice, the amplitude, frequency and duration of needle rotation also depend on the patient's constitution, the conditions of the illness, the feature of acupoints and the therapeutic requirements. These two methods can be used alone or in combination.

临床上，不管提插还是捻转，手法幅度的大小、频率的高低和操作时间的长短等，应根据患者的体质、病情和腧穴的部位以及医者所要达到的目的而灵活掌握。而且这两种基本手法，既可单独应用，也可配合运用。

2 Auxiliary manipulation

2 辅助手法

2.1 Stroking

2.1 循法

Stroke or gently pat the skin around the acupoints or along the meridian course (Fig. 4-19).

用手指指腹或指尖沿针刺穴位所属经脉循行路线，

This manipulation promotes the circulation of qi and blood, and activate meridian qi to help conducting needling sensaiton.

进行上下左右轻轻地循按或叩打的方法(图 4-19)。此法可推动气血,激发经气,促使针感传导。

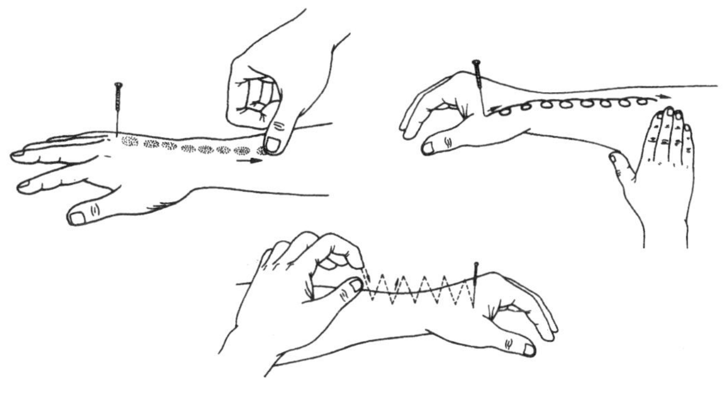

Fig.4-19 Stroking

图 4-19 循法

2.2 Scraping

After the needle reaches the desired depth, the needle handle is scraped with the nail. Hold the needle tail with the thumb or index finger, and scrape the handle slightly with the nail of the index finger or thumb from below to above; or hold the needle root with the thumb and middle finger, and scrape the needle handle with the nail of the index finger, from above to below(Fig. 4-20). This manipulation is used to stimulate the meridian qi to promote the needling sensation.

2.2 刮法

用指甲刮动针柄的方法。以拇指(或食指)抵住针尾,用食指(或拇指)指甲从下向上刮动针柄,或以拇指、中指夹持针根部,食指由上向下地刮动针柄(图 4-20)。此法可激发经气,促使得气。

2.3 Flicking

When the needle arrives at the required depth, gently flick the handle of the needle with the index finger whose nail is under the thumb belly, causing the needle to tremble. The flicking force should be gentle lest the needle flit(Fig. 4-21). This manipulation may stimulate meridian qi to promote the needling sensation.

2.3 弹法

用拇指指腹轻叩食指指甲,然后食指弹出触碰针柄,使针振动的方法。但用力不可过猛,以免针被弹飞(图 4-21)。此法有激发经气,促使得气的作用。

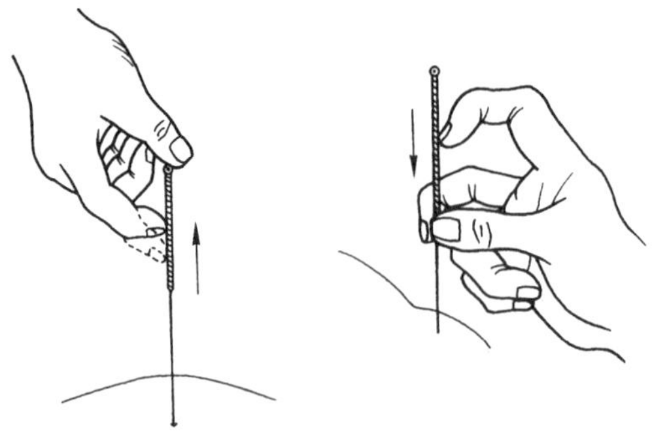

Fig.4-20　Scraping

图 4-20　刮法

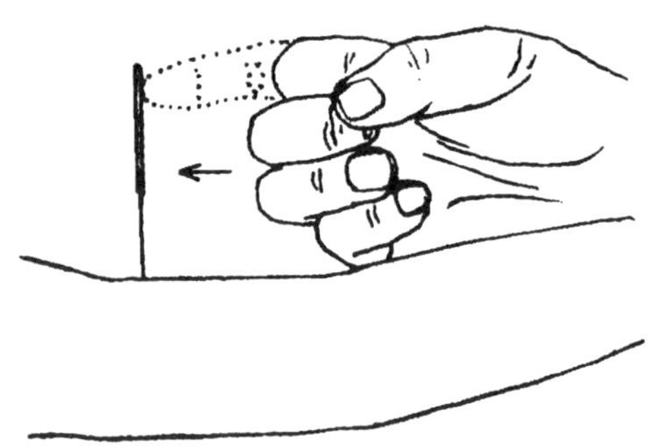

Fig.4-21　Flicking

图 4-21　弹法

2.4 Shaking

Hold the needle handle with the thumb and index fingers to shake the handle left side and right side. If the needle is inserted upright, shaking the needle may can stimulate meridian qi and enhance needling sensation(Fig. 4-22(1)); if the needle is horizontally inserted, shaking the needle can spread the needling sensation along the direction the needle-tip pointing(Fig. 4-22(2)).

2.4 摇法

用拇、食指持针柄，将针轻轻摇动的方法。若直立针身而摇，可激发经气，加强针感(图 4-22(1))。若卧针而摇，可促使针感向针尖方向传导(图 4-22(2))。

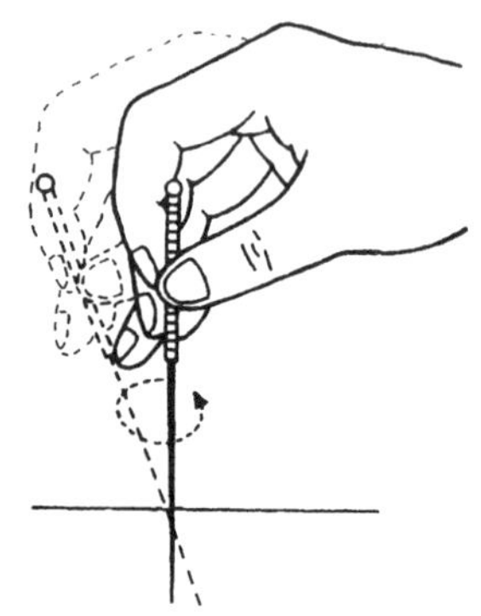

Fig.4-22(1)　Vertical shaking

图 4-22(1)　直针而摇

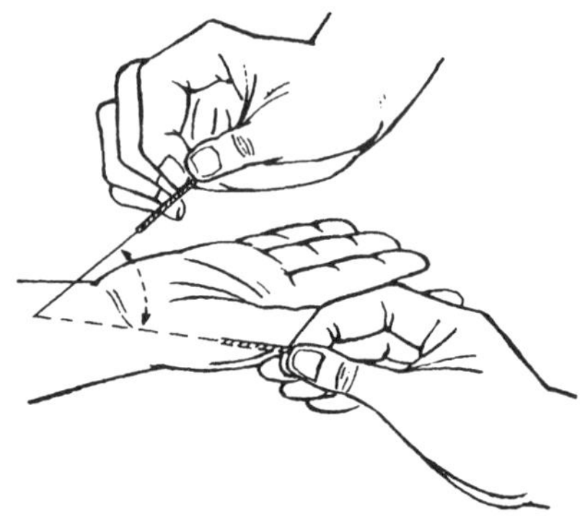

Fig.4-22(2)　Horizontal shaking

图 4-22(2)　卧针而摇

2.5 Flying

Hold the needle handle with the thumb and in-

2.5 飞法

用拇、食指持针柄，小幅

dex finger, and swiftly twist the handle several times in a small amplitude, then free the needle repeatedly, just like a bird flying its wings (Fig. 4-23). This method may promote "De Qi" to strengthen the needling sensation.

度地捻转针柄数次,然后在食指向前转动时顺势张开五指,如此反复,状如飞鸟展翅(图 4-23)。此法可促使得气,加强针感。

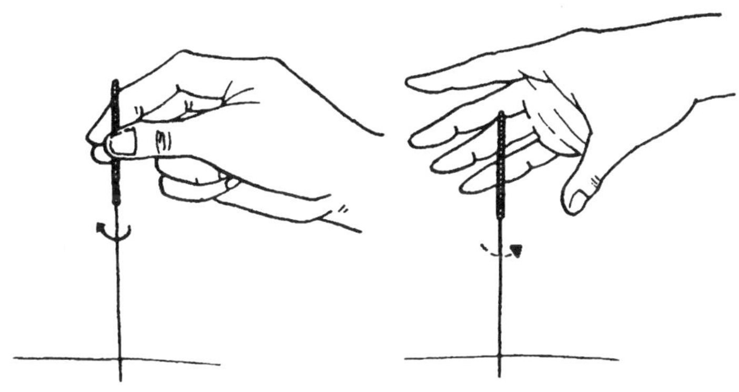

Fig.4-23 Flying

图 4-23 飞法

2.6 Trembling

Hold the needle handle with the thumb and index finger, and swiftly lift-thrust and rotate the needle in a smaller amplitude and higher frequency so as to vibrate the needle. This method is used to promote "De Qi", the arrival of qi (Fig. 4-24).

2.6 震颤法

用拇、食指持针柄,进行幅度小、频率高的提插捻转,使针身产生轻微震颤的手法,以促使得气(图 4-24)。

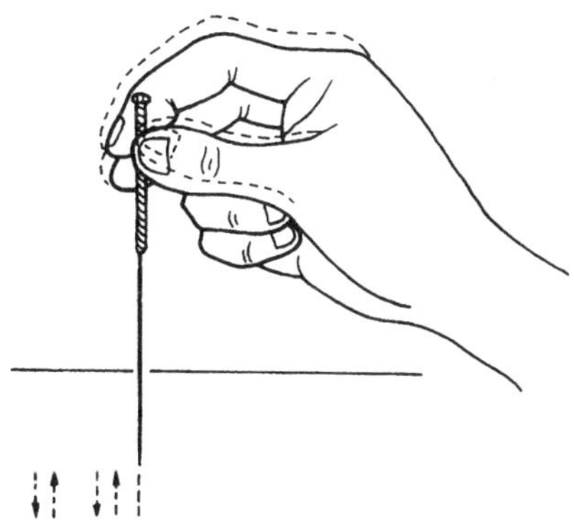

Fig.4-24 Trembling

图 4-24 震颤法

Section 6 De Qi

第6节 得气

De Qi, also known as needling sensation, refers to the reaction of the meridian qi in the area after acupuncture and certain lifting-thrusting and rotating manipulations. The needling sensation may be evaluated from two aspects, i. e. the localized sensation of the patient and the needle-beneath sensation of the acupuncturist. When the qi arrives, the patient may experience soreness, numbness, distension, heaviness or feverish, and itchiness around the acupoint, which may also spread to other places along the course of the meridian. At the same time, the acupuncturist may feel sinking, tightness, heaviness and fullness under the needle-tip, as *Ode to the Standard of Mystery*(Biao You Fu) stated, "De Qi is felt as a fish biting at the hook and pulling the line downwards".

得气，亦称为“针感”。是指针刺入腧穴后，通过提插、捻转等行针手法，使针刺部位产生经气感应。针下是否得气，可以从两个方面分析判断，即患者对针刺的感觉和医者刺手下的感觉。当针刺腧穴得气时，患者会在针刺部位出现酸、麻、重、胀或热、痒等感觉，这种感觉有时不仅仅局限在针刺部位，还会沿着一定部位、向一定方向扩散传导。在患者出现针感的同时，医者往往也会感到针下有沉、重、紧、涩的感觉，《标幽赋》对此有相应的描述“气之至也，如鱼吞钩饵之浮沉”。

De Qi is of vital importance in the acupuncture process and the key to the therapeutic outcomes. Just as stated in Ling Shu, "The essentials of acupuncture is to gain 'De Qi' and achieve good results". Generally speaking, a quick De Qi suggests a quick good effect from treatment, while a slow De Qi means a slow result; absence of qi may lead to no effect.

得气是针灸治疗过程中非常重要的环节，是决定治疗效果的关键，正如《灵枢·九针十二原》所说“刺之要，气至而有效”。一般而言，针刺得气或得气快，治疗作用就好，取效也快；针刺不得气或得气慢，则疗效出现慢，治疗效果也差或无治疗效果。

In acupuncture practice, if there is no needling

在临床上针刺若不得

sensation, the cause must be found out, such as inaccurate location of the acupoint, inappropriate angle and depth of the needling, or declined meridian qi. Then measures should be taken, i.e. to readjust the location of acupoint, the angle and depth of needling, or give herbs effective to enrich meridian qi. Also, the needle may be retained in the acupoint to await the arrival of qi; or manipulative techniques such as lifting-thrusting, rotating, stroking, flicking and scraping are adopted to activate meridian qi and accelerate qi arrival.

气,多因医者取穴不准,针刺角度、深度不当,或因患者经气衰弱等所致。所以不得气时应首先找出经气不至的原因,然后有针对性地采取相应举措,或重新取穴针刺,或调整针刺角度、深度,或通过药物补益经气等。也可采用将针留置在所刺腧穴之内,等候经气到来的候气法,或使用提插、捻转及弹、循、刮等以激发经气,促使经气到来的催气法。

Section 7 Techniques of Reinforcing and Reducing

第 7 节 毫针补泻

1 Fundamental reinforcing-reducing techniques

1.1 Reinforcing-reducing technique by rotating needle

When the needling sensation is gained, the needle is rotated with the thumb forwards more forcefully and quickly and backwards less forcefully and quickly, namely left rotation, which is named reinforcing technique(Fig. 4-25); while the needle is rotated with the thumb backwards more forcefully and quickly and forwards less forcefully and quickly, namely right rotation, which is named reducing technique(Fig. 4-26).

1 基本补泻手法

1.1 捻转补泻

针下得气后,当行捻转补法时则大指向前转时用力重、速度快,拇指向后转时用力轻、速度慢,即左转为主(图 4-25);而行捻转泻法时则拇指向后转时用力重、速度快,拇指向前转时用力轻、速度慢,即右转为主(图 4-26)。

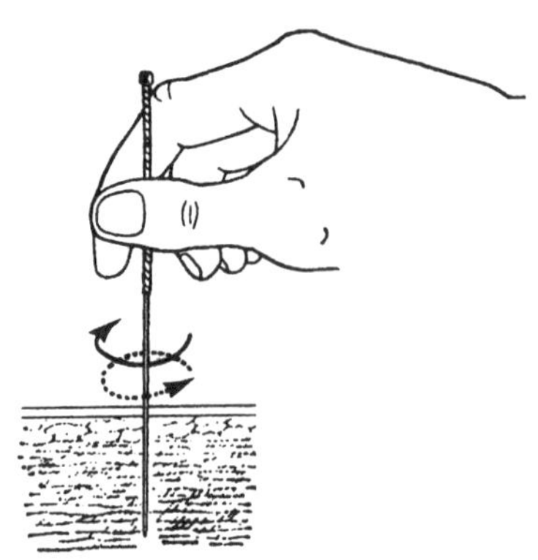

Fig.4-25　Reinforcing technique by rotating

图 4-25　捻转补法

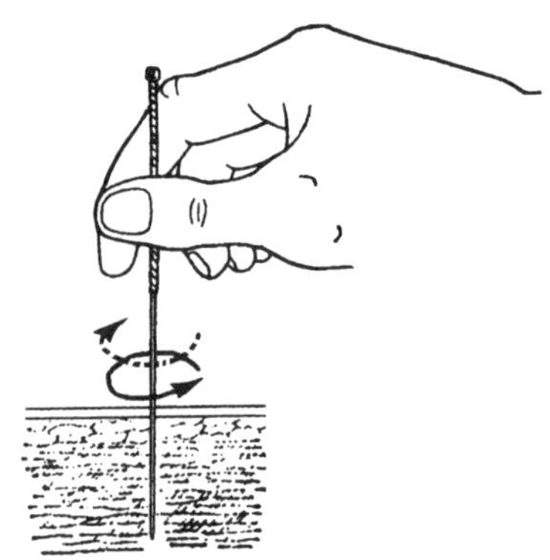

Fig.4-26　Reducing technique by rotating

图 4-26　捻转泻法

1.2　Reinforcing-reducing technique by lifting-thrusting needle

When the needling sensation is gained, reinforcing is performed by thrusting the needle forcefully and quickly, and lifting the needle gently and slowly (Fig.4-27); while reducing technique is performed by lifting the needle forcefully and quickly, and thrusting the needle gently and slowly(Fig.4-28).

1.2　提插补泻

针下得气后，如行提插补法，则下插时用力重、速度快，上提时用力轻、速度慢，即重插轻提(图 4-27)；如行提插泻法，则上提时用力重、速度快，下插时用力轻、速度慢，即重提轻插(图 4-28)。

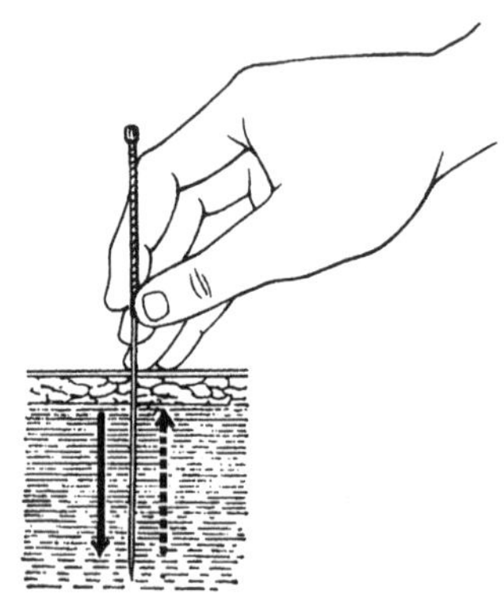

Fig.4-27　Reinforcing technique by lifting and thrusting

图 4-27　提插补法

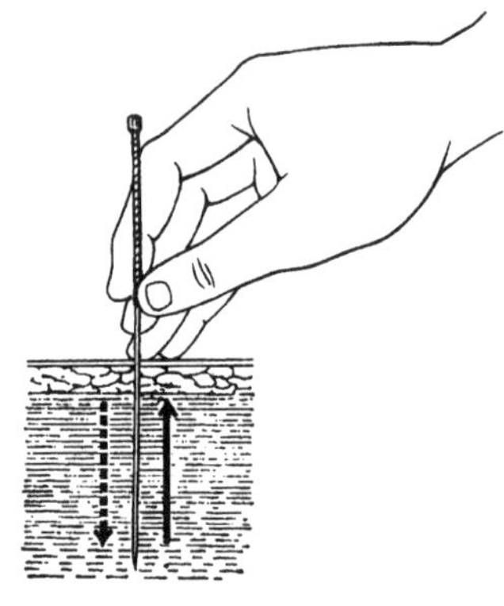

Fig.4-28　Reducing technique by lifting and thrusting

图 4-28　提插泻法

2 Other reinforcing-reducing techniques

2.1 Reinforcing-reducing technique by rapid and slow insertion and withdrawal

The reinforcing technique is performed by slowly inserting the needle to the expected depth, and by quickly withdrawing the needle beneath the skin when the needle retention is over. The reducing technique is performed by quickly inserting the needle to the desired depth and by slowly withdrawing the needle beneath the skin when the needle retention is over.

2.2 Reinforcing-reducing technique by needling along or against meridian course

The reinforcing technique is performed by directing the needle tip along the course of the meridian; whilst reducing technique is performed by directing the needle tip against the course of the meridian.

2.3 Reinforcing-reducing technique through patient's respiration

Reinforcing technique is performed by inserting the needle when the patient breathes in and withdrawing the needle when the patient breathes out; reducing technique is performed by inserting the needle when the patient breathes out and withdrawing the needle when the patient breathes in.

2.4 Reinforcing-reducing technique by keeping puncture-hole open or closed

Reinforcing technique is performed by pressing the puncture-hole instantly after the needle is withdrawn; while reducing technique is performed by not pressing the puncture-hole, or even shaking the needle to enlarge the hole on withdrawal of the needle.

2 其他补泻手法

2.1 疾徐补泻

进针后徐徐刺入欲达深度，留针结束后疾速退针至皮下，即徐进疾出，为补法。反之，进针后疾速刺入欲达深度，留针结束后徐徐退针至皮下，即疾进徐出为泻法。

2.2 迎随补泻

进针时针尖随着经脉循行去的方向刺入，即顺经而刺为补法；相反，针尖迎着经脉循行来的方向刺入，即逆经而刺为泻法。

2.3 呼吸补泻

随患者呼气时进针，留针结束则随患者吸气时出针即呼进吸出为补法；反之，吸气时进针，呼气时出针即吸进呼出为泻法。

2.4 开阖补泻

出针后迅速按压针孔为补法；出针后不立即按压针孔，甚至出针时边摇边退，摇大针孔，此为泻法。

2.5 Even reinforcing-reducing technique

After the needling sensation is gained, lift and thrust and rotate the needle at a moderate speed.

3 Influential factors of reinforcing-reducing techniques

3.1 Functional state

Acupuncture may exert bidirectional benign regulatory functions on human body. When the human body is under differing pathological conditions, acupuncture at one acupoint may exert similar or even opposite effects. Acupuncture may function to reinforce the body when it is in deficiency condition, or to reduce the body when it is in excess condition. For instance, in the treatment of exogenous fever, acupuncture at Dazhui(GV 14) may act to reduce excess by clearing heat; and it can reinforce lung deficiency to relieve cough. Therefore, the reinforcing-reducing effects of acupuncture are in close relationship with the healthy qi of human body, the functional state of human body.

3.2 Feature of acupoints

Each acupoint has its relative specificity. Some acupoints function to tonify deficiency, and others function to reduce the excess. For example, acupoints Zusanli(ST 36), Guanyuan(CV 4) and Qihai (CV 6) function to reinforce the body and are indicated for deficiency conditions; whilst acupoints Shaoshang(LU 1), Shixuan(EX UE11) and Shuigou (GV 26) function to reduce pathogens and are indicated for excess conditions. Thereby, the reinforcing-reducing effects of acupuncture are closely re-

2.5 平补平泻

得气后施以均匀的提插、捻转手法即为平补平泻。

3 影响针刺补泻的因素

3.1 功能状态

针刺具有双向的良性调节作用，人体处在不同的病理状态下，针刺同样的穴位可以产生不同甚至相反的作用。若机体处于虚惫状态而呈虚证时，针刺可以起到补虚的作用；若机体处于邪盛而表现为实证，针刺又可以起到泻实的作用。比如感冒发热，针刺大椎穴可以清热祛邪，起到泻的作用，如果肺虚咳嗽，同样可以针刺大椎穴来益肺止咳，起到补的作用。因而针刺补虚泻实的效果，与机体正气的盛衰，即机体的功能状态有密切关系。

3.2 腧穴特性

腧穴的功能具有相对的特异性。有的腧穴适宜于补虚，而有些腧穴适宜于泻实。如足三里、关元、气海等具有强壮作用，多用于补虚；而少商、十宣、人中(水沟)等具有祛邪作用，多用于泻实。所以，针刺补泻的效果与腧穴的特性也有密切关系。

lated to the relative specificity of acupoints.

3.3 Manipulative techniques

The reinforcing-reducing technique is the chief measure to regulate the excess or deficiency conditions of human body, and the important process to achieve reinforcing or reducing effects. Hence, proper and skillful manipulation of the reinforcing-reducing technique plays a vital role in gaining satisfactory reinforcing or reducing results.

3.3 施术手法

针刺补泻手法，是对机体不同虚实状态进行治疗的主要手段，也是取得补泻效果的重要元素。所以，想要取得满意的补泻效果，补泻手法的运用或补泻手法操作得当至关重要。

Section 8 Retaining and Withdrawing Needles

第8节 留针与出针

1 Needle-retaining method

Retaining the needle means to keep the needle in acupoint after it is inserted into the acupoint and manipulated. The needle-retaining time depends on the individual condition, 20～30 minutes in general. The purpose is to await qi arrival or prolong stimulation, so as to enhance acupuncture actions and enable further continuous manipulation to increase and consolidate the therapeutic effects.

1 留针法

将针刺入腧穴并施行手法得气后，使针留置于穴内一定时间称为留针。留针时间的长短，应根据具体情况而定，一般为20～30分钟。留针的目的是为了候气之需，或为延续刺激，加强针刺作用，以及为了便于继续行针施术，提高治疗效果。

2 Needle-withdrawing method

Withdrawing the needle refers to the usual method of removing the needle after the manipulation, or else after it has been retained. In withdrawing the needle, press the skin around the acupoint by a cotton ball with the thumb and index fingers of the left hand, and lift the needle beneath the skin with the right hand. Then, withdraw the needle quickly and press the hole with a dry cotton ball

2 出针法

出针法是留针结束后，将针拔出的操作方法。出针时，一般先以左手拇、食指持消毒干棉球轻压被刺腧穴旁皮肤，右手将针缓慢退至皮下，然后迅速拔出，再用左手所持干棉球按压穴位片刻。如有补泻，则出针的快慢及

to prevent bleeding. If reinforcing-reducing techniques are performed by rapid or slow insertion and withdrawal, or by keeping the puncture-hole open or closed, the techniques are conducted as above mentioned. After withdrawing the needles, the number of the needles should be checked to make sure that all needles are removed.

出针后是否按压穴孔，需视补泻不同而定。出针之后，还应核对针数，防止遗漏。

Section 9　Prevention and Management of Possible Accidents

第9节　异常情况的处理与预防

Although acupuncture is safe, some accidents may happen owing to careless or improper manipulation, or shortage of a comprehensive knowledge of anatomy.

针刺治病，虽较安全，但如操作不慎，或针刺手法不当，或对人体解剖部位缺乏了解等，则会出现一些异常情况。

1　Fainting

Fainting refers to loss of consciousness in acupuncture treatment.

Symptoms: Sudden onset of spiritlessness, dizziness and vertigo, sallow complexion, nausea and vomiting, profuse cold sweating on head, palpitation and cold limbs, dropped blood pressure, or even coma, falling to the ground, cyanosis of the lips and nails, and fecal and urinary incontinence.

Causes: Nervousness, weak or delicate constitution, or excessive fatigue and hunger, or profuse sweating, diarrhea and bleeding, or too forceful manipulation.

Management: Stop needling and withdraw all needles at once. Help the patient lie down and keep the head horizontal. In mild cases, the symptoms

1　晕针

晕针是在针刺过程中患者发生的晕厥现象。

症状：患者突然出现精神疲倦，头晕目眩，面色苍白，恶心欲吐，头出冷汗，心慌肢冷，血压下降，甚或神志昏迷，扑倒在地，唇甲青紫，二便失禁。

原因：患者精神紧张，体质虚弱，或过于疲劳、饥饿，或大汗、大泻、大出血之后，或医者针刺手法过重。

处埋：立即停止针刺，将针全部起出。再使患者平卧，头部放平。轻者休息片

will disappear after a short rest; in severe cases, nail or puncture Shuigou(GV 26), Suliao(GV 25) and Neiguan(PC 6); other comprehensive rescues can be given if necessary.

刻,症状即可缓解。重者用手掐或针刺人中(水沟)、素髎、内关等穴。必要时,配合其他急救措施。

Prevention: Firstly, an explanation of acupuncture procedure should be given to new patients who have never been needled before or to those who are nervous, in order to remove their worry about acupuncture. Meanwhile, prescribe fewer acupoints, puncture the patients gently and give lying posture. If they feel hungry, tired and thirsty, they should eat, rest and drink before acupuncture. During the acupuncture procedure, the acupuncturist should concentrate his attention on watching the patients' complexion and mental state, and inquire his/her feelings. If the first sign of fainting appears, quick measures should be taken to prevent it.

预防: 对初次接受针刺治疗或精神过于紧张的患者应先做好解释,消除对针刺的顾虑,同时选穴宜少,手法要轻,并给予卧位治疗。若饥饿、疲劳、大渴时,应令进食、休息、饮水后再予针刺。医者在针刺过程中要注意观察患者的神色,留针期间要不时询问患者,如有不适等晕针现象,可及时发现和处理,以尽量避免严重情况出现。

2 Stuck needle

In the manipulation or retention of the needles, the acupuncturist may feel a stuck sensation around the needle and find it difficult to rotate, lift and thrust, or withdraw; while the patient may feel pain.

2 滞针

滞针是指在行针或起针时医者感觉针下涩滞,捻转、提插、出针均感困难,而患者则感觉疼痛的现象。

Symptoms: The needle is found to be impossible or difficult to rotate, lift, thrust or withdraw; forceful manipulation may make the patient feel sever pain.

现象: 针在体内难以捻转、提插和出针,若勉强行使,则患者痛不可忍。

Causes: This may arise from nervousness. When the needle is inserted into the acupoint, the local muscles may contract violently; or it may be caused by improper manipulation, such as rotating the needle only in one direction, resulting in the needle being entwined in muscle fibers.

原因: 患者精神紧张,当针刺入腧穴后,局部肌肉强烈收缩,或行针手法不当,单向捻转致肌纤维缠绕针体。

Management: If the needle is stuck due to the contraction of the muscles, massage, stroke or pat the skin around the acupoint, or pluck the needle handle to ease the muscular tension. It is caused by one-direction manipulation, rotate the needle in the opposite direction to loosen the muscle fibers.

处理：若由局部肌肉过度收缩引起，可循按、轻拍局部，或叩弹针柄，以缓解肌肉的紧张。若单向捻针而致者，可向相反方向将针捻回，使缠绕的肌纤维松弛。

Prevention: Nervous patients should be encouraged to relax and remove their worry about acupuncture. In rotating manipulation, the needle should not be rotated in one direction to avoid the needle being entwined by muscle fibers.

预防：对精神紧张者，应让患者放松，消除顾虑后再予针刺。行捻转手法时，不可单向捻针，以避免肌纤维缠绕针身。

3 Bent needle

3 弯针

Bent needle means that the needle bends when or after it is inserted into the acupoint.

弯针是指进针时或将针刺入腧穴后，针身在体内形成弯曲的现象。

Symptoms: The needling direction and angle are changed in inserting or retaining the needle. It is difficult to lift-thrust, rotate or withdraw the needle; at the same time, the patient feels pain.

现象：针柄改变了进针或留针时的方向和角度，提插、捻转及出针均感困难，患者感到疼痛。

Causes: This may result from unskillful manipulations, or from the needle striking hard tissues, or from sudden change of the patient's posture, or from muscular contraction or from foreign pressure on the needle handle.

原因：医者手法不熟练，针尖碰到坚硬组织器官，或进针后患者改变体位，或肌肉紧张收缩或因针柄受到某种外力碰撞。

Management: If the bent needle is caused by a change of the patient's posture and muscular contraction, turn him gently back to its original position, relax the local muscles and slowly withdraw the needle along the bending direction. Never try to withdraw the needle by force, or the needle may break.

处理：若由患者体位改变、肌肉紧张收缩所致，应使患者慢慢恢复原来体位，局部肌肉放松后，顺着弯曲方向将针缓缓取出，切忌强行拔针，以免针体折断。

Prevention: The needling manipulation cannot be performed too quickly and forcefully. In the retention of the needle, ask the patient not to move

预防：医者应避免手法过速、过猛。留针过程中，嘱患者不要随意变动体位，注

his body, pay attention to the puncturing area and prevent the needle handle from striking and compression by foreign objects.

意保护针刺部位，针柄不得受外物碰撞和压迫。

4 Broken needle

4 断针

Broken needle means that the needle has broken inside the body.

断针又称折针，是指针体折断在人体内。

Symptoms: The needle body is broken during manipulation or on withdrawal of the needle. The broken part is left exposed above the skin, or buried beneath the skin.

现象：行针时或出针后发现针身折断，其断端部分针身尚露于皮肤外，或断端全部没入皮肤之下。

Causes: This may be caused by poor quality needle or eroded needle body or root, or by forceful manipulation and muscular contraction, or by sudden change of the patient's posture in needle retention, or by improper management of bent needle or stuck needle.

原因：针具质量欠佳，针身或针根有损伤剥蚀；或行针时刺激过强，肌肉猛烈收缩；或留针时患者突然变更体位；或弯针、滞针未能正确处理等。

Management: Ask the patient to keep calm to prevent the broken part of the needle going deeper into the body. If the broken part is obviously exposed above the skin, remove it with fingers or forceps. If the broken part of the needle is slightly exposed above the skin, press the skin beside the puncture-hole with the thumb and index fingers of the left hand, then carefully remove the needle with forceps held by the right hand. If the broken needle is completely inside the body, it should be located with an X-ray and removed by operation.

处理：首先嘱患者镇静，以防断针向肌肉深部陷入。若残端部分针身明显显露于体外时，可用手指或镊子将针取出。若残端部分针身稍显露于皮肤处时，可用左手拇、食二指垂直向下按压针孔两旁，右手持镊子小心将针取出。若断针部分完全断入体内时，应在X线下定位，手术取出。

Prevention: Careful inspection of the needle should be made before treatment in order to reject the needles which do not conform to the specified requirements. The needle body should not be absolutely inserted into the body and a part should be exposed above the skin. Avoid manipulating the need-

预防：针前认真仔细地检查针具，对不符合质量要求的针具，应剔除不用。针刺时不宜将针身全部刺入腧穴，应留部分针身在体外。避免过猛、过强的行针。在

le too violently and forcefully. In the manipulation or retention of the needle, the patient should be asked not to change his posture. Correctly manage the stuck and bent needle, and never try to withdraw the needle with too much force.

行针或留针时，应嘱患者不要变换体位。对于滞针、弯针等应及时正确地处理，不可强行硬拔。

5 Hematoma

Hematoma refers to a swelling around the punctured area due to subcutaneous bleeding.

Symptoms: Local swelling, distention and pain after withdrawing the needle, followed by bluish or purplish skin.

Cause: This may be caused by injuring the blood vessels.

Management: In mild cases of small amount of subcutanous bleeding, the small hematoma will disappear by its absorption. In severe cases of local swelling, severe pain and larger hematoma, apply cold compress to stop bleeding and then apply hot compress to dissipate the stagnated blood.

Prevention: Examine the needle carefully to avoid hooked needle; pay attention to the regional anatomy and avoid injuring the blood vessels; press the puncture-hole with a sterilized cotton ball as soon as the needle is withdrawn, for a longer period at the acupoints susceptible to bleeding, such as those on the head.

5 血肿

血肿是指针刺部位出现的皮下出血而引起肿痛的现象。

现象：出针后，针刺部位肿胀疼痛，继则皮肤呈现青紫色。

原因：刺伤血管。

处理：少量的皮下出血、皮下小血肿可以自行吸收消退。若局部肿胀疼痛较剧，血肿较大，可先作冷敷止血后，再做热敷，以促使局部瘀血消散吸收。

预防：仔细检查针尖有无钩毛，熟悉人体解剖部位，避开血管针刺，出针时立即用消毒干棉球按压针孔片刻，对容易出血部位（如头部）的穴位，适当延长按压时间。

Section 10 Precautions in Acupuncture

第10节 针刺注意事项

1 Preventing fainting

For patients who are hungry and tired, the needling should not be given instantly; for those

1 防止晕针

患者在过于饥饿、疲劳时，不宜立即进行针刺。对

who are nervous or weak in constitution, gentle needling manipulations should be given in a supine position.

于精神过度紧张、体质虚弱的患者,针刺手法不宜过强,并尽量选用卧位。

2 Contraindicated sites

The contraindicated sites include: ① Needling should not be given at nipples and navel; ②needling should not be given at the acupoints on the vertex of children when the fontanelle is not yet closed; ③needling should not be given at the acupoints on the abdomen and lower back or those acupoints effective to activate blood flow in the pregnant women or in the women during menstrual periods; ④it is not suitable to puncture the acupoints on an area where there is an infection, ulcer scar or lumps of unknown origin.

2 忌刺部位

忌刺部位包括:①乳中、脐中等穴不宜针刺;②小儿囟门未合时,头顶部的腧穴不宜针刺;③孕妇或妇女经期,其腹部、腰骶部腧穴以及通经活血的腧穴,不宜针刺;④皮肤有感染、溃疡、瘢痕以及不明原因肿块的部位,不宜针刺。

3 Contraindicated constitution

Acupuncture is indicated for a wide range of disorders. But it is contraindicated for those who have susceptibility to spontaneous hemorrhage or continuous bleeding after injury.

3 忌刺体质

毫针的适应证相当广泛,但常有自发性出血的患者,或损伤后出血不易止住的患者,不宜针刺。

4 Avoiding visceral injury

The acupoints located on the chest, flank, loin and back should not be punctured perpendicularly or deeply so as to prevent injuring the lung, heart, spleen, liver and kidneys; the acupoints around or above the navel should be punctured slowly to prevent injuring the intestine; the acupoints on the lower abdomen should be punctured after the bladder is emptied; when the acupoints on the nape, such as Fengfu (GV 16) and Yamen(GV 15), and on the governor vessel are punctured, attention should be paid to the needling angle and depth to prevent injuring the medulla oblongata and spinal marrow.

4 避免损伤内脏

对胸、胁、腰、背脏腑所居之处的腧穴,不宜直刺、深刺,防止刺伤肺、心、脾、肝、肾等脏器;脐周或脐上腹部穴位,入皮后下针应慢,避免伤及肠道;脐下腹部穴位,宜排空膀胱后再予针刺;针刺项部的风府、哑门和脊椎部的督脉腧穴,要注意掌握一定的角度、深度,以免伤及延髓和脊髓。

Chapter 5 Moxibustion

第5章 灸法

Moxibustion is a therapeutic method in which moxa wool or other ignitible materials are made into certain shapes and then ignited to fumigate or iron some parts of the body to balance the visceral functions via the heat and medications.

灸法是指利用艾绒或其他可燃药材，做成一定形状，点燃后熏灼或温熨体表一定部位，通过灸火的热力和药物的作用，调整经络脏腑功能，达到防治疾病的一种治疗方法。

Section 1 Functions of Moxibustion

第1节 灸法的作用

1 Warming meridian and expelling cold

Moxibustion functions to warm yang and expel cold, and unblock meridians and collaterals, and is indicated for arthritis, sciatic, menstrual cramps and common cold due to invasion of cold factors.

1 温经散寒

灸法具有温阳散寒、疏通经络的功能。临床上可以治疗寒邪为患之关节炎、坐骨神经痛、痛经、感冒等。

2 Supporting yang to arrest collapse

Moxibustion functions to return yang and arrest collapse, lift yang and stem sinking. It is often applied to treat coma due to yang-qi collapse, and prolapse of the stomach, uterus and anus due to pectoral Qi insufficiency and yang-qi collapse.

2 扶阳固脱

灸法有回阳固脱、升阳举陷的功用。可用灸法来治疗阳气虚脱而导致的昏迷，以及中气不足、阳气下陷而引起的胃下垂、子宫下垂、脱肛等疾病。

3 Dissipating blood-stasis and resolving masses

Moxibusiton acts to relieve toxin and swelling and resolve blood-stasis and masses by activating qi

3 消瘀散结

灸能使气机通畅、营卫和调，从而达到解毒消肿、化

movement and harmonizing nutrient and defense phases. Therefore, it is employed to treat mastitis, parotitis and lymph node tuberculosis due to unobstructed flow of qi and blood, and accumulation of blood and toxin.

瘀散结的效果。所以常可用于气血不畅、瘀毒互结之疾，如乳腺炎、腮腺炎、淋巴结结核等。

4 Preventing diseases and keeping healthy

Moxibustion can stimulate the healthy qi of human body to boost the resistance against diseases, functioning to prevent diseases, maintain health care and extend life span.

4 防病保健

灸法可以激发人体的正气，增强机体的抗病能力，具有预防疾病、养生保健、延年益寿等作用，是中医治未病的重要手段。

Section 2 Classification of Moxibustion

第 2 节 灸法的种类

There are many kinds of moxibustion methods from the perspectives the material and manipulation. The moxibustion methods in common use are illustrated in Table 5-1.

由于施灸材料的不同以及操作方法的差异，灸法种类很多，常用的灸法见表 5-1。

Table 5-1 Common moxibustion methods

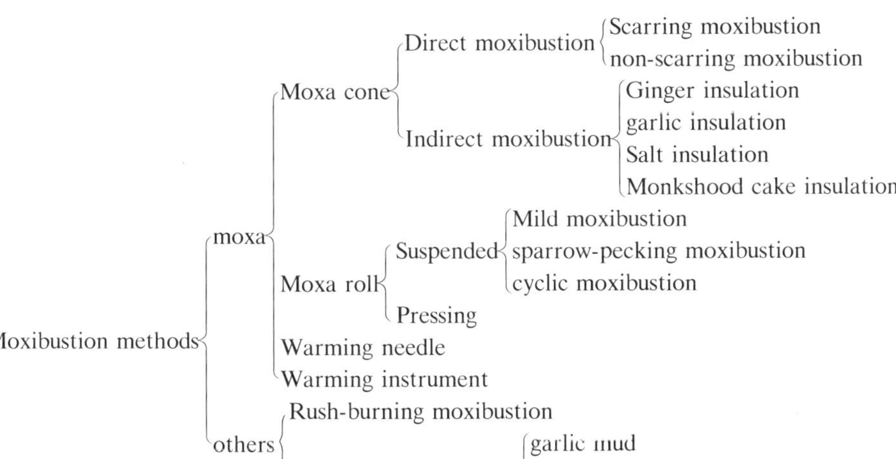

表 5-1　常用灸法

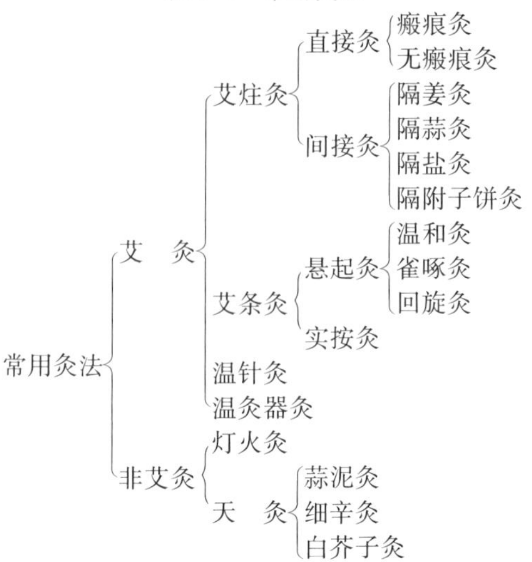

1　Moxibustion

1.1　Moxa cone

Moxibustion with moxa cones is a moxibustion method in which moxa wool is kneaded and shaped into cones of different sizes in diameter that are placed on the body surface and ignited. One cone of moxibustion is called one *zhuang*. The small cone is of soybean size, the middle cone of half size of jujube core, and the big cone of half size of the olive (Fig.5-1). Moxibustion with moxa cone may be divided into direct and indirect one.

1　艾灸

1.1　艾炷灸

艾炷灸，是把艾绒制作成大小不同的圆锥形艾炷，置于施灸部位，点燃施灸的方法。每燃烧完一个艾炷，称为一壮。施灸用的艾炷小者如黄豆大，中等如半截枣核大，大者如半截橄榄大（图5-1）。艾炷灸可分为直接灸和间接灸两类。

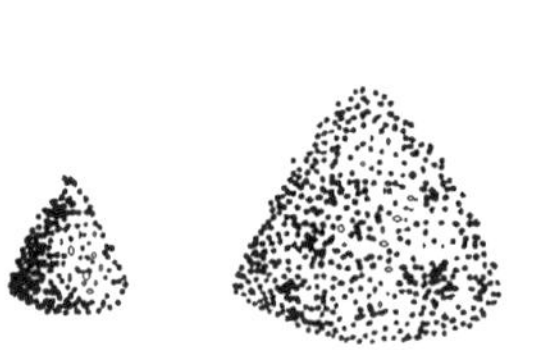
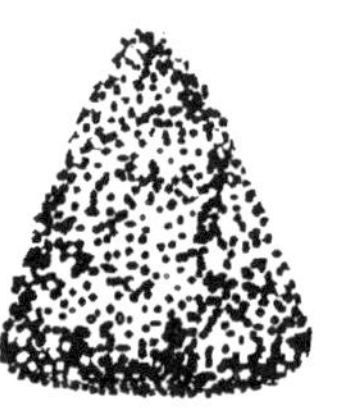
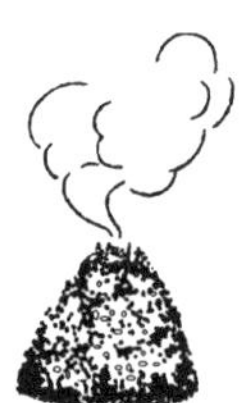

Fig.5-1　Moxa cone (small, middle, big)

图5-1　艾炷(小、中、大)

1.1.1　Direct moxibustion　Moxikustion with a

1.1.1　直接灸　即将艾炷

moxa cone placed directly on the acupoint and ignited is called direct moxibustion(Fig. 5-2). According to the presence of scar after moxibustion, direct moxibustion is classified into scarring moxibustion and non-scarring moxibustion.

直接置于皮肤上施灸的一种方法(图 5-2)。根据灸后穴位皮肤有无遗留瘢痕,又分为无瘢痕灸和瘢痕灸两种。

1.1.1.1 Non-scarring moxibustion Clinically, the middle and big cones are used. Place a moxa cone on the acupoint and ignite it from its top. When three-fifths of the cone is burnt, and the patient feels scorching, remove the cone with the forceps and put on another one. Generally, 3～5 cones of moxibustion is performed till the local skin turns reddened. This moxibustion is indicated for prolapse of anus, arthritis and thymion.

1.1.1.1 无瘢痕灸 又称非化脓灸,临床上多用中、大艾炷。操作时将艾炷放置于皮肤上,从上端点燃,当燃剩 2/5 左右,患者感到灼痛时,用镊子将艾炷夹去,换炷再灸,一般灸 3～5 壮,以局部皮肤红晕为度。此法可用于脱肛、关节炎和皮肤疣等。

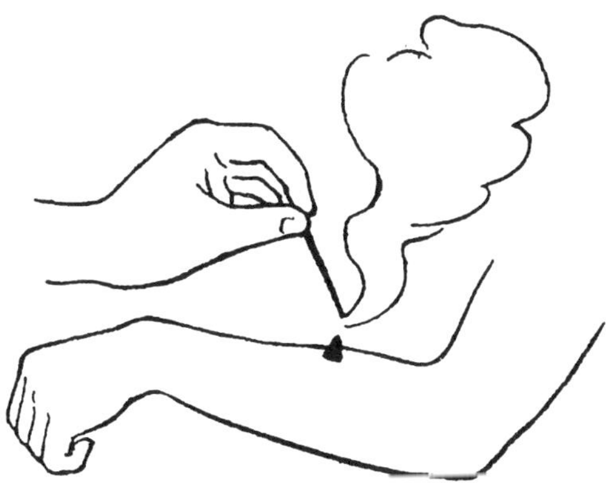

Fig.5-2 Direct moxibustion

图 5-2 直接灸

1.1.1.2 Scarring moxibustion Clinically, small cones are applied. Prior to moxibustion, apply a little garlic juice to the acupoint in order to increase the adhesion of the moxa to the skin. Then put the cone on the acupoint and ignite it from its top till it completely burns out; then remove the ash and put on another one, 5～7 cones in all. About five days

1.1.1.2 瘢痕灸 又称化脓灸,临床上多用小艾炷。施灸前先在施术部位上涂以少量大蒜液,以增加黏附和刺激作用,然后放置艾炷,从上端点燃,每壮艾炷必须燃尽,然后除去灰烬,易炷再

after moxibustion, the skin begins to fester and produce post-moxibustion sore; in about 45 days, the sore is healed and a scar is left behind. Clinically, this moxibusiton is indicated for asthma, chronic bronchitis, chronic enterogastritis and lung tuberculosis, etc.

灸,可灸5～7壮。灸后5天左右局部出现无菌性化脓形成灸疮，45天左右愈合,留有瘢痕。临床常用于治疗哮喘、慢性支气管炎、慢性肠胃炎、肺结核等。

1.1.2 Indirect moxibustion Moxibustion with some medicine separating the moxa cone and the skin is known as indirect mixbustion(Fig.5-3).

1.1.2 间接灸 又称隔物灸,即在艾炷与皮肤之间隔垫某种药物而施灸的一种方法(图5-3)。

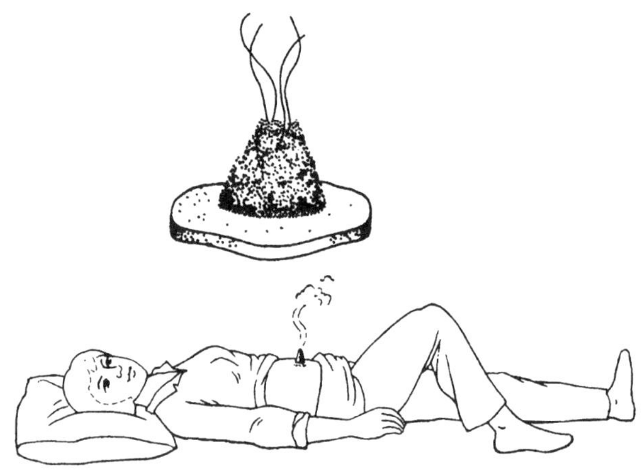

Fig.5-3 Indirect moxibustion

图5-3 间接灸

1.1.2.1 Moxibustion with ginger Cut a slice of fresh ginger 2～3 cm in diameter and 0.3～0.5 cm in thickness, puncture holes in it and place it on the acupoint selected. On the top of the piece of ginger, a middle or big cone is placed and ignited. When it burns out, remove the cone and put on another one. Generally 3～5 cones are given till the skin turns flushed. This moxibustion functions to warm yang and expel cold, downbear adversity and stop vomiting, and is indicated for vomiting, abdominal

1.1.2.1 隔姜灸 用新鲜生姜切成直径2～3厘米,厚0.3～0.5厘米的薄片,中间以针穿刺数孔,上置中、大艾炷,放在施灸部位,然后点燃,当艾炷燃尽后,可易炷再灸。一般灸3～5壮,以皮肤红晕为度。此法有温阳散寒、降逆止呕的作用,对受寒引起的呕吐、腹痛、泄泻和关

pain, diarrhea and joint pain due to pathogenic cold.

节痛疗效较好。

1.1.2.2 Moxibustion with garlic Cut a slice of fresh garlic 0.3～0.5 cm in thickness, and puncture holes in it, and put it on the acupoint. On the top of the garlic slice, place a moxa cone on the slice and ignite it; generally 3～5 cones of moxibustion is applied. This moxibustion functions to relieve swelling and dissipate masses, and is indicated for scrofula, mastitis and ulcers with boils.

1.1.2.2 隔蒜灸 用独头大蒜切成厚 0.3～0.5 cm 的薄片，中间以针穿刺数孔，上置艾炷放在施灸部位，然后点燃，一般灸 3～5 壮。此法有消肿散结的作用，多用于治疗淋巴结结核、乳腺炎、未溃疮疡等。

1.1.2.3 Moxibustion with salt Fill the umbilicus with dry pure salt, and place a small moxa cone on the salt and ignite it, 3～5 cones in general. This moxibusiton functions to return yang, rescue adversity and arrest collapse, and is clinically applied to treat diarrhea, menstrual cramps and collapse syndrome in stroke.

1.1.2.3 隔盐灸 用纯净干燥的食盐填于脐部，使其与脐平，上置小艾炷施灸，一般灸 3～5 壮。此法有回阳、救逆、固脱之功，临床常用于治疗腹泻、痛经、中风脱证等。

1.1.2.4 Moxibustion with monkshood cake Grind the monkshood into powder, and mix the powder with millet wine to make monkshood cake about 3 cm in diameter and 0.8 cm in thickness. Puncture holes in the cake and place it on the acupoint or diseases area. On the top of the cake, place a moxa cone and ignite it. This moxibustion functions to warm and enrich kidney yang, and is indicated for impotence, premature ejaculation, seminal emission, diarrhea and persistent unhealed ulcers due to declined kidney yang.

1.1.2.4 隔附子饼灸 将附子研成细末，以黄酒调和制成直径约 3 厘米、厚约 0.8 厘米的附子饼，中间以针穿刺数孔，上置艾炷，放在腧穴或患处，点燃施灸。此法有温补肾阳的功效，多用于治疗命门火衰而致的阳痿、早泄、遗精、泄泻和疮疡久溃不敛等病。

1.2 Moxibustion with moxa roll

In this moxibustion, one end of a moxa roll is ignited and pointed to the acupoint or treatment area. In the light of the presence of medication, the moxa roll falls into pure roll and medicated roll. The moxibustion manipulation is divided into sus-

1.2 艾条灸

即将艾条一端点燃，对准穴位或患处施灸的一种方法。根据艾条中是否掺合其他药物而有清艾条和药艾条之分。艾条灸按操作方法可

pended moxibustion and pressing moxibustion.

分为悬起灸和实按灸。

1. 2. 1　Suspended moxibustion　Ignite one end of a moxa roll and then direct it over the treatment site to perform moxibustion. There are three manipulations in suspended moxibustion.

1. 2. 1　悬起灸　将艾条点燃的一端悬于应灸部位上方施灸。具体操作方法有3种。

1. 2. 1. 1　mild-warm moxibustion　Ignite one end of a moxa roll and apply it over the acupoint or treatment area at a distance of 2～3 cm, causing a mild warmth without burning sensation. Carry on 10～15 minutes till the local skin turns red(Fig. 5-4). Clinically, mild-warm moxibustion is sometimes conducted with a moxa box.

1. 2. 1. 1　温和灸　将艾条的一端点燃，对准应灸的腧穴或患处，距皮肤2～3厘米处进行熏烤，使患者局部有温热感而无灼痛为宜，一般每穴灸10～15分钟，至皮肤红晕为度（图5-4）。临床上有时采用温灸盒来施行温和灸。

1. 2. 1. 2　Sparrow-pecking moxibustion　Ignite one end of a moxa roll and apply it over the acupoint at a varying distance between the roll and skin, moving the roll slowly down and up, just like a sparrow pecking food(Fig. 5-5).

1. 2. 1. 2　雀啄灸　艾条点燃的一端与施灸部位的皮肤并不固定在一定的距离，而是缓缓而下，在接近皮肤时再缓缓而上，如此一上一下地移动施灸，像鸟雀啄食一样（图5-5）。

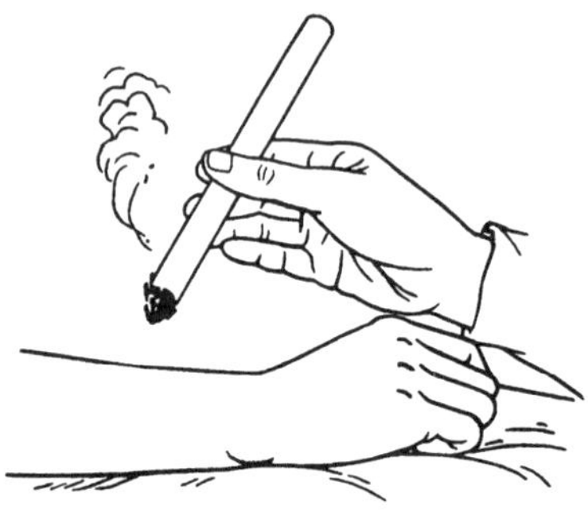

Fig.5-4　Mild-warm moxibustion

图5-4　温和灸

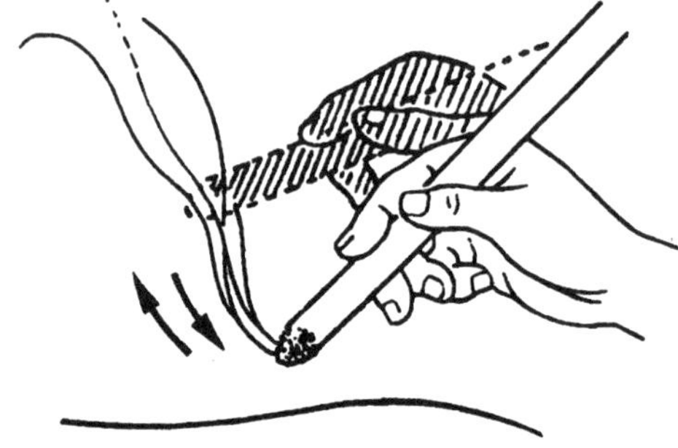

Fig.5-5　Sparrow-pecking moxibusiton

图5-5　雀啄灸

1. 2. 1. 3　Circular moxibustion　Ignite one end of a moxa roll and apply it over the acupoint at a fixed distance, moving it left side and right side or circu-

1. 2. 1. 3　回旋灸　艾条点燃的一端与施灸部位的皮肤虽保持一定的距离，但并不

larly(Fig. 5-6).

固定在一个点上，而是向左右方向移动或反复旋转地施灸(图 5-6)。

1.2.2 Pressing moxibustion Prior to moxibustion, place several layers of cotton cloth over the treatment area. Ignite one end of a moxa roll and press it on the treatment area, lift and press again. Repeat this procedure 6～9 times to make the heat penetrate into the deep tissues(Fig. 5-7). This moxibustion is indicated for arthritis and cervical spondylosis.

1.2.2 实按灸 施灸时，先在施灸处垫上绵布数层，将艾条的一端点燃，趁热按到施术部位上，然后提起，再点按、提起，如此反复 6～9 次，使热力透达深部。适用于关节炎、颈椎病等(图 5-7)。

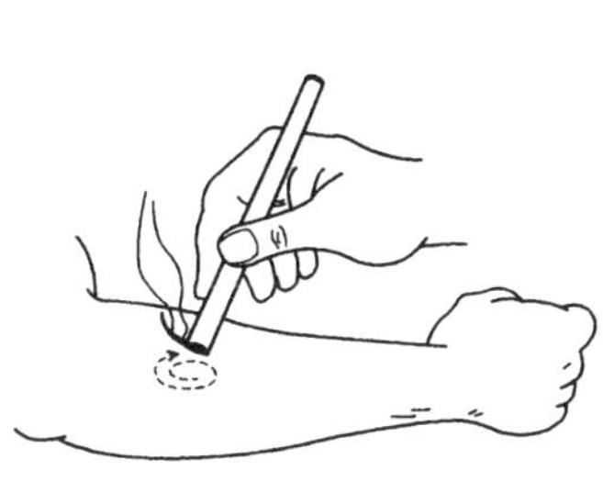

Fig.5-6 Circular moxibustion

图 5-6 回旋灸

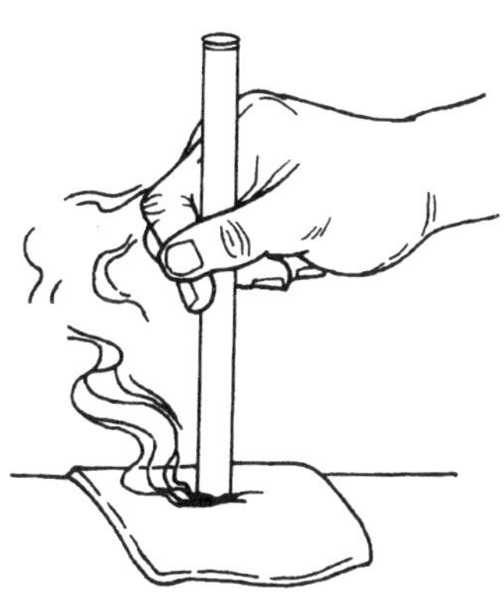

Fig.5-7 Pressing moxibustion

图 5-7 实按灸

1.2.3 Moxibustion with warming needle This moxibustion is a method combining the needling with moxibustion. In the retention of the needle, the moxa cone is around the needle tail, and ignite the moxa cone. When the cone burns out, remove the ash and give another cone, 3～5 cones in general (Fig. 5-8). Besides, a section of two-centimeter-long moxa roll may be inserted into the needle tail and ignited to conduct moxibustion. This moxibustion is suitable for some disorders necessary for both

1.2.3 温针灸 是针刺与艾灸相结合的一种方法。在针刺留针期间，用艾绒在针尾上搓捏制作橄榄形的艾炷，点燃施灸，燃尽后除去灰烬，可灸 3～5 壮(图 5-8)。也可取一段长约 2 厘米的艾条插在针柄上点燃施灸。适用于既需要针刺留针，又须施灸的疾病，如肩周炎、膝关

needling and moxibustion, such as shoulder periarthritis, knee arthritis and external humeral epicondylitis.

节炎、肱骨外上髁炎等。

1.2.4 Moxibusiton with moxa device In this moxibustion, various apparatus may be applied on the treatment area. For example, a small metal box is commonly used; inside the box there exists a smaller pot full of small holes around. In moxibustion, appropriate amount of moxa wool is put into the pot and ignite the wool, and apply the box on the treatment area for 15～20 minutes till the skin turns flushed(Fig.5-9). This moxibustion is primarily indicated for some disorders on the abdomen and back, such as abdominal pan, diarrhea and lumbago.

1.2.4 温灸器灸 利用各种温灸器具在应灸部位施灸的方法。如常用的温灸筒，其筒内套有小筒，小筒四周有孔。施灸时，将适量艾绒放入温灸筒的小筒内点燃，在应灸部位灸15～20分钟，皮肤呈现红晕即可(图5-9)。多用于灸治腹部、背部的一般常见病，如腹痛、腹泻、腰痛等。

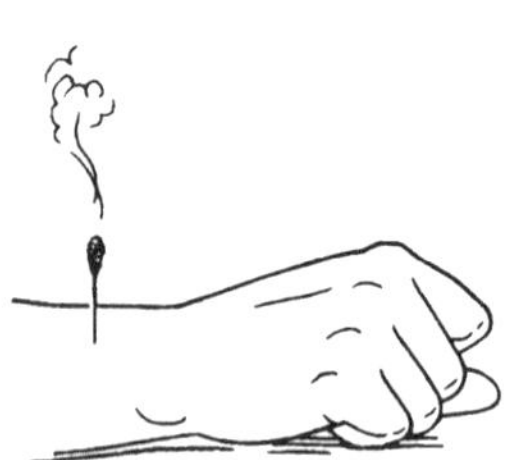

Fig.5-8 Moxibustion with warming needle

图5-8 温针灸

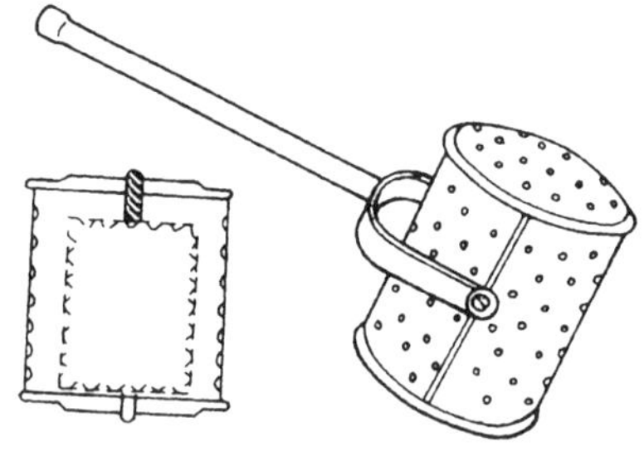

Fig.5-9 Moxibustion with moxa device

图5-9 温灸器灸

2 Non-moxa moxibustion

2.1 Rush-burning moxibustion

This moxibustion is performed by soaking a 10 cm rush in oil for 3～4 cm, then ignite the rush and place it directly on the acupoint. When the rush touches the acupoint, lift it swiftly and the sound of band may be heard(Fig.5-10). This moxibustion is usually applied to treat parotitis, tonsillitis and infantile convulsion, etc.

2 非艾灸

2.1 灯火灸

即取长约10厘米的灯芯草，将一端浸入麻油或其他植物油中，浸渍长3～4厘米，取出点燃，快速触点穴位，迅即提起，可闻及“啪”的一声(图5-10)。主要用于腮腺炎、扁桃体炎、小儿惊风等。

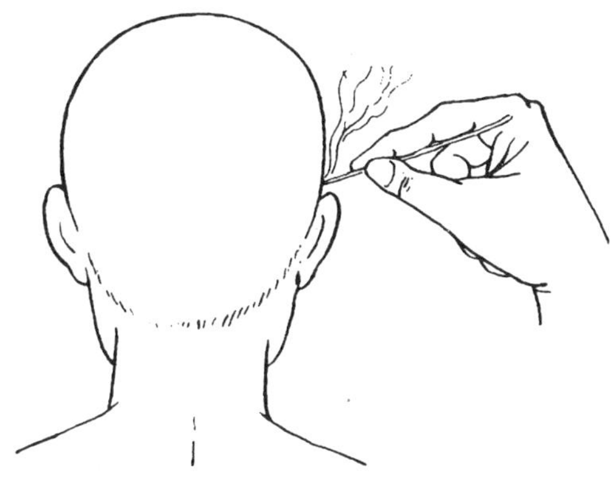

Fig.5-10 Rush-burnimg moxibustion

图 5-10 灯火灸

2.2 Vesiculating moxibustion

In vesiculating moxibustion, some irritating medicines are applied on the acupoints to cause local blisters or flush. The commonly used medicines include garlic mud, siebold wildginger and mustard seed.

2.2.1 Moxibustion with garlic mud Smash the garlic into mud and then apply the mud on the acupoints. For example, moxibustion with garlic mud on Yongquan(KI 1) can treat bloody coughing and nasal bleeding; moxibustion with garlic mud on Hegu(LI 4) can treat tonsillitis.

2.2.2 Moxibustion with siebold wildginger Grind siebold wildginger into powder. Add small amount of vinegar to the powder to make herbal paste, and then apply the herbal paste on the acupoints. For example, moxibustion with siebold wildginger on Yongquan(KI 1) or Shenque(CV 8) can treat childhood stomatitis.

2.2.3 Moxibustion with mustard seed Grind mustard seed into powder. Add small amount of water

2.2 天灸

又称穴位敷贴、穴位发泡疗法。将一些具有刺激性的药物，敷贴于穴位处，致局部皮肤起泡，或仅使局部充血潮红。常用的有蒜泥灸、细辛灸、白芥子灸等。

2.2.1 蒜泥灸 将大蒜捣烂如泥，取适量贴敷于穴位上。如敷涌泉穴治疗咯血、鼻出血，敷合谷穴治疗扁桃体炎等。

2.2.2 细辛灸 取细辛适量，研为细末，加醋少许调和成糊状，敷于穴位上。如敷涌泉或神阙穴可治小儿口腔炎等。

2.2.3 白芥子灸 将白芥子适量，研成细末，用水调和

to the powder to make herbal paste, and then apply the herbal paste on the acupoints or diseased sites. This moxibustion can treat arthritis, facial paralysis and asthma, etc.

成糊状，根据疾病敷贴于相应腧穴或患处，可用于治疗关节炎、面神经炎、哮喘等。

Section 3 Moxibustion Sensation and Reinforcing-Reducing Moxibusiton

第3节 灸感和灸法补泻

1 Moxibustion sensation

Moxibustion sensation refers to the subjective feelings in the moxibustion process, mainly displaying burning pain or burning heat and warmth. The moxibustion sensation not only lodges in the local area, but also penetrates into the deeper tissues, or spreads about, or transmits along the meridians. Appearance of moxibustion sensation helps improve clinical efficacy.

1 灸感

灸感是指在施灸过程中患者的自我感受。主要表现为灼痛或灼热、温热的感觉。这种感觉不仅局限在施灸局部皮肤，有时向组织深部透达，或向四周扩散，或沿着经络向一定方向传导。灸感的获得，有利于提高治疗效果。

2 Reinforcing-reducing moxibustion

Apart from the correct acupoints, the reinforcing-reducing effects of moxibustion also depend on appropriate reinforcing-reducing manipulations. As Ling Shu states, "the reinforcing method of moxibustion is to wait for the fire of the ignited cone to die out by itself, without being extinguished artificially. The reducing method is to blow on the ignited cone, and then put another cone on top to extinguish it." In other words, reinforcing moxibustion is performed by natural ignition of the cone and dying out of cone fire; and the reducing moxibustion is performed by roaring fire and quick ignition.

2 灸法补泻

灸法补泻效应的产生，除了选择合理的穴位外，还须采用正确的补泻方法。《灵枢·背腧》说："以火补者，毋吹其火，须自灭也；以火泻者，疾吹其火，传其艾，须其火灭也。"即补法时，点燃后不吹艾火，待其火力由小到大，缓慢燃尽；泻法时，点燃后吹旺艾火，快速燃尽。

Section 4 Precautions in Moxibustion

第4节 施灸的注意事项

1 Moxibustion sequence

In general, first apply moxibustion to the upper body, then to the lower body; first to the back, then to the chest and abdomen; first to the trunk, then to the limbs; first to the yang meridians, then to the yin meridians.

2 Contraindications

It is not advisable to apply moxibustion to a excess syndrome or fever due to yin deficiency. If necessary, the acupoint should be selected prudently and moxibustion intensity should be properly prescribed.

3 Contraindicated areas

Scarring moxibustion should not be applied to the face, nipples, and areas near large blood vessels. The abdominal and lumbosacral regions of women in pregnancy and during menstrual periods are not indicated for the use of moxibustion.

4 Management after moxibustion

If local small blisters are caused by over-stimulation by moxibustion, take care not to break them, they will be absorbed and heal by themselves. Large blisters should be punctured with sterilized filiform needle and drain the fluid. Put some gentian violet over the lesion. After scarring moxibustion is performed, the moxibustion sore should be kept from infection.

1 施灸的顺序

一般先灸上部，后灸下部；先灸后背，后灸胸腹；先灸躯干，后灸四肢；先灸阳经，后灸阴经。

2 慎灸病证

实热证、阴虚发热者，慎用灸法。如需施灸，须注意施灸穴位的选择，掌握好施灸的剂量。

3 忌灸部位

颜面、乳头和有大血管分布的部位，不宜采用瘢痕灸。孕妇和经期患者的腹部和腰骶部不宜施灸。

4 灸后的处理

施灸过量，局部出现小水泡，可任其自然吸收。如水泡较大，可用消毒毫针刺破水泡，放出水液，再涂以龙胆紫。瘢痕灸后，则应防止灸疮部位感染。

Chapter 6 Other Therapies

第 6 章 其他疗法

Section 1 Cupping Method

第 1 节 拔罐法

Cupping is a therapy in which a cup is attached to the skin surface, causing local congestion and stagnated blood through the negative pressure created by introducing heat in the form of an ignited material, in an attempt to preventing and treating diseases.

Cupping was also known as the horn method in ancient times since the animal horns are used as tool, when it was recorded in *Fifty-Two prescriptions* unearthed from Mawangdui Tombs of the Han Dynasty. It was principally used to stuck out blood and pus to treat skin ulcers. Gradually, the indications of cupping methods are expanded to many disorders in internal medicine, gynecology, pediatrics, traumatology and dermatology.

拔罐法是以罐为工具，利用燃火、抽气等方法排出罐内空气，造成负压，使之吸附于应拔部位，使局部皮肤充血、瘀血，以达到防治疾病目的的方法。

拔罐法古称“角法”，因其以兽角制成角杯作为拔罐工具。早在马王堆汉墓出土的帛书《五十二病方》中就有相关文字记载。起初主要用于吸血排脓，治疗外科疮疡等病证。其后治疗范围逐渐扩大至内、妇、儿、伤、皮肤等各科病证。

1 Types of cups

1 罐的种类

1.1 Bamboo cup

1.1 竹罐

Cut a section of good bamboo 3～5 cm in diameter and 6～10 cm in length(Fig. 6-1). The bamboo cup is light, economical, free from being dam-

用直径 3～5 厘米坚固的竹子截成 6～10 厘米长的竹筒(图 6-1)。这种罐的优点是

aged and applicable in medicinal boiling. But it is not transparent, and the changes inside the jar are invisible.

轻巧价廉,不易摔破,可用于药煮。缺点是质地不透明,难以观察罐内皮肤的变化情况。

1.2 Glass jar

This jar is made of glass and round like a ball, with different sizes(Fig. 6-1). It is transparent, so the changes of the skin inside the jar can be observed. But it is cold in attaching the skin and also easily broken.

1.2 玻璃罐

用玻璃制成,形如球状,有大小不等型号(图 6-1)。其优点是材质透明,使用时可直接观察罐内局部皮肤的变化。其缺点是触肤冰凉,容易摔碎。

1.3 Air-extracting cup

This kind of cup is made of transparent plastics or organic glasses, and attached with are-extracting device(Fig. 6-1). This cup is convenient for use, forceful in attaching to the skin and not easily broken.

1.3 抽气罐

用透明塑料或有机玻璃制成带有抽气装置的罐具(图 6-1)。使用方便,吸附力强,不易破碎。

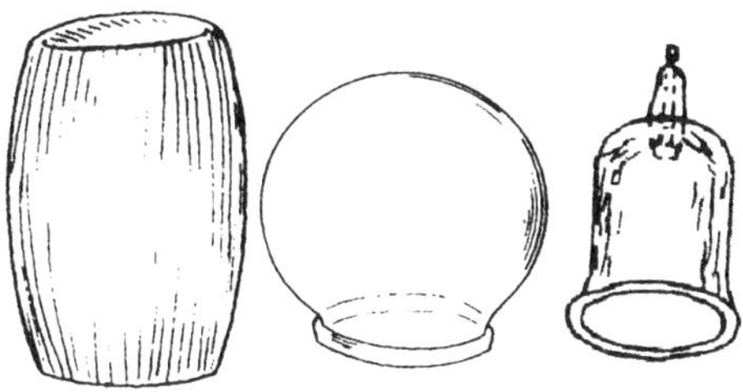

Fig.6-1 Cups

图 6-1 罐具

2 Methods

The air inside the cup is extracted to cause negative pressure, which enable the cup to be attached to the skin.

2 罐的吸附方法

罐的吸附方法是指排出罐内空气,产生负压,使之吸附在拔罐部位的方法。

2.1 Cupping with fire

Attach the cup to the skin by applying fire inside the cup to cause negative pressure.

2.1 燃火法

利用燃烧时火的热力排出罐内空气,形成负压,将罐吸在皮肤上。

2.1.1 Fire-twiddling method Grip a dry cotton ball with forceps and soak it into 95% alcohol, and

2.1.1 闪火法 用持针钳或镊子夹干棉球浸入 95%的乙

then squeeze the alcohol. Ignite the cotton ball and put it into the cup and stay there for 1～3 seconds, and then place the cup on the selected site as quickly as possible(Fig. 6-2). This cupping is most commonly used.

醇后取出，挤去多余酒精，点燃棉球，将其伸入罐内停1～3秒再抽出，并迅速将罐扣在应拔的部位上(图6-2)。此为临床最常用的拔罐方法。

2. 1. 2 Fire-throwing method Throw a piece of ignited paper into the cup, then rapidly place the mouth of the cup firmly against the skin at the selected area(Fig. 6-3).

2. 1. 2 投火法 将纸片燃着后投入罐内，迅速将罐扣在应拔的部位上(图6-3)。

2. 1. 3 Cotton-sticking method Stick a piece of cotton ball with 95% alcohol to the internal surface of the cup, ignite the cotton, then rapidly put the cup onto the given site.

2. 1. 3 贴棉法 用浸有95%乙醇棉花一小块，紧贴在罐具内壁，用火点燃后，迅速扣在应拔的部位上。

2. 1. 4 Alcohol method Drop 1～3 drops of 95% alcohol into the cup, let it evenly spread about the internal surface, ignite the alcohol, then place the cup rapidly onto the required site.

2. 1. 4 滴酒法 在罐内滴入95%乙醇1～3滴，转动罐具使其均匀地布于罐壁，用火点燃，迅速将罐扣在应拔的部位上。

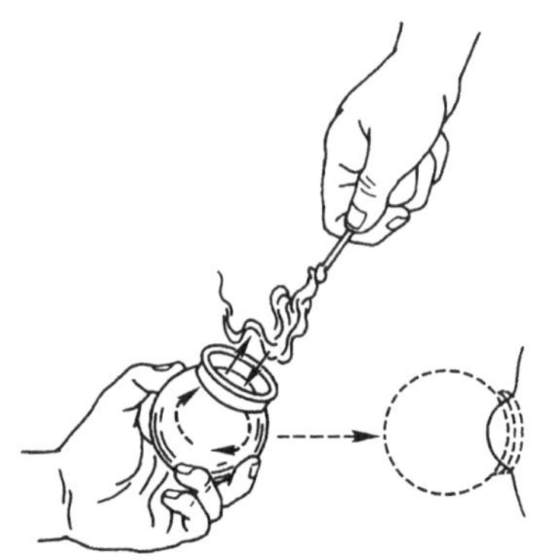

Fig.6-2 Fire-twiddling method

图6-2 闪火法

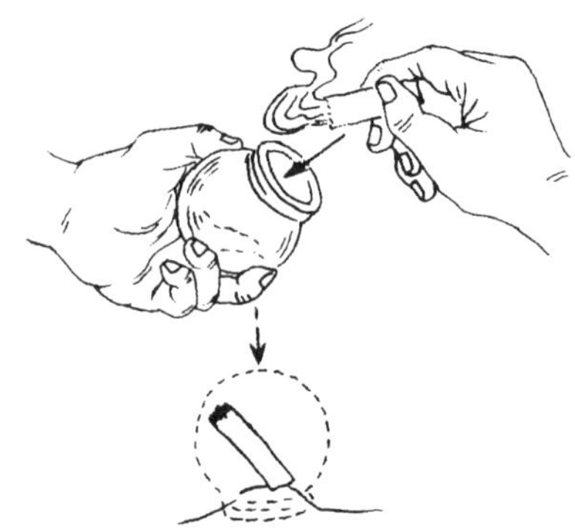

Fig.6-3 Fire-throwing method

图6-3 投火法

2.2 Cupping after boiling

In this cupping method, heat is used to discharge the air inside the cup to cause negative pressure, and place the cup on the affected site. The

2.2 水煮法

利用热气排出罐内空气，形成负压，使罐吸附在皮肤上的方法。一般多采用竹

bamboo cup is usually employed. Specifically, the bamboo cup is put into the water or medicinal fluid, boil for 1～2 minutes; then grip the cup with forceps with the opening downwards to dry the water, then rapidly place the cup on the affected site. If medicinal fluid is used, the medicine is selected according to the individual condition.

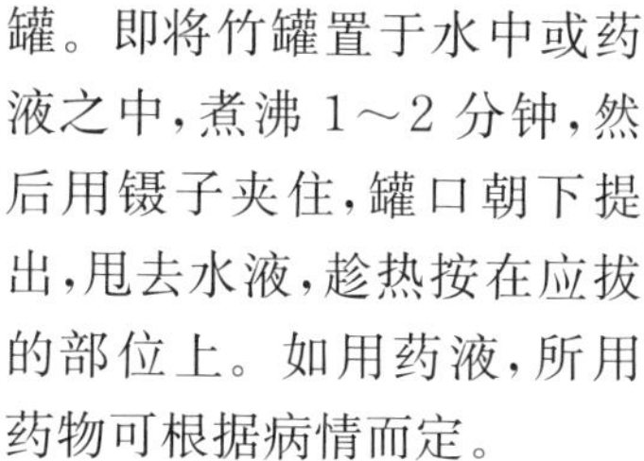

罐。即将竹罐置于水中或药液之中，煮沸 1～2 分钟，然后用镊子夹住，罐口朝下提出，甩去水液，趁热按在应拔的部位上。如用药液，所用药物可根据病情而定。

2.3 Air-extracting method

The cup is firstly covered on the selected area, extract the air inside the cup to cause negative pressure to enable the cup to firmly attach to the skin (Fig.6-4).

2.3 抽气法

先将抽气罐紧扣在应拔部位上，然后用抽气筒抽出罐内空气，使其产生负压，即能吸住(图 6-4)。

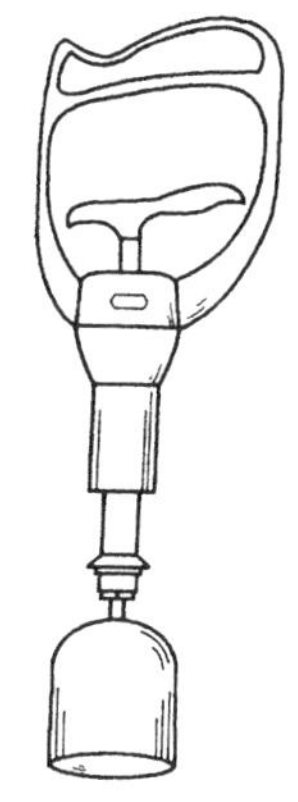

Fig.6-4 Air-extracting method

图 6-4 抽气法

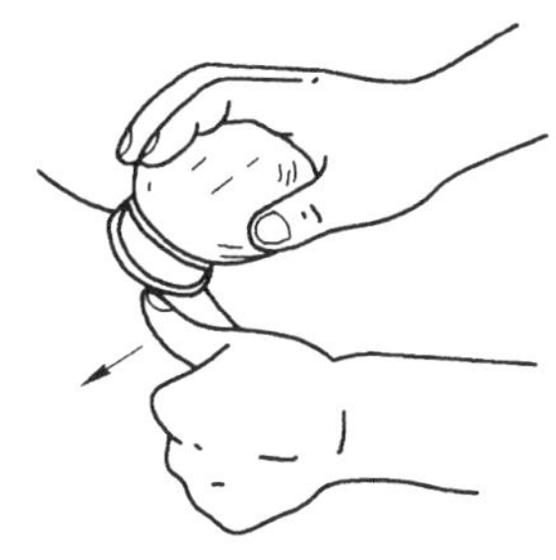

Fig.6-5 Cup-withdrawing method

图 6-5 起罐法

3 Cupping time and removal

3.1 Cupping time

The cupping time depends on the suction force, cupping areas and individual conditions, generally 10～15 minutes. Too forceful suction and long-term cupping may result in local blisters.

3 留罐时间和起罐方法

3.1 留罐时间

留罐时间主要根据吸力的大小、拔罐的部位及病情的需要等来决定，一般为 10～15 分钟。如罐具吸力大而留罐时间过长，可能导致拔罐局部起泡。

3.2 Withdrawal of the cup

Hold the cup with the left hand, and press the skin around the rim of the cup with the right hand to allow air in, thus the cup can be removed (Fig.6-5). Don't try to lift the cup fairly to avoid pain.

3.2 起罐方法

起罐时一般用左手握住罐底稍倾斜上提,同时右手拇指或食指在罐口旁边皮肤上往下按压,使空气进入罐内,即可将罐取下(图 6-5)。切不可强行上提拉拔,以免疼痛。

4 Clinical application of cupping methods

4.1 Cup-retaining method

After cupping, the cup is retained at the site for 10～15 minutes, and then remove the cup. This is the most commonly used method.

4.2 Mobile cupping

Before cupping, apply some lubricating oil on the skin of the affected site. Put the cup on the skin and then push the cup with the right hand upwards and downwards, back and forth, till the skin turns flushed, congested or even blood stasis is created; then the cup is removed(Fig. 6-6). This cupping method is mainly applied on large area where the muscles are thick, such as the back and thigh.

4 拔罐的临床应用

4.1 留罐法

即拔罐后将罐留置于施术部位 10～15 分钟,然后将罐取下。临床最为常用。

4.2 走罐法

即先在走罐部位涂一些油膏等润滑剂,再将罐拔住,然后用手握住罐子,上下往返推移,至所拔皮肤潮红、充血或瘀血时,将罐起下(图 6-6)。一般用于面积较大、肌肉丰厚的部位,如腰背部、大腿部等。

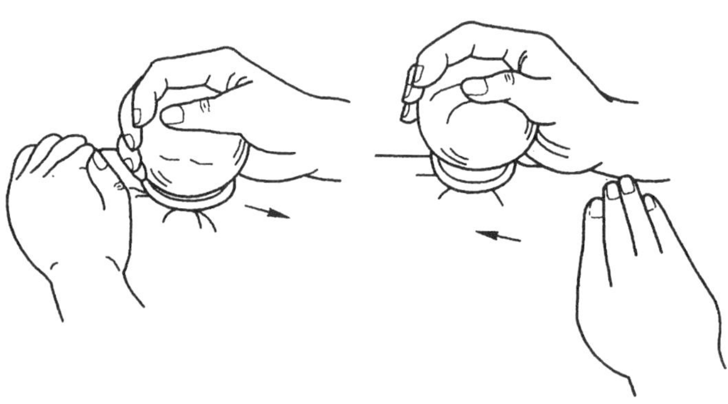

Fig.6-6 Mobile cupping

图 6-6 走罐

4.3 Flashing cupping

In this cupping method, put the cup on the skin and then remove it at once. Repeat this procedure 7～9 times until the skin turns flushed. It is often used to treat numbness of local skin, and in children who do not coordinate with cupping.

4.3 闪罐法

此法是用闪火法将罐拔住后，又立即取下，再迅速拔住，如此反复操作 7～9 次，直至皮肤潮红。多用于局部肌肤麻木的病证，以及如小儿等不配合留罐的患者。

4.4 Blood-letting cupping

First sterilize the area for cupping. Then prick the area with a three-edged needle or tap the skin with a dermal needle, and adopt cupping to promote blood-letting. This cupping is suitable for neurodermatitis, sprain and mastitis.

4.4 刺血拔罐法

即在应拔罐部位的皮肤消毒后，用三棱针点刺或用皮肤针叩刺后，再吸拔罐具，以加强放血治疗的作用。多用于神经性皮炎、扭伤、乳腺炎等。

4.5 Cupping while needling

This is a method combining needling and cupping. After qi arrives, the needle is retained and place the cup over the needle for 10～15 minutes, then remove the cup and needle. This method is indicated for shoulder periarthritis, sciatica and menstrual cramps(Fig. 6-7).

4.5 留针拔罐法

此法是将针刺和拔罐相结合应用的一种方法。即针刺得气后留针时，以针为中心拔罐，留置约 10～15 分钟，然后起罐出针。可用于肩周炎、坐骨神经痛、痛经等(图 6-7)。

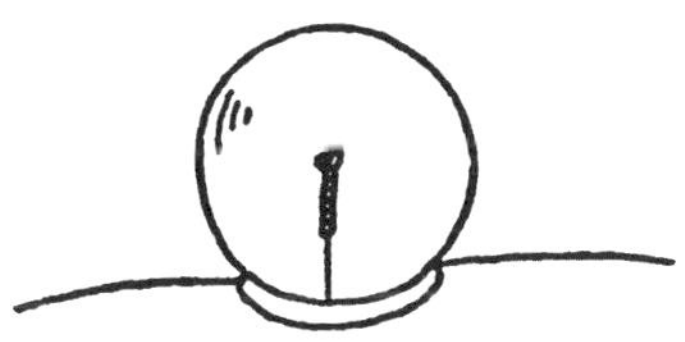

图 6-7 留针拔罐

Fig.6-7 Cupping while needling

5 Functions and indications

Cupping methods function to disperse wind and expel cold, unblock meridians and collaterals, activate qi-blood flow, relieve swelling and ease pain, and drain toxin and pus. Cupping methods have a

5 拔罐的作用和适应范围

拔罐法具有祛风散寒、通经活络、行气活血、消肿止痛、拔毒排脓等作用，其适应范围较为广泛，如关节炎、肩

wide variety of indications, such as arthritis, shoulder periarthritis, cervical spondylosis, sciatica, sprain of soft tissues, common cold, acute and chronic bronchitis, bronchial asthma, insomnia, acute and chronic enterogastritis, menstrual cramps, enuresis and urticaria.

周炎、颈椎病、坐骨神经痛、软组织扭伤以及感冒、急慢性支气管炎、支气管哮喘、失眠、急慢性肠胃炎、痛经、遗尿、荨麻疹等病证。

6　Precautions in cupping

Clinical precautions include following aspects: ①Cupping should be applied on the area with plump muscles; the area which is not flat or hairy is not suitable for cupping. ②Cups of different sizes are used according to the requirements of the area. If several cups are used, the cups should not be too close to result in pain. ③In fire cupping, the manipulation should be quick and stable enough to prevent from burning the skin and make the cup suck tightly. ④For women in pregnancy or during menstrual period, cupping cannot be performed on the abdomen and lower back.

6　拔罐的注意事项

临床上应注意以下事项：①拔罐时一般要选择肌肉丰满的部位，若骨骼凸凹不平、毛发较多的部位均不适宜拔罐。②拔罐时要根据所拔部位的面积大小而选择大小适宜的罐具。若拔罐数目较多时，罐具之间不宜紧紧挨着，以免牵拉皮肤产生疼痛。③火罐操作时动作要稳而快，既要防止烫伤皮肤，又要避免吸附无力，罐具脱落。④孕妇及经期患者的腹部、腰骶部不宜拔罐。

Section 2　Three-edged Needle Therapy, Dermal Needle Therapy, Intradermal Therapy, Electroacupuncture Therapy

第2节　三棱针法、皮肤针法、皮内针法、电针法

1　Three-edged needle therapy

The three-edged needle therapy is a therapeutic method in which a three-edged needle is used to puncture certain part of the body to let blood in or-

1　三棱针法

是指用三棱针刺破人体的一定部位，放出适量血液，达到治疗疾病目的的一种疗

der to prevent and treat diseases. The needle is of different sizes and three-edged in its body and sharp in the tip, so it was known as "feng zhen"(ensiform needle) in ancient times(Fig. 6-8).

法。三棱针有大小不同型号,针体呈三棱形,针尖锋利,古称"锋针"(图 6-8)。

1.1 Needle-holding posture

Hold the needle handle with the thumb and index finger of one hand, and support the lower end of the body with the middle finger, with 2～3 mm exposed to the tip(Fig. 6-9).

1.1 持针姿势

拇指和食指相对持捏针柄,中指指腹抵住针身下端,露出针尖 2～3 毫米(图 6-9)。

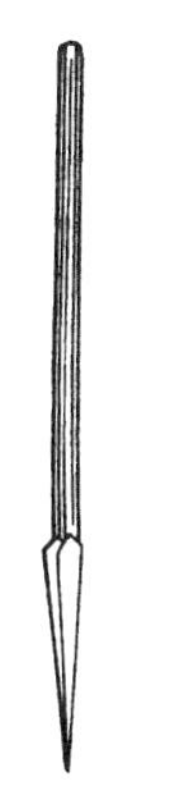

Fig.6-8 Three-edged needle

图 6-8 三棱针针具

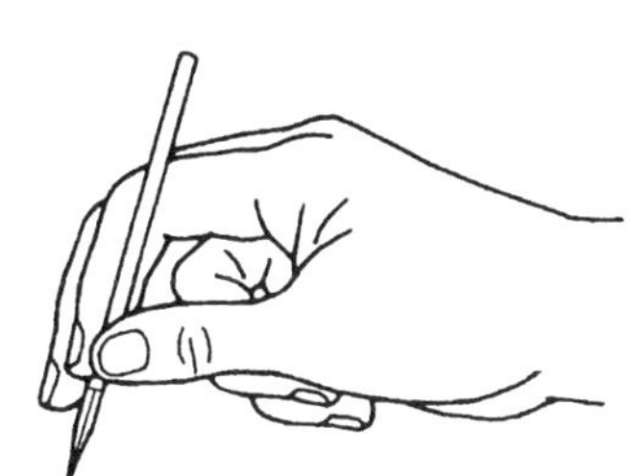

Fig.6-9 Holding the three-edged needle

图 6-9 三棱针持针姿势

1.2 Needling techniques

1.2.1 Spot pricking Before needling, heavy massage is given to the area around the acupoint to induce local congestion. Routine disinfection is given by cotton ball of 75% alcohol. Then hold the needle with the right hand, prick swiftly 2～3 mm deep, accurately at the acupoint, and withdraw the needle immediately. Then squeeze out a few drops of blood by pressing or cupping(Fig. 6-10). This technique is applied to let blood at acupoints, such as Shixuan (EX-UE 11), twelve Jing-Well acupoints, Erjian (EX-HN 6) and Dazhui(GV 14).

1.2 操作方法

1.2.1 点刺法 针刺前,在针刺部位上下推按,使血液积聚于针刺部位,用 75% 乙醇棉球消毒,右手持针对准穴位,速进速出,深 2～3 毫米,然后挤压针孔周围或加拔火罐,使出血少许(图 6-10)。此法多用于穴位放血,如十宣、十二井穴、耳尖、大椎等穴。

1.2.2　Clumpy pricking　Clumpy pricking means giving multiple punctures around the diseased area. According to the area of diseased site, several or decades of punctures are given from the outer margin to the center of the diseased site (Fig. 6-11). This technique is used to let blood in the diseased area, such as local hematoma and neurodermatitis.

1.2.2　散刺法　是对病变局部进行点刺的一种方法。根据病变部位大小的不同，可刺数针或数十针，由病变外缘环形向中心点刺（图6-11）。此法多用于病变局部放血，如扭伤局部瘀血肿胀、神经性皮炎等。

1.2.3　Collateral pricking　This is a blood-letting method by directly puncturing the superficial veins. Bind the upper end of puncture site with rubber band, disinfect the site with cotton of 2% iodine and 75% alcohol; puncture the visible veins to let out proper amount of blood, remove the needle instantly and press the punctured hole with a sterilized cotton ball (Fig. 6-12). This technique is employed to prick the veins in cubital fossa and popliteal fossa to treat summer-heat fever, hypertension and acute lumbar sprain, etc.

1.2.3　刺络法　是直接刺破显现静脉的一种放血方法。先用橡皮管结扎在针刺部位上端，再先后用2%碘酒棉球和75%乙醇棉球消毒，然后对准显现的静脉刺入，随即将针退出，使其流出适量血液，最后用消毒棉球按压针孔（图6-12）。此法多用于肘窝、腘窝等处静脉，可治疗中暑发热、高血压、急性腰扭伤等。

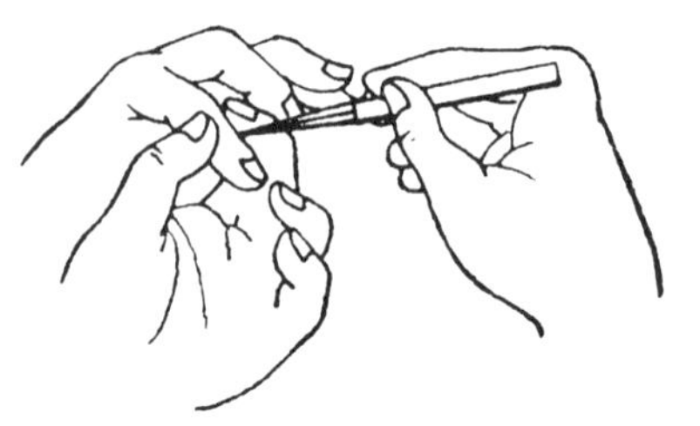

Fig.6-10　Spot pricking

图6-10　点刺法

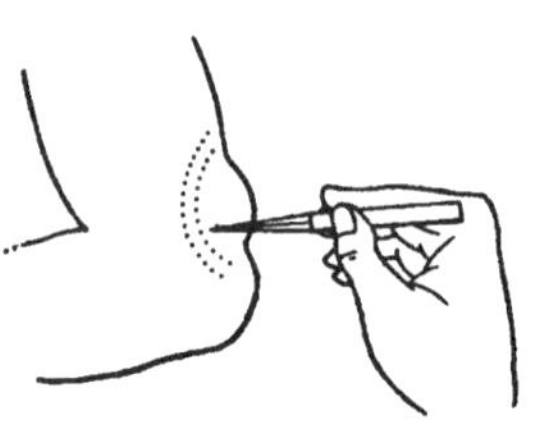

Fig.6-11　Clumpy pricking

图6-11　散刺法

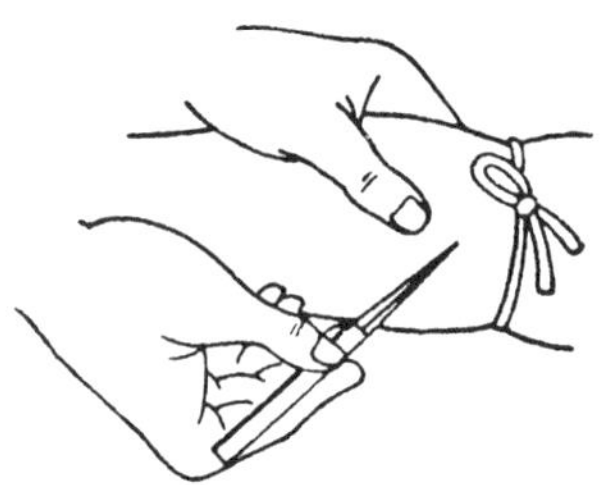

Fig.6-12　Collateral pricking

图6-12　刺络法

1.3　Indications

The three-edged needle therapy functions to unblock meridian and collateral, relieve swelling and ease pain, clear heat and relieve toxin, arouse consciousness and open orifices. It is frequently applied in the treatment of excess syndrome, heat syndrome,

1.3　适应范围

三棱针疗法具有通经活络、消肿止痛、清热解毒、醒神开窍等作用，适应范围较为广泛，凡各种实证、热证、瘀证、痛证及急症等均可应

blood-stasis, pain condition and acute condition, such as coma, high fever, summer-heat, hypertension, headache, trigeminal neuralgia, sprain, shoulder periarthritis, urticaria, acute pharyngolarynitis, styes, etc.

用。如昏厥、高热、中暑、高血压、头痛、三叉神经痛、扭伤、肩周炎、荨麻疹、急性咽喉炎、麦粒肿等。

1.4 Precautions

Clinic precautions include follwowing aspects: ①Before letting blood especially more blood, make necessary explanation to the patient; ②strict disinfection should be applied to prevent infection; ③ manipulative techniques should be gentle, accurate and swift, and not be too forceful to injure other tissues and large arteries; ④this method is not applied in those with the susceptibility to sponta-neous bleeding.

1.4 注意事项

临床应注意以下事项：①放血前尤其血量较大时，应先对患者做必要的解释工作。②严格消毒，防止感染。③操作时手法宜轻、准、快，不可用力过猛，损害其他组织，更不可伤及动脉。④凡有自发出血倾向或出血后不止的患者，不宜使用本法。

2 Dermal needle therapy

Dermal needles are used to stimulate certain parts of the body or acupoints, as a result to prevent or treat diseases.

The dermal needle is made of several short needles in the shape of the seedpod of a lotus inlaid into one end of a plastic handle, thus they are also known as the plum-blossom needle or seven-star needle. This instrument may have one or two heads(Fig. 6 13).

2 皮肤针法

皮肤针法就是运用皮肤针来刺激人体的一定部位或穴位，以达到防治疾病目的的一种治疗方法。

皮肤针是由多根短针集成一束，均匀镶嵌在如莲蓬状的针盘上，并固定在富有弹性的针柄上而制成的，又名“梅花针”或“七星针”(图 6-13)。

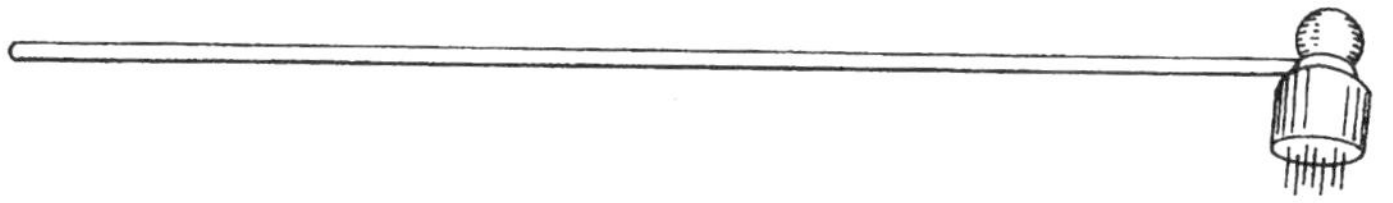

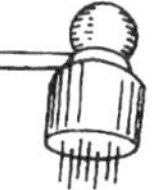

Fig.6-13 One-head needle Two-head needle

图 6-13 皮肤针

2.1 Manipulation methods

2.1.1 Disinfection The treatment areas must be cleaned with 75% alcohol cotton.

2.1.2 Needle holding Hold the posterior part of

2.1 操作方法

2.1.1 消毒 用 75%的乙醇棉球擦拭叩刺部位。

2.1.2 持针 右手拇指指

the handle with the thumb and the index finger of the right hand, with the other three fingers flexed naturally(Fig. 6-14).

腹和食指第一节桡侧缘握住针柄后段,其余三指自然屈曲(图 6-14)。

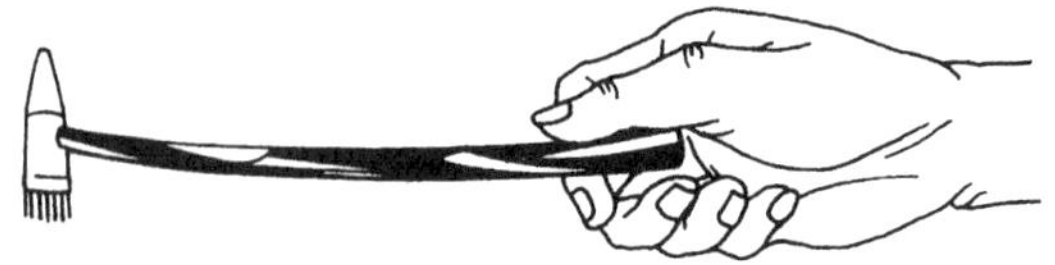

Fig.6-14　Holding the dermal needle

图 6-14　皮肤针持针

2. 1. 3　Manipulation　In tapping, three tips are offered: swiftly tap the skin with a light, flexible movement of the wrist; tap vertically on the skin, up and down; the tapping velocity and strength should be uniform.

2. 1. 3　操作　叩刺操作时有三个要点:运用腕部的弹力,使针尖叩刺皮肤后,立即弹起;叩刺时针尖与皮肤必须垂直,即直上直下;叩刺的速度和力度要均匀。

2.2　Stimulating intensity

The stimulating intensity differs from the areas to be tapped, body constitutions, and the condition of a disease. Thus the stimulating intensity is categorized into mild intensity, moderate intensity and strong intensity.

2.2　刺激强度

刺激的强度,是根据叩刺部位、患者体质和病情的不同来决定,一般可分轻、中、重三种。

2. 2. 1　Mild stimulation　It is applied by light tapping until the local skin becomes slightly reddened and congested; it is indicated for the aged and children, deficiency cases, chronic cases, and the disorders on the head and face.

2. 2. 1　轻度刺激　用力小,以叩刺部位皮肤出现轻微潮红、充血为度。适用于头面部、老弱幼儿患者,以及虚证、久病者。

2. 2. 2　Strong stimulation　It is applied by heavy tapping until slight bleeding appears on the local skin; it is indicated for the patients with strong constitutions and acute cases, and in excess cases, and for the disorders on the back and buttocks.

2. 2. 2　重度刺激　用力大,以叩刺部位皮肤有出血为度。适用于背部、臀部、年轻体壮患者,以及实证、新病者。

2. 2. 3　Moderate stimulation　It is applied by moderate tapping, until the local skin turns flushed, but

2. 2. 3　中等刺激　用力介于轻刺激与重刺激之间,以

without bleeding; it is indicated for most parts of body and patients.

叩刺部位皮肤出现明显潮红,但还没出血为度,适用于一般部位、一般患者。

2.3 Areas to be tapped

2.3 叩刺部位

2.3.1 Tapping along the course of meridian This is a method of tapping which is applied along the courses of the meridians, usually along the governor vessel and bladder meridian of foot-taiyang on the back, and along the yin or yang meridians on the limbs. For example, rheumatoid arthritis can be treated by tapping the back along the governor vessel and bladder meridian.

2.3.1 循经叩刺 是指沿着经脉循行路线进行叩刺的一种方法,常用于项背腰骶部的督脉和足太阳膀胱经,以及四肢部的三阴和三阳经。如类风湿关节炎可选择背部的督脉和足太阳膀胱经进行循经叩刺。

2.3.2 Tapping the prescribed acupoints This is a method on the basis of the main therapeutic actions of acupoints. The prescribed acupoints are usually the specific acupoints and Ashi acupoints. For example, external humeral epicondylitis is usually treated by tapping Quchi(LI 11) and Ashi acupoints.

2.3.2 穴位叩刺 是指在穴位上进行叩刺的一种方法,主要是根据穴位的主治作用,选择适当的穴位予以叩刺治疗,临床常用于各种特定穴、阿是穴等。如肱骨外上髁炎,可于曲池、阿是穴进行叩刺。

2.3.3 Local tapping Local tapping means tapping an affected area. For example, neurodermatitis and alopecia areata are often treated by tapping the local lesions.

2.3.3 局部叩刺 是指在患病局部进行叩刺的一种方法,如神经性皮炎、斑秃等,可予局部叩刺。

2.4 Indications

2.4 适应范围

A wide variety of illnesses are amenable to dermal needle therapy, such pain conditions as migraine, intercostal neuralgia, sciatica and dysmenorrheal; skin disorders such as neurodermatitis, alopecia areata and acne; and neurasthenia, chronic enterogastritis, rheumatoid arthritis and myopia.

皮肤针的适应范围很广,如偏头痛、肋间神经痛、坐骨神经痛、痛经等各种痛证;神经性皮炎、斑秃、痤疮等皮肤疾患;神经衰弱、慢性肠胃炎、类风湿关节炎、近视等。

2.5 Precautions

2.5 注意事项

Clinical precautions include following aspects:

施行皮肤针时应注意以

①The tips of the needles should be level with each other and not hooked, and the head and handle of the needle should be firmly jointed. ②When tapping, the tips of the needles should swiftly strike the skin at right angles to the surface to avoid causing any pain. ③ Tapping is contraindicated for the places where there are ulcers, inflammation or wounds. ④Tapping is contraindicated for those patients with disturbance of blood coagulation. ⑤After heavy tapping, the blood should be cleared and the skin surface cleaned and sterilized again to prevent infection.

下问题：①针尖有无钩毛，针面是否平齐，针头和针柄连接处是否牢固；②叩刺时动作要轻捷，正直无偏斜，以免造成患者疼痛；③局部有溃疡、炎症、损伤等处不宜叩刺；④凝血功能障碍者不宜使用本法；⑤如叩刺后局部有出血，应进行清洁和消毒，防止感染。

3　Intradermal needle therapy

The intradermal needle is also known as the "embedded needle". In this therapy, a specific small needle is inserted into the skin and fixed or retained for there for a certain period of time in order to give the skin regions a week but long-term stimulation, with the purpose of preventing and treating diseases.

Intradermal needle falls into two types in shape. The grain-like needle is a needle with a head like a grain of wheat, and the needle body and handle are in a same horizon(Fig. 6-15); the thumbtack needle is a needle with a head like a thumbtack, and the needle body and hand are in vertical direction(Fig. 6-16).

3　皮内针法

皮内针法又称"埋针法"，是将特制的小型针具刺入并固定于腧穴部位的皮内或皮下，作较长时间留针给穴位以弱而长时间的刺激，从而达到治疗疾病目的的一种疗法。

皮内针的针具有两种。颗粒型，又称麦粒型，其针柄呈环形，针身与针柄处于同一平面(图 6-15)；图钉型，又称揿钉型，其针柄呈环形，针身与针柄呈垂直状(图 6-16)。

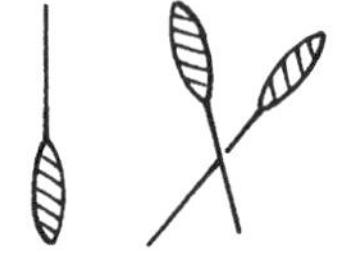

Fig.6-15　Grain-like needle

图 6-15　麦粒型

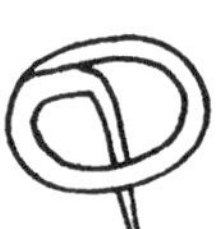

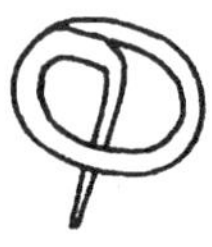

Fig.6-16　Thumbtack needle

图 6-16　图钉型

3.1　Manipulation

3.1.1　Grain-like needle　Stretch the skin around

3.1　操作方法

3.1.1　颗粒型皮内针法

the acupoint with the thumb and index finger of one hand, and hold the needle handle with forceps by the other hand and insert it horizontally into the acupoint; then fix the needle handle on the skin with adhesive tape of 10 mm×10 mm(Fig.6-17).

一手拇指、食指将穴位处皮肤向两侧撑开绷紧，另一手用镊子夹住针柄，对准腧穴，沿皮下横向刺入，然后用10毫米×10毫米的胶布将针柄固定于皮肤内(图6-17)。

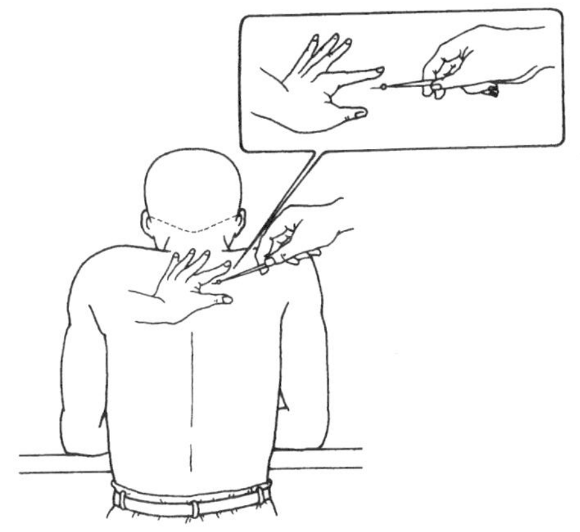

Fig.6-17 Insertion of grain-like needle

图6-17 颗粒型皮内针法

3.1.2 Thumbtack needle Hold the needle handle with the forceps and insert the needle accurately into the acupoint vertically; then fix the needle handle on the skin with adhesive tape of 10 mm × 10 mm; or the needle handle is stuck with a small square of adhesive tape, hold the needle with forceps or fingers, and then insert the needle into the acupoint.

3.1.2 揿钉型皮内针法 用镊子夹住针柄，对准腧穴，垂直刺入，然后用10毫米×10毫米的胶布将针柄固定于皮肤。也可将针柄先贴在小方块胶布上，用镊子或手执胶布直压揿入所刺穴位。

3.2 Needle-embedding time

The duration of needle embedding varies with the individual conditions, 2～3 days in general, and one week in the longest duration. In the hot days, the needle should not be retained over 2 days to prevent infection. During the retention of the needle,

3.2 埋针时间

皮内针可根据病情决定其留针时间的长短，一般为2～3天，最长可达1周。若天气炎热，留针时间不宜超过2天，以防感染。在留针

press the needle for 1～2 minutes every four hours to strengthen stimulation and enhance clinical efficacy.

3.3 Indications

The intradermal needle therapy is often applied to treat painful diseases and chronic conditions with repeated attacks, such as neurogenic headache, biliary colic, arthritis, neuroasthenia, hypertension, asthma, menstrual cramps, irregular menstruation, childhood enuresis, simple obesity, and withdrawal symptoms of smoking and toxification, etc.

3.4 Precautions

Clinic precautions include following aspects: ①The needle should not be embedded around the joints to influence the joint movement; ②after embedding, if local pain is felt, the needle should be taken out and embedded again at other acupoints; ③ during the retention of the needle, keep the needling area from contact with water in order to prevent infection; ④in hot weather with massive sweating, the needle should not be embedded for long periods.

4 Electroacupuncture therapy

Electroacupuncture is a therapeutic method in which a small electrical charge is applied to the needles already in acupoints where De Qi has been gained, with the purpose of treating and preventing diseases. This therapy combines the stimulation of both needling and electricity.

4.1 Manipulation

Before use of the electro-stimulator, first turn it off, and turn the output to zero. After the needling sensation is gained, apply two electrodes of the electro-stimulator onto the handles of two needles

期间，每隔 4 小时用手按压埋针处 1～2 分钟，以加强刺激，提高疗效。

3.3 适应范围

皮内针法临床多用于一些经常发作的疼痛性疾病和慢性疾病，如神经性头痛、胆绞痛、关节炎、神经衰弱、高血压、哮喘、痛经、月经不调、小儿遗尿，以及单纯性肥胖症、戒烟、戒毒等。

3.4 注意事项

临床应注意以下问题：①关节附近不宜埋针，以免影响关节活动；②埋针后，如患者感觉局部疼痛，应将针取出重埋，或改选其他穴位；③埋针期间，针处不可着水，避免感染；④热天出汗较多，埋针时间不要过长。

4 电针法

电针是在针刺得气后，将电针仪输出的脉冲电流通过毫针输入人体，以达到防治疾病的一种疗法。具有针刺和电生理效应的双重作用。

4.1 操作方法

使用前先关闭仪器电源开关，把输出电位器调至“0”位。针刺得气后，将一个输出端的两根导线接在同侧肢

on the same side. Turn the power on, select a desired wave-form and frequency, and slowly increase output to the patient's tolerance. Apply electricity generally for 20～30 minutes. If the needling sensation is felt decreasing, a certain increase in the output can be made; otherwise the electricity can be turned off for 1～2 minutes and then applied again to ensure an adequate intensity of stimulation. When the given treatment time is up, turn the output back to zero and turn off the electro-stimulator; then take the electrodes off and withdraw the needles.

体一对穴位的两个针柄上，然后打开电源开关，选好波形和频率，慢慢调大输出电流量至患者能耐受的程度。通电时间一般 20～30 分钟。如通电期间感觉刺激减弱时，可适当加大输出电流量，或暂时断电 1～2 分钟后再行通电。当达到预定时间后，先将输出电位器退回"0"位，然后关闭电源开关，取下针柄上的导线，最后将针取出。

4.2 Wave forms

4.2.1 Continuous wave Continuous wave is a consecutive pulsation with the same frequency (Fig. 6-18). It is categorized into dense wave and sparse wave in accordance with its frequency. The continuous wave with the frequency over 30 Hz is called dense wave; this wave can reduce the stress functioning of the nervous system to tranquilize and ease pain, and relieve muscular and vascular contraction; therefore it is often used to treat pain conditions and insomnia, and relieve muscular and vascular contraction. The continuous wave with the frequency less than 30 Hz is called sparse wave; this wave can cause muscular contraction and increase the tension of muscles and ligaments to restore the functions of the muscles and nerves; hence it is often used for limb paralysis, and the injury of the muscles, joints, ligaments and tendons.

4.2.2 Sparse-dense wave This is a wave-form with the alternate appearance of dense wave and sparse wave (Fig. 6-19). This wave can promote metabo-

4.2 波形意义

4.2.1 连续波 连续波是一种时间间隔不变的连续脉冲(图 6-18)。根据频率的不同又可分为密波和疏波。频率高于 30 Hz 的连续波称为密波，能降低神经应激功能。有镇静、止痛、缓解肌肉和血管痉挛等作用，常用于治疗各种痛证、失眠、肌肉和血管痉挛等。频率低于 30 Hz 的连续波则称为疏波，能引起肌肉收缩，提高肌肉韧带的张力，促进神经肌肉功能的恢复。常用于治疗肢体瘫痪及各种肌肉、关节、韧带、肌腱的损伤等。

4.2.2 疏密波 疏密波是密波和疏波交替出现的一种波形(图 6-19)，能促进代谢，

lism, accelerate blood circulation, improve nutrition supply and remove inflammatory edema, and is thus employed to treat sprains of soft tissues, arthritis, facial palsy, sciatic and local congelation, etc.

促进血液循环，改善组织营养，消除炎性水肿。常用于软组织损伤、关节炎、面神经炎、坐骨神经痛、局部冻伤等。

4.2.3 Intermittent wave This wave occurs at regular intervals(Fig. 6-20). This wave can enhance the excitation of muscular tissues and produce good contraction of the striated muscles, and is thus used to treat limb paralysis.

4.2.3 断续波 断续波是指波形有节律的时断时续(图6-20)，能提高肌肉组织的兴奋性，对横纹肌有良好的刺激收缩作用。常用于治疗肢体瘫痪。

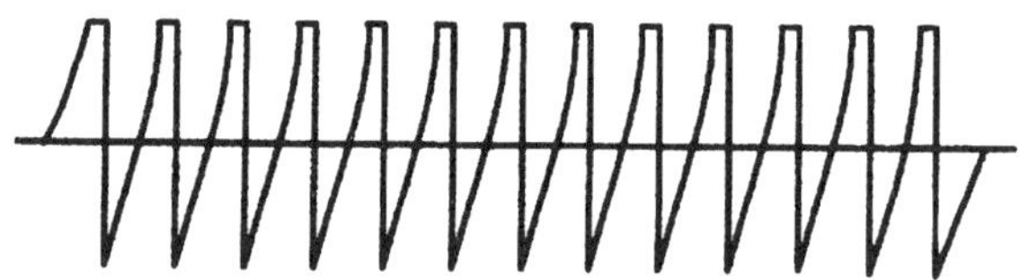

Fig.6-18 Waves of electroacupuncture

图 6-18 电针波形

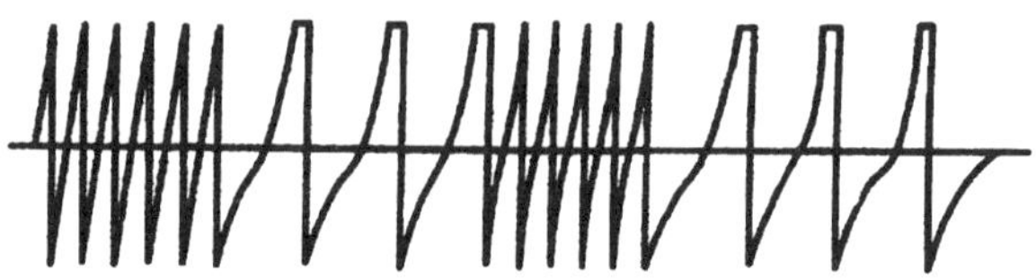

Fig.6-19 Sparse-dense wave

图 6-19 疏密波

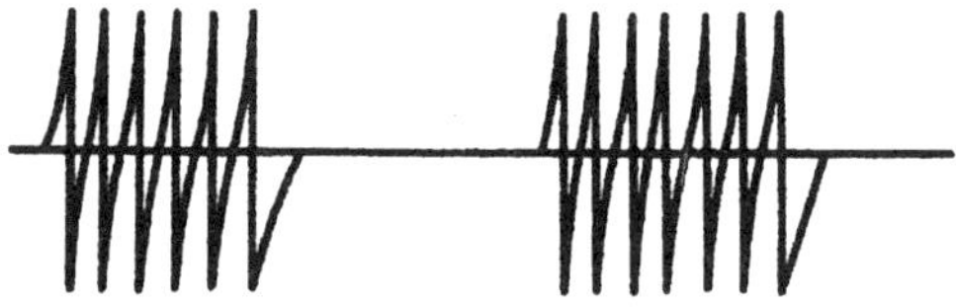

Fig.6-20 Intermittent wave

图 6-20 断续波

4.3 Indications

Electroacupuncture is indicated for a wide variety of diseases, especially in nervous system and for pain conditions, such as migraine headache, trige-minal neuralgia, sciatic, toothache, menstrual cramps, facial neuritis, multiple neuritis, myasthenia gravis, cerebral vascular accidents, spinal injury, arthritis, neuroasthenia and enuresis; it is also used in acupuncture anesthesia.

4.3 适应范围

电针可广泛用于各科疾病,尤其适用于神经系统疾病和各种痛证,如偏头痛、三叉神经痛、坐骨神经痛、牙痛、痛经、面神经炎、多发性神经炎、重症肌无力、脑血管意外、脊髓损伤、关节炎、神经衰弱、遗尿等。还常用于针刺麻醉。

4.4 Precautions

Clinic precautions include following aspects: ①Check the electro-stimulator before use to ensure that it is well functioned and absolutely turned off; ②the output current should be increased slowly, not suddenly, to prevent electrical accidents; ③electro-acupuncture should not be applied at two acupoints respectively on each side of the body in order to prevent the electrical current passing the heart; ④electro-acupuncture should not be applied in those with cardiac pacemaker and in the abdomen and back regions in the pregnant women.

4.4 注意事项

临床应注意以下问题:①电针器在使用前须检查性能是否良好,各开关是否处于关闭状态;②调节电流输出量应缓慢,不可突然增强,以免发生意外;③一个输出端的两根导线不宜接在机体左右的两个穴位上,以避免电流通过心脏;④安装心脏起搏器的患者以及孕妇的腹部、腰骶部不宜使用电针。

Section 3 Scalp Acupuncture

第3节 头针

Scalp acupuncture is a therapeutic method which applies acupuncture at the specific areas of the scalp to treat and prevent diseases.

The development of scalp acupuncture is in close relationship with the theories of meridian and acupoint. Apart from the numerous acupoints on the head, the yang meridians of the hand and foot

头针,是在头部特定的刺激线进行针刺以防治疾病的一种方法。

头针的发展与经络腧穴理论密切相关。头部除有丰富的穴位外,十二经脉中手足六阳经皆上循于头面,六

go up to the head, the hand-shaoyin meridian and foot-jueyin meridian also ascend to the head and face, and other yin meridians connect with the head via the meridian divergencies. This lays the theoretical foundation for scalp acupuncture.

阴经中手少阴与足厥阴经直接循行于头面部，其余阴经则通过经别与头部发生间接联系。由此奠定了头针疗法的理论基础。

1　Locations and indications of the areas

1　头针治疗线的定位和主治

The therapeutic lines in scalp acupuncture are all on the scalp. The scalp is divided, according to the anatomical terminology of the skull, into 4 regions(frontal region, parietal region, temporal region and occipital region) and 14 standard lines.

头针治疗线均位于头皮部位，按颅骨的解剖名称分额区、顶区、颞区、枕区 4 个区，14 条标准线。

1.1　Therapeutic lines on frontal region

1.1　额区治疗线

1.1.1　Middle Line of the Forehead (MS 1)

1.1.1　额中线

Location: On the anterior part of the head, the line 1 cun in length downwards along the governor vessel from Shenting(GV 24)(Fig. 6-21).

定位：在头前部，从督脉神庭穴向下引一条长1 寸的线(图 6-21)。

Indications: Epilepsy, mental disorders, insomnia, and headache.

主治：癫痫、精神失常、失眠、头痛等。

1.1.2　Lateral Line 1 of the Forehead (MS 2)

1.1.2　额旁 1 线

Location: On the anterior part of the head, the line 1 cun in length downwards along the bladder meridian from Meichong(BL 3)(Fig. 6-21).

定位：在头前部，从膀胱经眉冲穴向下引一条长 1 寸的线(图 6-21)。

Indications: Coronary heart disease, bronchial asthma, and bronchitis.

主治：冠心病、支气管哮喘、支气管炎等。

1.1.3　Lateral Line 2 of the Forehead (MS 3)

1.1.3　额旁 2 线

Location: On the anterior part of the head, the line 1 cun in length downwards along the gallbladder from Toulinqi(GB 15)(Fig. 6-21).

定位：在头前部，从胆经头临泣穴向下引一条长 1 寸线(图 6-21)。

Indications: Acute and chronic gastritis, ulcers of the stomach and duodenum, liver and gallbladder diseases.

主治：急慢性胃炎、胃和十二指肠溃疡、肝胆疾病等。

1.1.4 Lateral Line 3 of the Forehead (MS 4)

Location: On the anterior part of the head, the line 1 cun in length downwards along the sto-mach meridian from the site 0.75 cun medial to Touwei(St 8)(Fig.6-21).

Indications: Functional uterine bleeding, prolapse of uterus, impotence, seminal emission, and enuresis.

1.1.4 额旁3线

定位: 在头前部,从胃经头维穴内侧0.75寸起向下引一条长1寸的线(图6-21)。

主治: 功能性子宫出血、子宫脱垂、阳痿、遗精、遗尿等。

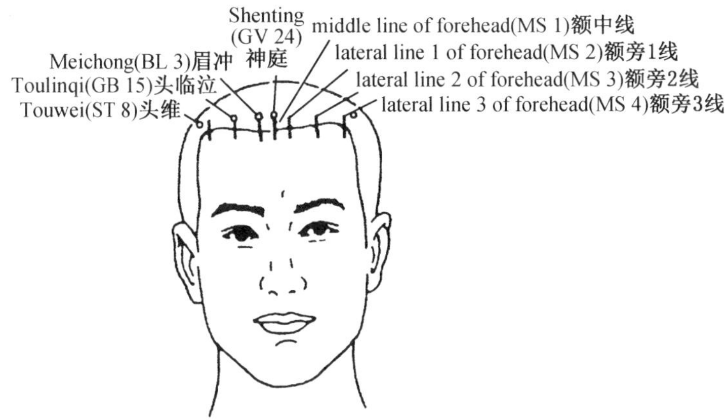

Fig.6-21 Therapeutic lines on frontal region

图6-21 额区治疗线

1.2 Therapeutic lines on parietal region

1.2.1 Middle Line of the Vertex (MS 5)

Location: On the vertex of the head, the line on the governor vessel between Baihui(GV 20) and Qianding(GV 21)(Fig.6-22).

Indications: Paralysis, numbness and pain in the lower back and legs, cortical polyuria, prolapse of rectum, enuresis, hypertension and vertex pain.

1.2.2 Lateral Line 1 of the Vertex (MS 8)

Location: On the vertex of the head, the line 1.5 cun in length on bladder meridian between Tongtian(BL 7) and Luoque(BL 8)(Fig.6-22).

1.2 顶区治疗线

1.2.1 顶中线

定位: 在头顶部,从督脉百会穴至前顶穴之间的连线(图6-22)。

主治: 腰腿瘫痪、麻木、疼痛,以及皮质性多尿、脱肛、遗尿、高血压、头顶痛等。

1.2.2 顶旁1线

定位: 在头顶部,从膀胱经通天穴向后引一条长1.5寸的直线到络却穴(图6-22)。

Indications: Paralysis, numbness and pain in the lower back and legs.

主治: 腰腿瘫痪、麻木、疼痛等。

1.2.3 Lateral Line 2 of the Vertex (MS 9)

1.2.3 顶旁2线

Location: On the vertex of the head, the line 1.5 cun in length on the gallbladder meridian between Zhengying(GB 17) and Chengling(GB 18)(Fig. 6-22).

定位: 在头顶部,从胆经正营穴向后引一条长1.5寸的直线到承灵穴(图6-22)。

Indications: Paralysis, numbness and pain in the upper limbs.

主治: 上肢瘫痪、麻木、疼痛等。

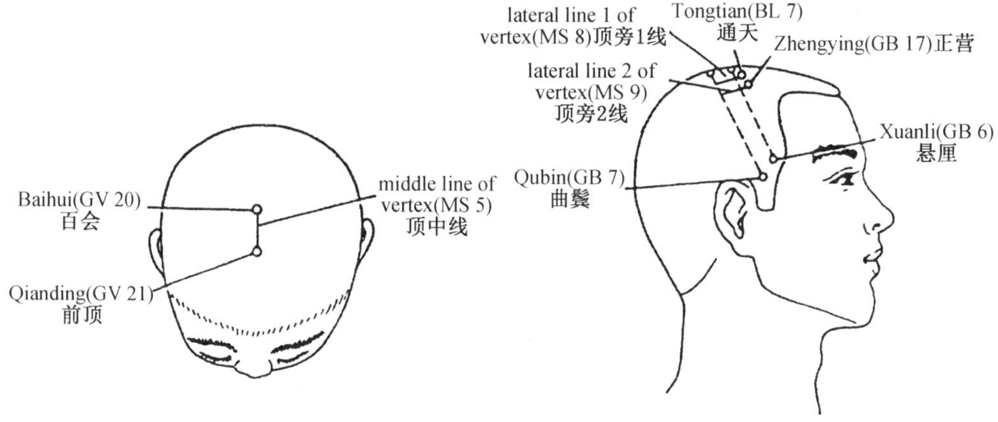

Fig.6-22 Therapeutic lines on the parietal region

图6-22 顶区治疗线

1.2.4 Anterior Oblique Line of the Vertex-Temporal (MS 6)

1.2.4 顶颞前斜线

Location: On the vertex and temporal region of the head, the line between Baihui(GV 20) and Xuanli(GB 6)(Fig. 6-23).

定位: 在头顶、头侧部,头部经外奇穴前神聪至胆经悬厘穴之间的连线(图6-23)。

Indications: The whole line is divided into five equal sections. The upper one-fifth section is effective for paralysis in the contralateral legs and trunk, the middle two-fifths section for paralysis in the contralateral arm, and lower two-fifths section for contralateral central facial palsy, aphemia and cere-

主治: 全线分为5等份,上1/5治疗对侧下肢和躯干瘫痪,中2/5治疗对侧上肢瘫痪,下2/5治疗对侧中枢性面瘫、运动性失语、脑动脉粥样硬化等。

bral arteriosclerosis.

1.2.5 Posterior Oblique Line of the Vertex-Temporal (MS 7)

Location: On the vertex and temporal region of the head, the line between Baihui(GV 20) and Qubin(GB 7)(Fig.6-23).

Indications: The whole line is divided into five equal sections. The upper one-fifth section is effective for sensory abnormality in the contralateral legs and trunk, the middle two-fifths section for sensory abnormality in the contralateral arm, and lower two-fifths section for contralateral facial sensory abnormality.

1.2.5 顶颞后斜线

定位: 在头顶、头侧部，督脉百会至胆经曲鬓穴之间的连线(图 6-23)。

主治: 全线分为 5 等份，上 1/5 治疗对侧下肢和躯干感觉异常；中 2/5 治疗对侧上肢感觉异常；下 2/5 治疗对侧头面部感觉异常。

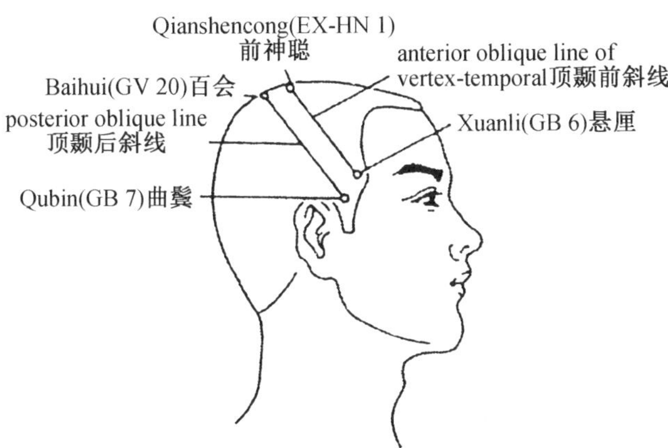

Fig.6-23 Therapeutic lines on the temporal region

图 6-23 顶颞区治疗线

1.3 Therapeutic lines on the temporal region

1.3.1 Anterior Temporal Line (MS 10)

Location: On the temporal area of the head, the line between Hanyan(GB 4) and Xuanli(GB 2) (Fig.6-24).

Indications: Migraine headache, aphemia, peripheral facial palsy and oral diseases.

1.3 颞区治疗线

1.3.1 颞前线

定位: 在头的颞部，胆经颔厌穴至悬厘穴的连线(图 6-24)。

主治: 偏头痛、运动性失语、周围性面神经麻痹以及口腔疾病等。

1. 3. 2　Posterior Temporal Line (MS 11)

Location: On the temporal area of the head, the line between Shuaigu(GB 8) and Qubin(GB 7) (Fig. 6-24).

Indications: Migraine headache, tinnitus, deafness and dizziness.

1. 3. 2　颞后线

定位: 在头的颞部,胆经率谷穴至曲鬓穴的连线(图 6-24)。

主治: 偏头痛、耳鸣、耳聋、眩晕等。

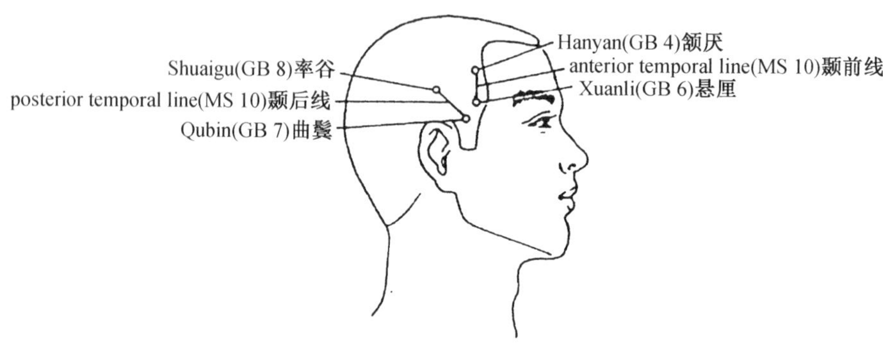

Fig. 6-24　Therapeutic lines on parietal region

图 6-24　颞区治疗线

1. 4　Therapeutic lines on the occipital region

1. 4. 1　Upper Middle Line of the Occipital Region (MS 12)

Location: On the posterior part of the head, the line 1.5 cun in length between Naohu(GV 17) and Qiangjian(GV 18)(Fig. 6-25).

Indications: Optic atrophy, cataract, and myopia.

1. 4. 2　Upper Lateral Line of the Occipital Region (MS 13)

Location: On the posterior part of the head, the line 1.5 cun in length upwards from the site 0.5 cun lateral to Naohu(GV 17)(Fig. 6-25).

Indications: Cortical visual disorder, optic atro-

1. 4　枕区治疗线

1. 4. 1　枕上正中线

定位: 在后头部,督脉脑户穴至强间穴之间长1.5寸的连线(图 6-25)。

主治: 视神经萎缩、白内障、近视眼等眼病。

1. 4. 2　枕上旁线

定位: 在后头部,由督脉脑户穴旁开 0.5 寸起,向上引一条长 1.5 寸的直线(图 6-25)。

主治: 皮质性视力障碍、

phy, cataract, and myopia.

视神经萎缩、白内障、近视眼等眼病。

1.4.3 Lower Lateral Line of the Occipital Region (MS 14)

Location: On the posterior part of the head, the line 2.0 cun in length downwards from Yuzhen (BL 9)(Fig.6-25).

Indications: Equilibrium disturbance due to cerebellar diseases, and posterior headache.

1.4.3 枕下旁线

定位: 在后头部,从膀胱经玉枕穴向下引一条长2寸的直线(图6-25)。

主治: 小脑疾病引起的平衡障碍、后头痛等。

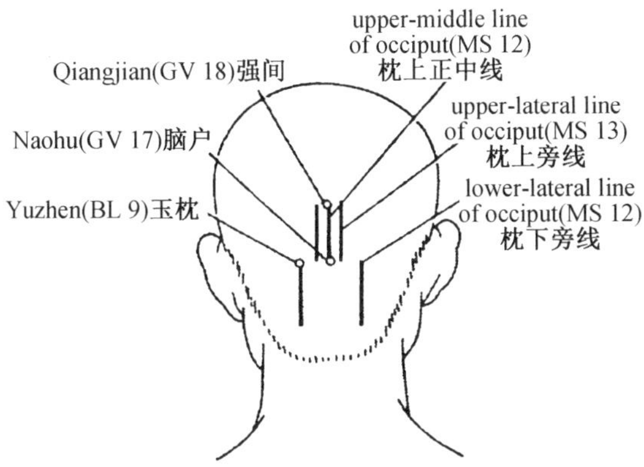

Fig.6-25 Therapeutic lines on the occipital region

图6-25 枕区治疗线

2 Indications

Scalp acupuncture is primarily indicated for cerebral diseases, such as hemiparalysis and limb numbness and aphasia due to cerebral vascular accidents, and cortical polyuria, cortical visual disturbance, epilepsy, childhood cerebral paralysis, low intelligence in children, chorea and shaking palsy; as well as mental disorders, headache, insomnia, hypertension, coronary heart disease, bronchitis, ulcers in the stomach and duodenum, impotence, prolapse of uterus, enuresis, sciatic, myopia and

2 头针的适应范围

头针主要用于治疗脑源性疾病,如脑血管意外而致的偏瘫、肢体麻木、失语,以及皮质性多尿、皮质性视力障碍、癫痫、小儿脑瘫、小儿弱智、舞蹈病、震颤麻痹等。此外,也可治疗精神病、头痛、失眠、高血压、冠心病、支气管炎、胃和十二指肠溃疡、阳痿、子宫脱垂、遗尿、坐骨

rhinitis.

神经痛、近视眼、鼻炎等各科疾病。

3 Manipulations

3　头针的操作方法

3.1 Posture and sterilization

Sitting position is often selected for the convenience to locate scalp acupoints and perform manipulations. Before acupuncture, the hair is separated to expose the scalp acupoints, and then sterilized with cotton ball of 75% alcohol.

3.1　体位和消毒

为便于头针的定位和操作，一般多取坐位。针刺前拨开头发、暴露头皮，用 75% 的乙醇棉球消毒头针刺激线的进针点。

3.2 Insertion of the needle

Select the filiform needles of the varying length from the therapeutic lines, and swiftly insert the needles beneath the scalp at the angle of 30°. When the needle tips reach the subgaleal layer and the practitioner feels decreasing resistance under his finger, further insert the needles horizontally to the desired location.

3.2　进针

根据治疗线的长度选择相应型号的毫针，针尖与头皮呈 30°夹角快速将针刺入头皮下。当针尖达到帽状腱膜下层时，指下感到阻力减小，然后使针与头皮平行沿着治疗线继续推进至所需的位置。

3.3 Rotation of the needle

In scalp acupuncture, the handle of the needle is held by the palmar surface of the thumb and the radial surface of the index finger(Fig. 6-26). The needle is rotated by bending and extending the index finger rapidly and continuously at the frequency of 200 times per minute for 2～3 minutes. The needle is then retained for 20～30 minutes, during which the needle is rotated 2～3 times. For those with hemiplagia, they are encouraged to exercise the paralyzed limbs(passive exercise in severe cases) during the need-ling retention to enhance clinical efficacy.

3.3　捻针

一般以拇指指腹和食指第一节的桡侧面夹持针柄，通过食指掌指关节快速的连续屈伸，使针身左右转动（图 6-26），频率达每分钟 200 次左右，持续捻转 2～3 分钟，留针 20～30 分钟。留针期间可行捻转手法 2～3 次。偏瘫等运动障碍患者留针期间嘱其活动肢体，重症患者可作被动活动，有助于提高治疗效果。

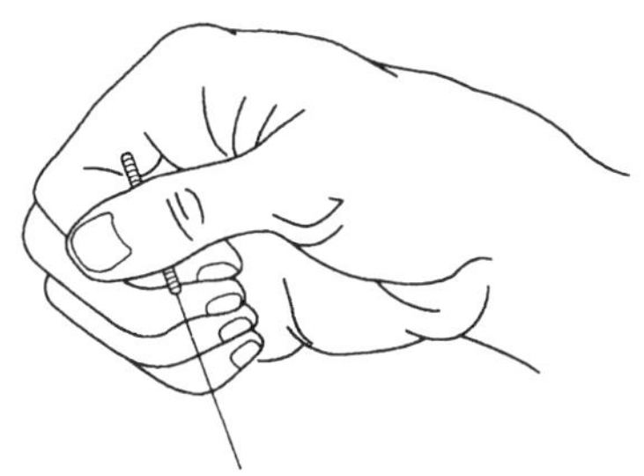

Fig.6-26 Needling rotation in scalp acupuncture

图 6-26 头针捻针

3.4 Withdrawal of the needle

Hold dry sterilized cotton ball against the acupoints by the pressing hand, and gently rotate the needle outwards under the skin by the puncturing hand. Quickly withdraw the needle and press the puncture hole with the cotton ball for 1～2 minutes to avoid bleeding.

4 Precautions in scalp acupuncture

Clinic precautions include following aspects: ①Since the scalp is covered by the hair, careful and strict disinfection should be done before needling to prevent infection; ②scalp acupuncture often produces strong stimulation, so sitting position is advisable to prevent fainting; ③scalp acupuncture is not recommended for infants because their cranial sutures have not ossified completely, or for those with defected skull; ④patients with cerebral hemorrhage are not advisable to undergo scalp acupuncture until the pathological condition and blood pressure are stably controlled.

3.4 起针

押手持消毒干棉球固定穴旁头皮，刺手夹持针柄轻轻捻转针身，缓慢将针退至皮下，然后快速出针，再用消毒干棉球按压针孔 1～2 分钟，以防出血。

4 头针的注意事项

临床应注意以下问题：①因头发遮盖头皮，所以消毒要仔细、严格，以防感染；②头针刺激较强，又常采用坐位，须防止晕针；③婴儿由于颅骨骨缝没有完全闭合，或者颅骨有缺损的患者，不宜采用头针治疗；④脑溢血患者，须待病情及血压稳定后方可进行头针治疗。

Section 4 Ear Acupuncture

第4节 耳针

Ear acupuncture is a therapy used in the treatment and prevention of diseases by stimulating certain points on the auricle with needles or other devices. This therapy, with broad indications, not only produces good therapeutic results, but also provides significant diagnositc references.

耳针是用针刺等方法刺激耳郭穴位以防治疾病的一种方法。其治疗范围广泛，不但对于疾病的治疗有特殊效果，而且对疾病的诊断亦有一定的参考意义。

1 Relationship between the ear with meridians and zang-fu organs

1 耳与经络脏腑的关系

1.1 Relationship between the ear and meridians

1.1 耳与经络的关系

The hand-taiyang meridian, hand and foot shaoyang meridians as well as hand-yangming meridian all enter into the ear; foot-yangming meridian ascends to the preauricular region and the foot-taiyang meridian reaches the upper corner of the ear. The yin meridians do not directly enter into the ear, but they can also communicate with the ear via their meridian divergencies which connect with the yang meridians. Therefore, the twelve meridians can directly or indirectly reach the ear, just as Ling Shu says: "All meridians converge at the ear."

手太阳、手足少阳经脉及手阳明络脉均入耳中；足阳明、足太阳经脉分别上耳前、至耳上角；六阴经虽不直接入耳，但都通过经别离、入、出、合与阳经相合，而与耳相联系。因此，十二经脉或直接或间接上达于耳部。故《灵枢·口问》曰："耳者，宗脉之所聚也。"

1.2 Relationship between the ear and zang-fu organs

1.2 耳与脏腑的关系

As recorded in Nei Jing and Nan Jing, the ear is in close relationship with the zang-fu organs in physiology and pathology. Ling Shu said: "Ear is one tissue of kidney system." Su Wen states, "Liver disorders can make the ear fail to hear." Nan Jing said: "Lung governs the sound and then ensure the ear to hear." *Standards of Diagnosis and Treatment* (Zheng Zhi Zhun Sheng) said: "Kidney opens into

据《内经》《难经》等记载，耳与脏腑在生理、病理上密切相关。《灵枢·五阅五使》曰："耳者，肾之官也。"《素问·脏气法时论》指出："肝病者……耳无所闻。"《难经·四十难》曰："肺主声，故令耳闻声。"《证治准绳·杂

the ears and the heart helps the ear." *Corrected Massage Techniques*(Li Zheng An Mo Yao Shu) divides the auricle into five parts: "The upper ear communicates with the heart, the lower ear with the kidney, the posterior-interior ear with the lung, the posterior-exterior ear with the liver, and the middle ear with the spleen."

病》曰:"肾为耳窍之主,心为耳窍之客。"《厘正按摩要术》则将耳郭分为心肝脾肺肾五部:"耳上属心……耳下属肾……耳后耳里属肺……耳后耳外属肝……耳后中间属脾。"

2 Anatomical terminolgy of auricular surface

2 耳郭表面解剖

2.1 Anatomical terminolgy of auricular anterior surface(Fig.6-27)

2.1 耳郭前面的表面解剖(图 6-27)

Helix The curling prominent brim of the auricle.

耳轮 耳郭卷曲的游离部分。

Helix tubercle The small bulge at the posterior-superior aspect of the helix.

耳轮结节 耳轮后上部的膨大部分。

Helix cauda The inferior part of the helix that forms the junction of the helix and the earlobe.

耳轮尾 耳轮向下移行于耳垂的部分。

Helixcrus A transverse ridge of the helix continuing backwards into the ear cavity in the center of the ear.

耳轮脚 耳轮深入耳甲的部分。

Antihelix The elevated ridge anterior to and parallel to the helix. The Y-shaped ridge located at the upper part of the helix.

对耳轮 与耳轮相对呈"Y"字形的隆起部,由对耳轮体、对耳轮上脚和对耳轮下脚三部分组成。

Antihelix body The main part of the antihelix that extends in a vertical direction.

对耳轮体 对耳轮下部呈上下走向的主体部分。

Superior antihelix crus The upward branch of the antihelix.

对耳轮上脚 对耳轮向上分支的部分。

Inferior antihelix crus The anterior branch of the antihelix.

对耳轮下脚 对耳轮向前分支的部分。

Triangular fossa The triangular depression circumscribed by the superior antihelix crus, the inferior antihelix crus, and the anterior portion of the helix.

三角窝 对耳轮上、下脚与相应耳轮之间的三角形凹窝。

Scapha The depression between the antihelix and helix.

耳舟 耳轮与对耳轮之间的凹沟。

Tragus　The small curved flap or eminence anterior to the auricle.

Supratragic notch　The depression between the upper border of the tragus and the helix crus.

Antitragus　The small tubercle inferior to the tragus, superior to the earlobe and opposite to tragus.

Intertragic notch　The depression between the tragus and the antitragus.

Antitragus-helix notch　The depression between the helix and antitragus.

Earlobe　The lowest part of the auricle where there is soft and fleshy tissue with no cartilage.

Concha　The hollow area formed by parts of the helix and antihelix, antitragus and the orifice of the external auditory meatus. It is composed of cymba concha and cavum concha.

Cymba concha　The concha superior to the helix crus.

耳屏　耳郭前方呈瓣状的隆起。

屏上切迹　耳屏与耳轮之间的凹陷处。

对耳屏　对耳轮下方、耳垂上方,与耳屏相对的瓣状隆起。

屏间切迹　耳屏和对耳屏之间的凹陷处。

轮屏切迹　对耳轮与对耳屏之间的凹陷处。

耳垂　耳郭下部无软骨的部分。

耳甲　部分耳轮和对耳轮、对耳屏及外耳门之间的凹窝。由耳甲艇、耳甲腔两部分组成。

耳甲艇　耳轮脚以上的耳甲部。

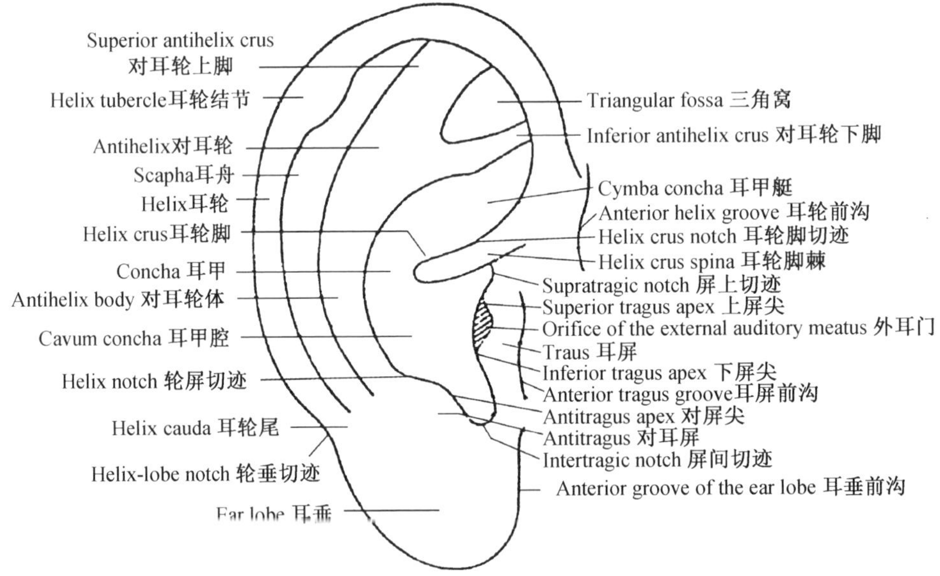

Fig.6-27　Surface anatomy of anterior auricle

图 6-27　耳郭前面的表面解剖

Cavum concha The concha inferior to the helix crus.

Orifice of the external auditory meatus The opening in front of the cavum concha.

2.2 Anatomical terminolgy of auricular posterior surface(Fig.6-28)

Posterior helix The flat part of the back of the helix.

Posterior helix cauda The flat part of the back of the helix cauda.

Posterior earlobe The flat part of the back of the earlobe.

Scapha eminence The eminence of the back of the helix notch.

Triangular fossa eminence The eminence of the back of the triangular fossa.

Cavum concha eminence The eminence of the back of the cavum concha.

Cymba concha eminence The eminence of the back of the cymba concha.

Superior antihelix crus groove The hollow groove of the back of the superior antihelix crus.

Inferior antihelix crus groove The hollow groove of the back of the inferior antihelix crus.

Antihelix groove The hollow groove of the back of the antihelix body.

Helixcrus groove The hollow groove of the back of the helix crus.

Antitragus groove The hollow groove of the back of the antitragus.

Upper ear root The highest part of the auricle connecting with the head.

Lower ear root The lowest part of the auricle connecting with the head.

耳甲腔 耳轮脚以下的耳甲部。

外耳门 耳甲腔前方的孔窍。

2.2 耳郭背面的表面解剖(图 6-28)

耳轮背面 耳轮背部的平坦部分。

耳轮尾背面 耳轮尾背部的平坦部分。

耳垂背面 耳垂背部的平坦部分。

耳舟隆起 耳舟在耳背呈现的隆起。

三角窝隆起 三角窝在耳背呈现的隆起。

耳甲艇隆起 耳甲艇在耳背呈现的隆起。

耳甲腔隆起 耳甲腔在耳背呈现的隆起。

对耳轮上脚沟 对耳轮上脚在耳背呈现的凹沟。

对耳轮下脚沟 对耳轮下脚在耳背呈现的凹沟。

对耳轮沟 对耳轮体在耳背呈现的凹沟。

耳轮脚沟 耳轮脚在耳背呈现的凹沟。

对耳屏沟 对耳屏在耳背呈现的凹沟。

上耳根 耳郭与头部相连的最上部。

下耳根 耳郭与头部相连的最下部。

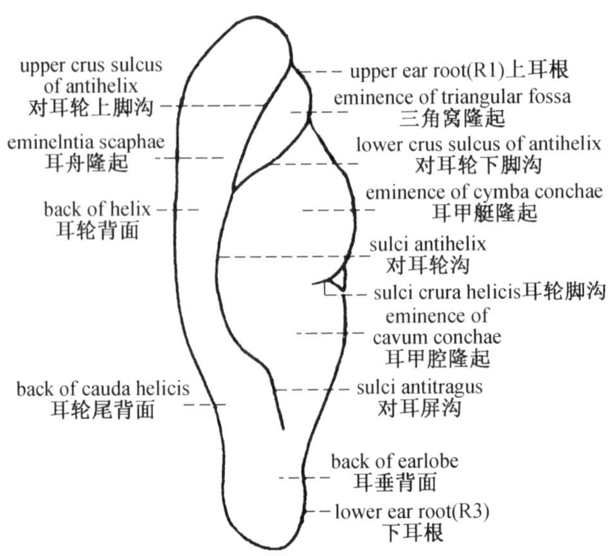

Fig.6-28　Surface anatomy of posterior auricle

图 6-28　耳郭背面的表面解剖

3　Distribution of auricular acupoints

Auricular acupoints are distributed on the ear like the points on the picture of an upside-down fetus, with the head downwards and hip upwards. The acupoints related to the head and face are distributed on the earlobe; the acupoints related to the upper limbs are distributed on the scapha; the acupoints related to the lower limbs are distributed on the superior and inferior antihelix crus; the acupoints related to the trunk are distributed on the antihelix body; the acupoints related to the organs in the chest are distributed on the cymba concha; the acupoints related to the organs in the abdomen are distributed on the cavum concha; the acupoints related to the pelvic cavity are distributed on the triangular fossa; and the acupoints related to the digestive tract are distributed around the helix crus (Fig.6-29).

3　耳穴的分布

耳穴在耳郭的分布犹如一个倒置在子宫内的胎儿，头部朝下、臀部朝上。其分布规律是：与头面相应的穴位分布在耳垂，与上肢相应的穴位分布在耳舟，与下肢相应的穴位分布在对耳轮上、下脚，与躯干相应的耳穴分布在对耳轮体，与胸腔内脏相应的穴位分布在耳甲腔，与腹腔内脏相应的耳穴分布在耳甲艇，与盆腔相应的耳穴分布在三角窝，与消化道相应的耳穴分布在耳轮脚周围（图 6-29）。

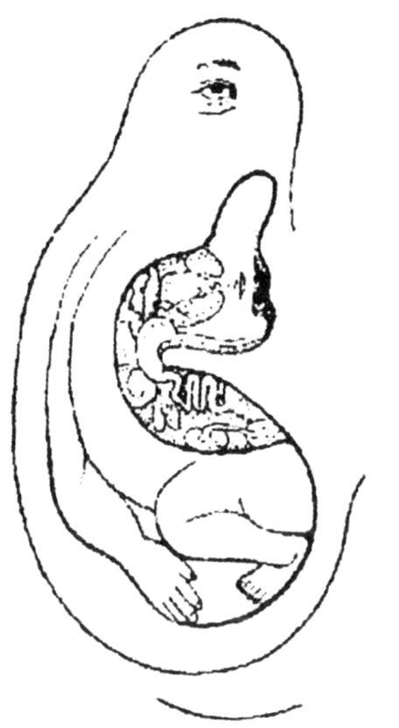

Fig.6-29 Schematic distribution of auricular acupoints

图 6-29 耳穴分布规律示意图

4 Location and indications of auricular acupoints

4.1 Acupoints on the helix

4.1.1 Regions on the helix(Fig. 6-30) The helix is divided into 12 regions. The helix crus is called helix region 1; the helix between helix crus notch and the upper border of the inferior antihelix crus is divided into three equal parts, and respectively called helix region 2, helix region 3 and helix region 4 from the top to the bottom; the helix between the upper border of the inferior antihelix crus and the anterior border of the superior antihelix crus is called helix region 5; the helix between the anterior border of the superior antihelix crus and ear apex is called helix region 6; the helix between the ear apex and the upper border of the helix tubercle is called helix region 7; the helix between the upper and lower borders of the helix tubercle is called helix region

4 耳穴的定位和主治

4.1 耳轮穴位

4.1.1 耳轮分区(图 6-30) 耳轮分为 12 个区。耳轮脚为耳轮 1 区;耳轮脚切迹到对耳轮下脚上缘之间耳轮分为三等份,自下而上依次为耳轮 2 区、3 区、4 区;对耳轮下脚上缘到对耳轮上脚前缘之间的耳轮为耳轮 5 区;对耳轮上脚前缘到耳尖之间的耳轮为耳轮 6 区;耳尖到耳轮结节上缘为耳轮 7 区;耳轮结节上缘到耳轮结节下缘为耳轮 8 区;耳轮结节下缘到轮垂切迹之间的耳轮分为四等份,自上而下依次为

8; the helix between the lower border of the helix tubercle and helix-lobe notch is divided into four equal parts, and respectively called helix region 9, helix region 10, helix region 11 and helix region 12 from the top to the bottom.

耳轮 9 区、10 区、11 区和 12 区。

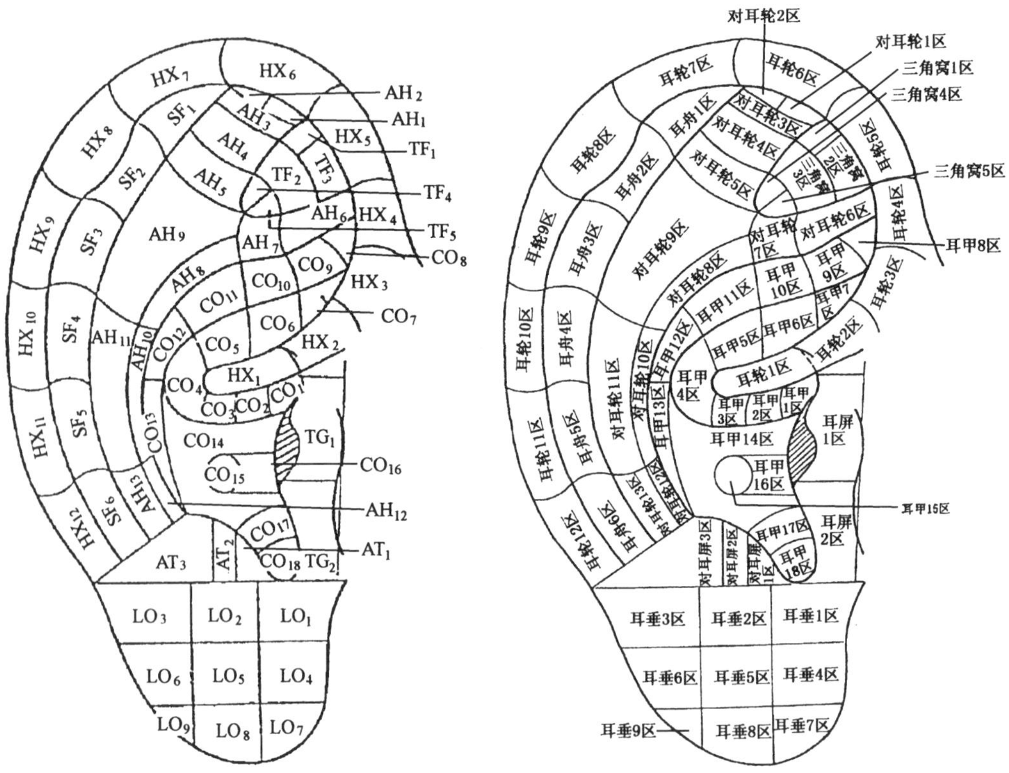

Fig.6-30　Region distributien of the auricle

图 6-30　耳郭分区图

4.1.2　Location and indications (Fig.6-31)

(1) Middle ear (HX_1)

Location: On the helix crus, in helix region 1.

4.1.2　耳轮穴位的定位和主治(图 6-31)

(1) 耳中

定位: 在耳轮脚处,即耳轮 1 区。

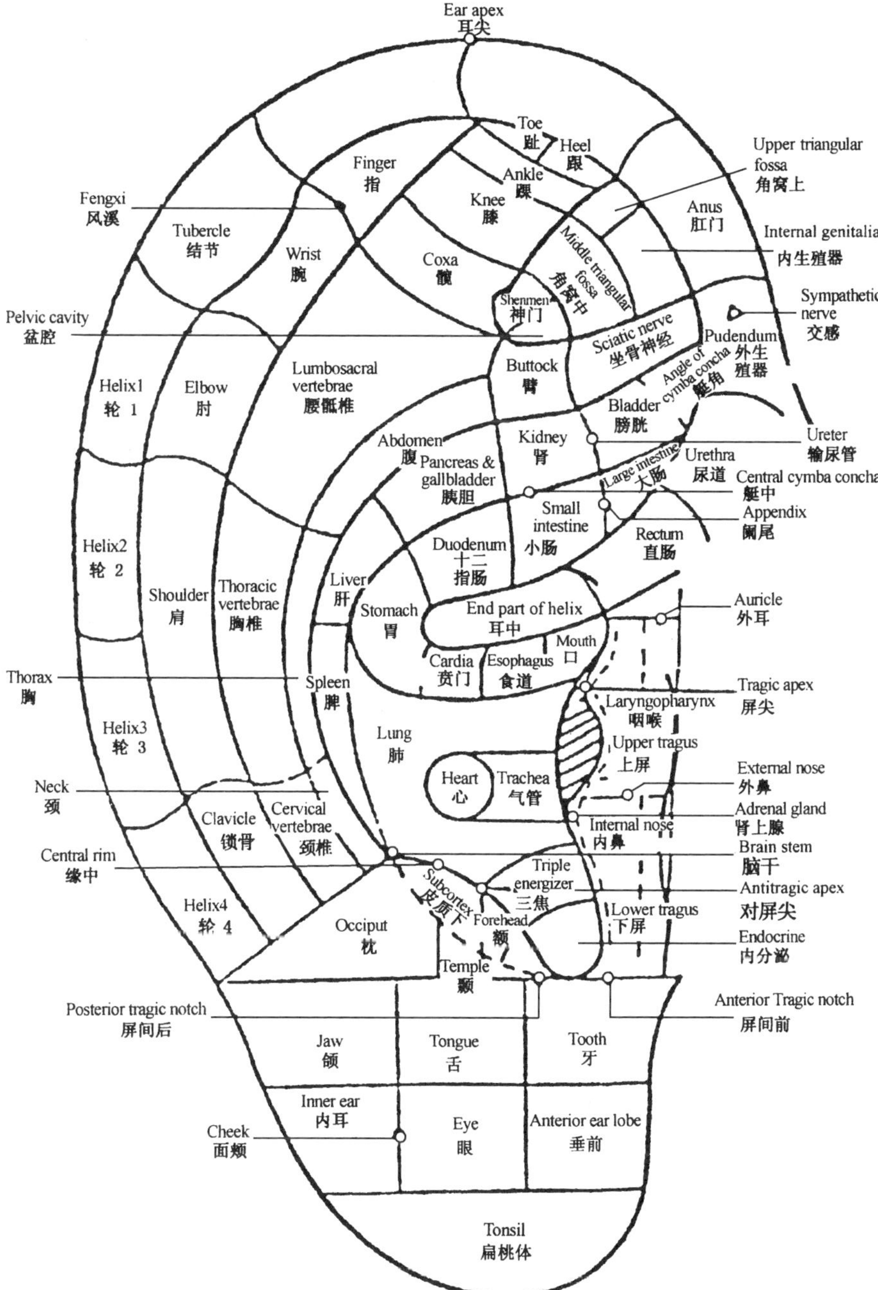

Fig.6-31 Location of auricular acupoints

图 6-31 耳穴定位图

Indications: Hiccup, urticaria and childhood enuresis.

主治：呃逆，荨麻疹，小儿遗尿。

(2) Rectum (HX_2)

(2) 直肠

Location: On the helix anterio-superior to the spine of the helix crus, namely in helix region 2.

定位：在耳轮脚棘前上方的耳轮处，即耳轮 2 区。

Indications: Diarrhea, constipation, prolapse of rectum and hemorrhoids.

主治：腹泻，便秘，脱肛，痔疮。

(3) Urethra (HX_3)

(3) 尿道

Location: On the helix above Zhichang(HX_2), namely in helix region 3.

定位：在直肠上方的耳轮处，即耳轮 3 区。

Indications: Infection of urinary tract, enuresis and urinary retention.

主治：尿路感染，遗尿，尿潴留。

(4) Extermal Genitalia (HX_4)

(4) 外生殖器

Location: On the helix anterior to the inferior antihelix crus, namely in helix region 4.

定位：在对耳轮下脚前方的耳轮处，即耳轮 4 区。

Indications: Vaginitis, testitis, scrotal eczema and impotence.

主治：阴道炎，睾丸炎，阴囊湿疹，阳痿。

(5) Anus (HX_5)

(5) 肛门

Location: On the helix anterior to the triangular fossa, namely in helix region 5.

定位：在三角窝前方的耳轮处，即耳轮 5 区。

Indications: Prolapse of rectum, hemorrhoids and anal fissure.

主治：脱肛，痔疮，肛裂。

(6) Ear Apex (HX_6, HX_7i)

(6) 耳尖

Location: At the apex where the ear is folded forwards, at the junction of the helix regions 6 and 7.

定位：在耳郭向前对折的上部尖端处，即耳轮 6、7 区交界处。

Indications: High fever, hypertension, stye, acute conjunctivitis, and toothache.

主治：发热，高血压，麦粒肿，急性结膜炎，牙痛。

(7) Tubercle (HX_8)

(7) 结节

Location: On the helix tubercle, namely in the helix region 8.

定位：在耳轮结节处，即耳轮 8 区。

Indications: Dizziness, headache and hypertension.

主治：头晕，头痛，高血压。

(8) Lunyi (HX_9)

Location: On the helix inferior to the helix tubercle, namely in helix region 9.

Indications: Fever, tonsillitis, and infection of upper respiratory tract.

(9) Luner(HX_{10})

Location: On the helix inferior to Lunyi (HX_9), namely in the helix region 10.

Indications: Fever, tonsillitis, and infection of upper respiratory tract.

(10) Lunsan(HX_{11})

Location: On the helix inferior to Luner (HX_{10}), namely in helix region 11.

Indications: Fever, tonsillitis, and infection of upper respiratory tract.

(11) Lunsi(HX_{12})

Location: On the helix inferior to Lunsan (HX_{11}), namely in helix region 12.

Indications: Fever, tonsillitis, and infection of upper respiratory tract.

4.2 Acupoints on the scapha

4.2.1 Regions on the scapha (Fig. 6-30) The scapha is divided into six regions. The scapha is divided into six equal parts, and respectively called scapha region 1, 2, 3, 4, 5 and 6 from the top to the bottom.

4.2.2 Location and indications (Fig. 6-30)

(1) Finger(SF_1)

Location: The upper part of scapha, namely in scapha region 1.

Indications: Paronychia, and numbness and pain in the fingers.

(8) 轮 1

定位: 在耳轮结节下方的耳轮处,即耳轮 9 区。

主治: 发热,扁桃体炎,上呼吸道感染。

(9) 轮 2

定位: 在轮 1 下方的耳轮处,即耳轮 10 区。

主治: 发热,扁桃体炎,上呼吸道感染。

(10) 轮 3

定位: 在轮 2 下方的耳轮处,即耳轮 11 区。

主治: 发热,扁桃体炎,上呼吸道感染。

(11) 轮 4

定位: 在轮 3 下方的耳轮处,即耳轮 12 区。

主治: 发热,扁桃体炎,上呼吸道感染。

4.2 耳舟穴位

4.2.1 耳舟分区(图 6-30) 耳舟分为 6 个区。将耳舟分为六等份,自上而下依次为耳舟 1 区、2 区、3 区、4 区、5 区和 6 区。

4.2.2 耳舟穴位的定位和主治(图 6-30)

(1) 指

定位: 在耳舟上方处,即耳舟 1 区。

主治: 甲沟炎,手指麻木和疼痛。

(2) Wrist(SF_2)

Location: Inferior to Zhi (SF_1), namely in scapha region 2.

Indications: Wrist sprain and pain.

(2) 腕

定位: 在指区的下方处，即耳舟2区。

主治: 腕关节扭伤,腕部疼痛。

(3) Fengxi(SF_1, SF_{2i})

Location: Anterior to the helix tubercle, at the junction of SF_1 and SF_2, namely at the junction of scapha regions 1 and 2.

Indications: Urticaria, skin itchiness, and allergic rhinitis.

(3) 风溪

定位: 在耳轮结节前方，指区与腕区之间，即耳舟1区、2区交界处。

主治: 荨麻疹、皮肤瘙痒症、过敏性鼻炎。

(4) Elbow(SF_3)

Location: Inferior to Wan (SF_2), namely in scapha region 3.

Indications: External and internal humeral epicondylitis.

(4) 肘

定位: 在腕区的下方处，即耳舟3区。

主治: 肱骨外上髁炎、肱骨内上髁炎。

(5) Shoulder(SF_4, SF_5)

Location: Inferior to Zhou (SF_3), namely in scapha regions 4 and 5.

Indication: Shoulder periarthritis.

(5) 肩

定位: 在肘区的下方处，即耳舟4区、5区。

主治: 肩关节周围炎。

(6) Clavicle(SF_6)

Location: Inferior to Jian(SF_4, SF_5), namely in scapha region 6.

Indication: Shoulder periarthritis.

(6) 锁骨

定位: 在肩区的下方处，即耳舟6区。

主治: 肩关节周围炎。

4.3 Acupoints on the antihelix

4.3.1 Regions on the antihelix(Fig. 6-30) The antihelix is divided into 13 regions. The superior antihelix crus is divided into three parts: upper part, middle part and lower part; the lower part is antihelix region 5; the middle part is antihelix region 4; the upper part is subdivided into two equal areas, the lower half is antihelix 3, and the upper half falls into two parts: the posterior area is antihelix region 2 and the anterior area is antihelix region 1. The in-

4.3 对耳轮穴位

4.3.1 对耳轮分区(图6-30) 对耳轮分为13个区。对耳轮上脚分为上、中、下3等份,下1/3为对耳轮5区，中1/3为对耳轮4区;再将上1/3分为上、下二等份,下1/2为对耳轮3区,再将上1/2分为前后两等份,后1/2为对耳轮2区,前1/2为对耳轮1

ferior antihelix crus is divided into three equal parts: the anterior and middle parts are named antihelix region 6, and the posterior part is named antihelix region 7. The area between the antihelix body at the junction of superior and inferior crus and helix notch is divided into five equal parts; the antihelix body along the concha is divided into anterior one-fourth part and posterior three-fourths part; the anterior-superior two-fifths part is named antihelix region 8, posterior-superior two-fifths part is named antihelix region 9, and anterior-middle two-fifths part is named antihelix region 10, posterior-middle two-fifths part is named antihelix region 11, anterior-inferior one-fifth part is named antihelix region 12, and the posterior-inferior one-fifth part is named antihelix region 13.

区。对耳轮下脚分为前、中、后三等份，中、前 2/3 为对耳轮 6 区，后 1/3 为对耳轮 7 区。将对耳轮体从对耳轮上、下脚分叉处至轮屏切迹分为五等份，再沿对耳轮耳甲缘将对耳轮体分为前 1/4 和后 3/4 两部分，前上 2/5 为对耳轮 8 区，后上 2/5 为对耳轮 9 区，前中 2/5 为对耳轮 10 区，后中 2/5 为对耳轮 11 区，前下 1/5 为对耳轮 12 区，后下 1/5 为对耳轮 13 区。

4.3.2 Location and indications(Fig.6-31)

4.3.2 对耳轮穴位的定位和主治(图 6-31)

(1) Heel(AH_1)

Location: In the anteriosuperior part of the superior antihelix crus, namely in the antihelix region 1.

Indication: Heel pain.

(1) 跟

定位： 在对耳轮上脚前上部，即对耳轮 1 区。

主治： 足跟痛。

(2) Toe(AH_2)

Location: In the posteriosuperior part of the superior antihelix crus, namely in the antihelix region 2.

Indications: Paronychia, and toe pain.

(2) 趾

定位： 在对耳轮上脚后上部，即对耳轮 2 区。

主治： 甲沟炎，趾部疼痛。

(3) Ankle(AH_3)

Location: Inferior to Zhi(AH_3) and Gen(AH 2), namely in the antihelix region 3.

Indication: Ankle sprain.

(3) 踝

定位： 在趾、跟区下方处，即对耳轮 3 区。

主治： 踝关节扭伤。

(4) knee(AH_4)

Location: On the middle one-third of superior

(4) 膝

定位： 在对耳轮上脚中

antihelix crus, namely in the antihelix region 4.

Indications: Knee arthritis, and knee pain.

(5) Hip(AH_5)

Location: On the lower one-third of superior antihelix crus, namely in the antihelix region 5.

Indications: Hip pain, sciatica, and lumbosacral pain.

(6) Sciatic Nerve(AH_6)

Location: On the anterior two-thirds of inferior antihelix crus, namely in the antihelix region 6.

Indications: Sciatic and paralysis of the lower limbs.

(7) Sympathesis(AH_{6a})

Location: At the junction of the end of the inferior antihelix crus and the medial margin of the helix, in the front end of antihelix region 6.

Indications: Gastrointestinal spasm, angina pectoris, arrhythmia, biliary colic, ureterolith, dysfunction of autonomic nerves.

(8) Buttooks(AH_7)

Location: On the posterior one-third of the inferior antihelix crus, namely in the antihelix region 7.

Indications: Sciatic, and breech fascitis.

(9) Abdomen(AH_8)

Location: On the upper two-fifths of the antihelix body, namely in the antihelix region 8.

Indications: Abdominal pain, abdominal distension, diarrhea, acute lumbar sprain, menstrual cramps, and postpartum pain due to uterine contraction.

(10) Lumbosacral Vertebrae(AH_9)

1/3 处,即对耳轮 4 区。

主治: 膝关节炎,膝部疼痛。

(5) 髋

定位: 在对耳轮上脚的下 1/3 处,即对耳轮 5 区。

主治: 髋关节疼痛,坐骨神经痛,腰骶部疼痛。

(6) 坐骨神经

定位: 在对耳轮下脚的前 2/3 处,即对耳轮 6 区。

主治: 坐骨神经痛,下肢瘫痪。

(7) 交感

定位: 在对耳轮下脚末端与耳轮内缘相交处,即对耳轮 6 区前端。

主治: 胃肠痉挛,心绞痛,心律失常,胆绞痛,输尿管结石,自主神经功能紊乱。

(8) 臀

定位: 在对耳轮下脚的后 1/3 处,即对耳轮 7 区。

主治: 坐骨神经痛,臀筋膜炎。

(9) 腹

定位: 在对耳轮体前部上 2/5 处,即对耳轮 8 区。

主治: 腹痛,腹胀,腹泻,急性腰扭伤,痛经,产后宫缩痛。

(10) 腰骶椎

定位: 在腹区后方,即对

Location: Posterior to Fu(AH_8), namely in the antihelix region 9.

Indication: Lumbosacral pain.

(11) Chest (AH_{10})

Location: On the middle two-fifths part of the front antihelix body, namely in the antihelix region 10.

Indications: Chest pain, chest fullness, intercostal neuralgia, and mastitis.

(12) Thoracic Vertebrae(AH_{11})

Location: Posterior to Xiong(AH_{10}), namely in the antihelix region 11.

Indications: Chest pain, breast distention and pain before menstruation, mastitis, and insufficient lactation after birth.

(13) Neck(AH_{12})

Location: On the inferior one-fifth of the front antihelix body, namely in the antihelix region 12.

Indications: Stiff neck, and neck pain.

(14) Cervical Vertebrae(AH_{13})

Location: Posterior to Jing(AH_{12}), namely in the antihelix region 13.

Indications: Stiff neck, and cervical spondylosis.

4.4 Acupoints on the triangular fossa

4.4.1 Regions on the triangular fossa(Fig. 6-30)

There are five regions on the triangular fossa. The part between the medial side of helix and the junction of superior and inferior antihelix crus is divided into three equal regions: anterior, middle and posterior regions; the middle region is named triangular fossa region 3; the anterior region is then subdivided into three equals: upper, middle and lower, the upper one-third is named triangular fossa region 1,

耳轮9区。

主治: 腰骶部疼痛。

(11) 胸

定位: 在对耳轮体前部中2/5处,即对耳轮10区。

主治: 胸痛,胸闷,肋间神经痛,乳腺炎。

(12) 胸椎

定位: 在胸区后方,即对耳轮11区。

主治: 胸痛,经前乳房胀痛,乳腺炎,产后泌乳不足。

(13) 颈

定位: 在对耳轮体前部下1/5处,即对耳轮12区。

主治: 落枕,颈项疼痛。

(14) 颈椎

定位: 在颈区后方,即对耳轮13区。

主治: 落枕、颈椎综合征。

4.4 三角窝穴位

4.4.1 三角窝分区(图6-30) 三角窝分为5个区。将三角窝由耳轮内缘至对耳轮上、下脚分叉处分为前、中、后三等份,中1/3为三角窝3区;再将前1/3分为上、中、下三等份,上1/3为三角窝1区,中、下2/3为三角窝2区;再将后1/3分为上、下

the middle and lower one-third is named triangular fossa region 2; the posterior one-third is then subdivided into two equals: the upper and lower section; the upper section is named triangular fossa region 4, and the lower section is named triangular fossa region 5.

4.4.2 Location and indications (Fig.6-31)

(1) Upper Triangular Fossa(TF_1)

Location: On the upper part of the anterior one-third of the triangular fossa, namely in the triangular fossa region 1.

Indication: Hypertension.

(2) Internal Gentalia(TF_2)

Location: On the middle and lower parts of the anterior one-third of the triangular fossa, namely in the triangular fossa region 2.

Indications: Functional uterine bleeding, menstrual cramps, irregular menstruation, infertility, impotence, seminal emission and premature ejaculation.

(3) Midde Triangular Fossa(TF_3)

Location: On the middle one-third of the triangular fossa, namely in the triangular fossa region 3.

Indication: Asthma.

(4) Shenmen (TF_4)

Location: On the upper part of the posterior one-third of the triangular fossa, namely in the triangular fossa region 4.

Indications: Insomnia, sleepiness, epilepsy, hypertension, pain condition, neurasthenia, depression, and withdrawal syndrome.

(5) Pelvic cavity(TF_5)

Location: On the lower part of the posterior

二等份,上 1/2 为三角窝 4 区,下 1/2 为三角窝 5 区。

4.4.2 三角窝穴位的定位和主治(图 6-31)

(1) 角窝上

定位: 在三角窝前1/3的上部,即三角窝 1 区。

主治: 高血压。

(2) 内生殖器

定位: 在三角窝前1/3的中、下部,即三角窝 2 区。

主治: 功能性子宫出血,痛经,月经不调,不孕,阳痿,遗精,早泄。

(3) 角窝中

定位: 在三角窝中1/3处,即三角窝 3 区。

主治: 哮喘。

(4) 神门

定位: 在三角窝后1/3的上部,即三角窝 4 区。

主治: 失眠,多梦,癫痫,高血压,痛证,神经衰弱,抑郁症,戒断综合征。

(5) 盆腔

定位: 在三角窝后1/3的

one-third of the triangular fossa, namely in the triangular fossa region 5.

Indications: Pelvic inflammation, and appendagitis.

下部，即三角窝 5 区。

主治：盆腔炎，附件炎。

4.5 Acupoints on the tragus

4.5 耳屏穴位

4.5.1 Regions on the tragus(Fig.6-30) There are four regions on the tragus. The lateral side of the tragus is divided into two equals of the upper and lower, the upper is named tragus region 1 and the lower is named tragus region 2. The medial side of tragus is also divided into two equals of the upper and lower, the upper is named tragus region 3 and the lower is named tragus region 4.

4.5.1 耳屏分区(图 6-30)

耳屏分为 4 个区。耳屏外侧面分为上、下二等份，上部为耳屏 1 区，下部为耳屏 2 区。耳屏内侧面分为上、下 2 等份，上部为耳屏 3 区，下部为耳屏 4 区。

4.5.2 Location and indications (Fig.6-31)

4.5.2 耳屏穴位的定位和主治(图 6-31)

(1) Upper Tragus(TG_1)

Location: On the upper half of the lateral side of the tragus, namely in the tragus region 1.

Indications: Pharyngitis.

(2) Lower Tragus(TG_2)

Location: On the lower half of the lateral side of the tragus, namely in the tragus region 2.

Indication: Rhinitis.

(3) External Ear(TG_{1u})

Location: Anterior to the superior tragic notch near the helix, namely on the upper edge of TG_1.

Indications: Otitis extena, otitis media, and tinnitus.

(4) Tragic Apex(TG_{1p})

Location: At the top of the upper tragus, posterior to TG_1.

Indications: Toothache, and squint.

(5) External Nose(TG_1, TG_{2i})

Location: In the middle of the lateral side of the

(1) 上屏

定位：在耳屏外侧面上 1/2 处，即耳屏 1 区。

主治：咽炎。

(2) 下屏

定位：在耳屏外侧面下 1/2 处，即耳屏 2 区。

主治：鼻炎。

(3) 外耳

定位：在屏上切迹前方近耳轮部，即耳屏 1 区上缘处。

主治：外耳道炎，中耳炎，耳鸣。

(4) 屏尖

定位：在耳屏游离缘上部尖端，即耳屏 1 区后缘处。

主治：牙痛，斜视。

(5) 外鼻

定位：在耳屏外侧面中

tragus, between TG_1 and TG_2.

Indication: Rhinitis.

(6) Adrenal Qland (TG_{2p})

Location: On the lower end of the free edge of the tragus, posterior to TG_2.

Indications: Low blood pressure, rheumatoid arthritis, mumps, dizziness, asthma and shock.

(7) Throat(TG_3)

Location: On the upper half of the medial side of the tragus, namely in the TG_3.

Indications: Hoarse voice, pharyngitis, tonsillitis and asthma.

(8) Internal Nose(TG_4)

Location: On the lower half of the medial side of the tragus, namely in the TG_4.

Indications: Rhinitis, maxillary sinusitis and nasal bleeding.

(9) Anterior Intertragus(TG_{2b})

Location: On the lowest part of the front of the intertragic notch, on the inferior edge of TG_2.

Indications: Pharyngitis, and stomatitis.

4.6 Acupoints on the antitragus

4.6.1 Regions on the antitragus(Fig.6-30) There are four regions on the antitragus. Make two vertical lines respectively from the antitragus apex and the midpoint between antitragus apex and helix notch to divide the lateral side of the antitragus into three regions: the anterior region, middle region and posterior region; the anterior region is named antitragus region 1, the middle region is named antitragus region 2 and the posterior region is named antitragus region 3; the medial side is named anti-

部,即耳屏1、2区之间。

主治: 鼻炎。

(6) 肾上腺

定位: 在耳屏游离缘下部尖端,即耳屏2区后缘处。

主治: 低血压,风湿性关节炎,腮腺炎,眩晕,哮喘,休克。

(7) 咽喉

定位: 在耳屏内侧面上1/2处,即耳屏3区。

主治: 声音嘶哑,咽炎,扁桃体炎,哮喘。

(8) 内鼻

定位: 在耳屏内侧面下1/2处,即耳屏4区。

主治: 鼻炎,上颌窦炎,鼻出血。

(9) 屏间前

定位: 在屏间切迹前方耳屏最下部,即耳屏2区下缘处。

主治: 咽炎,口腔炎。

4.6 对耳屏穴位

4.6.1 对耳屏分区(图6-30) 对耳屏分为4个区。由对屏尖及对屏尖至轮屏切迹连线之中点,分别向耳垂上线作两条垂直线,将对耳屏外侧面及其后部分为前、中、后3区,前为对耳屏1区,中为对耳屏2区,后为对耳屏3区。耳屏内侧面为对耳屏4区。

tragus region 4.

4.6.2 Location and indications (Fig.6-31)

(1) Forehead(AT_1)

Location: On the front part of the lateral side of the antitragus, namely in the antitragus region 1.

Indications: Front headache, dizziness, insomnia and dreaminess.

(2) Posterior Intertragus(AT_{1b})

Location: Posterior to the intertragic notch and anterior-lower antitragus, on the lower edge of the antitragus region 1.

Indication: Prosopantritis.

(3) Temple(AT_2)

Location: In the middle of the lateral side of the antitragus, namely in the antitragus region 2.

Indications: Migraine headache, and dizziness.

(4) Occiput(AT_3)

Location: Posterior to the lateral side of the antitragus, namely in the antitragus region 3.

Indications: Back headache, dizziness, epilepsy, asthma and neurasthenia.

(5) Subcortex(AT_4)

Location: On the medial side of the antitragus, namely in the antitragus region 4.

Indications: Pain condition, insomnia, neurasthenia, depression, gastric ulcer, and false myopia.

(6) Antitragic Apex(AT_1, AT_2, AT_{4i})

Location: On the tip of the free edge of the antitragus, at the junction of antitragus regions 1, 2 and 4.

Indications: Asthma, mumps, testitis, epididymitis, and neurodermatitis.

4.6.2 对耳屏穴位的定位和主治(图 6-31)

(1) 额

定位: 在对耳屏外侧面的前部,即对耳屏 1 区。

主治: 前头痛,头晕,失眠,多梦。

(2) 屏间后

定位: 在屏间切迹后方,对耳屏前下部,即对耳屏 1 区下缘处。

主治: 额窦炎。

(3) 颞

定位: 在对耳屏外侧面的中部,即对耳屏 2 区。

主治: 偏头痛,头晕。

(4) 枕

定位: 在对耳屏外侧面的后部,即对耳屏 3 区。

主治: 后头痛,头晕,癫痫,哮喘,神经衰弱。

(5) 皮质下

定位: 在对耳屏内侧面,即对耳屏 4 区。

主治: 痛证,失眠,神经衰弱,抑郁症,胃溃疡,假性近视。

(6) 对屏尖

定位: 在对耳屏游离缘的尖端,即对耳屏 1、2、4 区交点处。

主治: 哮喘,腮腺炎,睾丸炎,附睾炎,神经性皮炎。

(7) Middle Border(AT_2, AT_3, AT_{4i})

Location: On the free edge of the antitragus, at the midpoint between the antitragic apex and helix notch, at the junction of the antitragus regions 2, 3 and 4.

Indications: Enuresis, aural vertigo, diabetes insipidus, and functional uterine bleeding.

(8) Brain stem(AT_3, AT_{4i})

Location: On the helix notch.

Indications: Dizziness, back headache, and false myopia.

4.7 Acupoints on the concha

4.7.1 Regions on the concha(Fig.6-30) There are 18 regions on the concha. On the medial edge of the helix, point A is made at the junction of the middle and upper one-third of the line between helix notch and inferior antihelix crus; on the concha, point D is made at the crossing site between the line level with the end of helix crus and antihelix concha; point B is made at the junction of the middle and posterior one-third of the line between the end of helix crus and point D; point C is made at the junction of one-fourth and three-fourths of posterior edge of the opening of the external auditory canal. Draw a curving line from points A to B similar to the curve of the edge of the cymba concha; draw another curving line from points B to C similar to the curve of the lower edge of the inferior helix crus.

Divide the region between the front section of B-C line and the lower edge of inferior helix crus into three equal parts; the anterior one-third is named concha region 1, the middle one-third is named concha region 2, and the posterior one-third

(7) 缘中

定位： 在对耳屏游离缘上，对屏尖与轮屏切迹之中点处，即对耳屏 2、3、4 区交点处。

主治： 遗尿，内耳性眩晕，尿崩症，功能性子宫出血。

(8) 脑干

定位： 在轮屏切迹处。

主治： 眩晕，后头痛，假性近视。

4.7 耳甲穴位

4.7.1 耳甲分区(图 6-30)

耳甲分为 18 个区。在耳轮内缘上，设耳轮脚切迹至对耳轮下脚间中、上 1/3 交界处为 A 点；在耳甲内，由耳轮脚消失处向后作一水平线与对耳轮耳甲缘相交，设交点为 D 点；设耳轮脚消失处至 D 点连线的中、后 1/3 交界处为 B 点；设外耳道口后缘上 1/4 与下 3/4 交界处为 C 点。从 A 点向 B 点作一条与对耳轮耳甲艇缘弧度大体相仿的曲线；从 B 点向 C 点作一条与耳轮脚下缘弧度大体相仿的曲线。

将 BC 线前段与耳轮脚下缘间分成三等份，前 1/3 为耳甲 1 区、中 1/3 为耳甲 2 区、后 1/3 为耳甲 3 区。ABC 线前方，耳轮脚消失处

is named concha region 3. Before the A–B–C line, the ending area of the helix crus is named concha region 4. Divide the region between the front section of A–B line, the upper border of helix crus and medial edge of some helix into three equals; the posterior one-third is named concha region 5, the middle one-third is named concha region 6 and the anterior one-third is named concha region 7. Draw a line between the junction at the anterior and middle one-third of inferior antihelix crus and point A, and the cymba concha before the line is named concha region 8. Divide the concha region 8 after the front section of the A–B line and the lower border of the inferior antihelix crus into two equals, the anterior half is named concha region 9 and the posterior half is named concha region 10. Cymba concha superior to the back section of the A–B line divides the posterior border of concha region 10 and B–D line into two equals, the upper half is named concha region 11 and the lower half is named concha region 12. Draw a line between the helix notch and point B; the concha after this line and under B–D line is named concha region 13. Centered by the midpoint of the cavum concha, circled by the radius one-half of the distance between the midpoint of the B–C line, then the circular area is named concha region 15. Make two tangent lines at the highest and lowest points of concha region 15, and the part between the two lines is named concha region 16. The part around the concha regions 15 and 16 is named concha region 14. Connect the lowest point of external acoustic pore and the midpoint of the concha edge of the antitragus, and then divide the cavum concha below the line into two equals, the upper half is

为耳甲 4 区。将 AB 线前段与耳轮脚上缘及部分耳轮内缘间分成三等份，后 1/3 为 5 区、中 1/3 为 6 区、前 1/3 为 7 区。将对耳轮下脚下缘前、中 1/3 交界处与 A 点连线，该线前方的耳甲艇部为耳甲 8 区。将 AB 线前段与对耳轮下脚下缘间耳甲 8 区以后的部分，分为前、后二等份，前 1/2 为耳甲 9 区，后 1/2 为耳甲 10 区。在 AB 线后段上方的耳甲艇部，将耳甲 10 区后缘与 BD 线之间分成上、下二等份，上 1/2 为耳甲 11 区、下 1/2 为耳甲 12 区。由轮屏切迹至 B 点作连线，该线后方、BD 线下方的耳甲腔部为耳甲 13 区。以耳甲腔中央为圆心，圆心与 BC 线间距离的 1/2 为半径作圆，该圆形区域为耳甲 15 区。过 15 区最高点及最低点分别向外耳门后壁作两条切线，切线间为耳甲 16 区。15，16 区周围为耳甲 14 区。将外耳门的最低点与对耳屏耳甲缘中点相连，再将该线以下的耳甲腔部分为上、下二等份，上 1/2为耳甲 17 区、下 1/2 为耳甲 18 区。

named concha region 17 and the lower half is named concha region 18.

4.7.2 Location and indications (Fig.6-31)

(1) Mouth(CO_1)

Location: At the anterior one-third below the helix crus, namely in the concha region 1.

Indications: Facial paralysis, stomatitis, cholecystitis, periodontitis, and withdrawal syndrome.

(2) Esophagus(CO_2)

Location: At the middle one-third below the helix crus, namely in the concha region 2.

Indications: Esophagitis, and esophagism.

(3) Cardia(CO_3)

Location: At the posterior one-third below the helix crus, namely in the concha region 3.

Indications: Cardiospasm, and nervous vomiting.

(4) Stomach(CO_4)

Location: At the end of the helix crus, namely in the concha region 4.

Indications: Gastrospasm, gastritis, gastric ulcers, indigestion, nausea and vomiting, frontal headache, toothache, and insomnia.

(5) Duodenum(CO_5)

Location: On the posterior one-third of the helix crus and A-B line, namely in the concha region 5.

Indications: Duodenal ulcer, cholecystitis, cholelithiasis, and pylorospasm.

(6) Small Intestine(CO_6)

Location: On the middle one-third of the helix

4.7.2 耳甲穴位的定位和主治(图 6-31)

(1) 口

定位: 在耳轮脚下方前1/3处,即耳甲1区。

主治: 面瘫,口腔炎,胆囊炎,胆石症,牙周炎,戒断综合征。

(2) 食管

定位: 在耳轮脚下方中1/3处,即耳甲2区。

主治: 食管炎,食管痉挛。

(3) 贲门

定位: 在耳轮脚下方后1/3处,即耳甲3区。

主治: 贲门痉挛,神经性呕吐。

(4) 胃

定位: 在耳轮脚消失处,即耳甲4区。

主治: 胃痉挛,胃炎,胃溃疡,消化不良,恶心呕吐,前额痛,牙痛,失眠。

(5) 十二指肠

定位: 在耳轮脚及部分耳轮与AB线之间的后1/3处,即耳甲5区。

主治: 十二指肠溃疡,胆囊炎,胆石症,幽门痉挛。

(6) 小肠

定位: 在耳轮脚及部分

crus and A–B line, namely in the concha region 6.

耳轮与 AB 线之间的中1/3处,即耳甲 6 区。

Indications: Indigestion, abdominal pain, abdominal distention, tachycardia, and arrhythmia.

主治: 消化不良,腹痛,腹胀,心动过速,心律不齐。

(7) Large Intestine(CO_7)

(7) 大肠

Location: On the anterior one-third of the helix crus and A–B line, namely in the concha region 7.

定位: 在耳轮脚及部分耳轮与 AB 线之间的前1/3处,即耳甲 7 区。

Indications: Diarrhea, constipation, cough, toothache, and acne.

主治: 腹泻,便秘,咳嗽,牙痛,痤疮。

(8) Appendix(CO_6, CO_{7i})

(8) 阑尾

Location: At the conjunction of CO_6 and CO_7.

定位: 在小肠区与大肠区之间,即耳甲 6、7 区交界处。

Indications: Simple appendicitis, abdominal pain and diarrhea.

主治: 单纯性阑尾炎,腹痛,腹泻。

(9) Angle of Cymba Concha(CO_8)

(9) 艇角

Location: On the anterior part under the inferior antihelix crus, namely in the concha region 8.

定位: 在对耳轮下脚下方前部,即耳甲 8 区。

Indications: Prostatitis, and urethritis.

主治: 前列腺炎,尿道炎。

(10) Bladder(CO_9)

(10) 膀胱

Location: On the middle part under the inferior antihelix crus, namely in the concha region 9.

定位: 在对耳轮下脚下方中部,即耳甲 9 区。

Indications: Cystitis, enuresis, urinary retention, lumbago, sciatica, and back headache.

主治: 膀胱炎,遗尿,尿潴留,腰痛,坐骨神经痛,后头痛。

(11) Kidney(CO_{10})

(11) 肾

Location: On the posterior part under the inferior antihelix crus, namely in the concha region 10.

定位: 在对耳轮下脚下方后部,即耳甲 10 区。

Indications: Lumbago, tinnitus, neurasthenia, asthma, enuresis, seminal emission, impotence, premature ejaculation and irregular menstrua-tion.

主治: 腰痛,耳鸣,神经衰弱,哮喘,遗尿,遗精,阳痿,早泄,月经不调。

(12) Ureter(CO_9, CO_{10i})

(12) 输尿管

定位: 在肾区与膀胱区

Location: Between the CO_9 and CO_{10}, at the junction of concha regions 9 and 10.

之间，即耳甲9、10区交界处。

Indication: Urethral calculus.

主治: 输尿管结石。

(13) Pancrease and Gallbladder(CO_{11})

(13) 胰胆

Location: On the posteriosuperior part of cymba concha, namely in the concha region 11.

定位: 在耳甲艇的后上部，即耳甲11区。

Indications: Cholecystitis, cholelithiasis, ascariasis of the biliary tract, migraine headache, herpes zoster, otitis, and tinnitus.

主治: 胆囊炎，胆石症，胆道蛔虫症，偏头痛，带状疱疹，中耳炎，耳鸣。

(14) Liver(CO_{12})

(14) 肝

Location: On the posterioinferior part of the cymba concha, namely in concha region 12.

定位: 在耳甲艇的后下部，即耳甲12区。

Indications: Flank pain, dizziness, insom-nia, depression, premenstrual tension syndrome, irregular menstruation, climacteric syndrome, hypertension, myopia, and simple glaucoma.

主治: 胁痛，眩晕，失眠，抑郁症，经前期紧张综合征，月经不调，更年期综合征，高血压，近视眼，单纯性青光眼。

(15) Middle Cymba Concha(CO_6, CO_{10i})

(15) 艇中

Location: Between CO_6 and CO_{10}, at the junction of the concha regions 6 and 10.

定位: 在小肠区与肾区之间，即耳甲6、10区交界处。

Indications: Abdominal pain, abdominal distention, and ascariasis of the biliary tract.

主治: 腹痛，腹胀，胆道蛔虫症。

(16) Spleen(CO_{13})

(16) 脾

Location: Below the B-D line, on the posteriosuperior part of the cavum concha, namely in the concha region 13.

定位: 在BD线下方，耳甲腔的后上部，即耳甲13区。

Indications: Abdominal distension, diarr-hea, constipation, poor appetite, functional uterine bleeding, morbid leucorrhea, and auditory vertigo.

主治: 腹胀，腹泻，便秘，食欲不振，功能性子宫出血，白带过多，内耳性眩晕。

(17) Heart(CO_{15})

(17) 心

Location: In the depression of cavum concha, namely in the concha region 15.

定位: 在耳甲腔正中凹陷处，即耳甲15区。

Indications: Tachycardia, arrhythmia, angina

主治: 心动过速，心律不

pectoris, insomnia, neurasthenia, hysteria, and oral sores.

(18) Trachea(CO_{16})

Location: Between CO_{15} and the external auditory pore, namely in the concha region 16.

Indications: Asthma and bronchitis.

(19) Lung(CO_{14})

Location: In the cavum concha around the CO_{15} and CO_{16}, namely in the concha region 14.

Indications: Common cold, cough, asthma, chest fullness, hoarse voice, skin pruritus, urticaria, constipation and smoking withdrawal syndrome.

(20) Triple Energizer(CO_{17})

Location: On the part posterioinferior to external auditory pore, between CO_{14} and CO_{18}, namely in the concha region 17.

Indications: Constipation, abdominal distension, tinnitus, and pain on the lateral side of the upper limbs.

(21) Endocrine(CO_{18})

Location: Inside the intertragic notch and anterioinferior to the cavum concha, namely in the concha region 18.

Indications: Menstrual cramps, irregular menstruation, climacteric syndrome, acne, mala-ria, diabetes, and hypothyroidism or hyperthyroidism.

齐，心绞痛，失眠，神经衰弱，癔病，口舌生疮。

(18) 气管

定位： 在心区与外耳门之间，即耳甲 16 区。

主治： 哮喘，支气管炎。

(19) 肺

定位： 在心、气管区周围处，即耳甲 14 区。

主治： 感冒，咳嗽，哮喘，胸闷，声音嘶哑，皮肤瘙痒症，荨麻疹，便秘，戒断综合征。

(20) 三焦

定位： 在外耳门后下，肺与内分泌区之间，即耳甲 17 区。

主治： 便秘，腹胀，耳鸣，上肢外侧疼痛。

(21) 内分泌

定位： 在屏间切迹内，耳甲腔的前下部，即耳甲 18 区。

主治： 痛经，月经不调，更年期综合征，痤疮，间日疟，糖尿病，甲状腺功能减退或亢进症。

4.8 Acupoints on the earlobe

4.8.1 Regions on the earlobe (Fig. 6-30) There are 9 regions on the earlobe. Draw two parallel lines of equal distance respectively at the level with the upper line of the earlobe and the lowest point, and then draw two vertical lines with equal distance to

4.8 耳垂穴位

4.8.1 耳垂分区(图 6-30) 耳垂分为 9 个区。在耳垂上线至耳垂下缘最低点之间划两条等距离平行线，于上平行线上引两条垂直等分

divide the earlobe into nine regions. The upper three regions are respectively named earlobe regions 1, 2 and 3 from the front to the back; the middle three regions are respectively named earlobe regions 4, 5 and 6 from the front to the back; and the lower three regions are respectively named earlobe regions 7, 8 and 9 from the front to the back.

线，将耳垂分为9个区，上部由前到后依次为耳垂1区、2区、3区；中部由前到后依次为耳垂4区、5区、6区；下部由前到后依次为耳垂7区、8区、9区。

4.8.2 Location and indications(Fig.6-31)

4.8.2 耳垂穴位的定位和主治(图6-31)

(1) Tooth(LO_1)

Location: On the anteriosuperior part of the front earlobe, namely in the earlobe region 1.

Indications: Periodontitis, and low blood pressure.

(1) 牙

定位: 在耳垂正面前上部，即耳垂1区。

主治: 牙周炎，低血压。

(2) Tongue(LO_2)

Location: On the middle superior part of the front earlobe, namely in the earlobe region 2.

Indications: Glossitis, and stomatitis.

(2) 舌

定位: 在耳垂正面中上部，即耳垂2区。

主治: 舌炎，口腔炎。

(3) Jaw(LO_3)

Location: On the posteriosuperior part of the front earlobe, namely in the earlobe region 3.

Indications: Toothache, and inflammation of temporomandibular joint.

(3) 颌

定位: 在耳垂正面后上部，即耳垂3区。

主治: 牙痛，下颌关节炎。

(4) Anterior Earlobe(LO_4)

Location: On the anterior middle part of the front earlobe, namely in the earlobe region 4.

Indication: Neurasthenia and toothache.

(4) 垂前

定位: 在耳垂正面前中部，即耳垂4区。

主治: 神经衰弱，牙痛。

(5) Eye(LO_5)

Location: On the central part of the front earlobe, namely in the earlobe region 5.

Indications: Acute conjunctivitis, electric ophthalmia, stye, and false myopia.

(5) 眼

定位: 在耳垂正面中央部，即耳垂5区。

主治: 急性结膜炎，电光性眼炎，麦粒肿，假性近视眼。

(6) Internal Ear(LO_6)

Location: On the posterior middle part of the

(6) 内耳

定位: 在耳垂正面后中

front earlobe, namely in the earlobe region 6.

部,即耳垂6区。

Indications: Auditory vertigo, tinnitus, deafness and otitis media.

主治: 内耳性眩晕,耳鸣,耳聋,中耳炎。

(7) Cheek(LO_5, LO_{6i})

(7) 面颊

Location: Between the LO_5 and LO_6, at the junction of earlobe regions 5 and 6.

定位: 在耳垂正面眼区与内耳区之间,即耳垂5、6区交界处。

Indications: Facial palsy, trigeminal neuralgia, acne, verruca, facial spasms, and mumps.

主治: 面神经麻痹,三叉神经痛,痤疮,扁平疣,面肌痉挛,腮腺炎。

(8) Tonsil(LO_7, LO_8, LO_9)

(8) 扁桃体

Location: On the lower part of the front earlobe, namely in the earlobe regions 7, 8 and 9.

定位: 在耳垂正面下部,即耳垂7、8、9区。

Indication: Tonsillitis and pharyngitis.

主治: 扁桃体炎,咽炎。

4.9 Acupoints on the posterior surface of the ear

4.9 耳背穴位

4.9.1 Regions on the posterior surface of the ear (Fig.6-30) There are 5 regions on the posterior surface of the ear. Draw two horizontal lines respectively through the posterior surface of the ear corresponding to the junction of the superior and inferior crus of the antihelix and helix notch to divide the posterior surface of the ear into the upper, middle and lower parts; the upper part is named posterior region 1; the lower part is named posterior region 5; and the middle part is subdivided into three equals: the medial one-third is named posterior region 2, the middle one-third posterior region 3 and the lateral one-third posterior region 4.

4.9.1 耳背分区(图6-30) 耳背分为5个区。分别过对耳轮上、下脚分叉处耳背对应点和轮屏切迹耳背对应点作两条水平线,将耳背分为上、中、下3部,上部为耳背1区,下部为耳背5区,再将中部分为内、中、外三等份,内1/3为耳背2区、中1/3为耳背3区、外1/3为耳背4区。

4.9.2 Location and indications(Fig.6-31)

4.9.2 耳背穴位的定位和主治(图6-31)

(1) Heart(P_1)

(1) 耳背心

Location: On the upper part of the posterior surface of the ear, namely in the posterior region 1.

定位: 在耳背上部,即耳背1区。

Indications: Palpitation, insomnia, and dreami-

主治: 心悸,失眠,多梦。

ness.

(2) Lung(P_2)

Location: On the middle-medial part of the posterior surface of the ear, namely in the posterior region 2.

Indications: Asthma, and skin pruritus.

(2) 耳背肺

定位: 在耳背中内部，即耳背2区。

主治: 哮喘，皮肤瘙痒症。

(3) Spleen(P_3)

Location: At the center of the posterior surface of the ear, namely in the posterior region 3.

Indications: Stomachache, indigestion, poor appetite, and diarrhea.

(3) 耳背脾

定位: 在耳背中央部，即耳背3区。

主治: 胃痛，消化不良，食欲不振，腹泻。

(4) Liver(P_4)

Location: On the middle-lateral part of the posterior surface of the ear, namely in the posterior region 4.

Indications: Cholecystitis, cholelithiasis and flank pain.

(4) 耳背肝

定位: 在耳背中外部，即耳背4区。

主治: 胆囊炎，胆石症，胁痛。

(5) Kidney(P_5)

Location: On the inferior part of the posterior surface of the ear, namely in the posterior region 5.

Indications: Headache, dizziness, and neurasthenia.

(5) 耳背肾

定位: 在耳背下部，即耳背5区。

主治: 头痛，头晕，神经衰弱。

(6) Groove of Posterior Surface(GPS)

Location: In the groove of the antihelix and the grooves of the superior and inferior antihelix crus.

Indications: Hypertension, and skin pruritus.

(6) 耳背沟

定位: 在对耳轮沟和对耳轮上，下脚沟处。

主治: 高血压，皮肤瘙痒症。

(7) Upper Root of Auricle(R_1)

Location: At the top of the root of the ear.

Indication: Nasal bleeding.

(7) 上耳根

定位: 在耳根最上处。

主治: 鼻出血。

(8) Root of Auricular Vagus Norve(R_3)

Location: At the ear root on the posterior groove of the helix crus.

(8) 耳迷根

定位: 在耳轮脚后沟的耳根处。

Indications: Cholecystitis, cholelithiasis, ascariasis of the biliary tract, abdominal pain, diarrhea, nasal stuffiness, and tachycardia.

(9) Lower Root of Auricle(R_2)

Location: At the lowest part of the root of the ear.

Indications: Low blood pressure, paralysis of the lower limbs, and sequelae of infantile paralysis.

5 Clinical application of ear acupuncture

5.1 Indications

Ear acupuncture can be used to treat a wide variety of diseases in different fields, such as common cold, headache, dizziness, hypertension, arrhythmia, neurasthenia, asthma, acute and chronic enterogastritis, bacterial dysentery, cholecystitis, cholelithiasis, diabetes, sprain and contusion, sciatica, cervical spondylosis, shoulder periarthritis, urticaria, chloasma, acne, menstrual cramps, climacteric syndrome, mumps, hyperthyroidism or hypothyroidism, periodontitis, pharyngitis, tonsillitis, stye, obesity and withdrawal syndrome.

5.2 Principles of selecting ear acupoints

5.2.1 According to disease location When the body suffers from a disorder, the auricular acupoint related to the diseased organ is selected. For example, Stomach (CO_4) is selected for stomachache, Lung(CO_14) for cough, and Eye(LO_5) for myopia.

5.2.2 According to Chinese medical theory In the light of theories of the zang-fu and meridians, corresponding auricular acupoints may be selected. For example, Kidney(CO_10) may be selected for tinnitus, Lung (CO_14) for urticaria, Small Intestine

主治： 胆囊炎，胆石症，胆道蛔虫症，腹痛，腹泻，鼻塞，心动过速。

（9）下耳根

定位： 在耳根最下处。

主治： 低血压，下肢瘫痪，小儿麻痹后遗症。

5 耳针的临床应用

5.1 适应范围

耳针的临床治疗范围相当广泛，包括各科疾病，如感冒、头痛、头晕、高血压、心律不齐、神经衰弱、哮喘、急慢性肠胃炎、细菌性痢疾、胆囊炎、胆石症、糖尿病、扭挫伤、坐骨神经痛、颈椎病、肩周炎、荨麻疹、黄褐斑、痤疮、痛经、更年期综合征、腮腺炎、甲状腺功能亢进或低下、牙周炎、咽喉炎、扁桃体炎、麦粒肿、肥胖症和戒断综合征等。

5.2 选穴原则

5.2.1 按相应部位取穴 当机体患病时，可选取与病变部位相应的耳穴，如胃痛取“胃”穴；咳嗽取“肺”穴；近视眼取“眼”穴等。

5.2.2 按中医学理论取穴 根据脏腑、经络学说的理论，选取相应的耳穴，如耳鸣取“肾”穴；荨麻疹取“肺”穴；心动过速取“小肠”穴；坐骨

(CO_6) for tachycardia, and Bladder(coq). for sciatica.

5.2.3 According to western medicine In the light of the physiological and pathological knowledge in western medicine, relevant auricular acupoints may be selected. For example, Adrenal Gland(TG_{2P}) is selected for asthma, Endocrine(CO_{18}) for irregular menstruation, and Sympathesis(AH_{6a}) for gastric spasms.

5.2.4 According to clinical experi-ence Some empirical acupoints are selected in the light of the clinical experience. For example, Ear Apex(HX_6, HX_{7i}) is selected for stye, Shenmen(TF_1) for withdrawal syndrome, and Erbeigou(GPS) for hypertension.

5.3 Methods of manipulation

5.3.1 Detection of auricular acupoints When the internal organs or the body is diseased, some positive reactions may be found on the auricle by acupoints detection. These positive reactions can provide diagnostic evidence, and can also be employed as the therapeutic sites.

Observation by eyes Under natural light, observe the signs of morphological changes and discoloration on the auricle, such as papules, scaling, nodules, congestion, depressions or blisters.

Detection of the tender spot Find the tender spots or sensitive sites by gentle and even pressure with probing needle or filiform needle.

Detection by electric resistance The electro-detector may be applied to detect the electric resistance of the auricular acupoints. The lowered electric resis-tance of the auricular acupoints can be displayed by the monitor and indicator lamp or special sound.

神经痛取“膀胱”穴等。

5.2.3 按西医学理论取穴

根据西医学的生理、病理知识，选取相关耳穴，如哮喘取“肾上腺”穴；月经不调取“内分泌”穴；胃痉挛取“交感”穴等。

5.2.4 按临床经验取穴 根据临床实践经验，选取有效耳穴，如麦粒肿取“耳尖”穴；戒断综合征取“神门”穴；高血压取“耳背沟”等。

5.3 操作方法

5.3.1 耳穴探查 人体的内脏或躯体发病时，通过耳穴探查，往往可在耳郭的相应部位找出各种阳性反应。这些反应点既可作为辅助诊断的依据，也可作为治疗的刺激点。

望诊 在自然光线下，观察耳郭表面有无变形、变色等征象，如丘疹、脱屑、结节、充血、凹陷、小水疱等。

压痛 用探针或毫针针尾等，采用缓慢、均匀的压力寻找压痛点。

电阻测定 用电阻测定仪测定耳穴皮肤的电阻，低电阻的耳穴（良导电）可通过仪器的显示屏、指示灯或声音反映出来。

5. 3. 2 Stimulating methods

Filiform needle method Select the filiform needles of 0. 5 cun in length. Sterilize the acupoints first with 2% iodine and then 75% alcohol. Stabilize the auricle with the thumb and index finger of the left hand, with the middle finger against the posterior surface of the ear. Insert the needle into the acupoint with the right hand, with the needling depth of 0. 2～0. 3 cm to the cartilage. Generally, the needle is retained for 20～30 minutes, and the needle can be rotated to increase the needling sensation. Also electric stimulator may be used to give eletro-acupuncture.

Needle-embedding method After sterilization, thumbtack needle may be inserted into the auricular acupoint and then fix it with adhesive tape. Retain the needle for 2～3 days.

Pellet-pressing method Magnetic balls, cowherb seeds or rape seeds in the center of a small square of adhesive tapes of 0.5 cm×0. 5 cm are applied and fixed on the acupoints(Fig. 6-32). The patient is asked to press them 3～4 times a day till distending sensation appears. The other ear is alternately treated about three days later.

5. 3. 2 刺激方法

毫针法 针具选用 0.5 寸毫针。首先用 2% 碘酒消毒，再用 75% 乙醇脱碘，然后左手拇、食指固定耳郭，中指抵住针刺部位的背面，右手持针将针刺入耳穴，深度 0.2～0.3 厘米，以达软骨为准，一般留针 20～30 分钟。可使用捻转手法来加强针感。也可在针刺得气后接上电针仪，采用电针法。

埋针法 穴位消毒后，采用图钉形皮内针，刺入后用胶布将其固定，留针 2～3 天。

压丸法 将磁珠或王不留行或油菜籽等贴于 0.5 厘米×0.5 厘米的小方块胶布中央，然后敷贴于耳穴上并加以固定(图 6-32)。嘱患者每天自行按压该穴 3～4 次，有胀痛感为宜。3 天左右换另一侧耳穴治疗。

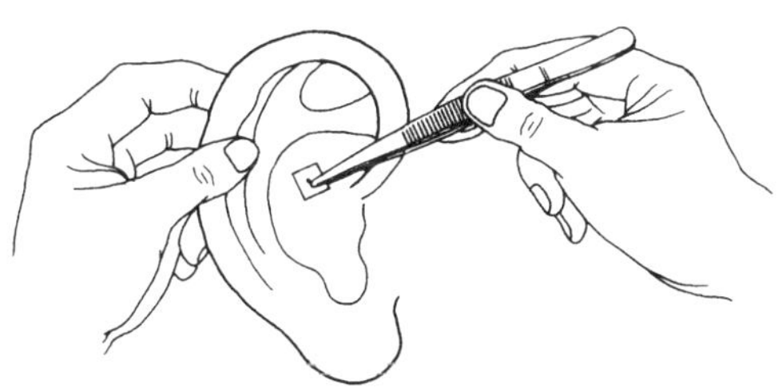

Fig.6-32 Pellet-pressing method

图 6-32 压丸法

5.4 Precautions

Clinic precautions include following aspects: ①Strict sterilization is especially required to prevent infection; ②for cases of sprain and motor impairment, during needling the patient is asked to exereise the affected site to increase clinical efficacy; ③attention should be paid to the possibility of the patient's fainting during needling; ④ear acupuncture is contraindicated for pregnant women who have a history of spontaneous abortion; ⑤ear acupuncture is not applied on the areas with eczema, inflammation, ulcers and congelation.

5.4 注意事项

临床应注意以下问题：①严格消毒，防止感染；②对扭伤和有运动障碍的患者，进针后宜适当活动患部，有助于提高疗效；③耳穴针刺时亦可发生晕针，应注意预防；④有习惯性流产史的孕妇应慎用针刺；⑤局部有湿疹、炎症、溃疡和冻伤的耳穴处禁针。

Part Two

Acupuncture Therapeutics

下 篇

针 灸 临 床

Chapter 1 General Introduction to Therapeutics

第1章 治疗总论

Section 1 Therapeutic Actions of Acupuncture and Moxibustion

第1节 针灸治疗作用

Treatment with acupuncture and moxibustion should be based upon Chinese medical theory and the four diagnostic methods, and proceed by adopting acupoints to prescribe acupuncture and moxibustion. Meridian differentiation in light of meridian theory by examining the meridians and acupoints plays a vital role in acupuncture practice. In the long-term medical practice, ancient physicians concluded that acupuncture functions to regulate yin and yang, unblock meridians and collaterals, reinforce the healthy qi and eliminate the pathogenic factors.

针灸治疗疾病，是在中医学理论指导下，通过四诊合参了解病情，根据辨证分析选取相应腧穴，进行针刺和艾灸治疗。诊察相应经络腧穴，依据经络理论进行经络辨证，对于针灸临床治疗非常重要。古代医家在长期的医疗实践中，总结出针灸具有调和阴阳、疏通经络、扶正祛邪的作用。

1 Regulating yin and yang

1 调和阴阳

In Chinese medicine, the physiological activities are thought to be the results of the balance between yin and yang in the human body. When the pathogenic factors such as six exogenous factors and seven emotions invade the human body, the relative balance between yin and yang is disturbed, leading

中医学认为，机体生理活动正常，是人体阴阳保持相互协调的结果。若因六淫七情等因素导致人体阴阳的偏盛偏衰，失去相对平衡，就会使脏腑经络功能活动失

to a dysfunction of zang-fu organs and meridians, thus diseases happen. Yin excess causes yang disorders and yang excess causes yin disorders. The essential principle of acupuncture treatment is to regulate yin and yang, restore the balance between yin and yang, and recover the normal functions of the zang-fu organs and meridians, hence to cure diseases.

常，从而引起疾病的发生。阴盛则阳病，阳盛则阴病。针灸治疗的根本原则，就是运用针灸方法调节阴阳的偏盛偏衰，可以使机体转归于阴阳平衡的状态，恢复脏腑经络的正常功能，从而达到治疗疾病的目的。

2 Unblocking meridians and collaterals

Meridians connect internally with the zang-fu organs and externally with the limbs and joints, and conduct qi and blood. Physiologically, the meridians conduct qi and blood to nourish the internal zang-fu organs and external striae. If the qi and blood flow smoothly, the zang-fu organs are well nourished, and the zang-fu organs can freely communicate with the body surface. If the meridians work abnormally and the circulation of qi and blood is blocked, the physiological functions are disturbed and pathological changes arise, consequently resulting in diseases. If the meridians are not free and the circulation of qi and blood is obstructed, such symptoms as pain and numbness appear. Acupuncture and moxibustion can unblock the meridians to promote the circulation of qi and blood, and diseases are cured.

2 疏通经络

经脉"内属于府藏，外络于支节"，其主要生理功能是运行气血，在正常状态下"内溉脏腑，外濡腠理"，气血运行通畅，则各脏腑器官得以营养，脏腑体表得以沟通。若经络功能失常，气血运行受阻，则会影响人体正常功能活动，进而出现病理变化，引起疾病的发生。经络不通，则气血运行受阻，其主要临床表现为疼痛、麻木等。针灸治疗可使经络通畅，促使气血正常运行，达到治疗疾病的目的。

3 Reinforcing healthy qi and eliminating pathogenic factors

The occurrence, development and prognosis of diseases are essentially a process of struggle between the healthy qi and pathogenic factors. When the healthy qi defeat the pathogenic factors, the conditions will be relieved; when the pathogenic factors

3 扶正祛邪

疾病的发生、发展及其转归的过程，实质上是正邪相争的过程。正盛邪祛则病情缓解，正虚邪盛则病情加重。《素问》说，"正气存内，

defeat the healthy qi, the conditions will be worsened. Su Wen states, "When the healthy qi is strong inside the body, the pathogenic factors cannot contract the body" "If the pathogenic factors contract, the healthy qi must be deficient." All the statements show that the occurrence of diseases depends on deficient healthy qi and vigorous pathogenic factors. Therefore, reinforcing the healthy qi and eliminating the pathogenic factors is the basic principle in acupuncture therapy. Therapeutically, the healthy qi should be reinforced and the pathogenic factors should be eliminated. Specifically, reinforcing method is employed for the conditions due to deficient healthy qi, and reducing method is employed for the conditions due to vigorous pathogenic factors; reinforcing and reducing methods in combination are indicated for the conditions due to simultaneous deficient healthy qi and vigorous pathogenic factors, however, the reinforcing method and reinforcing method should be adopted in light of the individual condition.

邪不可干""邪之所凑，其气必虚"。说明疾病的发生，是由于正气相对不足，邪气相对强盛所致。因此，增强正气、祛除邪气是针灸治病的基本原则。治疗上采用补虚泻实的方法，对于正气不足之虚证应予补法，邪气盛实之实证应用泻法；正虚与邪实并存者则须补泻并用，根据病情或以补虚为主兼以泻邪，或泻邪为主兼以补虚，或补泻并重。

Section 2 Therapeutic Principles of Acupuncture and Moxibustion

第 2 节 针灸治疗原则

The therapeutic principles of acupuncture and moxibustion are of great significance in the acupoint prescription and needling manipulation. There are a number of acupuncture and moxibustion methods in clinical practice, but in principle, they can be divided into four aspects: reinforcing deficiency and reducing excess, clearing heat and warming cold,

针灸的治疗原则对于针灸处方选穴以及操作方法的运用等具有重要指导意义。针灸临床的治疗方法很多，但从其治疗原则上看，可概括为补虚泻实、清热温寒、标本缓急和三因制宜四个方

treating *biao* or *ben* and emergent or chronic conditions, treating a disease according to its occurrence season, territory and individual constitution.

面。

1 Reinforcing deficiency and reducing excess

1 补虚泻实

Reinforcing deficiency and reducing excess is an essential principle in acupuncture practice, signifying that the deficiency conditions should be treated by reinforcing methods and excess conditions by reducing methods. Deficiency means healthy qi insufficiency and excess means pathogenic factors exuberance.

补虚泻实是指导针灸临床的基本原则，意即虚者补之、实者泻之。“虚”指正气不足，“实”指邪气盛。

1.1 Reinforcing deficiency

1.1 补虚

In acupuncture, reinforcing deficiency is performed principally by reinforcing its own meridian and the paired meridian, mother meridian and specific acupoints, as well as reinforcing techniques. The deficiency conditions of zang-fu organs are treated by needling its meridian acupoints, especially the Back-Shu acupoints and Yuan-Source acupoints, with reinforcing techniques; if its paired zang-fu organ is involved, the corresponding meridian acupoints may be used; furthermore, according to the mutual generation and restriction of the five elements, the mother meridian may be treated.

针灸补虚主要是通过补其本经、补其表里经和虚则补其母以及运用特殊穴等方法，并结合针刺手法之“补法”，达到“补虚”的目的。脏腑虚证，可选取其本经腧穴，尤其是相关的背俞穴和原穴，施行补法；若涉及与之相表里的脏腑，可选取与其相表里脏腑的经穴；还可根据五行生克理论，采取虚则补其母等方法。

1.2 Reducing excess

1.2 泻实

In acupuncture, reducing excess is performed principally by reducing its own meridian and paired meridian, son meridian and specific acupoints, as well as reducing techniques. The excess conditions of zang-fu organs are treated by needling its meridian acupoints, usually the He-Sea acupoints and Front-Mu acupoints, with reducing techniques. The excess conditions of acute onset can be treated by

针灸泻实主要通过采取泻其本经、泻其表里经和实则泻其子以及运用特殊穴等方法，结合针灸手法之“泻法”的施用，达到“泻实”的目的。脏腑实证，可选取本经腧穴，施以泻法治疗，常用本经合穴和本腑募穴；急症属

needling the Xi-Cleft acupoint and Jing-Well acupoint of its own meridian; when the condition is involved in its paired zang or fu organ, its paired meridian acupoints may be treated with reducing techniques. Moreover, according to the mutual generation and restriction of the five elements, the son meridian may be treated.

实者,可取本经郄穴和井穴,若涉及与之相表里的脏腑,可选取相表里经穴,并施以泻法治疗。此外,还可根据五行生克理论,采取实则泻其子的方法等。

1.3 Combination of reinforcing and reducing methods

In acupuncture practice, most conditions are of complex deficiency and excess, and their treatments should be administered by combined reinforcing and reducing methods. For example, liver-excess and spleen-deficiency syndrome displays liver-excess symptoms such as flank distention and pain, belching and acid regurgitation, as well as spleen-deficiency symptoms such as abdominal pain, poor appetite and loose stools; therapeutically, this syndrome should be treated by reducing the liver meridian and gallbladder meridian, and reinforcing the spleen meridian and stomach meridian. As a matter of fact, combined application of reinforcing and reducing methods is very common in clinical acupuncture; however, how to combine the reinforcing and reducing methods depends on the severity and urgency of the deficiency and excess conditions.

1.3 补泻兼施

在针灸临床上,最为多见的是虚实夹杂的病情,治疗上多补泻兼施。例如,肝实脾虚证,临床常见胁肋胀痛、嗳腐吞酸的肝实症状,又同时兼见腹痛、食欲不振、便溏等脾虚症状,治疗时应泻足厥阴经和足少阳经,补足太阴经和足阳明经。补泻兼施为针灸临床所常用,应根据虚实程度的轻重缓急,以决定补泻的多少先后。

2 Clearing heat and warming cold

The method of clearing heat and warming cold is performed by acupoint prescription, needling techniques, moxibustion methods and needle-retaining time.

2 清热温寒

临床上通过穴位的选择、手法的应用、不同针法灸法的实施,以及留针时间长短的控制等方法,来达到清热温寒的目的。

2.1 Clearing heat

Clearing heat is applicable for heat conditions. In general, heat-clearing method is characterized by superficial needling and rapid withdrawal, or pricking to bleed, swift manipulations, no retention of needles or reducing techniques. For instance, wind-heat condition should be treated by superficially needling Dazhui(CV 14), Quchi(LI 11), Hegu(LI 4) and Waiguan(TE 5) and the needles are quickly withdrawn to clear heat and relieve exterior conditions. If sore throat is accompanied, Shaoshang(LU 11) is pricked to bleed with a three-edged needle to help clear heat, relieve swelling and ease pain.

2.1 清热

"清热"是针对热性病证的治疗原则，一般以浅刺疾出，或点刺出血，手法轻快，不留针或针用泻法等来达到清泻热毒的目的。例如，风热感冒者，当取大椎、曲池、合谷、外关等穴浅刺疾出，可清热解表。若伴有咽喉肿痛者，可用三棱针在少商穴点刺出血，加强泻热、消肿、止痛的作用。

2.2 Warming cold

Warming cold is applicable for cold conditions. In general, cold-warming method is characterized by deep needling and long-term needle retention, reinforcing techniques and moxibustion methods. For instance, a cold pathogen in exterior and meridians can be removed by moxibustion methods; a cold pathogen in interior and zang-fu organs can be treated by deep needling with long-term needle retention, or heat-producing techniques, or moxibustion methods and needle-warming techniques.

2.2 温寒

"温寒"是针对寒性病证的治疗原则，一般以深刺、久留针，针用补法并加艾灸等以达到温经散寒的目的。例如：寒邪在表，留于经络者，可用艾灸法除之；若寒邪在里，凝滞脏腑，则宜深刺久留，或配合"烧山火"等手法，或加用艾灸、温针法等。

3 Treating *biao* or *ben*, urgency or chronic conditions

Biao and *ben*, urgency and chronic are relatively described, but they change in a complicated way in the process of diseases' occurrence and progression. In Su Wen, it states, "mastering the *biao* and *ben* of a disease, one can administer the treatment properly; if the *biao* and *ben* of a disease are not understood, the treatment won't help". This

3 标本缓急

标与本、缓与急是一个相对的概念，在疾病的发生、发展过程中，标本缓急复杂多变。《素问·标本病传论》曰："知标本者，万举万当，不知标本，是谓妄行。"强调了治疗疾病，掌握治标治本原

statement emphasizes the importance of mastering the *biao* and *ben* of a disease in the treatment of a disease.

则的重要性。

3.1 Ascertaining the root causes of a disease

Treating diseases should aim at removal of the causative factors. Clinical symptoms and signs are just the outer manifestations of a disease. Through syndrome differentiation and analysis of outer manifestations, the causative factors, affected location and pathogenesis can be ascertained. Then the therapeutic methods are established to treat the root causes of a disease. Take headache as an example, it results from many causes, such as exogenous factors, blood deficiency, blood stagnation, phlegm obstruction, qi depression and ascendant hyperactivity of liver yang; if just the local acupoints are used to ease pain, the headache may be relieved, but it can recur easily; so the causes of headache should be identified and different acupoints should be prescribed respectively to relieve exterior, enrich blood, activate blood and dissolve blood-stasis, resolve phlegm, regulate qi and alleviate depression, calm liver and subdue liver-yang; and the therapeutic outcomes will be better.

3.1 治病求本

治病求本是针对疾病的本质进行治疗。临床症状只是疾病反映于外的现象，通过辨证，由表及里，找出疾病发生的原因、部位和机制，抓住疾病的本质立法处方，以达到治病求本的目的。以头痛为例，可由多种原因引起，如外感、血虚、血瘀、痰阻、气郁、肝阳上亢等，仅用止痛的方法局部取穴治疗，虽可起到缓解疼痛的作用，但容易复发，必须针对引起头痛的原因，分别采取解表、养血、活血化瘀、化痰、理气解郁、平肝潜阳等法，选用相应穴位进行治疗，以使疗效更佳。

3.2 Treating the *biao* in urgency conditions

In pathogenesis, the *biao* and *ben* of a disease often exist simultaneously. If the *biao* aspect is more urgent than the *ben* aspect, the *biao* aspect may progress to be a critical condition in the case of unpunctual treatment; at this time, the *biao* aspect should be treated first and the *ben* aspect later. For instance, urinary and fecal retention due to other diseases should be treated immediately to relieve the retention, then the primary diseases are treated.

3.2 急则治标

标与本在病机上往往相互夹杂，若其证候表现为标病急于本病，如不及时处理，标病可能转为危重病证，此时应先治标病、后治本病。如治疗某些疾病引起的二便不通，则当先通其便，然后治其本病。

3.3 Treating the *ben* in remission conditions

In general, if a condition is stable, or it causes some non-lethal symptoms, or the *biao* aspect is relieved after treatment in the case of simultaneous *biao* and *ben* aspects, the *ben* aspect should be treated. Take dawn diarrhea due to kidney-yang deficiency as an example, diarrhea is the *biao* aspect and kidney-yang deficiency is the *ben* aspect; when diarrhea is relieved, the kidney-yang deficiency should be treated. This method is helpful for the chronic diseases and the remission conditions of acute diseases.

3.4 Simultaneously treating the *biao* and *ben* aspects

When the *biao* and *ben* aspects are moderate, they can be treated simultaneously. Take liver-spleen disharmony due to the liver failing to soothe as an example, when such symptoms as flank distention and pain, belching and acid regurgitation, poor appetite, vomiting and loose stools appear, its treatment should concentrate on soothing the liver qi, and harmonizing the spleen and stomach as well.

4 Treating a disease according to its occurrence season, territory and individual constitution

In the treatment of a disease, proper therapeutic methods should be formulated in accordance with its occurrence season and time, territory and individual constitution.

4.1 Treatment according to season

This refers to formulating proper treatment modalities in accordance with the occurrence seasons and treatment time of disorders. The alterna-

3.3 缓则治本

一般情况下，若本病病情稳定，或虽可引起其他病变，但无危急证候出现，或标本同病，标病经治疗缓解后，均可按“缓则治本”的原则予以处理。如肾阳虚引起的五更泻，泄泻是其症状为标，肾阳虚为本，标病缓解者，则应治疗本病。本法则对于慢性病和急性病的恢复期有重要指导意义。

3.4 标本兼治

当标病与本病处于俱缓或俱急的状态时，可采用标本兼治法。例如，由肝失疏泄而引起的脾胃不和，出现胁肋胀痛、嗳腐吞酸、食少呕吐、大便溏泄等症状，可在疏肝理气的同时兼调脾胃。

4 三因制宜

三因制宜，指因时、因地、因人制宜，即根据季节（包括时辰）、地理和治疗对象的不同情况而制定适宜的治疗方法。

4.1 因时制宜

因时制宜，即根据不同的季节和时辰特点，制定适宜的治疗方法。四时气候的

tion of seasons may have certain impact on the physiological functions and pathological changes of the human body. In the spring and summer, yang qi goes upwards and outwards, and the qi and blood of the human body flow to the body surface, so the pathogenic factors usually attack the body surface; in the autumn and winter, yin qi increases and the qi and blood of human body flow inside the body, so the pathogenic factors usually attack the interior of the body. Therapeutically, shallow needling is often performed in the spring and summer, and deep need-ling is often performed in the autumn and winter. In addition, the flow of qi and blood varies with the time within a day; acupuncture therapy emphasizes the relationship between acupoint selection and treatment time, namely the acupoints are selected according to the treatment time, such as midnight-noon ebb-flow method, eight methods of the mystic turtle, and the eight methods of flying and soaring, which are also the specific application of the principle of treatment according to time. Besides, this treatment principle also comprises the effective treatment time in acupuncture therapy; for example, menstrual cramps is generally treated before the coming menstruation.

变化，对人体的生理功能、病理变化均可产生一定的影响。春夏之季，阳气升发，人体气血趋向体表，病邪伤人亦多在浅表；秋冬之季，阴气渐盛，人体气血潜藏于内，病邪伤人亦多在深部。治疗上，春夏宜浅刺，秋冬宜深刺。人体气血流注呈现出与时辰变化相应的规律，针灸治疗注重取穴与时辰的关系，强调择时选穴，即根据不同的时辰选取不同的腧穴进行治疗。子午流注针法、灵龟八法、飞腾八法均是择时选穴治疗疾病的方法，也是因时制宜治疗原则的具体运用。此外，因时制宜还指应把握针灸的有效时机，如治疗痛经一般宜在月经来临前开始治疗等。

4.2 Treatment according to territory

This refers to formulating proper treatment modalities in accordance with the geographic territories of the disease occurrence. Because of the differing geographic environments, climate and living habits, the physiological activities and pathological features differ, and the treatment modalities vary. For example, in cold territories, moxibustion therapy is often used with bigger and more cones; where-

4.2 因地制宜

因地制宜，即根据不同的地理环境特点制定适宜的治疗方法。由于地理环境、气候条件和生活习惯的不同，人体的生理活动和病理特点也有区别，治疗方法亦有差异。如在寒冷的地区，治疗多用温灸，而且艾炷宜

as in the tropical territories, moxibustion therapy is infrequently used.

大、壮数宜多；在温热地区则反之。

4.3 Treatment according to individual constitution

4.3 因人制宜

This refers to formulating proper treatment modalities in accordance with the suffers' gender, age and body constitutions. Since the conditions of qi-blood and yin-yang are different in the individual body, the body bears various reactions and tolerance to the acupuncture stimulation, and the acupuncture methods differ. For example, the children may be treated with thin needles by shallow needling, with shorter retention of needle or even without retention of needle; while the elderly with weak constitutions is usually treated with mild needling techniques.

因人制宜，即根据患者的性别、年龄、体质等的不同特点制定适宜的治疗方法。因其体内气血阴阳状况存在差异，对针灸刺激的反应及耐受性亦存在差异，采用的针灸方法亦有区别。如小儿用针宜细，进针宜浅、留针时间宜短或不留针；年老体弱者针刺手法宜轻等。

Section 3 Acupuncture Prescriptions

第3节 针灸处方

Acupuncture prescription is the treatment regimen in acupuncture therapeutics, therefore, it is directly related to the therapeutic results. Clinically, acupuncture prescription should be made by selecting appropriate acupoints under the principle of syndrome differentiation and performing appropriate needling techniques.

针灸处方是针灸临床治疗的实施方案，处方得当与否，直接关系到治疗效果的好坏。根据辨证选取适当的腧穴，采用正确的刺灸方法，是针灸处方的主要内容。

1 Principles of acupoint selection

1 选穴原则

In acupuncture prescription, the acupoints are selected under the guidance of zang-fu theories and meridian theories, and according to the course of meridians; and some acupoints are selected in light

针灸处方中腧穴的选取，是在脏腑经络学说指导下，以循经取穴为主，并根据不同证候选取不同腧穴。选

of the symptoms. The principles of acupoint selection consist of three aspects: selecting local acupoints, selecting distal acupoints and selecting symptomatic acupoints.

穴原则主要包括近部取穴、远部取穴和随证取穴。

1.1 Selecting local acupoints

Selecting local acupoints means to select the acupoints near or around the affected areas. For example, Yingxiang(LI 20) and Yintang(EX-HN 3) are selected for nose problems, Jiache(ST 6) and Dicang(ST 4) for deviated mouth, Zhongwan(CV 12) and Liangmen(ST 21) for stomach disorders, and Fengchi(GV 20) for headache.

1.1 近部取穴

近部取穴是指选取病痛所在部位或邻近部位的腧穴。例如，鼻病取迎香、印堂，口㖞取颊车、地仓，胃病取中脘、梁门，头痛取风池等，皆属于近部取穴。

1.2 Selecting distal acupoints

Selecting distal acupoints means to select the acupoints far from the affected areas, particularly those acupoints below the elbows and knees. Based on the meridian distribution, those acupoints are not only indicated for the local disorders but also for the disorders along the meridian courses and far from the lesions. For instance, Hegu(LI 4) is selected to treat toothache; Chize(LU 5) and Yuji (LU 10) are selected to treat cough and hemoptysis; Zusanli(ST 36) is selected to treat stomachache.

1.2 远部取穴

远部取穴是指在距病位较远的部位选取腧穴的方法，多是取四肢肘膝关节以下的经穴。基于经络的联系，这些经穴不仅能治疗局部病证，而且还可以治疗本经循行所及的远隔部位的病证。例如：牙痛取合谷，咳嗽、咳血选尺泽、鱼际；胃脘痛取足三里等。

1.3 Selecting symptomatic acupoints

Selecting symptomatic acupoints means to select the acupoints indicated for the general symptoms or based on syndrome differentiation. The methods of selecting local or distal acupoints are suitable for diseases that are localized or have definite foci. However, some diseases are difficult to accurately determine their diseased sites in clinical practice, such as fever, insomnia, dreaminess, spontaneous sweating, night sweating, collapse, convulsion and coma. These diseases can be treated by selecting

1.3 随证取穴

随证取穴，是指针对某些全身症状或疾病的病机而选取腧穴。近部取穴和远部取穴适用于病痛部位明显或局限者，但临床上有许多疾病往往难以明确其病变部位，如发热、失眠、多梦、自汗、盗汗、虚脱、惊风、昏迷。对于这一类病证，可以根据中医辨证论治理论和腧穴主

acupoints on the basis of syndrome differentiation and the therapeutic properties of acupoints. For example, high fever can be treated by Dazhui(GV 14) and Quchi(LI 11); insomnia and dreaminess can be treated by Shenmen(HT 7) and Daling(PC 7); night sweating can be treated by Yinxi(HT 6) and Houxi(SI 3); collapse can be treated by Qihai(CV 6) and Guanyuan(CV 4); coma can be treated by Suliao(GV 25) and Shuigou(GV 26). Moreover, some acupoints are specially effective against certain diseases. For instance, chest stuffiness and shortness of breath due to qi problems can be treated by Danzhong(CV 17); blood deficiency and chronic bleeding can be treated by Geshu(BL 17); soreness and pain in the tendons and bones can be treated by Yanglingquan(GB 34).

治功能而选取适当腧穴。例如,治高热可选取大椎、曲池,治失眠多梦可选取神门、大陵,治盗汗可选取阴郄、后溪,治虚脱可选取气海、关元,治昏迷可选取素髎、水沟等。另外,有些腧穴对某些病证有特殊疗效,亦常选用,如属气病的胸闷、气促等取膻中,属血病的血虚、慢性出血等取膈俞,属筋病的筋骨酸痛等取阳陵泉,这些也都属随证取穴的范畴。

The methods above can be applied alone or in combination. For example, in treating asthma of excess syndrome, Danzhong(CV 17), Zhongfu(LU 1), Chize(LU 5) and Lieque(LU 7) are selected. In this prescription, there are the local acupoint Zhongfu(LU 1), the distal acupoints Chize(LU 5) and Lieque(LU 7), and the symptomatic acupoint Danzhong(CV 17)

上述取穴原则在临床上除可单独应用外,还常相互配合应用。例如,治疗哮喘实证,可选取膻中、中府、尺泽、列缺。其中取中府为近部取穴,取尺泽、列缺为远部取穴,取膻中为随证取穴。

2 Methods of acupoint combination

Acupoint combination means matching acupoints together with the same or similar therapeutic properties on the basis of the principles of selecting acupoints, so that they can cooperate with each other to potentiate their therapeutic effects. The methods of combining acupoints include combing acupoints of the involved meridian, combining acupoints of the exteriorly-interiorly paired meridians,

2 配穴方法

配穴方法是在选穴原则的基础上,选取两个以上具有协同作用的腧穴配伍应用的方法。配穴方法主要包括本经配穴、表里经配穴、上下配穴、前后配穴和左右配穴等。配穴时或使用将主治作用相同或相近的腧穴,或根

combining acupoints of the upper and lower parts of the body, combining acupoints in front and back, and combining contralateral acupoints. In acupoint combination, the acupoints with the same or similar therapeutic effect are applied, or the acupoints are selected in light of their indications or syndrome differentiation.

据病情或辨证配用有相应主治作用的腧穴。

2.1 Method of combining acupoints of the involved meridian

When one zang-fu organ or meridian is diseased, the acupoints of the involved meridian and zang-fu organ are prescribed. For instance, for coughing, Zhongfu(LU 1) as the local acupoint and of the Front-Mu acupoint of the lungs, Chize(LU 5) and Taiyuan(LU 9) as the distal acupoints of the involved lung meridian, are used.

2.1 本经配穴法

某一脏腑、经脉发生病变时，即选相应脏腑经脉的腧穴组成处方。如肺病咳嗽，可取局部腧穴肺募中府，同时远取本经之尺泽、太渊。

2.2 Method of combining acupoints of the exteriorly-interiorly paired meridians

When one zang-fu organ or meridian is diseased, the acupoints of its own meridian and its exteriorly-interiorly paired meridian are prescribed. For example, cough due to wind heat attacking the lungs can be treated by Chize(LU 5) as the lung meridian acupoint, and Quchi(LI 11) and Hegu(LI 4) as the large intestine acupoints. Combination of the Yuan-Source acupoints and Luo-Connecting acupoints is the specific application of this method.

2.2 表里经配穴法

某一脏腑、经脉有病，取其本经及表里经腧穴配合组成处方施治。如风热袭肺导致的感冒咳嗽，可选肺经的尺泽和大肠经的曲池、合谷，特定穴应用中的原络配穴法，也是本法在临床上的具体运用。

2.3 Method of combining acupoints of the upper and lower parts of the body

This method means the combined application of the acupoints above the waist and below the waist. For example, the stomach disorders can be treated by Neiguan(PC 6) as the acupoint above the waist and Zusanli(ST 36) as the acupoint below the waist;

2.3 上下配穴法

是指将腰部以上腧穴和腰部以下腧穴配合应用的方法，临床应用广泛。如治疗胃病取内关、足三里，治疗咽喉痛、牙痛取合谷、内庭，治

sore throat and toothache can be treated by Hegu (LI 4) as the acupoint above the waist and Neiting (ST 44) as the acupoint below the waist; prolapsed rectum and uterus can be treated by Baihui(GV 20) as the acupoint above the waist and Changqiang (GV 1) as the acupoint below the waist. Besides, the combined use of the eight Confluent acupoints is the specific application of this method.

疗脱肛、子宫下垂取百会、长强。此外，八脉交会穴配合应用等，也属于本法的具体应用。

2.4 Methods of combing acupoints in front and back of the body

This method is also known as "a method of combing back and belly, yin and yang acupoints". Front refers to the chest and abdomen, and back to the upper back and lower back. This method combines the acupoints in the front and back, and is often applied to treat the disorders of zang-fu organs. The "even-number needling method" and method of combining Front-Mu and Back-Shu acupoints, both mentioned in Ling Shu, are included. For instance, stomachache can be treated by Zhongwan(CV 12) and Liangmen(ST 21) as the front acupoints, and Weishu(BL 21) and Weicang(BL 50) as the back acupoints.

2.4 前后配穴法

前指胸腹，后指背腰。选取前后部位腧穴配合应用的方法称为前后配穴法，亦名腹背阴阳配穴法，治疗脏腑疾患常用此法。《灵枢·官针》所指“偶刺”法和俞募配穴法，均属本法范畴。例如，胃痛前取中脘、梁门，后取胃俞、胃仓。

2.5 Method of combining contralateral acupoints

This method combines the acupoints on the left and right sides of the body. In clinical application, bilateral acupoints are generally combined to enhance the clinical efficacy. This method is applicable for the disorders of zang-fu organs. For example, heart disorders can be treated by bilateral Xinshu(BL 15) and Neiguan(PC 6); stomach disorders can be treated by bilateral Weishu(BL 21) and Zusanli(ST 36). Bilateral acupoints, which do not

2.5 左右配穴法

是指选取肢体左右两侧腧穴配合应用的方法。临床应用时，一般左右穴同时取用，左右对称配穴，以加强协同作用，内脏疾患多用，如心病取双侧心俞、内关，胃病取双侧胃俞、足三里等，左右不同名腧穴也可并用。左右交叉配穴，多用于头面疾患。

bear the same name, can also be used in combination; but this method is principally applied for head disorders. For example, in the treatment of facial paralysis on the left side, left Jiache(ST 6) and Dicang(ST 4) are selected as the left-side acupoints, and right Hegu(LI 4) is selected as the right-side acupoint; in the treatment of headache on the left side, the left Touwei(ST 8) and Qubin(GB 7) are selected as the left-side acupoints, and right Yanglingquan(GB 34) and Xiaxi(GB 43) are selected as the right-side acupoints.

如:左侧面瘫,取左侧颊车、地仓,并配合右侧合谷等;左侧头角痛,取左侧头维、曲鬓,并配合右侧阳陵泉、侠溪等。

Section 4 Application of Specific Acupoints

第 4 节 特定穴的应用

Specific acupoints are mostly below the elbow and knee joints, and are frequently used in clinical practice. There exist some therapeutic features and rules in acupoints combination.

特定穴多位于肘膝关节以下,临床上最为常用,在选穴配伍上也有一定的特点和规律。

1 Clinical application of five Shu-Transport acupoints

1 五输穴的临床应用

The ancients drew an analogy between the meridian-qi circulation and water-flow stream. According to the volume of meridian qi and the depth of qi circulation within the body from the tips of the limbs to the elbow-knee joints, the five Shu-Transport acupoints are grouped under separate classifications, namely, the Jing-Well acupoint, Ying-Spring acupoint, Shu-Stream acupoint, Jing-River acupoint and He-Sea acupoint. The five Shu-Transport acupoints of the twelve main meridians are principally below the elbow and knee joints, totaling 60 in all.

古人把经气运行过程用自然界的水流由小到大、由浅入深的变化来形容,把五输穴按井、荥、输、经、合的顺序,从四肢末端向肘膝方向依次排列。十二经脉的五输穴均位于四肢肘膝关节以下,人体共有五输穴 60 个。五输穴具有自身的五行属性,按“阴井木”“阳井金”的阴阳五行学说归类,十二经

The five Shu-Transport acupoints correspond respectively to the five elements: the Jing-Well acupoints of the yin meridians correspond to the mood, while the Jing-Well acupoints of the yang meridians correspond to the metal. The names and five-element correspondence of the five Shu-Transport acupoints of the twelve main meridians are detailed in Tables 7-1 and 7-2.

脉五输穴穴名及其五行属性详见表 7-1、表 7-2。

Table 7-1 The names and five-element correspondence of the five Shu-Transport acupoints of the six yin meridians

Six yin meridians		Well (mood)	Spring (fire)	Stream (earth)	River (metal)	Sea (water)
Hand Meridians	Lung (metal)	Shaoshang (LU 11)	Yuji (LU 10)	Taiyuan (LU 9)	Jingqu (LU 8)	Chize (LU 5)
	Pericardium (minister fire)	Zhongchong (PC 9)	Laogong (PC 8)	Daling (PC 7)	Jianshi (PC 5)	Quze (PC 3)
	Heart (fire)	Shaochong (HT 9)	Shaofu (HT 8)	Shenmen (HT 7)	Lingdao (HT 4)	Shaohai (HT 3)
Foot Meridians	Spleen (earth)	Yinbai (SP 1)	Dadu (SP 2)	Taibai (SP 3)	Shangqiu (SP 5)	Yinlingquan (SP 9)
	Liver (wood)	Dadun (LR 1)	Xingjian (LR 2)	Taichong (LR 3)	Zhongfeng (LR 4)	Ququan (LR 8)
	Kidney (water)	Yongquan (KI 1)	Rangu (KI 2)	Taixi (KI 3)	Fuliu (KI 7)	Yingu (KI 10)

表 7-1 六阴经五输穴及与五行配属表

六阴经		井(木)	荥(火)	输(土)	经(金)	合(水)
手三阴	肺(金)	少商	鱼际	太渊	经渠	尺泽
	心包(相火)	中冲	劳宫	大陵	间使	曲泽
	心(火)	少冲	少府	神门	灵道	少海
足三阴	脾(土)	隐白	大都	太白	商丘	阴陵泉
	肝(木)	大敦	行间	太冲	中封	曲泉
	肾(水)	涌泉	然谷	太溪	复溜	阴谷

Table 7-2　The names and five-element correspondence of the five Shu-Transport acupoints of the six yang meridians

Six yang meridians		Well (metal)	Spring (water)	Stream (mood)	River (fire)	Sea (earth)
Hand meridians	Large intestine (metal)	Shangyang (LI 1)	Erjian (LI 2)	Sanjian (LI 3)	Yangxi (LI 5)	Quchi (LI 11)
	Triple energizer (minister fire)	Guanchong (TE 1)	Yemen (TE 2)	Zhongzhu (TE 3)	Zhigou (TE 6)	Tianjing (TE 10)
	Small intestine (fire)	Shaoze (SI 1)	Qiangu (SI 2)	Houxi (SI 3)	Yanggu (SI 5)	Xiaohai (SI 8)
Foot meridians	Stomach (earth)	Lidui (ST 45)	Neiting (ST 44)	Xiangu (ST 43)	Jiexi (ST 41)	Zusanli (ST 36)
	Gallbladder (Wood)	Zuqiaoyin (GB 44)	Xiaxi (GB 43)	Zulinqi (GB 41)	Yangfu (GB 38)	Yanglingquan (GB 34)
	Bladder (water)	Zhiyin (BL 67)	Zutonggu (BL 66)	Shugu (BL 65)	Kunlun (BL 60)	Weizhong (BL 40)

表7-2　六阳经五输穴及与五行配属表

六　阳　经		井(金)	荥(水)	输(木)	经(火)	合(土)
手三阳	大肠(金)	商阳	二间	三间	阳溪	曲池
	三焦(相火)	关冲	液门	中渚	支沟	天井
	小肠(火)	少泽	前谷	后溪	阳谷	小海
足三阳	胃(土)	厉兑	内庭	陷谷	解溪	足三里
	胆(木)	足窍阴	侠溪	足临泣	阳辅	阳陵泉
	膀胱(水)	至阴	足通谷	束骨	昆仑	委中

The indications of the five Shu-Transport acupoints were not totally identical in ancient literature. In Ling Shu, it was recorded that the Jing-Well acupoints were used to treat the disorders of the zang organs, the Ying-Spring acupoints, Shu-Stream acupoints and Jing-River acupoints were used to treat meridian-relevant disorders, and the He-Sea acupoints were used to treat the disorders of the fu organs. Nan Jing states that "The Jing-Well acupoints are indicated for fullness in the chest, the

古代文献对五输穴主治作用的记载不尽相同。据《灵枢》记载，井穴适用于与脏有关的病证，荥穴、输穴及经穴适用于与经脉有关的病证，合穴适用于与腑有关的病证。《难经·六十八难》说："井主心下满，荥主身热，输主体重节痛，经主喘咳寒热，合主逆气而泄。"临床上，

Ying-Spring acupoints for febrile diseases, the Shu-Stream acupoints for body heaviness and painful joints, the Jing-River acupoints for cough and asthma, chills and fever, and the He-Sea acupoints for diarrhea due to qi adversity". Clinically, the Jing-Well acupoints are used to treat coma, the Ying-Spring acupoints to treat febrile diseases, the Shu-Stream acupoints to treat joint pain, the Jing-River acupoints to treat cough and asthma, and the He-Sea acupoints to treat the disorders of the fu-organs.

井穴可用来治疗神志昏迷，荥穴可用来治疗热病，输穴可用来治疗关节痛，经穴可用来治疗喘咳，合穴可用来治疗六腑病证等。

According to the correspondence of the five elements between the five Shu-Transport acupoints and the zang-fu organs, Nan Jing puts forward an acupuncture treatment principle of "reinforcing the mother in deficiency and reducing the son in excess". Based on the generating relationship between the five elements, in deficiency conditions the mother acupoint is selected and in excess conditions the son acupoint is selected. For example, the lung pertains to the metal element, and so for the deficiency condition of the lung meridian, Taiyuan(LU 9), the earth acupoint of the lung meridian, is selected; and for the excess condition of the lung meridian, Chize(LU 5), the water acupoint of the lung meridian, is selected; this is a method of selecting mother or son acupoint on the diseased meridian. Furthermore, the mother or son acupoint of the mother or son meridian can be selected; for instance, the lung pertains to the metal element, so the excess condition of lung meridian can be treated by selecting Yingu(KI 10), the water acupoint of the kidney meridian, the son meridian; in the case of lung deficiency, Taibai(SP 3), the earth acupoint of the spleen meridian, the mother meridian, is selected.

五输穴的五行属性与脏腑的五行属性相合，《难经》提出"虚者补其母，实者泻其子"的针灸治疗原则。按五输穴五行属性以生我者为母、我生者为子的原则进行选穴，虚证选用母穴，实证选用子穴。这就是临床上所称的补母泻子法，如肺属金，虚则取太渊(土)，实则取尺泽(水)等，这是本经子母补泻取穴。除本经子母补泻取穴外，还有他经子母补泻取穴。肺属金，如肺实证可取其子经肾经(水)的阴谷(水)，肺虚证取其母经脾经(土)太白(土)，即为他经子母补泻取穴。

In addition, the qi-blood circulation along the five Shu-Transport acupoints is in close association with the alternation of Two-Hourly period. The ancient physicians, on the basis of the combination of the five Shu-Transport acupoints with yin-yang and five elements, associate the Heavenly Stems and Earthly Branches with zang-fu organs to create a special time-dependent needling therapy, which is named as ebb-midday needling therapy(*Ziwu Liuzhu* method).

另外，十二经脉五输穴的气血流注与时辰密切相关，古代医家以五输穴配合阴阳五行为基础，运用天干地支配合脏腑，总结出一种特殊的择时选穴治疗疾病的方法，即子午流注针法。

2　Clinical application of Back-Shu and Front-Mu acupoints

2　俞募穴的临床应用

The Back-Shu acupoints are the places on the back where the qi of the zang-fu organs is infused, while the Front-Mu acupoints are the places on the chest and abdomen where the qi of zang-fu organs converges. Each zang-organ and fu-organ has its own Front-Mu and Back-Shu acupoints(Table 7-3).

俞募穴是背俞穴和募穴的合称。背俞穴是脏腑之气输注之处，均位于背腰部；募穴是脏腑之气汇集之处，位于胸腹部。每一脏腑各有一背俞穴和一募穴，详见 7-3 表。

Table 7-3　The Back-Shu and Front-Mu acupoints of zang-fu organs

Acupoint	Lung	Pericardium	Heart	Liver	Spleen	Kidney
Back-Shu acupoint	Feishu (BL 13)	Jueyinshu (BL 14)	Xinshu (BL 15)	Ganshu (BL 18)	Pishu (BL 20)	Shenshu (BL 23)
Front-Mu acupoints	Zhongfu (LU 1)	Danzhong (CV 17)	Juque (CV 14)	Qimen (LR 14)	Zhangmen (LR 13)	Jingmen (GB 25)
Acupoint	Stomach	Gallbladder	Bladder	Large intestine	Triple energizer	Small intestine
Back-Shu acupoint	Weishu (BL 21)	Danshu (BL 19)	Pangguangshu (BL 28)	Dachangshu (BL 25)	Sanjiaoshu (BL 22)	Xiaochangshu (BL 27)
Front-Mu acupoint	Zhongwan (CV 12)	Riyue (GB 24)	Zhongji (CV 3)	Tianshu (ST 25)	Shimen (CV 5)	Guanyuan (CV 4)

表 7-3　脏腑俞募穴

俞/募	肺	心包	心	肝	脾	肾
俞穴	肺俞	厥阴俞	心俞	肝俞	脾俞	肾俞
募穴	中府	膻中	巨阙	期门	章门	京门
俞/募	胃	胆	膀胱	大肠	三焦	小肠
俞穴	胃俞	胆俞	膀胱俞	大肠俞	三焦俞	小肠俞
募穴	中脘	日月	中极	天枢	石门	关元

When pathological change occurs in a certain zang-organ or fu-organ, tenderness or sensitive reaction may appear at its own Back-Shu acupoint or Front-Mu acupoint. Therefore, these acupoints can help diagnose the disorders of zang-fu organs by observing or palpating the abnormal changes at these acupoints, and treat the disorders of the relevant zang-fu organs by needling and moxbustion at these acupoints. The Back-Shu acupoints are located on the yang aspect of body, which is an important place where yin diseases run into the yang; the Front-Mu acupoints are on the yin aspect of the body, which is an important place for yang diseases running into the yin. Generally speaking, the disorders of the zang-organs and in excess are treated by the Back-Shu acupoints, while the disorders of the fu-organs and in excess are treated by the Front-Mu acupoints. For example, zang-organs deficiency is usually treated by the corresponding Back-Shu acupoints with reinforcing techniques; fu-organs excess is usually treated by the Front-Mu acupoints with reducing techniques. Moreover, the Back-Shu acupoints and Front-Mu acupoints can also be used to treat the disorders of the tissues and organs related to their respective organs. For example, Ganshu (BL 18) can be used to treat the eye disorders and tendon disorders; Shenshu (BL 23) can be used to treat ear disorders.

某一脏腑发生病变时，常在其相应的俞募穴处出现疼痛或过敏等病理性反应。因此，临床上可通过观察、触扪俞募穴处的异常变化，来诊断相应脏腑疾病，又可利用针刺、艾灸作用于俞募穴来治疗相应脏腑疾病。俞为阳，是阴病行阳的重要处所；募为阴，是阳病行阴的重要处所。一般而言，脏病、虚证多取俞穴，腑病、实证多取募穴。例如：五脏虚损，取相应背俞穴以补之；六腑实满，取相应腹募穴以泻之。此外，俞募穴还可治疗与相应脏腑所属组织器官的病证，如取肝俞治疗目疾、筋病等，取肾俞治疗耳疾等。

3 Clinical application of Yuan-Source and Luo-Connecting acupoints

3 原络穴的临床应用

The Yuan-Source acupoints and Luo-Connecting acupoints can be used alone or in combination. The combination of the Yuan-Source acupoint of a

原穴和络穴在临床上既可单独应用，也可相互配合应用。本经原穴与其相表里

meridian with the Luo-Connecting acupoint of its exteriorly-interiorly paired meridian is termed "Yuan and Luo combination". When a pair of exteriorly-interiorly paired meridians are diseased, the first diseased meridian is thought to be the host and its Yuan-Source acupoint is selected; while the secondly diseased meridian is thought to be the guest and its Luo-Connecting acupoint is selected. Thus, Yuan and Luo combination is also called "host and guest combination", which is an exterior-interior acupoint combination. For example, if the lung meridian is diseased first, its Yuan-Source acupoint Taiyuan(LU 9) is selected; the large intestine is diseased secondly, its Luo-Connecting acupoint Pianli (LI 6) is selected. Alternatively, if the large intestine meridian is diseased first, its Yuan-Source acupoint Hegu(LI 4) is selected; the lung meridian is diseased secondly, its Luo-Connecting acupoint Lieque(LU 7) is selected. The Yuan-Source acupoints and Luo-Connecting acupoints of the twelve main meridians are presented in Table 7-4.

经的络穴相互配合应用时，称为"原络配穴"。若相表里脏腑经络同病，先病者为主，取本经的原穴（主穴），后病者为客，取相表里经的络穴（客穴），故原络配穴又称"主客原络配穴"，属表里配穴法的一种。如肺经先病，即先取肺经的原穴太渊；大肠后病，再取大肠经的络穴偏历。反之，若大肠先病，即先取大肠经的原穴合谷；肺经后病，再取肺经的络穴列缺。十二经原穴、络穴见表 7-4。

Table 7-4　The Yuan-Source acupoints and Luo-Connecting acupoints of the twelve main meridians

Meridian	Yuan-Source acupoint	Luo-Connecting acupoint	Meridian	Yuan-Source acupoint	Luo-Connecting acupoints
Lung meridian	Taiyuan (LU 9)	Lieque (LU 7)	Large intestine meridian	Hegu (LI 4)	Pianli (LI 6)
Pericardium meridian	Daling (PC 7)	Neiguan (PC 6)	Triple energizer meridian	Yangchi (TE 4)	Waiguan (TE 5)
Heart meridian	Shenmen (HT 7)	Tongli (HT 5)	Small intestine meridian	Wangu (SI 4)	Zhizheng (SI 7)
Spleen meridian	Taibai (SP 3)	Gongsun (SP 4)	Stomach meridian	Chongyang (ST 42)	Fenglong (ST 40)
Liver meridian	Taichong (LR 3)	Ligou (LR 5)	Gallbladder meridian	Qiuxu (GB 40)	Guangming (GB 37)
Kidney meridian	Taixi (KI 3)	Dazhong (KI 4)	Bladder meridian	Jinggu (BL 64)	Feiyang (BL 58)

表 7-4 十二经脉原络穴

经脉	原穴	络穴	经脉	原穴	络穴
手太阴肺经	太渊	列缺	手阳明大肠经	合谷	偏历
手厥阴心包经	大陵	内关	手少阳三焦经	阳池	外关
手少阴心经	神门	通里	手太阳小肠经	腕骨	支正
足太阴脾经	太白	公孙	足阳明胃经	冲阳	丰隆
足厥阴肝经	太冲	蠡沟	足少阳胆经	丘墟	光明
足少阴肾经	太溪	大钟	足太阳膀胱经	京骨	飞扬

4 Clinical application of eight Confluent acupoints

The eight Confluent acupoints are mostly around the wrist and ankle, and can be used either alone or in combination to treat the disorders of the extra vessel with which it communicates. For example, Houxi (SI 3), which communicates with the governor vessel, can be used to treat the stiffness and pain along the spinal column, and opisthotonos; Gongsun(SP 4), which communicates with the thoroughfare vessel, is effective for qi adversity and convulsion in the chest and abdomen. Alternatively, two of these acupoints can be used in combination to treat the disorders in the sites where their communicative vessels reach. These eight Confluent acupoints are classified into four groups, with one acupoint on the hand and the other on the leg in each group. These acupoints are indicated for a wide variety of disorders along their own meridians or their communicative vessels. For example, Gongsun(SP 4) communicates with the thoroughfare vessel and Neiguan(PC 6) communicates with the yin link vessel, and these two acupoints can be used in combination to treat the diseases in the heart,

4 八脉交会穴的临床应用

八脉交会穴多位于腕踝部上下，临床可单独应用治疗各自相通奇经的病证。如：脊柱强痛、角弓反张等督脉病证，可取通于督脉的后溪穴；胸腹气逆而拘急的冲脉病证，可取通于冲脉的公孙穴；也可两穴配伍，治疗两脉相合部位病证。8 个腧穴分为 4 组，均为固定的手足两穴配伍，临床应用范围广泛，可治疗本经及相关奇经循行联系部位的病证。如：公孙通冲脉，内关通阴维脉，两穴配伍可治疗冲脉与阴维脉相合部位（心、胸、胃部）病证；后溪通督脉，申脉通阳蹻脉，两穴配合可以治疗督脉与阳蹻脉相合部位（目锐眦、颈项、身、肩部）病证。这属“上下配穴法”的范畴。八脉交会穴配合关系及治疗部位

chest and stomach, where these two extra vessels reach; Houxi(SI 3) communicates with the governor vessel and Shenmai(BL 62) communicates with the yang heel vessel, and these two acupoints can be used in combination to treat the diseases in the inner canthus, neck, ear and shoulder where these two vessels reach. The latter use of combined acupoints is also included in the category of the so-called "matching of upper and lower acupoints". The ways of combining the Confluent acupoints and their therapeutic application are presented in Table 7-5.

见表7-5。

Table 7-5　The eight Confluent acupoints

Acupoint	Indication	Common condition
Gongsun (SP 4)	Disorders of the thoroughfare vessel	Heart, chest, stomach
Neiguan(PC 6)	Disorders of the yin link vessel	
Houxi(SI 3)	Disorders of the governor vessel	Inner canthus, neck, ear, shoulder
Shenmai (BL 62)	Disorders of the yang heel vessel	
Zulinqi(GB 41)	Disorders of the belt vessel	Outer canthus, retroauricle, cheek, neck, shoulder
Waiguan(TE 5)	Disorders of the yang link vessel	
Lieque(LU 7)	Disorders of the conception vessel	Lung system, throat, chest and diaphragm
Zhaohai(KI 6)	Disorders of the yin heel vessel	

表7-5　八脉交会穴

穴名	主治	相配合主治
公孙	冲脉病证	心、胸、胃
内关	阴维脉病证	
后溪	督脉病证	目内眦、颈项、耳、肩
申脉	阳跷脉病证	
足临泣	带脉病证	目锐眦、耳后、颊、颈、肩
外关	阳维脉病证	
列缺	任脉病证	肺系、咽喉、胸膈
照海	阴跷脉病证	

5 Clinical application of eight Influential acupoints

The eight Influential acupoints have special therapeutic functions for the disorders of their corresponding zang-fu organs and tissues, and are thus indicated for their relevant conditions. For example, for disorders of the fu-organs the Influential acupoint of fu-organ, Zhongwan(CV 12), is used; for blood-stasis conditions, Geshu(GB 17), the Influential acupoint of the blood, is used; for tendon disorders, Yanglingquan(GB 34), the Influential acupoint of the tendons, is used; for vessel disorders, Taiyuan(LU 9), the Influential acupoint of the vessels, is used. The eight Influential acupoints and their corresponding organs and tissues are presented in Table 7-6.

5 八会穴的临床应用

八会穴对各自相应的脏腑、组织等病证具有特殊治疗作用，临床上用于治疗这些相关病证。如：腑病，可取腑之会穴中脘；瘀血证，可取血之会穴膈俞；筋病，可取筋之会穴阳陵泉；脉病，可取脉之会穴太渊等。八会穴与有关脏腑组织的对应关系见表7-6。

Table 7-6 The eight Influential acupoints

Influential acupoint	Tissue	Influential acupoint	Tissue
Zhangmen(LR 13)	Zang-organs	Yanglingquan(GB 34)	Tendons
Zhongwan(CV 12)	Fu-organs	Taiyuan(LU 9)	Vessels
Danzhong(CV 17)	Qi	Dazhu(BL 11)	Bones
Geshu(GB 17)	Blood	Juegu(GB 39)	Marrow

表 7-6 八会穴

八会穴	脏腑组织	八会穴	脏腑组织
章门	脏会	阳陵泉	筋会
中脘	腑会	太渊	脉会
膻中	气会	大杼	骨会
膈俞	血会	绝骨	髓会

6 Clinical application of Xi-Cleft acupoints

Clinically, the Xi-Cleft acupoints are often used in treating the acute diseases of their corre-

6 郄穴的临床应用

临床上郄穴常用于治疗本经循行部位及其所属脏腑

sponding meridians and zang-fu organs. Specifically, the Xi-Cleft acupoints of the yin meridians are effective for bleeding conditions, whereas those of the yang meridians are effective for acute pain conditions. For example, hemoptysis results from the lung disorders and can thus be treated by Kongzui (LU 6), the Xi-Cleft acupoint of the lung meridian; acute stomachache can be treated by Liangqiu (ST 34), the Xi-Cleft acupoint of the stomach meridian. Apart from the single use of the Xi-Cleft acupoints, they are often used in combination with the eight Influential acupoints, which is termed as "Cleft-Influential acupoints combination". For example, combined use of Kongzui(LU 6), the Xi-Cleft acupoint of the lung meridian, and Geshu(BL 17), the Influential acupoint of the blood, is quite effective for hemoptysis due to lung diseases; combined use of Liangqiu(ST 34), the Xi-Cleft acupoint of the stomach meridian, and Zhongwan(CV 12), the Influential acupoint of fu-organs, is quite effective against acute stomachache. The Xi-Cleft acupoints are presented in Table 7-7.

的急性病证。其中，阴经郄穴多治血证，阳经郄穴多治急性痛症。例如：治疗肺病咳血，可取肺经郄穴孔最；治疗急性胃脘痛，可取胃经郄穴梁丘等。郄穴除单独使用外，常与八会穴配合使用，故有"郄会配穴"之称。如孔最配血会膈俞治疗肺病咳血效果尤佳，梁丘配腑会中脘治疗急性胃脘痛疗效更显著。各经郄穴见表 7-7。

Table 7-7　The Xi-Cleft acupoints

Meridian	Acupoint	Meridian	Acupoint
Lung meridian	Kongzui(LU 6)	Large intestine meridian	Wenliu(LI 7)
Pericardium meridian	Ximen(PC 4)	Triple energizer meridian	Huizong(TE 7)
Heart meridian	Yinxi(HT 6)	Small intestine meridian	Yanglao(SI 6)
Spleen meridian	Diji(SP 8)	Stomach meridian	Liangqiu(ST 34)
Liver meridian	Zhongdu(LR 6)	Gallbladder meridian	Waiqiu(GB 36)
Kidney meridian	Shuiquan(KI 5)	Bladder meridian	Jinmen(BL 63)
Yin link vessel	Zhubin(KI 9)	Yang link vessel	Yangjiao(GB 35)
Yin heel vessel	Jiaoxin(KI 8)	Yang heel vessel	Fuyang(BL 59)

表 7-7 郄穴

经 脉	郄 穴	经 脉	郄 穴
手太阴肺经	孔最	手阳明大肠经	温溜
手厥阴心包经	郄门	手少阳三焦经	会宗
手少阴心经	阴郄	手太阳小肠经	养老
足太阴脾经	地机	足阳明胃经	梁丘
足厥阴肝经	中都	足少阳胆经	外丘
足少阴肾经	水泉	足太阳膀胱经	金门
阴维脉	筑宾	阳维脉	阳交
阴蹻脉	交信	阳蹻脉	跗阳

7 Clinical application of Lower He-Sea acupoints

In Ling Shu, it states that "disorders of the six fu-organs can be treated by selecting their Lower He-Sea acupoints". It is showed that the Lower He-Sea acupoints are the primary acupoints effective for the six fu-organs disorders. For example, Zusanli(ST 36) is indicated for stomachache, Xiajuxu (ST 39) for diarrhea, Shangjuxu(ST 37) for appendicitis and dysentery, Yanglingquan (GB 34) for gallbladder pain, Weiyang (BL 39) and Weizhong (BL 40) for difficulty in urination and enuresis due to triple energizer qi failing to transform. The Lower He-Sea acupoints of the six fu-organs are shown in Table 7-8.

7 下合穴的临床应用

《灵枢·邪气藏府病形》提出"合治内府"的理论，说明下合穴是治疗六腑病证的主要穴位。如足三里治胃脘痛，下巨虚治泄泻，上巨虚治肠痈、痢疾，阳陵泉治胆痛，委阳、委中治三焦气化失常而引起的癃闭、遗尿等。六腑与下合穴关系见表 7-8。

Table 7-8 The Lower He-Sea acupoints of the six fu-organs

Fu-organ	Stomach	Large intestine	Small intestine	Triple energizer	Bladder	Gallbladder
Lower He-Sea acupoint	Zusanli (ST 36)	Shangjuxu (ST 37)	Xiajuxu (ST 39)	Weiyang (BL 39)	Weizhong (BL 40)	Yanglingquan (GB 34)

表 7-8　六腑下合穴

六腑	胃	大肠	小肠	三焦	膀胱	胆
下合穴	足三里	上巨虚	下巨虚	委阳	委中	阳陵泉

8　Clinical application of Crossing acupoints

The Crossing acupoints are mostly situated on the trunk and head. Ninety-five Crossing acupoints were recorded in *A-B Classie of Acupuncture and Moxikustion* (Zhen Jiu Jia Yi Jing). Because the Crossing acupoints are located at the intersection of two or more meridians, these acupoints are indicated for the disorders of their own meridians and the intersecting meridians. For example, Sanyinjiao(SP 6) pertains to the spleen meridian and is also the Crossing acupoint of the three foot yin meridians, so it can be used not only to treat the disorders of the spleen meridian, but also to treat the disorders of the liver meridian and the kidney meridian; Guanyuan(CV 4) and Zhongji(CV 3) are the acupoints of the conception vessel, and are also the Crossing acupoints of the conception vessel and three foot yin meridians, so it can be used to treat the diseases of the conception vessel, but also to treat the disorders of the three yin meridians of the foot.

8　交会穴的临床应用

交会穴大多位于躯干和头面部，《针灸甲乙经》记载有 95 个。由于有数条经脉相会，可治疗本经和交会经病证，临床上常用来治疗多经病证。如：三阴交既是足太阴脾经腧穴，又是足三阴经交会穴，故不仅可治脾经病证，也可治足厥阴肝经、足少阴肾经病证；关元、中极既是任脉腧穴，又是任脉、足三阴经之交会穴，故不仅能治疗任脉病证，也可治疗足三阴经病证。

Chapter 2 Treatment of Common Diseases

第 2 章 治疗各论

Section 1 Internal Diseases

第 1 节 内科病证

Wind Stroke

Wind stroke, known as "zu zhong" in Chinese, is a disease primarily manifested by sudden falling down with loss of consciousness, accompanied by deviated mouth, slurred speech, and hemiplegia, or just by deviated mouth and hemiplegia without sudden falling down. In Western medicine, this disease is mostly seen in acute cerebrovascular diseases, such as cerebral infarction, cerebral hemorrhage, cerebral embolism, and subarachnoid hemorrhage.

1 Etiology and pathogenesis

Wind stroke mainly results from such pathogenic factors as wind, fire, phlegm and blood stasis; and its focus lies in the brain, involving in the zang-fu organs, including the heart, liver, spleen, and kidney.

2 Syndrome differentiation

2.1 Meridian being attacked

Chief symptoms: Hemiplegia, deviated mouth,

中　风

中风又称"卒中",是以突然晕倒、不省人事,伴口角㖞斜、语言不利、半身不遂,或不经昏仆仅以口㖞、半身不遂为主的一种疾病。多见于西医学的急性脑血管病,如脑梗死、脑出血、脑栓塞、蛛网膜下腔出血等。

1 病因病机

中风的发生,风、火、痰、瘀是其主要病因,病位在脑府,病变涉及心、肝、脾、肾等脏腑。

2 辨证

2.1 中经络

主症:半身不遂,口角歪

slurred speech due to tongue stiffness.

The syndrome of wind-phlegm obstructing collaterals may be accompanied by numb limbs, dizziness and blurred vision, greasy tongue coating and wiry and slippery pulse. The syndrome of liver-yang hyperactivity may be accompanied by flushed complexion, reddened eyes, vertigo, headache, agitation and irritability, bitter taste in the mouth, dry throat, constipation, yellowish urine, red tongue with yellow coating, and wiry and forceful pulse. The syndrome of qi deficiency and blood stasis may be accompanied by weak limbs, half-body numbness, swelling and distension of the extremities, pale complexion, shortness of breath, lassitude, dark tongue with whitish coating, and thready and rough pulse.

斜，舌强语涩。

风痰阻络者，兼肢体麻木、头晕目眩、苔腻、脉弦滑。肝阳上亢者，兼面红目赤、眩晕头痛、心烦易怒、口苦咽干、大便干、小便黄、舌红苔黄、脉弦有力。气虚血瘀者，兼肢体软弱、偏身麻木、手足肿胀、面色淡白、气短乏力、舌暗苔白、脉细涩。

2.2 Zang-fu organs being attacked

Chief symptoms: Sudden falling down with loss of consciousness, daze and drowsiness, accompanied by hemiplegia, slurred speech due to stiff tongue, and deviated mouth.

The tense syndrome may be accompanied by locked jaw and clenched fists, flushed complexion, breathlessness, wheezing sputum in the throat, retention of urine and feces, and wiry slippery and rapid pulse. The flaccid syndrome may be accompanied by closed eyes and opened mouth, flaccid paralysis of the limbs, urinary incontinence, snoring, feeble breathing, cold limbs, and thready and weak pulse. If profuse sweating, reddish cheeks, and faint, floating or rootless pulse are present, they are the critical manifestations of outward collapse of genuine yang.

2.2　中脏腑

主症：突然昏仆、神志迷蒙、嗜睡，并见半身不遂、舌强语謇、口角㖞斜。

闭证者，兼牙关紧闭、两手握固、面赤气粗、喉中痰鸣、二便不通、脉弦滑而数。脱证者，兼目合口张、手撒遗尿、鼻鼾息微、四肢逆冷、脉象细弱等。如见汗出如油、两颧淡红、脉微欲绝或浮大无根，为真阳外越之危候。

3 Treatment

3.1 Essential treatment

3.1.1 Meridian being attacked

Principal acupoints: Upper limbs: Jianyu (LI 15), Quchi(LI 11), Shousanli(LI 10), Waiguan (TE 5), Hegu(LI4).

Lower limbs: Huantiao(GB 30), Yanglingquan (GB 34), Zusanli(ST 36), Jiexi(ST 41), Kunlun (BL 60).

Supplementary acupoints: Upper limbs: Jianliao (TE 14), Yangchi (TE 4), Houxi (SI 3). Lower limbs: Futu(ST 32), Yinshi(ST 33), Xuanzhong (GB 39). In the case of deviated mouth, add Dicang(ST 4), Jiache(ST 6), Chengjiang(CV 24), Hegu(LI 4) and Taichong(LR 3); in the case of slurred speech, add Lianquan(CV 23), Tongli(HT 5) and Yamen(GV 15); in the syndrome of wind-phlegm obstructing collaterals, add Fengchi(GB 20) and Fenglong(ST 40); in the syndrome of liver-yang hyperactivity, add Taichong(LR 3) and Taixi (KI 3); in the syndrome of qi deficiency and blood stasis, add Qihai(CV 6) and Sanyinjiao(SP 6).

Explanation: In this acupoints prescription, the acupoints of yangming meridians are mainly selected. Yangming meridians are of abundant qi and blood. If the qi and blood of yangming meridians flow smoothly, the healthy qi will be restored and normal functions of the body will be gradually recovered. In addition, other acupoints of the yang meridians on the limbs are selected in accordance with the pathways of their meridians to unblock meridians and collaterals.

3.1.2 Zang-fu organs being attacked

Principal acupoints: Tense syndrome: Shuigou

3 治疗

3.1 基本治疗

3.1.1 中经络

主穴：上肢的肩髃，曲池，手三里，外关，合谷。

下肢：环跳，阳陵泉，足三里，解溪，昆仑。

配穴：上肢取肩髎、阳池、后溪等穴，下肢取伏兔、阴市、悬钟等穴。口角㖞斜，加地仓、颊车、承浆、合谷、太冲；言语謇涩，加廉泉、通里、哑门；风痰阻络，加风池、丰隆；肝阳上亢，加太冲、太溪；气虚血瘀，加气海、三阴交。

方义：本方以阳明经穴为主，阳明经为多气多血之经，阳明经气血通畅，则正气得复，机体功能逐渐恢复。根据上下肢相应经脉循行，分别配以手足阳经的穴位，有疏通经络之效。

3.1.2 中脏腑

主穴：闭证取水沟，十二

(GV 26), twelve Jing-Well acupoints, Taichong (LR 3), Fenglong(ST 40), Laogong(PC 8).

井穴,太冲,丰隆,劳宫。

Flaccid syndrome: Guanyuan(CV 4), Shenque (CV 8).

脱证:取关元,神阙。

Supplementary acupoints: In the case of locked jaws, add Jiache(ST 6) and Xiaguan(ST 7); in the case of slurred speech, add Yamen(GV 15) and Lianquan(CV 23).

配穴: 牙关紧闭配颊车、下关;语言不利配哑门、廉泉。

Explanation: This acupoints prescription acts to pacify the liver and extinguish wind, clear fire and dissipate phlegm, and resuscitate unconsciousness and open blockage. The tense syndrome is caused by liver-yang hyperactivity and upward adversity of qi and blood, so the twelve Jing-Well acupoints are pricked to bleed, and Shuigou(GV 26) is punctured with reducing techniques to open blockage and resuscitate unconsciousness. The liver meridian goes up to the vertex, so Taichong(LR 3) is needled with reducing techniques to pacify the liver and suppress yang. Fenglong(ST 40), the Luo-Connecting acupoint of the stomach meridian, is used to remove turbidity and resolve phlegm. Laogong (PC 8), the Ying-Spring acupoint of the pericardium meridian of hand jueyin, is selected to clear heart heat. Guangyuan(CV 4) and Shenque(CV 8), two acupoints of the conception vessel, are treated by heavy moxibustion to revive yang and rectify adversity.

方义: 本方可平肝熄风、清火豁痰、开窍启闭。闭证乃由肝阳暴亢、气血上逆,取十二井穴点刺出血和泻水沟,具启闭、开窍、醒脑的作用。肝脉上巅,泻太冲以平肝潜阳。取胃经络穴丰隆,涤浊化痰。取手厥阴心包经荥穴劳宫清心泄热。取任脉穴关元、神阙,用大艾炷重灸回阳救逆。

3.2 Other therapies

3.2 其他治疗

Scalp acupuncture: Select the Anterior Oblique Line of the Vertex-Temporal (MS 6), Lateral Line 1 of Vertex (MS 8) and Lateral Line 2 of Vertex (MS 9), and horizontally insert the needles 1.5～2 cun beneath the scalp and rapidly rotate the needles for 2～3 minutes. The needles are retained for 30

头针: 选顶颞前斜线、顶旁1线及顶旁2线,选1.5～2寸毫针平刺入头皮下,快速捻转2～3分钟,留针30分钟,留针期间反复捻转2～3次。行针时和留针后嘱患者

minutes, and manipulated by rotating 2～3 times. During needle manipulation and retention, the patients are asked to exercise the affected limbs, consequently to promote the restoration of limb function.

活动患侧肢体，促进功能恢复。

Electroacupuncture: Choose two acupoints respectively on the upper limb and lower limb, or a pair of acupoints on the face. These acupoints are needled and the needles are retained when the needling sensation(De Qi) is induced. Then, the needles are connected with electroacupuncture instrument by an intermittent wave or sparse wave, with the electrical stimulation intensity adequate to induce slight muscular tremble. Each electroacupuncture stimulation lasts 20～30 minutes.

电针：在患侧上、下肢各选两个穴位或面部取一对穴位，针刺得气后留针，接通电针仪，采用断续波或疏波，以局部肌肉微颤为度，每次通电 20～30 分钟。

4　Remarks

4　按语

Acupuncture is quite effective in the treatment of wind stroke, especially in promoting the rehabilitation of limb movement, speech and swallowing function. The earlier acupuncture is performed, the better therapeutic outcome will be obtained. During treatment procedure, the patients should be instructed to practise functional exercises of the affected limbs.

针灸治疗中风疗效较满意，尤其对肢体运动、语言、吞咽功能的康复等有促进作用，针灸介入越早效果越好。治疗期间应指导患者进行瘫痪肢体的功能锻炼。

The prevention of wind stroke is very important. When there appear precursory signs of stroke, timely treatment must be administered immediately. In the acute stage of wind stroke, comprehensive treatments should be given in the case of high fever, coma, heart failure, intracranial hypertension, upper gastrointestinal hemorrhage, etc.

本病重在预防，出现中风先兆时，应及时进行治疗。中风急性期，出现高热、神昏、心力衰竭、颅内压增高、上消化道出血等情况时，应采取综合治疗措施。

Appendix: Pseudobulbar Paralysis

［附］　假性延髓麻痹

Pseudobulbar paralysis is a symptom of the injury in the bilateral cortico-bulbar tracts. It is com-

假性延髓麻痹又称假性球麻痹，是两侧皮质延髓束

monly seen in cerebral vascular accidents, amyotrophic lateral sclerosis and syphilitic cerebral arteritis. Chinese medicine holds that this disease is associated with heart dysfunction, or caused by pathogenic turbidity blocking brain collaterals, or results from throat malnutrition due to heart-spleen insufficiency, liver-kidney yin deficiency. It belongs to the categories of dysphagia, "Ye Ge" in Chinese medicine, or aphonia, "Yin Fei" in Chinese medicine.

损害所产生的症状。常见于脑血管意外、肌萎缩性侧索硬化、梅毒性脑动脉炎等病。中医学认为，本病与心之机能失常有关，或因邪浊阻滞脑络，闭阻喉窍；或心脾不足、肝肾阴虚，不能上承所致。本病归属中医学"噎膈""瘖痱"等范畴。

1　Clinical manifestations

Pseudobulbar paralysis is primarily manifested by upper motoneurons paralysis or incomplete paralysis of the muscles innervated by bulbar nerves, displaying dyskinesia of the soft palate, throat and tongue muscles, difficulty in swallowing, vocalization and speaking, absence of lingual amyotrophy and fibrillary tremor, presence of pharyngeal reflex, increased zygomatic reflex, and frequent forced crying and laughing. The somatosensory evoked potential may be abnormal.

1　临床表现

主要为延髓神经所支配的肌肉呈上运动神经元性瘫痪或不完全性瘫痪，出现软腭、咽喉、舌肌运动障碍，吞咽、发音、讲话困难，无舌肌萎缩及纤维性震颤，咽反射存在，下颌反射增强，常出现强哭强笑。诱发电位可有异常。

2　Treatment

Principal acupoints: Lianquan(CV 23), Yamen (GV 15), Tongli (HT5), Jianshi (PC 5), Shuigou (GV 26) and Fengchi (GB 20).

Supplementary acupoints: In the syndrome of wind-phlegm obstructing collaterals, add Taichong (LR 3) and Fenglong(ST 40). In the syndrome of blood stasis, add Xuehai (SP 10) and Geshu (BL 17). In the syndrome of scorching lung-heat, add Yuji(LU 10) and Shaoshang(LU 11). In the syndrome of heart-spleen insufficiency, add Zusanli(ST 36) and Sanyinjiao(SP 6). In the syndrome of liver-kidney yin deficiency, add Guanyuan(CV 4) and Taixi(KI 3).

2　治疗

主穴：廉泉，哑门，通里，间使，水沟，风池。

配穴：风痰阻络配太冲、丰隆；瘀血内停配血海、膈俞；肺热熏灼配鱼际、少商；心脾不足配足三里、三阴交；肝肾阴亏配关元、太溪。

3 Remarks

Acupuncture works well on pseudobulbar paralysis if proper needling techniques are performed. Nevertheless, if the needling depth is inadequate or the needling intensity is not strong enough, the therapeutic efficacy will be poor. The prognosis of pseudobulbar paralysis is excellent if the primary injury of the cortico-bulbar tract is controlled and improved; alternatively, the prognosis will be bad if the primary injury worsens or relapses.

3 按语

针灸治疗本病如方法得当，疗效较好。但如针刺深度不够，或手法操作刺激量不足，则疗效差。导致皮质延髓束损伤的原发病稳定并逐渐恢复时，预后良好。原发病加重或反复发作者，预后不佳。

Vertigo

Vertigo is a symptom that the eyes see stars and everything goes around. The location of vertigo is in the brain and the clear orifices. It falls into constant vertigo and paroxysmal vertigo. In mild case, vertigo only lasts for a short period of time and can be relieved by lying down with the eyes closed. In severe cases, the patients suffers from bodily movement with a constant rotary sensation like sitting in a sailing boat or a moving vehicle, even nausea and vomiting. Vertigo may be accompanied by other symptoms, which makes it lingering. Vertigo is often seen in such diseases as hypertension, cerebral arteriosclerosis, anemia, neurosis, aural vertigo and kinesia in Western medicine.

眩 晕

眩晕是自觉头晕眼花、视物旋转的一种症状。病位主要在脑髓清窍，有经常性和发作性之分。轻者发作短暂，平卧闭目片刻即安；重者如乘坐舟车，旋转起伏不定，甚则恶心呕吐，或兼见他证而迁延不愈，反复发作。眩晕可见于高血压、脑动脉硬化、贫血、神经衰弱、耳源性眩晕、晕动病等疾病。

1 Etiology and pathogenesis

The occurrence of vertigo is related to emotional disturbance(worry and anger), indulgence in fatty and sweet diets, and overstrain. Emotional disturbance, including agitation and great anger, may cause qi depression and subsequent transformed fire and liver-yang hyperactivity, which may disturb the

1 病因病机

眩晕起因与忧思恼怒、恣食肥甘、劳伤过度等有关。情志不舒，或急躁恼怒，气郁化火，肝阳暴亢，而致清窍被扰；恣食肥甘厚味，脾虚生湿，痰湿上蒙清窍；或体虚病

brain and clear orifices. Indulgence in fatty and sweet diets may result in spleen deficiency, in which phlegm-dampness produces and goes up to cloud the clear orifices. In constitutional weakness and after chronic illness, qi and blood are insufficient to nourish the brain. Overstrain may consume kidney-essence, which cannot produce marrow to fill up the brain. All the factors above may result in vertigo.

后，气血不足，清窍失养；或过劳耗伤肾精，脑髓不充，均可发为本病。

2 Syndrome differentiation

Chief symptoms: Dizziness and sparkling vision, vomiting, and even a tendency to fall down.

The syndrome of liver-yang hyperactivity may be accompanied by agitation and irritability, bitter taste in the mouth, tinnitus, red tongue with yellowish coating, and wiry pulse. The syndrome of phlegm-dampness accumulation may be accompanied by head heaviness as if wrapped, chest fullness and nausea, fat tongue with white greasy coating, and sluggish slippery pulse. The syndrome of kidney-essence deficiency may be accompanied by soreness and weakness in the loin and knees, seminal emission, light-colored tongue, and deep thready pulse. The syndrome of qi and blood deficiency may be accompanied by lassitude and fatigue, sallow complexion, light-colored tongue and thready pulse.

2 辨证

主症：头晕目眩，泛泛欲吐，甚则眩晕欲仆。

肝阳上亢者，兼急躁易怒、口苦、耳鸣、舌红苔黄、脉弦；痰湿中阻者，兼头重如裹、胸闷恶心、舌胖苔白腻、脉濡滑；肾精亏损者，兼腰膝酸软、遗精、舌淡、脉沉细；气血两虚者，兼神疲乏力、面色㿠白、舌淡、脉细。

3 Treatment

3.1 Essential treatment

Principal acupoints: Fengchi (GB 20), Baihui (GV 20), Neiguan (PC 6), Taichong (LR 3), and Taixi (KI 3).

Supplementary acupoints: In the syndrome of liver-yang hyperactivity, add Xingjian (LR 2) and Taixi (KI 3); in the syndrome of phlegm-dampness accumulation, add Fenglong (ST 40), Zhongwan

3 治疗

3.1 基本治疗

主穴：风池，百会，内关，太冲，太溪。

配穴：肝阳上亢加行间、太溪；痰湿中阻加丰隆、中脘、阴陵泉；气血两虚加足三里、脾俞、胃俞；肾精亏虚加

(CV 12) and Yinlingquan(SP 9); in the syndrome of qi and blood deficiency, add Zusanli (ST 36), Pishu(BL 20) and Weishu(BL 21); in the syndrome of kidney-essence deficiency, add Shenshu(BL 23), Ganshu(BL 18) and Sanyinjiao(SP 6).

肾俞、肝俞、三阴交。

Explanation: Fengchi(GB 20), an acupoint of the gallbladder meridian, and Taichong(LR 3), an acupoint of the liver meridian, are selected to clear liver and gallbladder, and suppress liver-yang hyperactivity. Baihui(GV 20) acts to elevate qi and blood, and regulate qi and blood flow in combination with Fengchi(GB 20). Neiguan(PC 6) is used to relieve chest fullness and regulate qi, harmonize the middle energizer, resolve phlegm and stop vomiting. Taixi(KI 3) and Taichong(LR 3) are used to nourish the liver and kidney, enrich blood and essence.

方义：取胆经风池和肝经太冲，清泻肝胆、平抑肝阳。百会提升气血，与风池合用可疏调头部气血。内关宽胸理气，和中化痰止呕。太溪、太冲滋补肝肾、养血益精。

3. 2 Other therapies

Scalp acupuncture: Select the Posterior Temporal Line(MS 11) and Middle Line of Vertex(MS 5), and quickly insert the needles beneath the scalp. The needles are rotated fast. The treatment is given once a day, 20 minutes per time. For severe cases, the needles may be retained for longer time.

3. 2 其他治疗

头针：选颞后线、顶中线，沿头皮刺入，快速捻转，每日 1 次，一般每次留针 20 分钟，严重者可延长留针时间。

4 Remarks

Acupuncture has excellent therapeutic effects on vertigo. However, the causative reasons, accurate diagnosis and underlying diseases should be considered as well. For paroxysmal vertigo, the patients are asked to close their eyes and calmly lie on their backs. If vomiting is accompanied, the vomitus should be prevented from entering the trachea.

4 按语

针灸治疗眩晕具有较好的临床疗效，但是应查明原因，明确诊断，注意原发病的治疗。眩晕发作时，嘱患者闭目或平卧，保持安静，如伴呕吐应防止呕吐物误入气管。

Appendix: Hypertension

Hypertension, the short form of essential hy-

[附] 高血压病

高血压病全称“原发性

pertension, is a common chronic condition where there is a persistent high arterial pressure at a state of rest (>140/90 mmHg or 18.6/12kPa). Hypertension belongs to the categories of "headache", "vertigo" and "liver wind" in Chinese medicine. It is often caused by imbalance between yin and yang in the liver and kidney, which mostly results from emotional disturbance, improper diets, internal deficiency and overstrain.

高血压病",是以安静状态下持续性动脉压增高(血压大于140/90毫米汞柱或18.6/12千帕)为主要表现的一种常见慢性疾病。本病归属于中医学"头痛""眩晕""肝风"等范畴。多因情志失调、饮食失节、内伤虚损等导致肝肾阴阳失调所致。

1　Clinical manifestations

1　临床表现

Headache and vertigo, distended head, blurred vision, tinnitus, palpitation, insomnia and amnesia.

The syndrome of liver-fire exuberance may manifest vertigo and headache, flushed complexion and reddened eyes, agitation, bitter taste in the mouth, red tongue with dry yellow coating, and wiry pulse. The syndrome of yin deficiency and yang hyperactivity may manifest vertigo and headache, tinnitus, palpitation and insomnia, burning sensation in the five centers, red tongue with less coating, and wiry thready and rapid pulse. The syndrome of phlegm-dampness accumulation may manifest headache and vertigo, chest fullness, diminished appetite, nausea and vomiting sputum, white greasy coating and slippery pulse. The syndrome of qi deficiency and blood stasis may manifest vertigo and headache, palpitation, shortness of breath, sallow complexion, dark-purplish tongue with possible ecchymosis, and thin rough pulse.

头痛头晕,头胀,眼花耳鸣,心悸失眠,健忘。肝火亢盛者,眩晕头痛,面红目赤,烦躁不安,口苦,舌红苔干黄,脉弦;阴虚阳亢者,眩晕头痛,耳鸣,心悸失眠,五心烦热,舌红少苔,脉弦细数;痰湿壅盛者,眩晕头痛,胸闷食少,呕恶痰涎,苔白腻,脉滑;气虚血瘀者,眩晕头痛,心悸气短,面色萎黄,舌质紫暗或有瘀点,脉细涩。

2　Treatment

2　治疗

2.1　Essential treatment

2.1　基本治疗

Principal acupoints: Baihui(GV 20), Quchi(LI 11), Taichong(LR 3), Hegu(LI 4), and Sanyinjiao (SP 6).

主穴:百会,曲池,太冲,合谷,三阴交。

Supplementary acupoints: In the syndrome of liver-fire exuberance, add Fengchi (GB 20) and Xingjian(LR 2); in the syndrome of yin deficiency and yang hyperactivity, add Taixi(KI 3), Ganshu (BL 18) and Shenshu(BL 23); in the syndrome of phlegm-dampness accumulation, add Fenglong(ST 40) and Zusanli(ST 36); in the syndrome of qi deficiency and blood stasis, add Qihai(CV 6) and Geshu (BL 17). In the presence of vertigo and head heaviness, add Baihui(GV 20) and Taiyang(EX-HN5); in the presence of palpitation, add Neiguan(PC 6) and Shenmen(HT 7).

配穴：肝火亢盛加风池、行间；阴虚阳亢加太溪、肝俞、肾俞；痰湿壅盛加丰隆、足三里；气虚血瘀加气海、膈俞。头晕头重加百会、太阳；心悸加内关、神门。

2.2 Other therapies

2.2 其他治疗

Three-edged needle therapy: Select 1～2 acupoints each time from the Ear Apex(Ex-HN 6), Dazhui (GV 14), Yintang($EX-HN_3$) and Quchi(LI 11). Prick the acupoints to bleed 3～5 drops.

三棱针：取耳尖、大椎、印堂、曲池等穴。每次选1～2穴，点刺出血3～5滴。

Ear acupuncture: Select 3～4 acupoints from the Groove of the Posterior Surface(PS), Ear Apex (HX_6, HX_{7i}), Sympathesis (AH_{6a}), Shenmen (TF 4) and Heart(CO_{15}). Puncturing, needle embedding or *Semen Vaccariae* (Wang Bu Liu Xing) sticking may be applied at these acupoints.

耳针：取耳背沟、耳尖、交感、神门、心等。每次选3～4穴，针刺或埋针，也可用王不留行贴压。

3 Remarks

3 按语

Acupuncture is effective in decreasing blood pressure in all stages of hypertension, especially for the first stage of hypertension. The clinical manifestations of all stages can be improved to a certain extent. For cases with hypertensive crisis that developed from persistent hypertension, medications in Chinese medicine and Western medicine should be administered in order to control the blood pressure in time. In the treatment of hypertension, strong stimulation by acupuncture and electro-acupuncture

针灸对各期高血压病均有降压作用，对1期高血压尤为明显。各期的临床症状可获得不同程度的改善，对顽固性高血压发展为高血压危象者，应与中西药物并用，以控制血压。对血压过高者，应避免强刺激。

is prohibited.

In secondary hypertension due to other diseases, the primary diseases should be treated actively. In ordinary time, patients with hypertension should avoid emotional irritation and overstrain, eat low-sodium food, and quit smoking and drinking alcohol.

对于其他原发疾病引起的继发性高血压,应积极治疗原发病。平素要求患者避免精神刺激,过度劳累,低盐清淡饮食,戒烟戒酒。

Headache

Headache is a type of disorder in which pain appears in head as the cardinal symptom in various acute and chronic diseases. Headache may be caused by all kinds of exogenous and endogenous factors, which result in dysfunction of the head meridians, qi and blood obstruction, or malnutrition of the brain. Headache is frequently seen in hypertension, vascular headache, neurological headahce, encephalitis, meningitis, acute cerebrovascular diseases and glaucoma, etc.

头 痛

头痛是以头部疼痛为主要表现的一类病证,各种外邪或内伤等因素均可使头部经络失调、气血不通或脑窍失养而导致头痛。本病多见于高血压、血管性头痛、神经性头痛、脑炎、脑膜炎、急性脑血管疾病、青光眼等病。

1 Etiology and pathogenesis

The causative factors of headache can be classified into exogenous and endogenous factors. For exogenous headache, pathogenic wind is the chief factor or in combination with other causes, which can attack the head and block the head meridians. For endogenous headache, the causes include emotional disturbance, improper diets, weak constitution, or chronic disorders. Liver depression may lead to liver-yang hyperactivity, which disturbs the clear orifices(brain); or the brain fails to be nourished due to weak constitution, kidney deficiency and qi-blood insufficiency; or indulgence in fatty and sweet foods may produce phlegm and dampness

1 病因病机

头痛的病因分为外感、内伤两方面。外感头痛主要由风邪或兼夹其他病邪,上犯清窍,阻遏经络而致头痛。内伤头痛可因情志、饮食、体虚、久病等所致;或肝郁不遂,肝阳上亢,清窍被扰;或体虚肾亏,气血不足,脑海失养;或过嗜肥甘,痰湿内生,脑络阻滞;或跌仆外伤,脑络瘀阻,均可导致内伤头痛。

in the body, which obstruct the brain collaterals; or falling down and external injury may cause blood stasis in the brain collaterals. All these factors result in endogenous headache.

2 Syndrome differentiation

2.1 Exogenous headache

Chief symptoms: Persistent headache radiating to the neck and back, acute onset, accompanied by exterior symptoms caused by exogenous factors.

The syndrome of wind cold may be accompanied by aversion to wind and cold, thin white coating and floating tight pulse. The syndrome of wind heat may be accompanied by distended head, fever, thirstiness with desire to drink, constipation, dark yellow urine, yellowish coating, and floating rapid pulse. The syndrome of wind dampness may be accompanied by heavy head as if wrapped, weakness and heaviness of the limbs, white greasy coating and sluggish pulse.

2.2 Endogenous headache

Chief symptoms: Lingering and mild headache with intermittent paroxysm.

The syndrome of liver-yang hyperactivity may be accompanied by distended head, sparkling vision, agitation and irritability, flushed complexion reddened eyes, bitter taste in the mouth, red tongue with thin yellowish coating, and wiry pulse. The syndrome of liver-kidney yin deficiency may be accompanied by vertigo, tinnitus, soreness and weakness in the loins and knees, red tongue with less coating, and wiry thready pulse. The syndrome of qi and blood deficiency may be accompanied by empty headache, vertigo, lassitude and fatigue, lusterless complexion, light-colored tongue with whitish coating, and weak thready pulse. The syndrome

2 辨证

2.1 外感头痛

主症：头痛连及项背，痛无休止，发病较急，兼见外感表证。

风寒头痛者，兼恶风畏寒、苔薄白、脉浮紧；风热头痛者，兼头胀发热、口干欲饮、大便干、小便黄、苔黄、脉浮数；风湿头痛者，兼头重如裹、肢体困重、苔白腻、脉濡。

2.2 内伤头痛

主症：头痛绵绵，时作时休，发病较缓。

肝阳上亢者，兼头胀目眩、心烦易怒、面红目赤、口苦、舌红苔薄黄、脉弦；肝肾阴虚者，兼头晕耳鸣、腰膝酸软、舌红苔少、脉弦细；气血亏虚者，兼头部空痛、头晕、神疲无力、面色不华、舌淡苔白、脉细弱；痰浊上蒙者，兼头昏蒙、胸脘闷胀、苔白腻、脉滑；瘀血阻络者，常有头部外伤史，迁延日久，兼痛处固定不移、痛如锥刺、舌紫暗或有瘀斑、苔薄、脉细涩。

of phlegm-turbidity may be accompanied by hazy dizziness, chest and abdominal fullness, white greasy coating and slippery pulse. The syndrome of blood stasis obstructing collaterals, often resulting from head trauma and lingering for a long time, may be accompanied by fixed pricking pain, dark-purplish tongue with possible petechia and thin coating, and thready rough pulse.

On basis of syndrome differentiation above, headache can be differentiated according to the meridian distribution. Pain in the forehead pertains to yangming headache, pain in the lateral side of the head to shaoyang headache, pain in the occipital region to taiyang headache, and pain at the vertex of the head to jueyin headache.

在以上辨证基础上，可根据头痛的部位进行经络辨证，前额痛为阳明头痛，侧头痛为少阳头痛，后枕痛为太阳头痛，巅顶痛为厥阴头痛。

3 Treatment

3 治疗

3.1 Essential treatment

3.1 基本治疗

3.1.1 Exogenous headache

3.1.1 外感头痛

Principal acupoints: Baihui (GV 20), Taiyang (EX-HN 5), Fengchi (GB 20), Lieque (LU 7) and Ashi acupoint.

主穴：百会，太阳，风池，列缺，阿是穴。

Supplementary acupoints: In the syndrome of wind cold, add Fengmen (BL 12); in the syndrome of wind heat, add Quchi (LI 11) and Dazhui (GV 14); in the syndrome of wind dampness, add Yinlingquan (SP 9).

配穴：风寒头痛者，加风门；风热头痛者，加曲池、大椎；风湿头痛者，加阴陵泉。

Explanation: Baihui (GV 20) and Taiyang (EX-HN5) act to promote qi flow in the head. Fengchi (GB 20), the Crossing acupoint of foot-shaoyang meridian and yang link vessel, functions to dispel wind and promote blood circulation, and unblock collaterals to relieve pain. Lieque (LU 7), the Luo-Connecting acupoint of the lung meridian, is used to disperse lung and unblock collaterals, which is indi-

方义：百会、太阳可疏导头部经气。风池为足少阳与阳维脉的交会穴，功长祛风活血、通络止痛。列缺为肺经络穴，可宣肺通络、兼治头项诸疾。阿是穴通经活络止痛。

cated for head and neck disorders. Ashi acupoints are selected to unblock meridians and collaterals to relieve pain.

3.1.2 Endogenous headache

Principal acupoints: Baihui(GV 20), Touwei (ST 8), Fengchi(GB 20), Zusanli(ST 36) and Ashi acupoints.

Supplementary acupoints: In the syndrome of liver-yang hyperactivity, add Taichong(LR 3) and Taixi(KI 3); in the syndrome of phlegm-turbi-dity, add Fenglong(ST 40) and Yinlingquan(SP 9); in the syndrome of blood stasis, add Sanyinjiao(SP 6) and Geshu(BL 17); in the syndrome of blood deficiency, add Xuehai(SP 10) and Pishu(BL 20); in the syndrome of kidney deficiency, add Taixi(KI 3) and Shenshu(BL 23).

Explanation: Baihui(GV 20) acts to regulate qi and blood to enrich brain morrow. Touwei(ST 8) is used to unblock head meridians. Fengchi(GB 20) is used to promote blood circulation and unblock meridians, clear head and brighten eyes. Zusanli(ST 36) is selected to supplement qi and blood, nourish brain and enrich marrow. Ashi acupoints are used to unblock collaterals and relieve pain.

In addition, in the case of yangming headache, add Touwei(ST 8) and Hegu(LI 4); in the case of shaoyang headache, add Shuaigu(GB 8) and Waiguan(TE 5); in the case of taiyang headache, add Tianzhu(BL 10) and Houxi(SI 3); in the case of jueyin headache, add Sishencong(EX-HN 1) and Taichong(LR 3).

3.2 Other therapies

Ear acupuncture: Select Subcortex(AT 4), Occiput(AT 3), Temple(AT 2), Forehead(AT 1),

3.1.2 内伤头痛

主穴：百会，头维，风池，足三里，阿是穴。

配穴：肝阳上亢者，加太冲、太溪；痰浊头痛者，加丰隆、阴陵泉；瘀血头痛者，加三阴交、膈俞；血虚头痛者，加血海、脾俞；肾虚头痛者，加太溪、肾俞。

方义：百会疏调气血以养脑髓。头维疏通头部经气。风池活血通经，清利头目。足三里补益气血，滋养脑髓。阿是穴通络止痛。

另外，阳明头痛者，加头维、合谷；少阳头痛者，加率谷、外关；太阳头痛者，加天柱、后溪；厥阴头痛者，加四神聪、太冲。

3.2 其他治疗

耳针：选皮质下、枕、颞、额、脑干、神门，每次选 2～3

Brain stem(AT 3, 4i) and Shenmen(TF 4). Two or three acupoints are treated each time by needling, or embedding needles or sticking *Semen Vaccariae* (Wang Bu Liu Xing). For obstinate headache, blood-letting can be applied by pricking the posterior auricular veins.

穴针刺,或埋针或贴压王不留行。对于顽固性头痛可在耳背静脉点刺出血。

4 Remarks

Acupuncture is quite effective for headache. However, the causes of headaches are complicated. If a headache is not relieved or even increasingly deteriorated after several acupuncture treatments, the causative factors should be found out and comprehensive treatments should be implemented.

In the presence of severe headache with meningeal irritation, such critical diseases as subarachnoid hemorrhage should be considered. For hypertensive headache, acupuncture with strong stimulation should be performed carefully.

4 按语

针灸治疗头痛有较好效果。头痛原因复杂,对于多次治疗无效,或头痛继续加重者,要进一步查明病因,采取综合治疗。

严重头痛伴脑膜刺激征者,应高度警惕蛛网膜下腔出血等重症。对高血压头痛患者应慎用强刺激。

Appendix: Migraine

A migraine is a neurovascular dysfunction mani fested by recurrent onset of lateral headache and often accompanied by nausea, vomiting and hypersensitivity to lights and sounds. Chinese medicine holds that the occurrence of migraine is associated with such factors as emotional disturbance. Hyperactive liver-yang goes up to disturb the clear orifices; or deficient spleen produces dampness, which may cloud the clear orifices; or in chronic conditions, the collaterals are involved and obstructed, thus migraine appears.

[附] 偏头痛

偏头痛是由于神经血管性功能失调所引起的疾病,以一侧头部疼痛反复发作,常伴有恶心、呕吐,对光及声音过敏等特点。中医学认为,本病多与情绪等相关。肝阳上亢,清窍被扰;或脾虚生湿,蒙蔽清窍;或久病入络,脉络痹阻而致痛。

1 Clinical manifestations

Migraine often happens in one side of the head, localized in the forehead, temple and occipital region. It may attack at any time, but frequently oc-

1 临床表现

多为一侧头痛,常局限于额部、颞部和枕部。任何时间可发作,但以早晨起床时多

curs in the morning when one gets up. The pain may last for hours to days. A typical migraine has precursory symptoms such as myopsis, visual field defects, unilateral or homonymous blindness. The pain may shift from one site to the other, even radiate to the neck and shoulders.

发,症状可持续数小时到数天。典型的偏头痛有先兆症状,如眼前闪烁暗点、视野缺损、单盲或同侧偏盲。发作时疼痛部位可向另一个部位转移,同时可放射至颈肩部。

2 Treatment

2 治疗

Principal acupoints: Ashi acupoint, Shuaigu (GB 8), Jiaosun(TE 20), Fengchi(GB 20), Hegu (LI 4), Taichong(LR 3) and Waiguan(TE 5).

主穴:阿是穴,率谷,角孙,风池,合谷,太冲,外关。

Supplementary acupoints: In the syndrome of liver-yang hyperactivity, add Sishencong(EX-HN 1) and Xingjian(LR 2); in the syndrome of phlegm-dampness, add Fenglong(ST 40) and Zusanli(ST 36); in the syndrome of blood stasis, add Xuehai (SP 10) and Geshu(BL 17).

配穴:肝阳上亢加四神聪、行间;痰湿偏盛加丰隆、足三里;瘀血头痛加血海、膈俞。

3 Remarks

3 按语

Acupuncture works excellently on migraine. But, treatment prior to its typical paroxysm works better. During treatment periods, the patients should guarantee adequate sleep and avoid excessive stress to reduce the frequency of its onset.

针刺治疗偏头痛有较好疗效,在典型发作前治疗,其疗效更明显。患者治疗期间要保证足够的睡眠,避免过度紧张以减少发作。

Facial Paralysis

面 瘫

Facial paralysis, also known as "deviation of the mouth and eyes", is a disease that is mainly manifested by deviated mouth and incomplete closure of the eyes. It may happen in patients at any ages during any seasons. It generally occurs in a sudden way and usually on one side of the face. Facial paralysis is peripheral facial palsy in Western medicine, Bell's palsy in particular.

面瘫是以口角歪斜、眼睑闭合不全为主症的一种病证,又称"口眼㖞斜"。本病可发生于任何年龄,无明显季节性,发病急速,以一侧面部发病多见。本病即西医学的周围性面神经麻痹,最常见于贝尔麻痹。

1 Etiology and pathogenesis

1 病因病机

Both hand and foot yang meridians go up to the

手足阳经均上头面部,

head and face. When the healthy qi is insufficient, meridians are empty, and body defense is weak, the exogenous wind may invade the meridians and collaterals on the face. This leads to meridian qi stagnation and malnutrition of the tendons and meridians, hence resulting in facial paralysis.

机体正气不足，脉络空虚，卫外不固，外感风邪，乘虚入中面部经络，致经气阻滞，筋脉失养而发生面瘫。

2 Syndrome differentiation

2 辨证

Chief symptoms: Upon waking up, there happenone-side facial weakness, numbness and paralysis, disappearance of wrinkles, enlarged rima oculi, flattened nasolabial groove, and drooping mouth-angle to the healthy side. The diseased face is unable to frown, raise the eyebrow, close the eyes, show the teeth, and blow out the cheeks. In some cases at the beginning of the disease, there may exist pain behind the ear, an impaired sense of taste of the front two-thirds of the tongue on the affected side, and hypersensitivity of hearing.

主症：睡眠醒来时出现一侧面部肌肉板滞、麻木、瘫痪，额纹消失，眼裂变大，鼻唇沟变浅，口角下垂歪向健侧，病侧不能皱眉、蹙额、闭目、露齿、鼓颊；部分患者初起时有耳后疼痛，还可出现患侧舌前2/3味觉减退或消失、听觉过敏等症。

The syndrome of wind cold is often seen in the early stage with the history of cold contraction, accompanied by light-colored tongue with thin whitish coating, and floating tight pulse. The syndrome of wind heat is also seen in the early stage, accompanied by fever, dry throat, red tongue with thin yellowish coating, and floating rapid pulse. The syndrome of qi-blood deficiency is mainly seen in the convalescent stage or in longstanding cases, accompanied by lassitude, pale complexion, vertigo, light-colored tongue with whitish coating, and weak thready pulse.

风寒证常见于发病初期，兼有面部受凉史，舌淡、苔薄白、脉浮紧；风热证常见于发病初期，兼发热、咽干、舌红、苔薄黄、脉浮数。气血不足见于恢复期或病程较长的患者，兼见肢体倦怠无力、面色淡白、头晕、舌淡、苔白、脉细弱。

3 Treatment

3 治疗

3.1 Essential treatment

3.1 基本治疗

Principal acupoints: Yangbai(GB 14), Sibai(ST 2), Taiyang(EX-HN_5), Jiache(ST 6), Dicang(ST 4), Hegu(LI 4), and Taichong(LR 3).

主穴：阳白，四白，太阳，颊车，地仓，合谷，太冲。

Supplementary acupoints: For the syndrome of wind cold, add Fengchi(GB 20); for the syndrome of wind heat, add Quchi(LI 11); for convalescent stage, add Zusanli(ST 36); for inability to raise the eyebrow, add Cuanzhu(BL 2) and Yuyao(EX-HN 4); for mastoid pain, add Yifeng(TE 17); for deviated mentolabial groove, add Shuigou(GV 26) and Chengjiang (CV 24); for flattened nasola bial groove, add Yingxiang(LI 20).

配穴:风寒证加风池;风热证加曲池。恢复期加足三里。抬眉困难加攒竹、鱼腰;乳突部疼痛加翳风;颏唇沟歪斜加水沟、承浆;鼻唇沟变浅加迎香。

Explanation: Yangbai(GB 14), Sibai(ST 2), Taiyang(EX-HN 5), Jiache(ST 6) and Dicang(ST 4) are on the face and act to free qi and blood, regulate tendons and unblock collaterals. Hegu(LI 4) and Taichong(LR 3) are distal to the face, and are applied with reducing techniques to disperse wind and unblock collaterals in the acute stage. Zusanli (ST 36) is needled with reinforcing techniques in the convalescent stage to supplement qi and blood.

方义:阳白、四白、太阳、颊车、地仓等面部腧穴可疏调局部筋脉气血,活血通络。合谷、太冲为循经远端选穴,急性期用泻法可祛风通络。在恢复期,加足三里用补法,可补益气血。

3.2 Other therapies

3.2 其他治疗

Dermal needle therapy: Tap Yangbai(GB 14), Quanliao(SI 18), Dicang(ST 4) and Jiache(ST 6) with plum-blossom needle until the regional area is flushed. The treatment is prescribed every day or once every other day. This method is suitable for facial paralysis in the convalescent stage.

皮肤针:用梅花针叩刺阳白、颧髎、地仓、颊车,以局部潮红为度,每日或隔日1次,适用于恢复期。

Bloodletting and cupping: Prick Yangbai (GB 14), Quanliao(SI 18), Dicang(ST 4) and Jiache(ST 6) with a three-edged needle, and then place cups on these acupoints for bloodletting. This method is given twice a week and indicated for facial paralysis in the convalescent stage or for longstanding cases.

刺络拔罐:用三棱针点刺阳白、颧髎、地仓、颊车,拔罐,每周2次,适用于恢复期或顽固性面瘫。

4 Remarks

4 按语

Acupuncture is the first choice for the treatment of peripheral facial paralysis and usually has

针灸治疗周围性面瘫为首选方法,具有很好的临床

excellent therapeutic outcomes. In the acute stage, fewer acupoints and gentle manipulations are advisable. For the syndrome of wind cold, moxibustion is conducted to obtain better results, and electroacupuncture is contraindicated. In some longstanding cases, there may display facial spasm due to muscular atrophy, deviation of the mouth to the affected side, even facial convulsion, which is known as inverse phenomena.

疗效。早期取穴宜少，手法宜轻；风寒证加灸效果更好，不宜使用电针。部分患者病程迁延日久，可因瘫痪肌肉出现挛缩，口角反牵向患侧，甚则出现面肌痉挛，形成“倒错”现象。

The prognosis of peripheral facial paralysis is closely related to the injury severity of the facial nerves. Generally speaking, facial paralysis caused by aseptic inflammation has a favorable prognosis, while that caused by viruses such as Hunter's facial palsy has a poor prognosis. If the paralysis has not recovered within 3 to 6 months, sequelae may be left in most situations.

周围性面瘫的预后与面神经的损伤程度密切相关，一般而言，由无菌性炎症导致的面瘫预后较好，而由病毒导致的面瘫（如亨特面瘫）预后较差，如果 3～6 个月内不能恢复，多留有后遗症。

During the treatment period, face masks and eye covers are to be used to prevent the face from the attack of wind and cold.

治疗期间面部应避免吹风受寒，可戴口罩、眼罩防护。

Facial Pain

面　痛

Facial pain is a disease primarily manifested by radiating, scorching and spastic pain in the eyes and cheeks. It often happens in one side of the face and in people at the ages of 40 to 60, most frequently in women. It is often seen in trigeminal neuralgia in Western medicine.

面痛是以眼、面颊部出现放射性、烧灼样抽掣疼痛为主症的疾病，又称“面风痛”“面颊痛”。多发于一侧，发病年龄以 40～60 岁多见，女性为主。本病见于西医学三叉神经痛。

1　Etiology and pathogenesis

1　病因病机

Facial pain usually results from exogenous pathogens and obstruction of qi and blood in the meridians, or from upward invasion of stagnant

本病主要由外感邪气，经络气血痹阻不通；或情志不调，郁热上冲；或阴虚阳

heat due to emotional disturbance, or from yang hyperactivity and rising fire due to yin deficiency. Trauma and blood stasis in long-term diseases can also cause facial pain.

亢，虚火上炎所致；或外伤、久病成瘀入络，而致面痛。

2 Syndrome differentiation

2 辨证

Chief symptoms: Sudden onset of severe facial pain, like sparkling, cutting, pricking or scorching, and facial convulsions. It may be accompanied by flushed complexion, lacrimation, and salivation, often evoked by speaking, swallowing, brushing teeth, washing face, cold stimulation, or emotional upset. The pain lasts for only several seconds or minutes. The frequency and times of its onset are not fixed; however, no symptom will present between attacks.

主症：面部疼痛突然发作，呈闪电样、刀割样、针刺样、电灼样剧烈疼痛，痛时面部肌肉抽搐，伴面部潮红、流泪、流涎、流涕等，常因说话、吞咽、刷牙、洗脸、冷刺激、情绪变化等诱发。持续数秒到数分钟，发作次数不定，间歇期无症状。

The syndrome of wind cold may be accompanied by a history of wind-cold contraction, aggravation by coldness and relief by warmth, presence of clear nasal discharge, whitish tongue coating, and floating tight pulse. The syndrome of wind heat may be accompanied by burning sensation in the painful areas, salivation, red eyes and lacrimation, thin yellowish coating and rapid pulse. The syndrome of stagnant heat in liver and stomach may be accompanied by agitation, irritability, thirstiness, constipation, red tongue with yellowish coating, and rapid pulse. The syndrome of yang hyperactivity due to yin deficiency may be accompanied by emaciation, and thready, rapid and feeble pulse. The syndrome of qi stagnation and blood stasis may be accompanied, usually with a history of trauma or in longstanding disorders, by a fixed pain, dark tongue with possible ecchymosis, and thready rough pulse.

感受风寒者，兼有感受风寒史，面痛遇寒则甚、得热则轻，鼻流清涕，苔白，脉浮紧；感受风热者，兼有痛处灼热感、流涎、目赤流泪、苔薄黄、脉数；肝胃郁热者，兼烦躁易怒、口渴便秘、舌红苔黄、脉数；阴虚阳亢者，兼形体消瘦、脉细数无力；气血瘀滞者，多兼有外伤史，或病变日久，痛点多固定不移、舌暗或有瘀斑、脉细涩。

According to the distribution courses of meridians, pain around eyes belongs to the disorders of foot-taiyang meridian, while pain in the upper and lower mandibles belongs to the disorders of hand-yangming meridian, foot-yangming meridian and hand-taiyang meridian.

根据经脉的分布，眼部痛主要属足太阳经病证；上颌、下颌部痛，主要属手足阳明和手太阳经病证。

3 Treatment

3 治疗

3.1 Essential treatment

3.1 基本治疗

Principal acupoints: Cuanzhu(BL 2), Sibai(ST 2), Xiaguan(ST 7), Dicang(ST 4), Jiache(ST 6), Hegu(LI 4), and Fengchi(GB 20).

主穴：攒竹，四白，下关，地仓，颊车，合谷，风池。

Supplementary acupoints: In the case of ophthalmic pain, add Sizhukong(TE 23), Yangbai(GB 14) and Yuyao(EX-HN 4); in the case of upper mandible pain, add Quanliao(SI 18) and Yingxiang (LI 20); in the case of lower mandible pain, add Chengjiang(CV 24) and Yifeng(TE 17). In the syndrome of wind cold, add Fengmen(BL 12) and Lieque(LU 7); in the syndrome of wind heat, add Quchi(LI 11) and Chize(LU 5); in the syndrome of stagnant heat in the liver and stomach, add Neiting (ST 44) and Taichong(LR 3); in the syndrome of yang hyperactivity due to yin deficiency, add Taichong(LR 3) and Taixi(KI 3); in the syndrome of qi stagnation and blood stasis, add Sanyinjiao(SP 6) and Geshu(BL 17).

配穴：眼部痛者，加丝竹空、阳白、鱼腰；上颌部痛者，加颧髎、迎香；下颌部痛者加承浆、翳风；风寒证者，加风门、列缺；风热证者，加曲池、尺泽；肝胃郁热者加内庭、太冲；阴虚阳亢者加太冲、太溪；气血瘀滞者加三阴交、膈俞。

Explanation: Cuanzhu(BL 2), Sibai(ST 2), Xiaguan(ST 7), Dicang(ST 4) and Jiache(ST 6) are selected to unblock the collaterals on the face. Hegu (LI 4), the Yuan-Source acupoint of the hand-yangming meridian, in combination with Taichong(LR 3) acts to disperse wind and unblock collaterals, relieve pain and muscular spasms. Fengchi(GB 20) is good at dispersing wind, unblocking collaterals and

方义：攒竹、四白、下关、地仓、颊车，疏通面部经络。合谷为手阳明经原穴，与太冲相配可祛风通络、止痛定痉；风池擅长祛风通络止痛。

relieving pain.

3.2 Other therapies

Ear acupuncture: Subcortex(AT 4), Cheek(LO 5,6i), Jaw(LO 3), Forehead(AT 1), and Shenmen (TF 4) are selected. Filiform needle acupuncture, needle-embedding or pressure with *Semen Vaccariae* (Wang Bu Liu Xing) may be applied at these acupoints.

Bloodletting and cupping: Prick Jiache (ST 6), Dicang(ST 4) and Quanliao(SI 18) with a three-edged needle, and then conduct cupping method on these acupoints to let blood. The treatment is given once every other day.

Intradermal needle therapy: Find the trigger points on the face, insert needles into them, and then fix them with plaster. The intradermal needles are embedded for 2 to 3 days and alternate with other needles.

4 Remarks

Trigeminal neuralgia is a persistent intractable disease. Acupuncture has definite analgesic effect, especially for primary trigeminal neuralgia. For secondary trigeminal neuralgia, it is advisable to find causative factors and treat the primary diseases.

3.2 其他治疗

耳针：选皮质下、面颊、颌、额、神门。毫针刺法，或用埋针法，或用王不留行压丸法。

刺络拔罐：选颊车、地仓、颧髎，用三棱针点刺，行闪罐法，隔日 1 次。

皮内针：在面部寻找扳机点，将揿针刺入，外以胶布固定，埋藏 2～3 日，更换揿针。

4 按语

三叉神经痛是一种顽固难治病证，针刺治疗有一定的止痛效果，对原发性三叉神经痛治疗效果较好，对继发性要查明原因，针对病因治疗。

Common Cold

Common cold, also called "Wind Contraction", is one of the frequent exogenous diseases caused by the invasion of wind. It is clinically characterized by nasal stuffiness, cough, chills and fever, and general discomforts. It may occur around the year, especially in the spring. The upper respiratory infection in Western medicine falls into the category

感　冒

感冒，又称"伤风"，是风邪侵袭人体所致的常见外感疾病。临床表现以鼻塞、咳嗽、恶寒发热、全身不适为特征。全年均可发病，尤以春季多见。西医学的上呼吸道感染属于中医学"感冒"范

of common cold in Chinese medicine.

畴。

1 Etiology and pathogenesis

Common cold principally results from the invasion of pathogenic factors when the body constitution is weak and body resistance decreases, giving rise to nasal stuffiness, cough, headache, chills and fever. When pathogenic wind cold attacks the body surface, the lungs fail to disperse and skin pores are obstructed; when pathogenic wind heat scorches the lung, the lung fails to depurate and descend, and the striae fails to discharge. The common cold is usually caused by pathogenic wind, probably mingled with dampness and summer-heat.

1 病因病机

主要由于体虚,机体卫外不固,邪气乘虚侵袭人体,引起鼻塞、咳嗽、头痛、恶寒发热等一系列肺卫症状。风寒束表,则肺气不宣、毛窍闭塞;风热灼肺,则肺失清肃、腠理疏泄。感冒以风邪多见,也常夹湿、夹暑等。

2 Syndrome differentiation

Chief symptoms: Chills and fever, headache, nasal stuffiness, nasal discharge, and floating pulse.

The syndrome of wind cold manifests severe chills, mild fever, absence of sweating, nasal stuffiness, thin snivel, cough, thin whitish coating, and floating tight pulse. The syndrome of wind heat manifests mild chills, severe fever, sweating, sore throat, thirstiness, thin yellowish coating, and floating rapid pulse. The syndrome of summer-heat and dampness manifests dull fever, difficulty in sweating, headache as if wrapped, chest fullness, poor appetite, whitish greasy coating and soggy pulse.

2 辨证

主症:恶寒发热,头痛,鼻塞流涕,脉浮。

感受风寒者,恶寒重、发热轻;无汗,鼻塞流清涕,咳嗽,苔薄白,脉浮紧;感受风热者,微恶风寒、发热重,有汗,咽喉肿痛,口渴,苔薄黄,脉浮数;感受暑湿者,身热不扬,汗出不畅,头痛如裹,胸闷纳呆,苔白腻,脉濡。

3 Treatment

3.1 Essential treatment

Principal acupoints: Lieque(LU 7), Hegu(LI 4), Dazhui(GV 14), and Fengchi(GB 20).

Supplementary acupoints: In the syndrome of wind cold, add Fengmen(BL 12) and Feishu(BL 13); in the syndrome of wind heat, add Quchi(LI 11). In the case of dampness, add Yinlingquan(SP

3 治疗

3.1 基本治疗

主穴:列缺,合谷,大椎,风池。

配穴:风寒感冒者,加风门、肺俞;风热感冒者,加曲池;夹湿者,加阴陵泉;夹暑者,加委中;体虚感冒者,加

9); in the case of summer-heat, add Weizhong(BL 40); in the case of weak constitution, add Zusanli (ST 36), in the case of nasal stuffiness, add Yingxiang(LI 20); in the case of headache, add Taiyang (EX-HN 5); in the case of sore throat, add Shaoshang(LU 11); in the case of general aching, add Shenzhu(GV 12).

足三里。鼻塞者,加迎香;头痛加太阳;咽喉疼痛者,加少商;全身酸楚者,加身柱。

Explanation: Common cold is caused by invasion of pathogenic factors into the lung and defensive qi. Lieque(LU 7), an acupoint of hand-taiyin meridian, and Hegu(LI 4), an acupoint of hand-yangming meridian, are selected to disperse pathogens and relieve exterior conditions. The governor vessel dominates yang qi of the entire body, so moxibustion is conducted on Dazhui(GV 14) to warm yang and disperse coldness, or bloodletting is performed at Dazhui(GV 14) to clear heat. Fengchi (GB 20) is selected to disperse coldness, brighten eyes and clear head.

方义: 感冒为外邪侵犯肺卫所致,故取手太阴经列缺、手阳明经合谷以祛邪解表。督脉主一身之阳气,灸大椎可通阳散寒,刺络出血可清泻热邪。取风池疏散风邪,清利头目。

3.2 Other therapy

3.2 其他治疗

Cupping: Select Dazhui(GV 14), Shenzhu(GV 12) and Feishu(BL 13), and perform cupping method on these acupoints for 10 minutes.

拔罐: 选大椎、身柱、肺俞,拔罐后留罐10分钟。

4 Remarks

4 按语

Acupuncture is effective for common cold. The common cold should be identified from the early symptoms of some infectious diseases.

针灸治疗感冒有一定的疗效,感冒应与某些传染病早期症状加以鉴别。

During the epidemic seasons of common cold, it is advisable to perform acupuncture on Zusanli(ST 36) to prevent from common cold.

在感冒流行季节,可针灸足三里等穴,有预防作用。

During treatment, patients are asked to take adequate rest, eat light food, and drink more water.

治疗期间应保证充足的休息,进食清淡食物,多饮开水。

Cough

Cough is the chief symptom of disorders of the respiratory system. According to its causative factors, cough can be classified into two categories: exogenous cough and endogenous cough. Exogenous cough results from invasion of external factors, and exogenous cough from a dysfunctions of zang-fu organs. In Western medicine, cough is frequently seen in upper respiratory tract infection, acute and chronic bronchitis, pneumonia and pulmonary tuberculosis.

1 Etiology and pathogenesis

Exogenous cough is caused by invasion of external wind-cold or wind-heat into the lung and defensive qi, resulting in the failure of the lung to disperse and depurate. Endogenous cough is caused by dysfunctions of zang-fu organs, such as the lung, spleen, liver and kidney.

2 Syndrome differentiation

2.1 Exogenous cough

Chief symptoms: Coughing with a short duration, accompanied by symptoms of exterior conditions.

The syndrome of exogenous wind cold manifests forceful cough, expectoration of thin white sputum, nasal stuffiness, snivel, chills and fever, aching limbs, thin whitish coating, and floating tight pulse. The syndrome of exogenous wind heat manifests cough with short breath, expectoration of sticky and yellow sputum, sore throat, general fever and sweating, slight aversion to wind, red tongue-tip with thin yellowish coating, and floating rapid pulse.

咳　嗽

咳嗽是肺系疾病的主要症状。根据发病原因，可分为外感咳嗽和内伤咳嗽两大类，外感咳嗽是由外邪侵袭引起的，内伤咳嗽则为脏腑功能失调所致。咳嗽多见于上呼吸道感染、急慢性支气管炎、肺炎、肺结核等病。

1 病因病机

外感咳嗽是外感风寒、风热之邪侵袭肺卫，肺气不宣，清肃失常，而致咳嗽；内伤咳嗽则为脏腑功能失调所致，肺、脾、肝、肾诸脏功能失调皆可导致咳嗽。

2 辨证

2.1 外感咳嗽

主症：咳嗽，病程较短，兼有表证。

外感风寒者，咳嗽声重，咯痰稀薄、色白，鼻塞流涕，恶寒发热，肢体酸楚，苔薄白，脉浮紧；外感风热者，咳嗽气粗，咯痰黏稠、色黄，咽痛，身热汗出，微恶风，舌红，苔薄黄，脉浮数。

2.2 Endogenous cough

Chief symptoms: Cough with a long duration, accompanied by symptoms related to zang-fu organs disorders.

The syndrome of phlegm-dampness blocking lungs manifests expectoration of profuse white sputum, stuffiness in the chest and epigastrium, abdominal distension, poor appetite, light-colored tongue with white greasy coating and soggy slippery pulse. The syndrome of liver-fire scorching lungs manifests difficult expectoration of scanty and sticky sputum, hypochondriac pain while coughing, red eyes, bitter taste in the mouth, red tongue tip and margin with dry thin yellow coating, and wiry rapid pulse. The syndrome of lung-yin deficiency manifests dry cough with scanty sputum or bloody sputum, afternoon flush and night sweats, emaciation, lassitude, red tongue with little coating, and thready rapid pulse.

2.2 内伤咳嗽

主症：咳嗽，病程较长，兼脏腑症状。

痰湿阻肺者，兼咳嗽痰多、色白，胸脘痞闷，腹胀纳差，舌淡苔白腻，脉濡滑；肝火灼肺者，兼气逆咳嗽，痰少而黏、不易咯吐，引胁作痛，目赤口苦，舌边尖红，苔薄黄少津，脉弦数；肺阴亏虚者，兼干咳少痰、咳声短，或痰中带血，潮热盗汗，形体消瘦，神疲乏力，舌红少苔，脉细数。

3 Treatment

3.1 Essential treatment

3.1.1 Exogenous cough

Principal points: Lieque(LU 7), Hegu(LI 4) and Feishu(BL 13).

Supplementary points: In the syndrome of externally contracted wind-cold, add Fengmen(BL 12) and Taiyuan(LU 9); in the syndrome of invasion of wind-heat, add Dazhui(GV 14) and Quchi(LI 11); and in the case of sore throat, add Shaoshang(LU 11) with pricking for bloodletting.

Explanation: Lieque(LU 7), the Luo-Connecting acuoint of the lung meridian, is selected to expel external wind and strengthen the lung in dispersing. Hegu(LI 4) and Lieque(LU 7), the combination of

3 治疗

3.1 基本治疗

3.1.1 外感咳嗽

主穴：列缺，合谷，肺俞。

配穴：风寒者，加风门、太渊；风热者，加大椎、曲池；咽喉痛者，加少商点刺放血。

方义：列缺为肺之络穴，祛风解表，使肺气通调，清肃有权；合谷与列缺原络相配，加强宣肺解表的作用；咳嗽

Yuan-Source acupoint and Luo-Connecting acupoint, are used to enhance the dispersing function of the lung. Because coughing is a disorder of the lung, Feishu(BL 13) is selected to regulate the functions of the lung.

病变在肺，取肺俞调理肺脏功能。

3.1.2 Endogenous cough

3.1.2 内伤咳嗽

Principal acupoints: Feishu (BL 13), Taiyuan (LU 9) and Sanyinjiao(SP 6).

主穴：肺俞，太渊，三阴交。

Supplementary acupoints: In the syndrome of phlegm-dampness blocking lungs, add Fenglong(ST 40) and Yinlingquan(SP 9); in the syndrome of liver-fire scorching lungs, add Xingjian(LR 2); in the syndrome of lung-yin deficiency, add Gaohuang(BL 43); and in the case of bloody cough, add Kongzui (LU 6).

配穴：痰湿蕴肺者，加丰隆、阴陵泉；肝火灼肺者，加行间；肺阴亏虚者，加膏肓；咯血者，加孔最。

Explanation: In endogenous cough, lung-yin is consumed, so Taiyuan (LU 9), the Yuan-Source acupoint of the lung meridian, and Feishu(BL 13), the Back-Shu acupoint of the lung, are selected to regulate lung-qi; Sanyinjiao(SP 6) is used to soothe liver and invigorate spleen, resolve phlegm and stop coughing.

方义：内伤咳嗽，肺阴耗伤，取肺经原穴太渊、背俞穴肺俞调理肺气，取三阴交疏肝健脾、化痰止咳。

3.2 Other therapy

3.2 其他治疗

External acupoint-application: Select Feishu(BL 13), Dingchuan(EX-B 1) and Fengmen(BL 12). Herbal paste may be prepared by using equal amounts of *Sinapis Semen Albae* (Bai Jie Zi), *Kansui Radix* (Gan Sui), *Asari Radix et Rhizoma* (Xi Xin), *Flos Caryophylli* (Ding xiang), *Atracylodis Rhizoma* (Cang zhu), and *Chuanxiong Rhizoma* (Chuan xiong). After grinding the herbs into powder and adding the groundmass to make herbal cakes. The herbal cakes are applied on above acupoints. It is advisable to adopt this method during

穴位贴敷：选肺俞、定喘、风门，用白芥子、甘遂、细辛、丁香、苍术、川芎等量，研成细粉，调成糊状，制成药饼，贴在穴位上。运用此法尤以三伏天为佳。

the Three Periods of Dog Days in the summer.

4 Remarks

Cough is frequently seen in many respiratory diseases, and acupuncture is effective in relieving cough. In clinical practice, clear diagnosis entails the use of medications if necessary.

4 按语

咳嗽见于多种呼吸系统疾病。针灸缓解咳嗽有一定疗效，临证必须明确诊断，必要时配合药物治疗。

Asthma

Asthma is a common disease marked by recurrent attacks of paroxysmal shortness of breath, wheezing in the throat, even with the mouth opened and shoulders raised, and inability to lie horizontally. Asthma can attack year-round, especially during cold seasons or drastic climate alternation. In Western medicine, it can be seen in bronchial asthma, chronic asthmatic bronchitis, emphysema and cardiac asthma.

哮 喘

哮喘是指突然发作的以呼吸急促，喉间哮鸣，甚则张口抬肩、不能平卧为主症的一种常见反复发作性疾患。本病一年四季均可发病，以寒冷季节和天气急剧变化时发病较多。哮喘多见于西医学支气管哮喘、慢性喘息性支气管炎、肺气肿、心源性哮喘等。

1 Etiology and pathogenesis

The basic cause of the disease is the internal retention of phlegm-fluid. Preference for fatty and sweet food may cause dysfunction of the spleen in transformation and transportation, resulting in retention of dampness and phlegm, which may block the air passages and thus induce asthma. In children, the asthma attacks are usually triggered by invasion of exogenous factors. In adults, its onset is triggered by evoking the latent phlegm in the lungs in the case of long-term illnesses and zang-fu organ dysfunction. In acute stage, asthma usually results from qi obstruction and phlegm accumulation, mani festing as an excess syndrome; in the remission stage, it results from lung-kidney deficiency due to its repeated onset.

1 病因病机

本病的基本病因为痰饮内伏。偏嗜肥甘厚味，致脾失健运，聚湿生痰，痰饮阻塞气道，发为痰鸣哮喘。小儿每因外感而发；成年者多由久病内伤，引动肺内伏痰而发病。发作期气阻痰壅，多为实证；缓解期由于反复发作，多见肺肾亏虚。

2 Syndrome differentiation

2.1 Excess syndrome

Chief symptoms: Asthma with harsh and deep breathing, preference for exhaling, forceful pulse, short duration, or in the acute stage.

The syndrome of wind cold manifests coughing and panting, chills, absence of sweating, headache, absence of thirst, thin white tongue coating and floating tight pulse. The syndrome of phlegm-heat obstructing the lung may manifest coughing and panting, chest fullness, or body feverishness, thirst, red tongue with yellowish greasy coating, and slippery rapid pulse.

2.2 Deficiency syndrome

Chief symptoms: Asthma with weak voice, dyspnea, weak constitution, feeble pulse, long duration and recurrent onset, or in the remission stage.

The syndrome of lung-qi deficiency manifests shortness of breath aggravated by exertion, sputum wheezing in the throat, fatigue, after-exercise sweating, light-colored tongue with thin whitish coating, and thready rapid pulse. The syndrome of kidney-qi deficiency manifests breathlessness with more exhalation and less inhalation, discontinuous breathing, after-exercise panting, weak and aching loin and knees, pale tongue with thin whitish coating, and deep thready pulse.

3 Treatment

3.1 Essential treatment

3.1.1 Excess syndrome

Principal acupoints: Lieque(LU 7), Chize(LU 5), Danzhong(CV 17), Feishu(BL 13), Dingchuan

2 辨证

2.1 实证

主症：哮喘声高气粗，呼吸深长，呼出为快，脉象有力，病程短，或当哮喘发作期。

风寒外袭者，兼咳嗽喘息、形寒无汗、头痛、口不渴、苔白薄、脉浮紧；痰热阻肺者，兼咳喘、胸中烦闷，或见身热口渴，舌红苔黄腻、脉滑数。

2.2 虚证

主症：哮喘声低气怯，气息短促，体质虚弱，脉弱无力，病程长，反复发作或当哮喘间歇期。

肺气虚者，兼喘促气短、动则加剧，喉中痰鸣，神疲乏力，动则汗出，舌淡苔白，脉细数；肾气虚者，呼多吸少、不得接续，动则喘甚，腰膝酸软，舌淡苔薄白，脉沉细。

3 治疗

3.1 基本治疗

3.1.1 实证

主穴：列缺，尺泽，膻中，肺俞，定喘。

(EX-B 1).

Supplementary acupoints: In the syndrome of wind cold, add Fengmen(BL 12); in the syndrome of wind heat, add Dazhui(GV 14) and Quchi(LI 11); in the syndrome of phlegm heat, add Fenglong (ST 40); in the case of severe dyspnea, add Tiantu (CV 22).

配穴：风寒者，加风门；风热者，加大椎、曲池；痰热者，加丰隆；喘甚者，加天突。

Explanation: Lieque (LU 7), an acupoint of hand-taiyin meridian, is selected to disperse lung-qi and dispel pathogenic factors. Chize(LU 5), the He-Sea acupoint of hand-taiyin meridian, is used to descend lung-qi adversity, resolve phlegm and suppress asthma. Danzhong(CV 17) is used to release chest and regulate qi movement. Feishu(BL 13), the Back-Shu acupoint of the lung, is selected to disperse lung and remove phlegm. Dingchuan(EX-B 1) is an empiric and effective acupoint against asthma.

方义：手太阴经列缺宣通肺气，祛邪外出。其合穴尺泽，肃肺化痰、降逆平喘。膻中可宽胸理气。取肺之背俞穴，以宣肺祛痰。定喘为平喘之经验效穴。

3.1.2 Deficiency syndrome

3.1.2 虚证

Principal acupoints: Feishu(BL 13), Gaohuangshu(BL 43), Shenshu(BL 23), Dingchuan(EX-B 1), Taiyuan(LU 9), Taixi(KI 3), Zusanli(ST 36).

主穴：肺俞，膏肓俞，肾俞，定喘，太渊，太溪，足三里。

Supplementary acupoints: In the syndrome of lung-qi deficiency, add Chize(LU 5) and Qihai(CV 6). In the syndrome of kidney-qi deficiency, add Yingu(KI 10) and Guanyuan(CV 4).

配穴：肺气虚者，加尺泽、气海；肾气虚者，加阴谷、关元。

Explanation: Acupuncture and moxibustion on Feishu(BL 13) and Gaohuangshu(BL 43) can supplement lung-qi and enrich lung-yin. Shenshu(BL 23) can stem the reception of kidney-qi. Combined use of Taiyuan(LU 9) and Taixi(KI 3), the Yuan-Source acupoints of lung meridian and kidney meridian, can supplement the lung-qi and kidney-qi. Zusanli(ST 36) can regulate the spleen and stomach, nourish the spleen to enrich the lung, as a re-

方义：肺俞、膏肓俞针灸并用，可补肺气、滋肺阴。肾俞以纳肾气。肺经原穴太渊配肾经原穴太溪，可补肺肾之气。足三里调脾胃、培土生金，以资肺气。定喘为平喘之经验效穴。

sult to produce lung-qi. Dingchuan(EX-B 1) is an empiric and effective acupoint against asthma.

3. 2 Other therapy

Application at acupoints: Select Feishu(BL 13), Gaohuangshu(BL 43) and Dingchuan(EX-B 1). Grind *Sinapis Semen Albae* (Bai Jie Zi, 30 g), *Kansui Radix* (Gan Sui, 15 g), and *Asari Radix et Rhizoma* (Xi Xin, 15 g) into powder, and mix the herbal powder with ginger juice into pastes, and shape them into small cakes. Then, apply the cakes on the above acupoints for 2～3 hours till the local skin turns flushed and slightly painful. In the case of local blistering, sterilize and prick the blisters, and then apply gentian violet on the affected areas.

3. 2 其他治疗

穴位贴敷：选肺俞、膏肓俞、定喘。常用白芥子 30 克，甘遂 15 克，细辛 15 克共为细末，用生姜汁调药粉成糊状，制成药饼敷于穴位上，贴 2～3 小时，以局部可有红晕微痛为度。若起泡，消毒后挑破，涂龙胆紫。

4 Remarks

Acupuncture can remarkably reduce the onset frequency of asthma in the remission stage. Treatment during the Three Periods of Dog Days in the summer has good preventive effects. For severe asthma or status asthmaticus, medications are recommended.

Asthma may be seen in many diseases. After relieving asthmatic paroxysm, the primary diseases should be treated accordingly. For cardiac asthma, acupuncture may be used as an adjunct therapy. Patients are asked to keep warm in the seasonal alternation and climate change. For those with allergic constitutions, it is advisable for them to stay away from allergens.

4 按语

针灸可明显减轻缓解期患者发作次数。在夏季三伏天治疗有很好的预防作用。对发作严重或哮喘持续状态，应配合药物治疗。

哮喘可见于多种疾病，发作缓解后，应积极治疗其原发病。对心源性哮喘，针刺只作辅助治疗。季节交替，气候变化时应注意保暖。属过敏体质者，注意避免接触致敏源。

Palpitation

Palpitation refers to an unduly rapid action of the heart which is felt by the patient and accompa-

心　悸

心悸是指患者自觉心中悸动、惊慌不安，甚则不能自

nied by nervousness and restlessness uncontrollable. It may be seen in some organic or functional diseases, such as coronary heart disease, hypertensive heart disease, arrhythmias, anemia, and cardiac neurosis.

主的一种病证。本病可见于某些器质性或功能性疾病，如冠心病、高血压性心脏病、心律失常，以及贫血、心脏神经官能症等病。

1 Etiology and pathogenesis

Palpitation often results from weak constitution, emotional disturbance and exertion, in which the heart is deprived of nourishment; or from the disturbance of the heart-spirit by pathogenic factors, followed by undue heartbeat.

1 病因病机

本证的发生常因久病体虚、情志所伤、劳倦等，使心失所养；或邪扰心神，致悸动不安，而发为本病。

2 Syndrome differentiation

Chief symptoms: Paroxysmal subjective feeling of an uncertain heartbeat, accompanied by terror, fright and restlessness, which are sometimes uncontrollable.

The syndrome of heart-gallbladder deficiency manifests palpitation induced by fright, accompanied by fatigue, light-colored tongue with thin coating, and wiry thready pulse. The syndrome of heart-spleen deficiency may be accompanied by dizziness and vertigo, poor appetite, lusterless complexion, pale tongue with thin whitish coating, and thready weak pulse. The syndrome of hyperactive fire due to yin deficiency may be accompanied by restlessness, insomnia, tinnitus and aching loin, dry mouth, red tongue with less coating, and thready rapid pulse. The syndrome of heart-vessel obstruction may be accompanied by chest oppression and paroxysmal heart pain, dark purple tongue with possible ecchymosis, and thready rough or irregular pulse. The syndrome of water-qi invading heart may be accompanied by chest oppression nad panting, inability to lie down, expectoration of profuse

2 辨证

主症：自觉心跳心慌，时作时止，常有善惊易恐、坐卧不安，甚则不能自主。

心虚胆怯者，常因惊恐而发，兼神疲乏力、舌淡苔薄，脉弦细；心脾两虚者，兼头晕目眩、纳差乏力、面色淡、舌淡苔白、脉细弱；阴虚火旺者，兼心烦少寐、耳鸣腰酸、口干、舌红少苔、脉细数；心脉瘀阻者，兼胸闷心痛阵发、舌紫暗或有瘀斑、脉细涩或结代；水气凌心者，兼胸闷气喘、不能平卧、咯吐泡沫痰涎、形寒肢冷、舌淡苔白滑、脉滑数。

frothy sputum, coldness in the body and limbs, pale tongue with whitish greasy coating, and slippery rapid pulse.

3 Treatment

3.1 Essential treatment

Principal acupoints: Neiguan(PC 6), Ximen(PC 4), Shenmen(HT 7), Xinshu(BL 15), Juque(CV 14).

Supplementary acupoints: In the syndrome of heart-gallbladder deficiency, add Danshu(BL 19) and Tongli(HT 5); in the syndrome of heart-spleen deficiency, add Pishu(BL 20) and Zusanli(ST 36); in the syndrome of hyperactive fire due to yin deficiency, add Shenshu(BL 23) and Taixi(KI 3); in the syndrome of heart-vessel obstruction, add Danzhong(CV 17) and Geshu(BL 17); in the syndrome of water-qi invading heart, add Shenque(CV 8) and Qihai(CV 6). In the case of susceptibility to fright, add Daling(PC 7); in the case of edema, add Shuifen(CV 9).

Explanation: Neiguan (PC 6) and Ximen(PC 4), the Luo-Connecting acupoint and Xi-Cleft acupoint of the pericardium meridian, are selected to regulate heart qi and move qi and blood. Shenmen (HT 7), the Yuan-Source acupoint of the heart meridian, is used to tranquilize the heart and subside palpitations. Combined use of Xinshu(BL 15) and Juque(CV 14), the Back-Shu acupoint and Front-Mu acupoint of the heart, are used to regulate qi activity in the heart. Combined use of these acupoints functions to suppress fright and calm spirit.

3.2 Other therapy

Ear acupuncture: Select Sympathesis(AH 6a), Shenmen(TF 4), Heart(CO 15), Spleen(CO 13), and Kidney(CO 10). Puncture these acupoints by

3 治疗

3.1 基本治疗

主穴: 内关,郄门,神门,心俞,巨阙。

配穴: 心虚胆怯者,加胆俞、通里;心脾两虚者,加脾俞、足三里;阴虚火旺者,加肾俞、太溪;心脉瘀阻者,加膻中、膈俞;水气凌心者,加神阙、气海。善惊者,加大陵;浮肿者,加水分。

方义: 心包经络穴内关、郄穴郄门可调理心气、疏导气血。心经原穴神门,宁心安神定悸。心之背俞穴心俞,配心之募穴巨阙,可调理心脏气机。诸穴配合以镇惊安神。

3.2 其他治疗

耳针: 选交感、神门、心、脾、肾,用毫针轻刺激。亦可用揿针埋藏或用王不留行

mild stimulation. Needle embedding or ear-pressure with *Semen Vaccariae*(Wang Bu Liu Xing) is applicable as well.

贴压。

4 Remarks

During the therapeutic period, patients should well regulate the minds and prevent from unfavorable emotional stimulation. The underlying primary diseases of palpitation should be actively treated.

4 按语

治疗过程中，要调节情志，防止不良情绪对心脏的影响。对可能引起心悸的原发性疾病积极治疗。

Insomnia

Insomnia, also known as sleeplessness, refers to the inability to have normal sleep, including difficulty in falling asleep, inadequate sleep, difficulty in staying asleep, or even inability to sleep all night in severe cases. It may be often seen in neurasthenia in Western medicine.

不 寐

不寐又称"失眠""不得卧"等，是以经常不能获得正常睡眠，或入睡困难，或睡眠时间不足，或睡眠不深，严重者彻夜不眠为特征的病证。本病可见于西医学神经衰弱等病。

1 Etiology and pathogenesis

Insomnia is related to emotional disturbance, improper diet, over-exertion and weak constitution. Over-thinking, anxiety and over-stress will impair the heart and spleen, causing inadequate production of qi and blood, followed by malnourishment of the heart-spirit. Fear, terror or sexual indulgence may impair the kidney, causing in-coordination between the heart and kidney, and disquieted heart spirit. Weak constitution, heart-gallbladder deficiency, improper diet followed by disharmony of the spleen and stomach may cause insomnia.

1 病因病机

本证与情志、饮食、劳倦、体虚等因素相关。思虑劳倦，损伤心脾，心神失养；或因惊恐、房劳伤肾，心肾不交，神志不宁；或因体质素弱，心虚胆怯，或饮食不节，脾胃不和均可导致失眠。

2 Syndrome differentiation

Chief symptoms: Difficulty in falling asleep or intermittent waking through the period of attempted sleep, and even inability to sleep all night.

2 辨证

主症：经常不易入睡，或寐而易醒，甚则彻夜不眠。

The syndrome of heart-spleen deficiency manifests palpitation, forgetfulness, dizziness and vertigo, lusterless complexion, fatigue, poor appetite, pale tongue with whitish coating, and thready weak pulse. The syndrome of heart-gallbladder qi-deficiency manifests susceptibility to fear and fright, pale tongue with whitish coating, and wiry thready pulse. The syndrome of in-coordination between the heart and kidney manifests restlessness, irritability, distension and fullness in the chest and flank, dizziness, tinnitus, seminal emission, night sweats, dry mouth, red tongue and thready rapid pulse. The syndrome of liver-yang hyperactivity manifests restlessness, irritability, distension and fullness in the chest and flank, red tongue with yellowish coating, and wiry rapid pulse. The syndrome of spleen-stomach disharmony manifests gastric fullness, belching with foul eructation and acid regurgitation, red tongue with thick greasy coating, and slippery rapid pulse.

心脾亏虚者，心悸健忘，头晕目眩，面色无华，神疲乏力，纳差，舌淡苔白，脉细弱；心胆气虚者，善惊多恐，舌淡苔白，脉弦细；心肾不交者，心烦不寐，头晕耳鸣，遗精盗汗，口干舌红，脉细数。肝阳上扰者，兼见心烦、急躁易怒、胸胁胀满、舌红苔黄、脉弦数；脾胃不和者，兼见脘闷噫气、嗳腐吞酸、舌红苔厚腻、脉滑数。

3 Treatment

3.1 Essential treatment

Principal acupoints: Shenmen(HT 7), Neiguan (PC 6), Sishencong(EX-HN 1), Zhaohai(KI 6), Shenmai(BL 62) and Anmian(EX).

Supplementary acupoints: In the syndrome of heart-spleen deficiency, add Xinshu(BL 15) and Pishu(BL 20); in the syndrome of heart-gallbladder qi-deficiency, add Xinshu(BL 15) and Danshu(BL 19); in the syndrome of in-coordination between the heart and kidney, add Taixi(KI 3) and Xinshu (BL 15); in the syndrome of liver-fire disturbing heart, add Xingjian(LR 2) and Xiaxi(GB 43); in the syndrome of phlegm-fire in the interior, add

3 治疗

3.1 基本治疗

主穴：神门，内关，四神聪，照海，申脉，安眠。

配穴：心脾两虚者，加心俞、脾俞；心胆气虚者加心俞、胆俞；心肾不交者，加太溪、心俞；肝火扰心者，加行间、侠溪；痰热内扰者，加丰隆、内庭；脾胃不和者，加公孙、足三里；神经衰弱者，加足三里、关元；失精者，加关元、志室；梦多者，加魄户、厉

Fenglong(ST 40) and Neiting(ST 44); in the syndrome of disharmony between the spleen and stomach, add Gongsun(SP 4) and Zusanli(ST 36). In the case of neurasthenia, add Zusanli(ST 36) and Guanyuan(CV 4); in the case of seminal emission, add Guanyuan(CV 4) and Zhishi(BL 52); in the case of dreaminess, add Pohu(BL 42) and Lidui(ST 45); in the case of dizziness and forgetfulness, add Yintang(EX-HN 3) and Fengchi(GB 20).

兑;头昏健忘,加印堂、风池。

Explanation: Since the heart houses the mind, Shenmen(HT 7), the Yuan-Source acupoint of the heart meridian, and Neiguan(PC 6), the Luo-Connecting acupoint of the pericardium meri-dian, are selected to calm the heart and tranquilize the mind. The brain is the palace where the mind dwells, so Sishencong(EX-HN 1) and Anmian(EX) are selected to calm down and tranquilize the spirit. Zhaohai(KI 6) and Shenmai(BL 62) are the Confluent acupoints respectively communicating with the yin heel vessel and yang heel vessel; dysfunction of the yang heel vessel will cause insomnia, hence these two acupoints are treated to harmonize the functions of the yin heel vessel and yang heel vessels. Anmian(EX) is an effective and empiric acupoint against insomnia.

方义: 心藏神,首选心经原穴神门、心包经络穴内关宁心安神。脑为元神之府,取四神聪、安眠镇静安神。照海、申脉为八脉交会穴,交通阴阳蹻脉,阳蹻脉功能亢盛则失眠,故补阴泻阳协调蹻脉功能。安眠为治疗失眠的经验效穴。

3.2 Other therapies

3.2 其他治疗

Ear acupuncture: Select Subcortex (AT 4), Heart(CO 15), Kidney(CO 10), Liver(CO 12) and Shenmen(TF 4). Needling, needle-embedding or ear-pressure with *Semen Vaccariae* (Wang Bu Liu Xing) is applicable as well.

耳针: 选皮质下、心、肾、肝、神门。毫针刺,或揿针埋藏,或王不留行贴压。

Cupping: Select the distribution course of the bladder meridian from the neck to the lumbar area. Fire cupping is done from the neck downwards along the course until the skin becomes flushed.

拔罐: 自项至腰部足太阳经背部侧线,用火罐自上而下行走罐,以背部潮红为度。

4 Remarks

Acupuncture is quite effective for insomnia, and excellent results will be achieved if acupuncture is performed in the afternoon or at night. Insomnia is in close association with emotional factors, so it is advisable to help with psychotherapy to release emotional distress. For the cases caused by other diseases, the primary diseases should be treated at the same time.

4 按语

针灸治疗不寐效果良好，尤其是在下午或晚间针灸效果更好。本病与情绪变化有关，要适当配合心理疏导，消除紧张情绪。由其他疾病引起不寐者，应同时治疗其原发病。

Chest Stuffiness

Chest stuffiness refers to the disorder that is chiefly manifested by stuffiness and pain in the chest, even the pain radiating to the back, and shortness of breath. In mild cases, there may only be chest fullness and difficulty in respiration; in severe cases, there may be squeezing pain in the chest, cold limbs and profuse sweating. It is often seen in coronary angina pectoris in Western medicine.

胸　痹

胸痹是指胸部闷痛，甚则胸痛彻背，气短为主的一种病证。轻者仅感胸闷，呼吸不畅；重者胸痛如绞，肢冷汗出。本病多见于西医学冠心病心绞痛等病。

1 Etiology and pathogenesis

The disease is caused by yang inactivity in the chest due to heart-lung qi deficiency in the elderly; or by phlegm-dampness accumulation due to spleen deficiency and invasion of cold pathogens, which then obstruct chest yang and cause chest stuffiness.

1 病因病机

本证多由年老心肺气虚，胸阳不振；或脾虚生湿，湿痰内蕴，寒邪内侵，痹阻胸阳所致。

2 Syndrome differentiation

Chief symptoms: Chest pain, stuffy pain in mild cases and squeezing pain in severe cases.

The syndrome of deficiency cold manifests chest pain radiating to the back, chest fullness, shortness of breath, aversion to cold, cold extremities aggravated by cold, white slippery or greasy

2 辨证

主症：胸部疼痛，轻者胸闷如塞，重者胸痛如绞。

虚寒证者，胸痛彻背，胸闷气短，恶寒肢冷，受寒痛甚，舌苔白滑或腻，脉沉迟；痰浊证者，胸闷而痛，气短喘

tongue coating, and deep slow pulse. The syndrome of phlegm turbidity manifests chest fullness and pain, shortness of breath, coughing with profuse white sticky sputum, white greasy tongue coating and slow pulse. The syndrome of blood stasis manifests stabbing pain in the chest, or paroxysmal colicky pain radiating to the back, purple lips, dark tongue, and thready rough or irregular pulse.

促,咳嗽,痰多黏腻色白,舌苔白腻,脉缓;瘀血证者,胸痛如刺,痛彻肩背,唇紫,舌质暗,脉细涩或结代。

3 Treatment

3 治疗

3.1 Essential treatment

3.1 基本治疗

Principal acupoints: Neiguan (PC 6), Xinshu (BL 15), Juque(CV 14), Danzhong(CV 17) and Ximen(PC 4).

主穴: 内关,心俞,巨阙,膻中,郄门。

Supplementary acupoints: In the case of aversion to cold, add Feishu(BL 13) and Fengmen(BL 12) by moxibustion; in the case of cold limbs, add Qihai (CV 6) or Guanyuan(CV 4) by moxibustion; in the case of phlegm turbidity, add Fenglong(ST 40) to resolve phlegm turbidity; in the case of blood stasis, add Geshu(BL 17) and Sanyinjiao(SP 6) to promote the flow of qi and blood; in the case of back pain, add Xinshu(BL 15); in the case of purple lips and tongue, add Shaochong(HT 9) and Zhongchong(PC 9) for bloodletting.

配穴: 恶寒者加灸肺俞、风门;肢冷者加灸气海或关元;痰浊者配丰隆化痰;瘀血者加膈俞、三阴交行气活血;背痛者加心俞;唇舌紫绀者可取少冲、中冲点刺出血。

Explanation: Neiguan (PC 6) and Ximen (PC 4), the Luo-Connecting acupoint and the Xi-Cleft acupoint of the pericardium meridian, are selected to activate blood and unblock collaterals to ease pain. Xinshu(BL 15) and Juque(CV 14), the Back-Shu acupoint and Front-Mu acupoint of the heart, are selected to regulate heart-qi, activate blood and unblock collaterals. Danzhong(CV 17), the Influential acupoint of qi, is used to free qi activity and relieve pain.

方义: 内关是心包经络穴,配心包经郄穴郄门,以活血通络而止痛。心之背俞穴配合募穴巨阙,可调理心气、活血通络。配气会膻中调畅气机而止痛。

3.2 Other therapy

Ear acupuncture: Select Heart(CO 15), Small Intestine(CO 6), Sympathesis(AH 6a), Subcortex (AT 4) and Chest(MA). Puncture these acupoints with strong stimulation. Each time, 3～5 acupoints are needled, and the needles may be retained for 1 hour.

3.2 其他治疗

耳针：取心、小肠、交感、皮质下、胸等穴，强刺激，每次选 3～5 穴，留针 1 小时。

4 Remarks

Acupuncture is quite effective in the relief of chest stuffiness. Severe chest pain, accompanied by cyanosis and coldness in the extremities, and profuse sweating, is frequently seen in such serious diseases as a cute myocardial infarction, and comprehensive treatment should be prescribed immediately.

4 按语

针灸治疗胸痹在缓解症状方面有较好的疗效。胸痹如心痛剧烈、手足青至节、汗出肢冷，多见于急性心肌梗死等严重疾患，应采取综合治疗。

Manic-depressive Syndrome

Manic-depressive syndrome is a mental disorder. Depressive disorder is marked by silence, reticence, apathy and incoherent speech, and pertains to a yin type; while the manic syndrome is marked by madness, restlessness, even abusing others and damaging objects, and pertains to a yang type. These two types are similar to each other in pathogenesis and may relate to each other, so they are collectively named as manic-depressive syndrome in Chinese medicine. It is mainly seen in young and middle-aged people and its occurrence is related to familial inheritance and usually evoked by violent mental irritations. Manic-depressive syndrome is frequently seen in the manic or depression type of schizophrenia in Western medicine.

癫　狂

癫狂是一种精神失常的病证。沉默静呆、表情淡漠、语无伦次者为癫证，属阴证；狂躁不安，甚则打人毁物者为狂证，属阳证。二者在病因和病机方面有相似之处，故临床上常癫狂并称。本证多见于青壮年，与家族遗传有一定关系，多以强烈的精神刺激为诱因。本病见于西医学狂躁型、抑郁型精神分裂症等。

1 Etiology and pathogenesis

Manic-depressive syndrome is caused by inter-

1 病因病机

本病由情志内伤所致，

nal emotional impairment. Depressive syndrome is due to malnourishment of the heart-spirit, which results from over-thinking and ensuing injury of the heart and spleen. Manic syndrome is caused by fire transformed from liver depression, which then consumes the fluid and produces phlegm-heat; or by upward disturbance of the heart-mind by stomach-fire with phlegm.

癫证多由思虑太过，耗伤心脾，心神失养所致；狂证多由肝郁化火，烁津成痰，痰热互结，或胃火夹痰，上扰心神而发。

2 Syndrome differentiation

2 辨证

2.1 Depressive syndrome

Chief symptoms: Mental depression, apathy, reticence, quietness and inactivity, and murmuring to oneself.

The syndrome of liver-qi depression may be accompanied by fullness in the chest and flank, pale tongue with thin whitish coating, and wiry pulse. The syndrome of phlegm-qi accumulation may be accompanied by lack of personal hygiene, poor appetite, red tongue with whitish greasy coating, and wiry slippery pulse. The syndrome of heart-spleen deficiency may be accompanied by susceptibility to fright, lassitude, poor appetite, and deep thready feeble pulse.

2.1 癫证

主症：精神抑郁，表情淡漠，沉默痴呆，静而少动，喃喃自语。

肝郁气滞者，兼胸胁胀满、舌淡苔薄、脉弦；痰气郁结者，兼秽洁不分、不思饮食、舌红、苔白腻、脉弦滑；心脾两虚者，兼心悸易惊、体倦纳差、脉沉细无力。

2.2 Manic syndrome

Chief symptoms: Agitation, vexation, shouting and cursing others, climbing walls, singing in public, running around, and even beating others.

The syndrome of spiritual disturbance by phlegm-fire may be accompanied by an angry look in the eyes, flushed complexion and red eyes, abnormally forceful physical strength, no appetite, insomnia, purple-red tongue with yellowish greasy coating, and wiry slippery and rapid pulse. The syndrome of yin consumption due to excess fire may be accompanied by the prolonged manic condition and

2.2 狂证

主症：喧闹躁动，叫骂不避亲疏，登高而歌，弃衣而走，甚者持物伤人。

痰火扰神者，兼两目怒视、面红目赤、气力逾常、不食不眠、舌红绛、苔黄腻或黄燥、脉弦大滑数；火盛伤阴者，兼狂病日久、呼之能止、形瘦面红而秽、舌红少苔、脉细数；气血瘀滞者，兼面色暗滞、头痛心悸、舌紫暗有瘀

manifested by talkativeness, emaciation, flushed and turbid complexion, red tongue with less coating, and thready rapid pulse. The syndrome of qi stagnation and blood stasis may be accompanied by dark and turbid complexion, headache and palpitation, dark purplish tongue with ecchymosis, and wiry thready rough pulse.

斑、脉弦涩。

3 Treatment

3.1 Essential treatment

3.1.1 Depressive syndrome

Principal acupoints: Neiguan (PC 6), Shuigou (GV 26), Fenglong(ST 40), Dazhui(GV 14), Taichong (LR 3) and Houxi(SI 3).

Supplementary acupoints: In the syndrome of liver-qi depression, add Xingjian (LR 2) and Danzhong(CV 17); in the syndrome of phlegm-qi accumulation, add Zhongwan(CV 12) and Zhigou (TE 6); in the syndrome of heart-spleen deficiency, add Xinshu(BL 15) and Pishu(BL 20). In the case of sudden crying or laughing, add Jianshi(PC 5) and Baihui(GV 20); in the case of poor appetite, add Zusanli(ST 36) and Gongsun(SP 4).

Explanation: Neiguan(PC 6), the Luo-Connecting acupoint of the pericardium meridian, is selected to regulate qi and move blood, calm the heart and tranquilize the mind. Dazhui(GV 14) and Shuigou(GV 26), two acupoints of the governor vessel that connects with the brain, are applied to awaken the brain. Houxi (SI 3), the Confluent acupoint communicatting with the governor vessel, is selected to tranquilize the mind. Taichong(LR 3) is selected to soothe the liver and regulate qi. Fenglong(ST 40) is used to remove dampness and resolve phlegm. Combined use of the above acupoints can achieve

3 治疗

3.1 基本治疗

3.1.1 癫证

主穴：内关，水沟，丰隆，大椎，太冲，后溪。

配穴：肝郁气滞者，加行间、膻中；痰气郁结者，加中脘、支沟；心脾两虚者，加心俞、脾俞；哭笑无常者，加间使、百会；纳呆者，加足三里、公孙。

方义：内关为心包经络穴，可理气活血、宁心安神。大椎、水沟乃督脉穴，督脉络脑，取之从阳引阴，醒脑开窍。后溪通于督脉，可宁神定志。太冲疏肝理气，丰隆除湿化痰。诸穴共用达理气豁痰、开窍醒神之功。

the effects of regulating qi and dissipating phlegm, awakening mind and arousing spirit.

3.1.2 Manic depression

Principal acupoints: Jiuwei(CV 15), Shangwan (CV 13), Neiguan(PC 6), Daling(PC 7), Shenmen (HT 7) and Zhongchong(PC 9).

Supplementary acupoints: In the syndrome of spiritual disturbance by phlegm-fire, add Neiting (ST 44), Quchi(LI 11) and Fenglong(ST 40); in the syndrome of yin consumption due to excess fire, add Xingjian(LR 2), Taixi(KI 3) and Sanyinjiao (SP 6); in the syndrome of qi stagnation and blood stasis, add Xuehai(SP 10) and Geshu(BL 17).

Explanation: Jiuwei(CV 15) and Shangwan(CV 13), two acupoints of the conception vessel, are selected to treat the disorders of the governor vessel. Neiguan(PC 6), Daling(PC 7), Zhongchong(PC 9) and Shenmen(HT 7) are used to purge the fire of the pericardium and heart meridians to tranquilize mind and calm heart.

3.2 Other therapy

Three-edged needle therapy: About 3 to 5 acupoints of Sun Zhenren's 13 Ghost Points are selected and pricked with three-edged needles to let 1~3 drops of blood. This treatment can be given once every other day.

4 Remarks

Acupuncture has definite effects on manic-depressive syndrome. During the period of treatment, patients must be closely monitored to prevent suicide, beat others and damage objects.

Manic-depressive syndrome is usually of a prolonged duration and recurs easily, especially after emotional irritation. Therefore, continuous treat-

3.1.2 狂证

主穴: 鸠尾,上脘,内关,大陵,神门,中冲。

配穴: 痰火扰神者,加内庭、曲池、丰隆;火盛伤阴者,加行间、太溪、三阴交;气血瘀滞者,加血海、膈俞。

方义: 鸠尾、上脘为任脉穴,以求从阴引阳。内关、大陵、中冲、神门清泻心包经、心经之火而安神宁志。

3.2 其他治疗

三棱针法: 选孙真人十三鬼穴,每次 3~5 个穴位,三棱针点刺出血 1~3 滴,隔日 1 次。

4 按语

针灸治疗本病有一定的疗效,在治疗过程中,要对患者进行严密监护,防止自杀及伤人毁物。

本病病程长,且易反复发作,尤其在精神刺激时更易复发。因此,病情缓解后

ment in remission stage is required to consolidate the therapeutic effects.

应继续巩固治疗。

Epilepsy

Epilepsy, also known as "Yang Xian Feng" in Chinese medicine, is a paroxysmal mental disease marked by sudden, short and repeated attacks, manifested by falling down in a fit, loss of consciousness, foam on the lips, convulsion with eyes turned upwards, or screaming. After some time, consciousness returns and the patient's condition becomes normal. It corresponds to the epileptic seizures in Western medicine.

痫　病

痫病俗称"羊痫风"，是一种发作性神志失常的疾病。本病以突然昏仆、口吐涎沫、两目上视、四肢抽搐、或有鸣声、醒后神志如常人为特征。本病相当于西医学的癫痫。

1　Etiology and pathogenesis

Epilepsy mostly relates to familiar heredity. It is caused by head injury when delivered, emotional disturbance and skull trauma, which may result in qi adversity and orifice obstruction by phlegm-turbidity.

1　病因病机

本病的发生多有家族遗传史，或因孕期生产中胎儿头部受损引起；亦有情志刺激、脑部外伤等，导致机体气机逆乱，痰浊阻窍而发病。

2　Syndrome differentiation

Chief symptoms: A grand mal seizure: Before onset, it may manifest dizziness, headache and chest distress as the precursor symptoms, and is followed by falling down in a fit, loss of consciousness, pallid complexion, upward staring of the eyes, clenched jaws, convulsion, foam on the mouth, even occasional screaming, urinary and fecal incontinence, awaking after a short time; after seizure, it is manifested by mental upset, fatigue and sleepiness. A petit mal seizure: epilepsy is manifested by sudden breakdown and transient loss of consciousness, and consciousness regain after a few seconds or minutes.

2　辨证

主症：大发作者表现为发作前常有头晕头痛、胸闷不舒等预兆，旋即突然昏仆，不省人事，面色苍白，两目上视，牙关紧闭，四肢抽搐，口吐白沫，甚则尖叫，二便失禁，短暂即清醒，发作后则觉精神恍惚，乏力欲寐。小发作者表现为动作突然中断，意识短暂丧失，多在数秒至数分钟即可恢复。

Epilepsy in the remission stage can be differentiated as follows. The syndrome of spirit disturbance by phlegm-fire is accompanied by vexation and irritability, bitter taste in mouth, dry throat, red tongue with yellowish greasy coating, and wiry slippery pulse. The syndrome of wind-phlegm blockage is preceded by dizziness, chest fullness, profuse sputum, red tongue with whitish greasy coating, and forceful wiry and slippery pulse. The syndrome of heart-spleen deficiency is accompanied by listlessness, fatigue, thin body, poor appetite, loose stools, pale tongue with whitish coating, and feeble pulse. The syndrome of liver-kidney yin deficiency is accompanied by dim complexion, dizziness and blurred vision, dry eyes, aching loins and knees, red tongue with less coating, and thready rapid pulse. The syndrome of blood stasis in brain collaterals is usually followed by a stroke or traumatic brain injury.

间歇期可按以下辨证：痰火扰神者，兼急躁易怒、口苦咽干、舌红、苔黄腻、脉弦滑；风痰闭阻者，发病前多有眩晕、胸闷、痰多、舌红、苔白腻、脉弦滑；心脾两虚者，兼神疲乏力、体瘦纳呆、大便溏薄、舌淡苔白、脉弱；肝肾阴虚者，兼面色晦暗、头晕目眩、两目干涩、腰膝酸软、舌红少苔、脉细数；中风或脑外伤后出现痫病者，为瘀阻脑络。

3 Treatment

3.1 Essential treatment

Principal acupoints: Acute stage: Neiguan(PC 6), Dazhui(GV 14), Baihui(GV 20), Houxi(SI 3), and Yaoqi(EX-B8).

Remission stage: Yintang(EX-HN 3), Jiuwei(CV 15), Jianshi(PC 5), Taichong(LR 3), and Fenglong (ST 40).

Supplementary acupoints: In the case of coma, add Shuigou(GV 26), Shixuan(EX-UE 11) and Yongquan(KI 1); for night seizure, add Zhaohai (KI 6); for daytime seizure, add Shenmai(BL 62); in the syndrome of spirit disturbance by phlegm-fire, add Shenmen(HT 7) and Neiting(ST 44); in the syndrome of wind-phlegm blockage, add Hegu

3 治疗

3.1 基本治疗

主穴：发作期：内关，大椎，百会，后溪，腰奇。

间歇期：印堂，鸠尾，间使，太冲，丰隆。

配穴：发作时见昏迷加水沟、十宣、涌泉；夜间发作加照海，白天发作加申脉；痰火扰神者，加神门、内庭；风痰闭阻者，加合谷、阴陵泉、风池；心脾两虚者，加心俞、脾俞、足三里；肝肾阴虚者，

(LI 4), Yinlingquan(SP 9) and Fengchi(GB 20); in the syndrome of the syndrome of heart-spleen deficiency, add Xinshu(BL 15), Pishu(BL 20) and Zusanli(ST 36); in the syndrome of liver-kidney yin deficiency, add Ganshu(BL 18), Shenshu(BL 23), Taixi(KI 3) and Sanyinjiao (SP 6); in the syndrome of blood stasis in brain collaterals, add Geshu(BL 17) and Neiguan(PC 6).

加肝俞、肾俞、太溪、三阴交；瘀阻脑络者，加膈俞、内关。

Explanation: Neiguan(PC 6), the Luo-Connecting acupoint of the pericardium meridian, can regulate the heart-mind. Dazhui (GV 14) and Baihui (GV 20) are the acupoints of the governor vessel; Houxi(SI 3) is the Confluent acupoint that communicates with the governor vessel, which enters and connects with the brain. These three acupoints are needled to arouse brain and induce resuscitation. Yaoqi(EX-B 8) is an empiric acupoint for epilepsy. Yintang(EX-HN 3) functions to regulate the spirit and restore consciousness. Jiuwei(CV 15), the Luo-Connecting acupoint of the conception vessel, can regulate yin and yang. Jianshi(PC 5), the Jing-River acupoint of the pericardium meridian, is applied to calm the heart-spirit, and regulate qi and blood. Taichong(LR 3) is applied to pacify and extinguish liver-wind. Fenglong (ST 40) is used to resolve phlegm-turbidity.

方义：内关为心包经络穴，可调理心神。大椎、百会为督脉穴，后溪通督脉，督脉入络脑，故针刺可醒脑开窍。腰奇是治疗本病的经验穴。印堂可调神开窍。鸠尾为任脉络穴，取之调理阴阳。间使为心包经经穴，可调心神、理气血。太冲平熄肝风。丰隆豁痰化浊。

3.2　Other therapy

Ear acupuncture: Select 2 to 3 acupoints out of Stomach(CO 4), Subcortex(AT 4), Shenmen (TF 4), Heart(CO 15), and Occiput (AT 3). Puncture two or three acupoints each time with filiform needles or apply ear-pressure with *Semen Vaccariae* (Wang Bu Liu Xing) at these acupoints.

3.2　其他治疗

耳针：选胃、皮质下、神门、心、枕。每次选 2～3 穴，毫针针刺，或用王不留行贴压。

4 Remarks

Acupuncture is effective in relieving the symptoms and reducing the onset frequency of epileptic seizures. For the secondary seizures, the primary causes should be ascertained and treatment should be aimed at its primary causes.

If the epileptic seizures persist or are accompanied by severe symptoms such as high fever or coma, a combined treatment should be applied.

4 按语

针灸治疗癫痫能改善症状,减少发作次数。对于继发性癫痫须明确诊断,积极治疗原发病。

对癫痫持续发作,或伴有高热、昏迷等危重症候的患者必须采取综合疗法。

Wasting-Thirsty Syndrome

Wasting-thirsty syndrome(“Xiao Ke” in Chinese) is a disease characterized by excessive drinking, excessive eating, excessive urination, thin body or sweet urine. According to its clinical symptoms, it falls into three types: upper, middle and lower wasting-thirsty syndromes. It is similar to diabetes mellitus in Western medicine.

消 渴

消渴是以多饮、多食、多尿、形体消瘦,或尿有甜味为特征的病证,临床上根据患者的症状不同,分为上、中、下三消。本病相当于西医学的糖尿病。

1 Etiology and pathogenesis

The general pathogenesis of the wasting-thirsty syndrome is yin deficiency and dry heat, which involves the lung, spleen and kidney respectively in the upper, middle and lower wasting-thirsty syndromes.

1 病因病机

本病主要病机是燥热和伤阴,病变涉及肺、脾、肾。上、中、下三消分别累及不同脏腑。

2 Syndrome differentiation

Chief symptoms: Excessive drinking, excessive eating, excessive urination, thin body or sweet urine.

The syndrome of lung heat consuming body fluids, known as upper wasting-thirsty syndrome, is accompanied by strong thirst and excessive drinking, dry mouth and tongue, red tongue tip and margins with thin yellowish coating, and forceful rapid

2 辨证

主症:多饮,多食,多尿,形体消瘦,或尿有甜味。

肺热津伤(上消)者,兼烦渴多饮、口干舌燥、舌边尖红、苔薄黄、脉洪数。胃热炽盛(中消)者,兼多食善饥、口渴尿多、形体消瘦、大便干

pulse. The syndrome of stomach heat, known as middle wasting-thirsty syndrome, is accompanied by an increased appetite and hunger, thirstiness and voluminous urine, emaciation, dry stools, yellowish coating and forceful slippery pulse. The syndrome of kidney-yin deficiency, known as lower wasting-thirsty syndrome, is accompanied by frequent urination and voluminous urine, murky and greasy urine, sweet urine, aching loins and knees, dizziness, vertigo, dry and itchy skin, red tongue with less coating, and thready rapid pulse. The syndrome of yin-yang deficiency is accompanied by frequent urination, murky and greasy urine, even urination right after drinking, pale complexion, dry ear helix, absence of warmth in the limbs, aversion to cold, impotence or irregular menstruation, pale tongue with dry whitish coating, and deep thready and weak pulse.

燥、苔黄,脉滑实有力。肾阴亏虚(下消)者,兼尿频尿多、混浊如膏脂或尿甜,腰膝酸软,头晕耳鸣,皮肤干燥、瘙痒,舌红苔少,脉细数;阴阳两虚者,兼小便频数、混浊如膏,甚至饮一溲一,面容憔悴,耳轮干枯,四肢欠温,畏寒怕冷,阳痿或月经不调,舌淡苔白而干,脉沉细无力。

3 Treatment

3.1 Essential treatment

Principal acupoints: Weiwanxiashu(EX-B 3), Feishu(BL 13), Pishu(BL 20), Shenshu(BL 23), Sanyinjiao(SP 6), and Taixi (KI 3).

Supplementary acupoints: In the upper wasting-thirsty syndrome, add Taiyuan(LU 9) and Shaofu (HT 8); in the middle wasting-thirsty syndrome, add Neiting(ST 44) and Diji(SP 8); in the lower wasting-thirsty syndrome, add Fuliu(KI 7) and Taichong(LR 3); in the syndrome of yin-yang deficiency, add Guanyuan(CV 3) and Mingmen(GV 4). In the case of dry mouth and thirst, add Lianquan(CV 23) and Chengjiang(CV 24); in the case of increased appetite and easy hunger, add Hegu(LI 4), Shangjuxu(ST 37), Fenglong(ST 40) and Zhongwan (CV 12); in the case of voluminous urine and night

3 治疗

3.1 基本治疗

主穴: 胃脘下俞,肺俞,脾俞,肾俞,三阴交,太溪。

配穴: 上消者,加太渊、少府。中消者,加内庭、地机。下消者,加复溜、太冲;阴阳两虚者,加关元、命门。烦渴、口干舌燥者,加廉泉、承浆;多食善饥者,加合谷、上巨虚、丰隆、中脘;多尿、盗汗者,加复溜、关元;视物模糊者,加光明、攒竹;皮肤瘙痒者,加风池、大椎、曲池、血海。

sweats, add Fuliu(KI 7) and Guanyuan(CV 4); in the case of blurred vision, add Guangming(GB 37) and Cuanzhu(BL 2); in the case of itchy skin, add Fengchi(GB 20), Dazhui(GV 14), Quchi(LI 11) and Xuehai(SP 10).

Explanation: Weiwanxiashu(EX-B 3) is an extra acupoint and empiric acupoint for wasting-thirsty syndrome. Feishu(BL 13) is used to enrich lung yin; Shenshu(BL 23) and Taixi(KI3) are used to enrich kidney yin; Sanyinjiao(SP6) acts to nourish the liver and kidney; Pishu(BL20) is used to enrich yin and produce fluids.

方义：胃脘下俞又名胰俞，为经外奇穴，是治疗本病的经验效穴。肺俞培补肺阴。肾俞、太溪滋补肾阴。三阴交滋补肝肾。脾俞健脾滋阴生津。

3.2 Other therapy

Ear acupuncture: Select 3 to 4 acupoints from Pancreas and Gallbladder(CO 11), Endocrine(CO 18), Kidney(CO 10), Triple Energizer(CO 17), Root of Ear Vagus(R 2), Shenmen(TF 4), Heart (CO 15), Liver(CO 12), Lung(CO 14), Apex of the Tragus (TG 1p), and Stomach(CO 4). Puncture these acupoints with filiform needles by mild stimulation, or embed the intradermal needles or apply *Semen Vaccariae*(Wang Bu Liu Xing) at these acupoints.

3.2 其他治疗

耳针：选胰胆、内分泌、肾、三焦、耳迷根、神门、心、肝、肺、屏尖、胃。每次3～4穴，毫针轻刺激，或用皮内针埋藏或用王不留行贴压。

4 Remarks

Acupuncture can be used as an adjunct therapy for wasting-thirsty syndrome. Combined acupuncture and medications can work excellently on this syndrome. Patients with this syndrome easily suffer from skin infection, therefore, in the performance of acupuncture, strict disinfection should be conducted and fewer acupoints are used. Patients are asked to actively regulate their diets, and participate in physical exercises.

4 按语

针灸可以作为糖尿病的辅助疗法，配合药物进行治疗，有较好的效果。糖尿病患者的皮肤容易化脓感染，针灸时注意严格消毒，用穴要少而精。患者应积极配合调整饮食，参加适量的体育锻炼。

Flank Pain

Flank pain refers to pain conditions in the hy-

胁 痛

胁痛是以一侧或两侧胁

pochondriac or costal regions on one or both sides. It is commonly seen in such liver-gallbladder diseases as acute or chronic hepatitis, acute or chronic cholecystitis and cholelithiasis, and intercostal neuralgia in Western medicine.

胁部疼痛为主要表现的病证。常见于西医学的急慢性肝炎、急慢性胆囊炎、胆石症等肝胆病变以及肋间神经痛等。

1　Etiology and pathogenesis

The liver meridian of foot-jueyin and gallbladder meridian of foot shaoyang distribute on both sides of the hypochondriac regions, so the occurrence of flank pain is mostly concerned with disorders of the liver and gallbladder. Flank pain may result from liver-qi depression, liver-gallbladder dampness-heat, blood-stasis in collaterals, and malnourishment due to liver-yin insufficiency.

1　病因病机

足厥阴肝经及足少阳胆经分布于两胁，胁痛的产生主要责之于肝胆。肝气郁滞，肝胆湿热，瘀血阻络，肝阴不足失养，均可导致胁痛。

2　Syndrome differentiation

Chief symptoms: Pain in the hypochondriac regions comes and goes.

The syndrome of liver-qi depression manifests flank distension and pain, wandering pain in the hypochondriac region which is relieved or aggravated by emotion, pain relief by belching or flatulence, poor appetite, abdominal fullness, thin whitish tongue coating, and wiry pulse. The syndrome of blood stasis in collaterals manifests fixed stabbing pain, aggravation during night, dark purplish tongue, and deep rough pulse. The syndrome of dampness-heat accumulation manifests dry mouth and bitter taste in the mouth, chest fullness and poor appetite, nausea, vomiting, dark yellow urine, or jaundice, yellowish greasy tongue coating, and wiry, slippery and rapid pulse. The syndrome of liver-yin deficiency manifests lingering dull constant pain in the hypochondriac regions, dry mouth and throat, dizziness, dry eyes, red tongue with less

2　辨证

主症：胁肋疼痛，常反复发作。

肝气郁结者，胁肋胀痛、走窜不定，疼痛每因情志变化而增减，得嗳气或矢气则舒，纳呆食少，脘腹胀满，苔薄白，脉弦；瘀血阻络者，胁肋刺痛、固定不移，入夜尤甚，舌质紫暗，脉沉涩；湿热蕴结者，口干苦，胸闷纳呆，恶心呕吐，小便黄赤，或有黄疸，舌苔黄腻，脉弦滑而数；肝阴不足者，胁肋隐痛，绵绵不休，口干咽燥，两目干涩，舌红少苔，脉弦细或细数。

coating, and thready wiry or rapid pulse.

3 Treatment

3.1 Essential treatment

Principal acupoints: Qimen (LR 14), Zhigou (TE 6), Yanglingquan (GB 34), and Zusanli (ST 36).

Supplementary acupoints: In the syndrome of liver-qi depression, add Xingjian (LR 2) and Taichong (LR 3) to soothe the liver and regulate qi; in the syndrome of blood stasis in the collaterals, add Geshu (BL 17) and Ashi acupoint point to dissolve blood-stasis and ease pain; in the syndrome of dampness-heat accumulation, add Zhongwan (CV 12) and Sanyinjiao (SP 6) to clear heat and disinhibit dampness; in the syndrome of liver-yin deficiency, add Ganshu (BL 18) and Shenshu (BL 23) to nourish the liver and kidney.

Explanation: The meridians of the liver and gallbladder supply the hypochondriac regions, so the local acupoint Qimen (LR 14) of the liver meridian and the distal acupoint Yanglingquan (GB 34) of the gallbladder meridian are used to free the qi movement of the liver and gallbladder, move qi and relieve pain; Zhigou (TE 6) is used to move qi in the triple energizer, and in combination with Zusanli (ST 36) to harmonize the stomach and relieve distension, and regulate qi activity.

3.2 Other therapies

Ear acupuncture: Select acupoints Liver (CO 12), Gallbladder (CO 11), Chest (AH 10) and Shenmen (TF 4). Puncture these acupoints by filiform needles or apply *Semen Vaccariae* (Wang Bu Liu Xing) at these acupoints.

Dermal needle therapy: Gently tap the affected

3 治疗

3.1 基本治疗

主穴: 期门，支沟，阳陵泉，足三里。

配穴: 肝气郁结加行间、太冲疏肝理气；瘀血阻络加膈俞、阿是穴化瘀止痛；湿热蕴结加中脘、三阴交清热利湿；肝阴不足加肝俞、肾俞补益肝肾。

方义: 肝胆经布于胁肋，故近取肝经期门、远取胆经阳陵泉疏利肝胆气机、行气止痛。取支沟以疏通三焦之气，配足三里和胃消痞、疏调气机。

3.2 其他疗法

耳针: 选肝、胆、胸、神门，毫针刺激，亦可用王不留行贴压。

皮肤针: 用皮肤针轻轻

areas in the flank and their corresponding Jiaji acupoint(EX-B 2) with dermal needle, and then cupping is applied. This therapy is indicated for the flank pain due to blood stasis.

叩刺胁肋部痛点及与痛点对应的夹脊穴，并加拔火罐。适用于瘀血疼痛。

4　Remarks

4　按语

Acupuncture works well on flank pain, especially on primary intercostal neuralgia. For flank pain due to herpes zoster, consecutive acupuncture treatment is necessary to relieve pain.

针灸治疗胁痛有较好的效果。对原发性肋间神经痛效果尤佳；对由带状疱疹而遗留的肋间神经痛，常需连续治疗才能止痛。

For acute flank pain, after pain relief by acupuncture, the primary causes should be identified and etiological treatments should be applied.

对于急性胁痛，用针刺止痛后应注意明确病因，以采取相应的治疗措施。

Stomachache

胃　痛

Stomachache, also known as epigastric pain, is characterized by repeated recurrence of pain in the upper abdominal region. Since the pain is near the cardiac region, it is also called "cardiac pain" "epigastric-cardiac pain" or "inferio-cardiac pain". Stomachache is commonly seen in acute or chronic gastritis, peptic ulcers, gastrointestinal neurosis in Western medicine.

胃痛，又称"胃脘痛"，是以上腹胃脘部反复性发作性疼痛为主的病证。由于疼痛位近心窝部，古人又称"心痛""胃心痛""心下痛"等。胃痛多见于急慢性胃炎、消化性溃疡、胃肠神经官能症等病。

1　Etiology and pathogenesis

1　病因病机

The common causes of stomachache include following aspects: pathogenic cold invades the stomach and then blocks qi movement; or improper food intake may injure the stomach and cause food retention; or qi depression may damage the liver, and liver qi then disturbs the stomach; or long-term blood-stasis accumulation may obstruct qi movement, then results in pain; or the spleen and stomach are weak and the stomach-yin is insufficient,

胃痛的常见原因有寒邪客胃，寒阻气机，或饮食伤胃、食滞不化，或气郁伤肝、肝气犯胃，或瘀血内结，以致气机阻滞，不通则痛，或因脾胃虚弱、胃阴不足，胃腑失于温煦或濡养而痛。

then the stomach fails to be warmed or nourished, causing stomach pain.

2 Syndrome differentiation

2.1 Excess syndrome

Chief symptoms: Sudden onset of severe pain in the epigastric area, aggravated by pressure and after meals.

The syndrome of pathogenic cold invading stomach manifests pain alleviated by warmth and aggravated by cold, preference for warm fluids, thin white tongue coating, and wiry tight pulse. The syndrome of food retention manifests fullness and distending pain, belching with bad odor, acid regurgitation, vomiting or pain relief after passing gas, thick and greasy tongue coating, and slippery pulse. The syndrome of liver-qi attacking stomach manifests distending pain radiating to the hypochondriac regions, belching, acid regurgitation, desire to sigh, pain triggered by emotional disturbance, thin whitish tongue coating, and wiry pulse. The syndrome of qi-blood stagnation manifests fixed pain, dark purplish tongue with possible petechia, and thready rough pulse.

2.2 Deficiency syndrome

Chief symptoms: Dull pain in the epigastric region, preference for local pressure, pain relief after eating.

The syndrome of spleen-stomach deficiency-cold is accompanied by watery vomiting, loose stools, fatigue and lassitude, pale tongue with thin coating, and feeble pulse. The syndrome of stomach-yin deficiency is accompanied by dull burning pain in the stomach, hunger but with no desire to eat, dry mouth and throat, constipation, red tongue

2 辨证

2.1 实证

主症：上腹胃脘部暴痛，痛势较剧，痛处拒按，食后痛增。

寒邪犯胃者，得温痛减、遇寒痛增，喜热饮，苔薄白，脉弦紧；饮食停滞者，胀满疼痛，嗳腐吞酸，呕吐或矢气后痛减，苔厚腻，脉滑；肝气犯胃者，胀痛连胁，嗳气吞酸，喜叹息，每因情志因素诱发，苔薄白，脉弦；气滞血瘀者，痛有定处，舌质紫暗或有瘀斑，脉细涩。

2.2 虚证

主症：胃脘部疼痛隐隐，痛处喜按，食后痛减。

脾胃虚寒者，兼吐清水，便溏，神疲乏力，舌淡苔薄，脉虚弱；胃阴不足者，胃脘灼热隐痛，饥不欲食，咽干口燥，大便干结，舌红少津，脉细数。

with little fluids, and thready rapid pulse.

3 Treatment

3.1 Essential treatment

Principal acupoints: Zusanli(ST 36), Zhongwan (CV 12), and Neiguan(PC 6).

Supplementary acupoints: In the syndrome of pathogenic cold invading stomach, add Weishu(BL 21); in the syndrome of food retention, add Xiawan (CV 10) and Liangmen(ST 21); in the syndrome of liver-qi attacking stomach, add Taichong(LR 3); in the syndrome of qi-blood stagnation, add Geshu(BL 17); in the syndrome of spleen-stomach deficiency-cold, add Pishu(BL 20) and Weishu(BL 21); in the syndrome of stomach-yin deficiency, add Sanyinjiao (SP 6) and Neiting(ST 44).

Explanation: Zusanli(ST 36) is the Lower He-Sea acupoint of the stomach and functions to treat stomach disorders; Zhongwan(CV 12), a local acupoint, is the Influential acupoint of the fu-organs and the Front-Mu acupoint of the stomach; combined use of these two acupoints can harmonize the stomach and stop pain. Neiguan(PC 6), the Confluent acupoint communicating with the yin link vessel, is the key acupoint in the treatment of stomachache.

3.2 Other therapies

Ear acupuncture: Select 2 to 3 acupoints from Stomach(CO 4), Liver(CO 12), Spleen(CO 13), Shenmen(TF 4), Sympathesis(AH 6a) and Duodenum(CO 5). Puncture these acupoints shallowly with filiform needles or apply ear-pressure with *Semen Vaccariae* (Wang Bu Liu Xing) at these acupoints.

Electro-acupuncture: Select Zusanli(ST 36) and

3 治疗

3.1 基本治疗

主穴: 足三里,中脘,内关。

配穴: 寒邪犯胃加胃俞;饮食停滞加下脘、梁门;肝气犯胃加太冲;气滞血瘀加膈俞;脾胃虚寒加脾俞、胃俞;胃阴不足加三阴交、内庭。

方义: 足三里是胃的下合穴,善治胃腑病证;中脘为腑会、胃之募穴,又为局部穴,两穴合用能和胃止痛。内关通于阴维脉,是治疗胃痛的要穴。

3.2 其他治疗

耳针: 选胃、肝、脾、神门、交感、十二指肠。每次选2~3穴,毫针浅刺,或用王不留行贴压。

电针: 选足三里、上巨

Shangjuxu(ST 37), and treat these two acupoints by strong stimulation at a dense wave.

虚。电针密波,较强刺激。

4 Remarks

Acupuncture works well on stomachache and such symptoms as epigastric fullness and distension, and nausea, especially on acute stomachache. Stomachache is sometimes similar to cardiac infarction or some severe digestive disorders, so the definite causes should be ascertained and corresponding treatments should be applied. Patients are advised to take regular diets, and avoid spicy foods and alcohol.

4 按语

针灸治疗胃脘疼痛以及上腹部胀满、恶心等症状效果较好,尤其对急性胃痛疗效显著。胃痛的临床表现有时可与心肌梗死或某些严重的消化系统疾病表现相似,应注意鉴别,明确病因后采取相应的治疗措施。嘱患者注意饮食规律,忌食刺激食物,忌饮烈酒。

Abdominal Pain

Abdominal pain refers to pain in the lower abdomen, below the epigastric region and above the upper border of the pubic bone. It is frequently encountered in the diseases in internal medicine, gynecology and surgery, especially in the digestive system and gynecological system.

腹 痛

腹痛指胃脘以下、耻骨毛际以上部位发生疼痛的病证。多见于内、妇、外科等疾病,而以消化系统和妇科疾病更为常见。

1 Etiology and pathogenesis

Invasion of exogenous cold may impair the yang-qi in the middle energizer; invasion of exogenous heat may mingle with the dampness and food and consequently result in qi obstruction. Spleen-yang inactivity may impair the spleen and stomach, leading to qi obstruetion; emotional depression may give rise to liver-qi adversity; or external trauma may cause qi and blood stagnation. All above causes may result in abdominal pain.

1 病因病机

外感寒邪,中阳受损;外感热邪,湿热食滞交阻于中,均可导致气机阻滞而发病。脾阳不振,脾胃损伤,气机不畅;情志抑郁,肝气横逆;或因外伤导致气滞血瘀,均可引发本病。

2 Syndrome differentiation

Chief symptoms: Acute abdominal pain is

2 辨证

主症:急性腹痛发病急

marked by abrupt onset of severe pain, and chronic abdominal pain by lingering intermittent pain.

The syndrome of cold accumulation manifests abrupt onset of intense abdominal pain which responds to warmth and gets worse by cold invasion, pale tongue with whitish coating, and deep tight pulse. The syndrome of dampness-heat accumulation manifests abdominal pain with refusal to pressure, abdominal distension and fullness, constipation or hesitate bowel movement, dark urine, red tongue with yellowish sticky coating, and slippery rapid pulse. The syndrome of qi and blood stagnation manifests abdominal distension and pain which radiates into the lateral abdomen and may be alleviated by belching or flatulence and worsened by anger, dark purplish tongue with possible petechia, and wiry rough pulse. The syndrome of spleen-yang inactivity manifests intermittent dull pain which may be relieved by pressure and aggravated by hunger and exertion, loose stools, lassitude and aversion to cold, pale tongue with thin whitish coating, and deep thready pulse.

骤,痛势剧烈。慢性腹痛病程较长,腹痛缠绵,时作时止。

寒邪内积者,腹痛暴急,喜温怕冷,多因感寒而发作,舌淡苔白,脉沉紧;湿热壅滞者,腹痛拒按,胀满不舒,大便涩滞不爽,小便短赤,舌红,苔黄腻,脉滑数;气滞血瘀者,脘腹胀痛,痛引少腹,得嗳气或矢气则痛减,遇恼怒则加剧,舌紫暗,或有瘀点,脉弦涩;脾阳不振者,腹痛缠绵,饥饿劳累后加剧,痛时喜按,大便溏薄,神疲怯冷,舌淡苔白,脉沉细。

3 Treatment

3.1 Essential treatment

Principal acupoints: Zusanli(ST 36), Zhongwan (CV 12), Tianshu(ST 25), Sanyinjiao(SP 6) and Guanyuan(CV 4).

Supplementary acupoints: In the syndrome of cold accumulation, add Shenque(CV 8) and Gongsun (SP 4); in the syndrome of dampness-heat accumulation, add Yinlingquan(SP 9) and Neiting(ST 44); in the syndrome of qi-blood stagnation, add Ququan(LR 8) and Xuehai(SP 10); in the syndrome of spleen-yang inactivity, add Pishu(BL 20),

3 治疗

3.1 基本治疗

主穴: 足三里,中脘,天枢,三阴交,关元。

配穴: 寒邪内积者,加灸神阙;湿热壅滞者,加配阴陵泉、内庭;气滞血瘀者,加曲泉、血海;脾阳不振者,加脾俞、胃俞、章门。

Weishu(BL 21) and Zhangmen(LR 13).

Explanation: Zusanli(ST 36) is the Lower He-Sea of the stomach and acts to treat epigastric and abdominal disorders. Zhongwan (CV 12) is the Front-Mu acupoint of the stomach and the Influential acupoint of the fu-organs; Tainshu(ST 25) is the Front-Mu acupoint of the large intestine; Guanyuan (CV 4) is the Front-Mu acupoint of the small intestine; these three acupoints are used to regulate qi of the fu-organs. Sanyinjiao(SP 6) functions to harmonize qi and blood in the three foot-yin meridians, thus the pain is relieved.

方义: 足三里为胃之下合穴,善治腹部疾病。中脘为腑会、胃之募穴,天枢为大肠募穴,关元为小肠募穴,三穴可通调腑气。三阴交通调足三阴经气血,通则不痛。

3.2 Other therapy

Ear acupuncture: Select 2 to 4 acupoints from Stomach(CO 4), Small Intestine(CO 6), Large Intestine(CO 7), Liver(CO 12), Spleen(CO 13), Sympathesis(AH 6a), and Shenmen(TF 4). Puncture these acupoints when pain experiences with moderate stimulation or apply ear-pressure with intradermal needles or *Semen Vaccariae*(Wang Bu Liu Xing)at these acupoints.

3.2 其他治疗

耳针: 选胃、小肠、大肠、肝、脾、交感、神门。每次取2～4穴,疼痛时用中强刺激,亦可耳穴埋针或王不留行贴压。

4 Remarks

Acupuncture is quite effective for abdominal pain. However, precise diagnosis must be established after pain is relieved, and treatment should be aimed at the primary diseases. During the treatment of acute abdominal pain with acupuncture, strict observation of the diseases is required, or else it can be transferred to surgery.

4 按语

针灸治疗腹痛有较好的效果,止痛以后应明确诊断,积极治疗原发病。对于急腹症引起的腹痛,针灸治疗时应严密观察病情变化,必要时转外科治疗。

Vomiting

Vomiting is a common clinical symptom, and can appear alone or as an accompanying symptom in

呕 吐

呕吐是临床常见病证,既可单独为患,亦可见于多

many diseases. Vomiting is often seen in acute and chronic gastritis, cardiospasm, pylorospasm, gastroneurosis and cholecystitis in Western medicine.

种疾病。呕吐可见于西医学的急慢性胃炎、贲门痉挛、幽门痉挛、胃神经官能症、胆囊炎等。

1 Etiology and pathogenesis

The stomach receives and processes water and foods, and its qi descends during normal function. When the stomach-qi goes upwards, vomiting experiences. Invasion of exogenous factors, improper diets or emotional injury may cause stomach-qi adversity and then result in vomiting.

1 病因病机

胃主受纳，腐熟水谷，以降为顺，若上逆则为呕吐。或感受外邪，或饮食不节，或情志内伤等原因，皆可导致胃气上逆，引起呕吐。

2 Syndrome differentiation

Chief symptoms: Excess syndrome of vomiting generally exhibits sudden attack, with profuse acid and fermented vomitus. Deficiency syndrome of vomiting displays lingering vomiting with a small amount of light vomitus.

The syndrome of cold invading the stomach manifests vomiting of thin water or sputum, loose stools, preference for warmth and aversion to cold, whitish tongue coating, and slow pulse. The syndrome of heat accumulation in the stomach manifests vomiting acid, foul, bitter vomitus, constipation, dry mouth and thirstiness, preference for coldness and aversion to warmth, yellowish tongue coating and rapid pulse. The syndrome of phlegm-fluids obstruction presents with watery vomitus, accompanied by epigastric fullness, poor appetite, white greasy tongue coating, and slippery pulse. The syndrome of liver-qi attacking the stomach manifests vomiting after emotional disturbance, acid regurgitation, belching, ordinary irritability, thin pale tongue and wiry pulse. The syndrome of spleen-stomach deficiency-cold manifests vomiting

2 辨证

主症：实证一般发病急，呕吐量多，吐出物多酸臭味。虚证病程较长，发病较缓，时作时止，吐出物不多，腐臭味不甚。

寒邪客胃者，呕吐清水或痰涎，大便溏薄，喜暖畏寒，苔白，脉迟；热邪内蕴者，呕吐酸苦热臭物，大便燥结，口干而渴，喜寒恶热，苔黄，脉数；痰饮内阻者，呕吐清水痰涎，脘闷纳差，苔白腻，脉滑；肝气犯胃者，每因精神不畅而发作，嗳气吞酸，平时多烦善怒，苔薄白，脉弦；脾胃虚寒者，饮食稍有不慎，呕吐即易发作，纳差便溏，倦怠乏力，舌淡苔薄，脉弱。

just after an inappropriate meal, susceptibility to vomiting, poor appetite, loose stools, lassitude, pale tongue coating, and feeble pulse.

3 Treatment

3.1 Essential treatment

Principal acupoints: Neiguan(PC 6), Zusanli (ST 36), and Zhongwan(CV 12).

Supplementary acupoints: In the syndrome of cold invading the stomach, add Shangwan(CV 13) and Weishu(BL 21); in the syndrome of heat accumulation, add Hegu(LI 4) and prick Jinjin(EX-HN 12) and Yuye(EX-HN 13) to bleed; in the syndrome of phlegm-fluids obstruction, add Danzhong (CV 17) and Fenglong(ST 40); in the syndrome of liver-qi attacking the stomach, add Yanglingquan (GB 34) and Taichong(LR 3); in the syndrome of spleen-stomach deficiency-cold, add Pishu(BL 20) and Weishu(BL 21). In the case of food retention, add Liangmen(ST 21) and Tianshu(ST 25); in the case of acid regurgitation and absence of vomitus, add Gongsun(SP 4).

Explanation: Neiguan(PC 6), the Luo-Connecting acupoint of the hand-jueyin meridian, functions to loosen chest and regulate qi, descend adversity and stop vomiting. Zusanli(ST 36), the He-Sea acupoint of the foot-yangming meridian, is used to regulate qi activity in the stomach and intestine, and descend stomach-qi. Zhongwan(CV 12), the Front-Mu acupoint of the stomach, can regulate qi and harmonize the stomach to stop vomiting.

3.2 Other therapy

Ear acupuncture: Select 3 to 4 acupoints from Stomach(CO 4), Cardia(CO 3), Esophagus (CO 2), Sympathesis(AH 6a), Shenmen(TF 4), Spleen

3 治疗

3.1 基本治疗

主穴：内关，足三里，中脘。

配穴：寒吐者，加上脘、胃俞；热吐者，加合谷，并可用金津、玉液点刺出血；痰饮内阻者，加膻中、丰隆；肝气犯胃者，加阳陵泉、太冲；脾胃虚寒者，加脾俞、胃俞。食滞者，加梁门、天枢；泛酸干呕者，加公孙。

方义：内关为手厥阴经络穴，宽胸理气，降逆止呕。足三里为足阳明经合穴，调理胃肠气机，通降胃气。中脘乃胃之募穴，理气和胃止呕。

3.2 其他治疗

耳针：选胃、贲门、食道、交感、神门、脾、肝。每次选3～4穴，毫针刺激，亦可耳穴

(CO 13), and Liver(CO 12). Puncture these acupoints with filiform needles, or embed intradermal needles or apply ear-pressure with *Semen Vaccariae* (Wang Bu Liu Xing) at these acupoints.

埋针或王不留行贴压。

4 Remarks

Acupuncture has a wonderful effect on vomiting. As for the treatment of morning sickness or vomiting due to drug reaction, refer to the therapies mentioned above. Treatment of vomiting due to severe obstruction in the upper digestive tract, tumors and cerebral diseases should aim at the primary diseases.

4 按语

针灸治疗呕吐效果良好,因妊娠或药物反应引起的呕吐,亦可参照本病治疗。对于上消化道严重梗阻、癌肿引起的呕吐以及脑源性呕吐,应重视原发病的治疗。

Diarrhea

Diarrhea refers to abnormally frequent and liquid or watery fecal discharges. In Western medicine, diarrhea is often seen in acute and chronic enteritis, gastrointestinal dysfunction, allergic enteritis, ulcerative colitis, etc.

腹　泻

腹泻又称“泄泻”,是指排便次数增多,粪便稀薄,甚至如水样的病证。腹泻多见于西医学的急慢性肠炎、胃肠功能紊乱、过敏性肠炎、溃疡性结肠炎等。

1 Etiology and pathogenesis

The main organs involved in diarrhea are the spleen, stomach, large intestine and small intestine. Acute diarrhea is mostly caused by exogenous cold-dampness or dampness-heat, and chronic diarrhea is usually caused by qi deficiency in the spleen and stomach due to longstanding disorders. Diarrhea can also result from liver-qi attacking the spleen, or insufficient kidney-yang failing to warm the spleen. Thus, spleen deficiency and dampness excess are the two most essential factors in causing diarrhea.

1 病因病机

腹泻的病位主要在脾、胃和大小肠。急性腹泻多由于感受寒湿或湿热之邪,慢性腹泻多为久病气虚,脾胃虚弱;亦有肝失疏泄,横逆乘脾,或命门火衰,不能温煦脾土。脾虚、湿盛是导致本病发生的重要因素。

2 Syndrome differentiation

Chief symptoms: Acute diarrhea is marked by

2 辨证

主症:急性腹泻发病急,

sudden onset, short-term duration, and increased frequency of fecal discharges, and scanty urine; chronic diarrhea is marked by lingering onset, long-term duration, usually evolution from acute diarrhea, and fewer frequency of fecal discharges.

病程短,大便次数显著增多,小便减少;慢性腹泻发病势缓,病程较长,多由急性腹泻迁延而来,便泻次数较少。

Acute diarrhea: The syndrome of exogenous cold-dampness invasion manifests loose stools with water and food, abdominal distension and pain, intestinal gurgling, absence of thirst, chills and preference for warmth, pale tongue with whitish and slippery coating, and slow pulse. The syndrome of exogenous dampness-heat invasion manifests yellowish and foul stools, burning sensation in the anus, abdominal pain, restlessness and thirst, scanty yellow urine, red tongue with yellowish greasy coating, and soggy rapid pulse. The syndrome of food retention manifests abdominal pain and intestinal gurgling, foul diarrhea with undigested food, relief after bowel movements, accompanied by belching, acid regurgitation, thick filthy or greasy tongue coating, and slippery pulse.

急性腹泻:感受寒湿者,大便清稀,水谷相杂,肠鸣胀痛,口不渴,身寒喜温,舌淡,苔白滑,脉迟;感受湿热者,大便色黄而臭伴有黏液,肛门灼热,腹痛,心烦口渴,小便短赤,舌红苔黄腻,脉濡数;饮食停滞者,腹痛肠鸣,大便恶臭,泻后痛减,伴有未消化的食物,嗳腐吞酸,舌苔垢浊或厚腻,脉滑。

Chronic diarrhea: The syndrome of spleen-stomach deficiency manifests loose stools with undigested food, intermittent onset or soon after eating fatty food, frequent bowel movements, sallow complexion, no desire to food, pale tongue with whitish coating, and feeble pulse. The syndrome of liver-qi stagnation manifests distension and fullness in the chest and hypochondriac regions, belching and diminished appetite, recurrence due to emotional disturbance or stress, thin red tongue and wiry pulse. The syndrome of kidney-yang deficiency manifests intestinal gurgling and diarrhea with abdominal pain just before dawn, relief after bowel movements,

慢性腹泻:脾胃虚弱者,大便溏薄,完谷不化,反复发作,稍进油腻食物,则大便次数增多,面色萎黄,不思饮食,舌淡苔白,脉无力;肝郁气滞者,平素多有胸胁胀闷,嗳气食少,每因抑郁恼怒或情绪紧张而发作,舌淡红,脉弦;肾阳不足者,常于黎明之前,腹部作痛,肠鸣即泻,泻后痛减,腰酸腿软,消瘦,舌淡苔白,脉沉细。

aching loins and knees, emaciation, pale tongue with whitish coating, and deep thready pulse.

3 Treatment

3.1 Essential treatment

Principal acupoints: Acute diarrhea: Tianshu (ST 25), Shangjuxu(ST 37), Yinlingquan(SP 9), and Shuifen(CV 9); chronic diarrhea: Shenque(CV 8), Tianshu(ST 25), Zusanli(ST 36), and Gongsun (SP 4).

Supplementary acupoints: In the syndrome of exogenous cold-damp invasion, add Shenque(CV 8); in the syndrome of exogenous dampness-heat invasion, add Neiting(ST 44); in the syndrome of food retention, add Zhongwan(CV 12); in the syndrome of spleen-stomach deficiency, add Pishu(BL 20) and Taibai(SP 3); in the syndrome of liver-qi stagnation, add Taichong(LR 3); in the syndrome of kidney-yang deficiency, add Shenshu(BL 23) and Mingmen(GV 4).

Explanation: Tianshu(ST 25), the Front-Mu acupoint of the large intestine, is used to regulate qi activity in the stomach and intestine. Shangjuxu(ST 37), the Lower He-Sea acupoint of the large intestine, is applied to unblock fu-organs, eliminate dampness and retention; Yinlingquan(SP 9) acts to nourish the spleen and resolve dampness. Shuifen (CV 9) induces diuresis to dry stools. Shenque(CV 8) is applied with moxibustion to warm and reinforce the original yang, strengthen body constitution to stem diarrhea. Zusanli(ST 36) and Gongsun (SP 4) can invigorate the spleen and stomach.

3.2 Other therapy

Ear acupuncture: Select 3 to 4 acupoints from Large Intestine(CO 7), Stomach(CO 4), Spleen

3 治疗

3.1 基本治疗

主穴：急性腹泻取天枢、上巨虚、阴陵泉、水分；慢性腹泻取神阙、天枢、足三里、公孙。

配穴：感受寒湿者，加灸神阙；感受湿热者，加内庭；饮食停滞者，加中脘；脾胃虚弱者，加脾俞、太白；肝郁者，加太冲；肾阳不足者，加肾俞、命门。

方义：天枢为大肠募穴，可调理肠胃气机。上巨虚为大肠下合穴，可通腑除湿导滞，取“合治内腑”之意。阴陵泉可健脾化湿。水分利小便而实大便。灸神阙可温补元阳，固本止泻。足三里、公孙健脾益胃。

3.2 其他治疗

耳针：选大肠、胃、脾、肝、肾、交感。每次选 3～4

(CO 13), Liver (CO 12), Kidney (CO 10), and Sympathesis (AH 6a). Puncture these acupoints with filiform needles, or embed intradermal needles or apply *Semen Vaccaiae* (Wang Bu Liu Xing) at these acupoints.

穴，毫针针刺。亦可耳穴埋针或王不留行贴压。

4 Remarks

Acupuncture has successful effect in relieving diarrhea. In practice, it is necessary to give intravenous drip of fluids in case of severe dehydration due to acute enteritis or ulcerative colitis. Patients are advised to take regular bland diets, and avoid raw, cold, spicy, oily and greasy food.

4 按语

针灸治疗腹泻有显著疗效。若急性胃肠炎或溃疡性结肠炎等因腹泻频繁而出现脱水现象者，应适当配合输液治疗。治疗期间应注意清淡饮食，忌食生冷、辛辣、油腻之品。

Constipation

Constipation refers to the condition in which the feces are hard and elimination from the bowels is difficult and infrequent. In Western medicine, habitual constipation, secondary constipation due to intestinal neurosis and weak constitution, anal fissure, hemorrhoids, proctitis and drug-induced constipation may be treated with the therapies in this section.

便 秘

便秘是指大便秘结不通，粪质干燥、坚硬，排便艰涩难下的病证。西医学的习惯性便秘，神经官能症、全身衰弱所致肠道蠕动减弱引起的便秘，或肛裂、痔疮、直肠炎等肛门直肠疾患引起的便秘，以及药物引起的便秘等均可参照本节治疗。

1 Etiology and pathogenesis

Constipation is mainly caused by the dysfunction of the large intestine movements. Costitutional yang hyperactivity may lead to accumulation of heat in the stomach and intestines; or endogenous heat consuming body fluids give rise to dryness and heat in the intestines; or emotional disturbances, such as anxiety and depression, or lack of movement can cause the descent of lung-qi and stagnation of intes-

1 病因病机

便秘主要为大肠传导功能失常所致。素体阳盛，胃肠积热；或邪热内燔，津液受烁，肠道燥热；或情志不畅，忧愁思虑过度；或久坐少动，肺气不降，肠道气机郁滞，而成实证便秘。久病体虚，气血两伤，气虚则大肠传导无

tinal qi activity; all these factors may lead to constipation of excess syndrome. In deficiency of qi and blood due to long-standing illnesses, qi fails to move the bowels and blood fails to nourish the large intestine; yang-qi insufficiency in the lower energizer and following cold accumulation results in retention of feces in the large intestine; all these factors may lead to constipation of deficiency syndrome.

力，血虚则肠失滋润；或下焦阳气不充，阴寒凝结，糟粕不行，凝结肠道而成虚证便秘。

2 Syndrome differentiation

Chief symptoms: Difficult defecation with discharge of dry and hard stools.

The syndrome of constipation due to heat manifests fullness and distending pain in the abdomen, red face and fever, dry mouth and vexation, foul breath, preference for cold drinks, red tongue with dry yellowish coating, and slippery rapid pulse. The syndrome of qi stagnation manifests urgency to defecate, frequent belching, fullness and distending pain in the abdomen, aggravation by emotional disturbance, fullness in the chest and hypochondria, bitter taste in the mouth, thin sticky tongue coating, and wiry pulse. The syndrome of qi deficiency manifests hard defecation followed by sweating and shortness of breath, normal stools, sallow complexion, pale tongue with thin coating, and feeble thready pulse. The syndrome of blood deficiency manifests sallow complexion, dizziness and palpitations, pale lips and thready pulse. The syndrome of cold accumulation manifests hard defecation and dry stools, accompanied by clear and profuse urine, pain and cold sensation in the abdomen, absence of warmth in the limbs, preference for warmth and aversion to cold, pale tongue with whitish coating, and deep slow pulse.

2 辨证

主症：大便秘结不通，排便艰涩难解。

热秘者，兼腹胀腹痛、面红身热、口干心烦、口臭、喜冷饮、舌红苔黄或黄燥，脉滑数；气秘者，欲便不得，兼嗳气频作、腹中胀痛，遇情志不舒则便秘加重，胸胁痞满，口苦，舌苔薄腻，脉弦；气虚便秘者，兼见临厕努挣、挣则汗出气短，便后疲乏，大便并不干硬，面色㿠白，舌淡嫩，苔薄，脉虚。血虚便秘者，兼见面色无华、头晕心悸、唇舌色淡，脉细；寒秘者，大便艰涩，排出困难，兼小便清长、腹中冷痛、四肢不温、畏寒喜暖、舌淡苔白、脉沉迟。

3 Treatment

3.1 Essential treatment

Principal acupoints: Tianshu (ST 25), Zhigou (TE 6), Shuidao(ST 28), Guilai(ST 29), and Fenglong (ST 40).

Supplementary acupoints: In the syndrome of heat accumulation, add Hegu(LI 4) and Neiting(ST 44); in the syndrome of qi stagnation, add Taichong(LR 3) and Zhongwan(CV 12); in the syndrome of qi deficiency, add Pishu(BL 20) and Qihai (CV 6); in the syndrome of blood deficiency, add Zusanli(ST 36) and Sanyinjiao(SP 6); in the syndrome of cold accumulation, add Shenque(CV 8) and Guanyuan(CV 4).

Explanation: Tianshu (ST 25), the Front-Mu acupoint of the large intestine, is used to free qi flow in the large intestine, and then ensure the normal movement of the bowels. Zhigou (TE 5) can promote qi flow in the triple energizer and unblock the bowels. Shuidao (ST 28), Guilai (ST 29) and Fenglong (ST 40) can regulate the spleen and stomach, relieve stagnation and unblock the fu-organs.

3.2 Other therapy

Ear acupuncture: Select acupoints of Large Intestine(CO 7), Rectum(HX 2), Sympathesis (AH 6a), and Subcortex(AT 4). Puncture these acupoints with filiform needles by moderate or mild stimulation, or embed intradermal needles or apply *Semen Vaccariae* (Wang Bu Liu Xing) at these acupoints.

4 Remarks

Acupuncture is quite effective against constipation. If the condition does not respond well to acupuncture treatments, it is necessary to find out the real causative factors. Patients should be advised to

3 治疗

3.1 基本治疗

主穴：天枢，支沟，水道，归来，丰隆。

配穴：热秘者，加合谷、内庭；气秘者，加太冲、中脘；气虚便秘者，加脾俞、气海；血虚便秘者，加足三里、三阴交；寒秘者，加神阙、关元。

方义：天枢为大肠募穴，疏通大肠腑气，腑气通则大肠传导功能正常。支沟宣通三焦气机，通调肠腑。水道、归来、丰隆，可调理脾胃、行滞通腑。

3.2 其他治疗

耳针：选大肠、直肠、交感、皮质下。毫针中等强度刺激或弱刺激，亦可耳穴埋针或王不留行贴压。

4 按语

针灸治疗便秘有较好疗效。如经治疗多次而无效，应查明原因。患者平时应坚持体育锻炼，多食蔬菜水果，

encourage regular physical exercise and more vegetables and fruits, and cultivate the habit of regular defecation.

养成定时排便的习惯。

Lumbago

腰 痛

Lumbago, known as lumbar pain, is a frequently encountered disease in which subjective pain is felt in the lumbar region. In Western medicine, it is often seen in injuries of the soft tissues of the lumbar region, muscular rheumatism, lumbar spondylotic diseases and some internal disorders.

腰痛又称“腰脊痛”，是以自觉腰部疼痛为主症的一类病证。本证常见于西医学的腰部软组织损伤、肌肉风湿、腰椎病变及部分内脏病变。

1 Etiology and pathogenesis

1 病因病机

Lumbago can be caused by invasion of either exogenous pathogenic factors or endogenous pathogenic factors. In exogenous pathogenic factors, exposure to wind and cold may affect the meridians and collaterals, leading to unsmooth flow of qi and blood. In endogenous pathogenic factors, over-exertion and falling down may injure the tendons and collaterals, causing qi and blood stagnation; weak constitution or kidney-essence deficiency may induce lumbago.

腰痛的发生，可由外感、内伤所致。外感风寒湿诸邪，浸渍经络，气血运行不畅；或劳累过度，闪挫跌仆，经筋络脉受损，均可致气滞血瘀；素体禀赋不足，或肾精亏虚，发为腰痛。

2 Syndrome differentiation

2 辨证

Chief symptoms: Aches or pains in the lower back.

主症：腰部疼痛。

The syndrome of invasion by exogenous pathogenic cold-dampness manifests the history of cold contraction in the lumbar region, aggravation by climate alternation or in rainy cloudy days, cold pain and heaviness of the lumbar area, muscular stiffness in the loins with limited movement, or pain radiating downwards to the buttocks and lower limbs. The syndrome of qi and blood stagnation

寒湿腰痛者，有腰部受寒史，逢天气变化或阴雨风冷时加重，腰部冷痛重着，或拘挛不可俯仰，或痛连臀腿；瘀血腰痛者，有腰部劳伤或陈伤史，劳累、晨起、久坐时加重，腰部两侧肌肉触之有僵硬感，痛处固定不移；肾虚

manifests the history of lumbar injury, aggravation by over-exertion, getting up, and long-term sitting, muscular stiffness in the lumbar regions, and fixed pain. The syndrome of kidney deficiency manifests chronic onset of dull pain, soreness in the lumbar regions, accompanied by lassitude and fatigue, pale tongue and thready pulse.

腰痛者,起病缓慢,腰痛隐隐,或酸多痛少,乏力易倦,舌淡,脉细。

3 Treatment

3.1 Essential treatment

Principal acupoints: Ashi acupoint, Dachangshu (BL 25), and Weizhong(BL 40).

Supplementary acupoints: In the syndrome of kidney deficiency, add Shenshu(BL 23), Mingmen (GV 4) and Zhishi(BL 52).

Explanation: Ashi acupoint and Dachangshu (BL 25) can promote qi and blood circulation of the affected meridians, collaterals and muscle sinews to relieve pain. Weizhong(BL 40), an acupoint of the meridian of foot-taiyang and an empiric acupoint for lumbar conditions, can regulate qi and blood circulation of the bladder meridian in the back.

3.2 Other therapies

Ear acupuncture: Needle Lumbosacral Vertebrae(AH 9), Kidney(CO 10) and Shenmen(TF 4) and simultaneously ask the patient to move the loin. Intradermal needles may be embedded or *Semen Vaccariae* (Wang Bu Liu Xing) may be applied at these acupoints.

Dermal needle therapy: The affected area is first pricked by a dermal needle and then cupped. This therapy is indicated for lumbago caused by cold-dampness invasion and blood stasis.

4 Remarks

The therapeutic results of acupuncture vary

3 治疗

3.1 基本治疗

主穴:阿是穴,大肠俞,委中。

配穴:肾虚腰痛者,配肾俞、命门、志室。

方义:阿是穴、大肠俞可疏通局部经脉、络脉及经筋之气血,通经止痛。委中为足太阳经穴,可疏调腰背部膀胱经之气血。

3.2 其他治疗

耳针:取患侧腰骶椎、肾、神门,毫针刺后嘱患者活动腰部;亦可用皮内针埋藏或王不留行贴压。

皮肤针:选择腰部疼痛部位,用梅花针叩刺出血,加拔火罐。适用于寒湿腰痛和瘀血腰痛。

4 按语

针灸治疗腰痛的疗效因

with the different causes. In general, acupuncture is most effective for lumbar sprain and muscular rheumatism, next for lumbar joints disorders and poor for lumbar ligament laceration. Treatment of lumbago due to pelvic disorders and kidney disorders should aim at its causative factors. Acupuncture therapy is contraindicated for lumbago caused by spinal tuberculosis and tumors.

病因不同而有差异。对腰肌劳损及肌肉风湿疗效最好，腰椎关节病疗效较好，而对腰部韧带撕裂疗效较差。对于盆腔疾患及肾脏疾患引起的腰痛应以治疗原发病为主。因脊柱结核、肿瘤等引起的腰痛，则不属针灸治疗范围。

Bi Syndrome

Bi syndrome is characterized by obstruction of qi and blood in the meridians and collaterals caused by invasion of pathogenic wind, cold and dampness, and manifests pain, heaviness and limited movement of the muscles, tendons and joints, and even swelling and hot sensation in the joints. Bi syndrome may be seen in rheumatic arthritis, rheumatoid arthritis, osteoarthritis, fibrositis and neuralgia, etc.

痹　证

痹证是由于风、寒、湿等外邪侵袭人体，闭阻经络，气血运行不畅所导致的肌肉、筋骨、关节发生疼痛、重着、屈伸不利，甚或关节肿大灼热等为主要临床表现的病证。常见于西医学的风湿性关节炎、类风湿关节炎、骨性关节炎、纤维组织炎和神经痛等病。

1　Etiology and pathogenesis

The intrinsic causes of Bi syndrome include constitution weakness, healthy qi deficiency and defensive qi insufficiency. Bi means obstruction. Invasion of exogenous pathogenic factors may result in obstruction in the muscles, joints, meridians and collaterals. According to the feature of pathogenic factors and clinical symptoms, Bi syndrome can be subdivided into wandering (wind) Bi syndrome, painful(cold) Bi syndrome and fixed(damp) Bi syndrome and heat Bi syndrome.

1　病因病机

素体虚弱，正气不足，卫外不固，是引起痹证的内在因素。痹有闭阻不通之义。感受外邪，易使肌肉、关节、经络痹阻而成痹证。根据病邪偏胜和症状特点，分为行痹（风痹）、痛痹（寒痹）、着痹（湿痹）和热痹。

2　Syndrome differentiation

Chief symptoms: Pains of muscles and joints with

2　辨证

主症：关节肌肉疼痛、屈

limited movement.

The wandering Bi syndrome manifests migrating pain, occasionally accompanied by chills and fever, pale tongue with thin whitish coating, and floating pulse. The painful Bi syndrome manifests severe pain in the fixed sites, which is alleviated by warmth and aggravated by cold, absence of local redness and heat, thin whitish tongue coating, and wiry tight pulse. The fixed Bi syndrome manifests soreness and pain, heavy sensation, swelling or numbness of the limbs and joints, which is aggravated by, or may recur in rainy and cloudy days, whitish sticky tongue coating, and soggy moderate pulse. The heat Bi syndrome manifests heat, swelling and burning pain of one or several joints with limited movement and refusal to pressure, accompanied by thirstiness, restlessness, yellowish tongue coating, and rapid slippery pulse.

伸不利。

行痹者,疼痛游走,痛无定处,时见恶风发热,舌淡苔薄白,脉浮;痛痹者,疼痛较剧,痛有定处,遇寒痛增,得热痛减,局部无红肿热胀,苔薄白,脉弦紧;着痹者,肢体关节酸痛,重着不移,肌肤麻木不仁,阴雨天加重或发作,苔白腻,脉濡缓;热痹者,关节局部灼热红肿,痛不可触,关节活动不利,可涉及单个或多个关节,并兼有口渴烦闷、苔黄、脉滑数等症状。

3 Treatment

3.1 Essential treatment

Principal acupoints: Ashi acupoint and local acupoints.

Supplementary acupoints: In the wandering Bi syndrome, add Geshu(BL 17) and Xuehai(SP 10); in the painful Bi syndrome, add Shenshu(BL 23) and Guanyuan(CV 4); in the fixed Bi syndrome, add Yinlingquan(SP 9) and Zusanli(ST 36); in the heat Bi syndrome, add Dazhui(GV 14) and Quchi (LI 11). Other acupoints may be applied in accordance with the distribution course of meridians which pass through the diseased location.

Explanation: Ashi acupoint are used to activate qi and blood circulation in the diseased meridians and collatertals, hence the meridians are unblocked

3 治疗

3.1 基本治疗

主穴: 阿是穴;局部腧穴。

配穴: 行痹者,配膈俞、血海;痛痹者,配肾俞、关元;着痹者,配阴陵泉、足三里;热痹者,配大椎、曲池。另可根据部位循经配穴。

方义: 疼痛局部循经取穴,旨在疏通局部经络气血,经络通则痹痛遂解。风邪胜

and Bi syndrome is improved. In the wandering Bi syndrome, Geshu(BL 17) and Xuehai(SP 10) are used to activate blood flow and disperse wind. In the painful Bi syndrome, Shenshu(BL 23) and Guanyuan(CV 4) are used to strengthen yang-qi and expel coldness; in the fixed Bi syndrome, Yinlingquan(SP 9) and Zusanli(ST 36) are used to nourish the spleen and eliminate dampness; in the heat Bi syndrome, Dazhui(GV 14) and Quchi(LI 11) are used to purge heat and disperse wind, regulate qi activity and relieve swelling of the joints.

为行痹，取膈俞、血海以活血祛风。寒邪胜为痛痹，取肾俞、关元，振奋阳气而祛寒邪。湿邪胜为着痹，取阴陵泉、足三里健脾利湿。热痹取大椎、曲池泻热疏风、利气消肿。

3.2 Other therapies

Cupping: Heavy tapping with a dermal need-le on the lateral sides of the spine or on the affected joints is often performed to induce slight bleeding, followed by cupping.

Electro-acupuncture: The same acupoints as described above are needled. When qi arrives after needle insertion, electricity is applied with continuous wave or sparse-dense wave at the patients' tolerance for 20 minutes. Treatment is given once a day or once every other day, and 10 treatments make up one course.

3.2 其他治疗

拔罐：用皮肤针重叩背脊两侧和关节病痛部位，使出血少许，加拔火罐。

电针：选取上述穴位，进针得气后加脉冲电刺激，以患者能耐受为度，采用连续波或疏密波，通电时间为 20 分钟，每日或隔日 1 次，10 次为 1 个疗程。

4 Remarks

Acupuncture is quite effective against Bi syndrome. In clinical practice, rheumatic arthritis and rheumatoid arthritis should be distinguished. As for rheumatoid arthritis, comprehensive treatments should be prescribed. For the patients with Bi syndrome, attention should be paid to keeping warm in an attempt to prevent from the invasion by pathogenic wind, cold and dampness.

4 按语

针刺治疗痹证有较好疗效。临床上应注意区分风湿性关节炎与类风湿关节炎，类风湿关节炎应综合治疗。患者平时应注意关节的保暖，避免风寒湿邪的侵袭。

Wei Syndrome

Wei syndrome is a condition marked by flaccidity, muscular atrophy, motor impairment or even paralysis of the limbs. Wei syndrome is seen in infectious multiple neuritis, motor neuronopathy, myasthenia gravis, myodystrophia and traumatic peripheral nerve impairment.

痿 证

痿证是指肢体痿软无力，肌肉萎缩，甚至运动功能丧失而成瘫痪之类的病证。痿证可见于西医学的感染性多发性神经根炎、运动神经元病、重症肌无力、肌营养不良及周围神经损伤等引起的肢体瘫痪。

1 Etiology and pathogenesis

Wei syndrome primarily results from attack of dampness-heat and toxin on the basis of healthy qi deficiency, or from consumption of qi and body fluids by heat after illnesses, or from exogenous dampness which transforms into heat and thus blocks the meridians and collaterals, or from endogenous dampness and ensuing heat due to spleen-stomach deficiency which then causes loosening and flaccidity of the tendons and muscles, or from malnutrition of the tendons and muscles due to liver-kidney insufficiency and essence-blood deficiency.

1 病因病机

多由正气不足，感受湿热毒邪，或病后余热燔灼，伤津耗气。外感湿邪浸淫，郁久化热，湿热闭阻经络；脾胃虚损，湿从内生，蕴湿积热，使筋脉肌肉弛纵不收；或肝肾不足，精血亏损，筋脉失养所致。

2 Syndrome differentiation

Chief symptoms: Weakness, muscular flaccidity or atrophy or paralysis of the limbs.

The syndrome of consumption of body fluids by lung heat manifests fever with perspiration, sudden onset of flaccid limbs after the fever has been subsided, vexation, thirst, yellow urine, red tongue with yellowish coating, and wiry rapid pulse. The syndrome of dampness-heat accumulation manifests progressive flaccid limbs, especially in the lower limbs, hot sensation in the affected limbs, dark urine, red tongue with yellowish sticky coating, and

2 辨证

主症：肢体软弱无力，肌肉弛缓，甚则萎缩或瘫痪。

肺热津伤者，兼发热多汗、热退后突然出现肢体软弱无力，心烦口渴，小便短黄，舌红，苔黄，脉细数；湿热浸淫者，兼肢体逐渐痿软无力、下肢为重，足胫热感，小便赤涩，舌红，苔黄腻，脉濡数；脾胃虚弱者，兼肢体痿软无力日久、食少纳呆、腹胀便

soggy rapid pulse. The syndrome of spleen-stomach deficiency manifests lingering limb flaccidity, poor appetite, abdominal fullness, loose stools, sallow complexion, pale tongue with whitish coating, and thready moderate pulse. The syndrome of liver-kidney insufficiency manifests limb flaccidity and muscular atrophy after prolonged illness, soreness and weakness in the loins and knees, tinnitus, dizziness, red tongue with less coating, and thready rapid pulse.

溏、面色少华、舌淡、苔白、脉细缓；肝肾亏虚者，兼病久肢体痿软不用、肌肉萎缩、腰膝酸软、头晕耳鸣、舌红绛、少苔、脉细数。

3 Treatment

3 治疗

3.1 Essential treatment

3.1 基本治疗

Principal acupoints: Upper limbs: Jianyu (LI 15), Quchi(LI 11), Hegu(LI 4) and Jiaji(EX-B 2) in the neck and chest.

主穴：上肢：肩髃，曲池，合谷，颈胸部夹脊穴。

Lower limbs: Biguan(ST 31), Fengshi(GB 31), Zusanli(ST 36), Yanglingquan(GB 34), Sanyinjiao (SP 6), and Jiaji(EX-B 2) in the lumbar region.

下肢：髀关，风市，足三里，阳陵泉，三阴交，腰部夹脊穴。

Supplementary acupoints: In the syndrome of consumption of body fluids by lung heat, add Chize (LU 5) and Feishu(BL 13); in the syndrome of dampness-heat accumulation, add Yinlingquan(SP 9) and Dazhui(GV 14); in the syndrome of spleen-stomach deficiency, add Pishu(BL 20), Weishu(BL 21) and Zhongwan(CV 12); in the syndrome of liver-kidney insufficiency, add Ganshu(BL 18) and Shenshu(BL 23).

配穴：肺热津伤者，配尺泽、肺俞；湿热浸淫者，配阴陵泉、大椎；脾胃虚弱者，配脾俞、胃俞、中脘；肝肾不足者，配肝俞、肾俞。

Explanation: The key to the treatment of Wei syndrome is to regulate the yangming meridian, tonify qi and blood, unblock the tendons and collaterals. In the light of the therapeutic principle of Su Wen that "Flaccidity condition should be treated by needling acupoints of the foot-yangming meridian", therefore, the acupoints of the yangming meridians

方义：治痿证重在调理阳明，补益气血，疏筋通络。根据《素问·痿论》"治痿独取阳明"的治疗原则，主要取上下肢阳明经穴位。夹脊穴为督脉之旁络，可调阴阳、行气血。

in the upper and lower limbs are used. Jiaji acupoints(EX-B 2), located laterally to the governor vessel, act to harmonize yin and yang, and activate qi and blood circulation.

3.2 Other therapies

Dermal needle therapy: Tap the acupoints above mentioned. The acupoints around the diseased areas should be tapped repeatedly till the diseased areas become hot or flushed. The treatment is given once every other day.

Electro-acupuncture: Needle the acupoints around the affected areas. When qi arrives, electricity is applied with an intermittent wave at the patients' tolerance. The treatment is given once a day and the needles are retained for 30 minutes each time. Ten treatments make up one course.

4 Remarks

Wei syndrome responds well to acupuncture treatment but may require long-term treatment since its long duration. Combination of acupuncture with such therapies as medications, massage and physiotherapy can enhance the clinical efficacy.

3.2 其他治疗

皮肤针: 叩刺上述穴位。病变部位腧穴需反复叩刺，以局部微热或充血为度，隔日1次。

电针: 在瘫痪肌肉处选取穴位，针刺得气后加脉冲电刺激，采用断续波，以患者能耐受为度，每日1次，每次留针30分钟，10次为1个疗程。

4 按语

针刺治疗痿证有较好的疗效。但本病疗程较长，须坚持治疗。同时可配合药物、推拿、理疗等以提高疗效。

Urinary retention

Urinary retention is a disorder which manifests difficulty in urination, dribbling urine, and even blockage of urine. It is frequently seen in organic and functional disorders in the urinary bladder, urethra and prostate gland.

1 Etiology and pathogenesis

Urinary retention results from accumulation of dampness-heat in the bladder, or from potent heat

癃 闭

癃闭是指排尿困难，点滴而下，甚至小便闭塞不通为主的疾患。癃闭可见于西医学的膀胱、尿道器质性和功能性病变及前列腺疾患等所造成的排尿困难和尿潴留。

1 病因病机

本病由膀胱湿热互结，或肺热壅盛，津液输布失常，

in the lungs failing to distribute body fluids, or from post-traumatic blood-stasis influencing the qi activity in the bladder, or from spleen-qi deficiency, or from insufficient kidney-yang failing to warm and activate yang-qi in the bladder.

或跌仆损伤，瘀滞经脉，影响膀胱气化而致小便不通；脾虚气弱，或命门火衰，不能温煦鼓舞膀胱气化，使膀胱气化无权，形成癃闭。

2 Syndrome differentiation

2 辨证

2.1 Excess syndrome

2.1 实证

Chief symptoms: Acute onset of urinary retention with severe pain in the lower abdomen.

主症：小便闭塞不通，小腹急痛，发病急。

The syndrome of dampness-heat accumulation in the bladder manifests scanty urine, difficult urination, or even dribbling urine or urinary retention, abdominal fullness, accompanied by bitter taste and stickiness in the mouth, thirst but without a desire to drink, slowed bowel movement, red tongue with yellowish greasy coating, and deep rapid pulse. The syndrome of lung heat manifests shortness of breath, dry throat, cough, red tongue with yellowish coating, and rapid pulse. The syndrome of liver-qi stagnation manifests urinary difficulty, distension and urgency in the lower abdomen, accompanied by bitter taste in the mouth, restlessness, irritability, distension and fullness in the hypochondriac region, red tongue with yellowish coating, and wiry pulse. The syndrome of post-traumatic blood-stasis manifests the history of traumatic injury, fullness and pain in the lower abdomen, purplish tongue and rough pulse.

湿热内蕴者，小便量少难出，严重时点滴不出，小腹胀满，兼口苦口黏、口渴不欲饮、大便不畅、舌红、苔黄腻、脉沉数；肺热壅盛者，兼呼吸急促、咽干、咳嗽、舌红苔黄、脉数；肝郁气滞者，小便不通或通而不畅，小腹胀急，兼口苦、多烦善怒、胁腹胀满、舌红、苔黄、脉弦；外伤血瘀者，兼有外伤或损伤病史、小腹满痛、舌紫暗、脉涩。

2.2 Deficiency syndrome

2.2 虚证

Chief symptoms: Chronic onset of dribbling urine and feeble urination.

主症：小便滴沥不爽，排出无力，发病缓。

The syndrome of spleen-qi deficiency manifests shortness of breath, poor appetite, sinking distention in the lower abdomen, pale tongue with whitish

脾虚气弱者，兼气短纳差、小腹坠胀、舌淡苔白、脉细弱；肾阳虚者，兼面色㿠白、

coating, and weak thready pulse. The syndrome kidney-yang deficiency manifests sallow comple-xion, listlessness, aching loins and knees, pale tongue with whitish coating, and deep, weak and thready pulse.

3 Treatment

3.1 Essential treatment

3.1.1 Excess syndrome

Principal acupoints: Zhibian(BL 54), Yinlingquan(SP 9), Sanyinjiao(SP 6), Zhongji(CV 3) and Pangguanshu(BL 28).

Supplementary acupoints: In the syndrome of dampness-heat accumulation, add Weiyang(BL 39); in the syndrome of lung heat, add Chize(LU 5); in the syndrome of liver-qi stagnation, add Taichong (LR 3) and Dadun(LR 1); in the syndrome of blood-stasis, add Qugu(CV 2), Ciliao(BL 32) and Xuehai(SP 10).

Explanation: Zhibian(BL 54), an acupoint of the bladder meridian, can restore the qi activity of the bladder. Yinlingquan(SP 9) functions to clear heat and disinhibit dampness to promote urination. Sanyinjiao(SP 6) can harmonize qi and blood of the three yin meridians of the foot to eliminate blood-stasis. Zhongji(CV 3), the Front-Mu acupoint of the bladder, and Pangguangshu(BL 28), the Back-Shu acupoint of the bladder, can improve qi activity of the bladder.

3.1.2 Deficiency syndrome

Principal acupoints: Zhibian(BL 54), Guanyuan (CV 4), Pishu(BL 20), Sanjiaoshu(BL 22) and Shenshu(BL 23).

Supplementary acupoints: In the syndrome of qi deficiency of the middle energizer, add Qihai(CV 6) and Zusanli(ST 36); in the syndrome of kidney-

神气虚弱、腰膝酸软、舌淡苔白、脉沉细无力。

3 治疗

3.1 基本治疗

3.1.1 实证

主穴：秩边，阴陵泉，三阴交，中极，膀胱俞。

配穴：湿热内蕴者，加委阳；邪热壅肺者，加尺泽；肝郁气滞者，加太冲、大敦；瘀血阻滞者，加曲骨、次髎、血海。

方义：秩边为膀胱经穴，可疏导膀胱气机。阴陵泉清热利湿而通小便。三阴交通调足三阴经气血，消除瘀滞。中极为膀胱募穴，配膀胱之背俞穴，俞募相配，促进气化。

3.1.2 虚证

主穴：秩边，关元，脾俞，三焦俞，肾俞。

配穴：中气不足者，加气海、足三里；肾气亏虚者，加太溪、复溜；无尿意或无力排

qi deficiency, add Taixi(KI 3) and Fuliu(KI 7); in the case of no desire to urination or feeble urination, add Qihai(CV 6) and Qugu(CV 2).

尿者,加气海、曲骨。

Explanation: Zhibian(BL 54), an acupoint of the bladder meridian, can restore the qi activity of the bladder. Guanyuan(CV 4), the Crossing acupoint of the conception vessel and the three yin meridians of the foot, acts to warm and tonify the lower energizer and improve qi activity of the bladder. Pishu(BL 20) and Shenshu(BL 23) function to nourish the spleen and kidneys. Sanjiaoshu(BL 22) can harmonize the triple energizer to improve qi activity of the bladder.

方义: 秩边为膀胱经穴,可疏导膀胱气机。关元为任脉与足三阴经交会穴,能温补下元,鼓舞膀胱气化。脾俞、肾俞补益脾肾。三焦俞通调三焦,促进膀胱气化功能。

3.2 Other therapy

3.2 其他治疗

Ear acupuncture: Select 3 to 5 acupoints from Kidney(CO 10), Bladder(CO 9), Lung(CO 14), Liver(CO 12), Spleen(CO 13), Triple Energizer (CO 17), Sympathesis(AH 6a), Shenmen(TF 4), Subcortex(AT 4), and Lumbosacral Vertebrae(AH 9). Needle these acupoints with filiform needles by moderate intensity, or embed intradermal needles or apply *Semen Vaccariae* (Wang Bu Liu Xing)at these acupoints.

耳针: 选肾、膀胱、肺、肝、脾、三焦、交感、神门、皮质下、腰骶椎。每次选3～5穴,毫针中强刺激,亦可用皮内针埋藏或用王不留行贴压。

4 Remarks

4 按语

Acupuncture therapy is quite effective for urinary retention, especially for that due to functional causes. Acupuncture treatment can prevent from pains of urine drainage and urinary infections. When the bladder is full, the acupoints on the lower abdomen should be punctured obliquely or transversely.

针灸治疗癃闭有一定效果,可以避免导尿的痛苦和泌尿道感染,尤其是对于功能性尿潴留,疗效更好。膀胱过度充盈时,下腹部穴位应斜刺或平刺。

Appendix 1 Prostatic Hyperplasia

[附1] 前列腺增生症

Prostatic hyperplasia, also known as enlargement of the prostate gland, is characterized by uri-

前列腺增生症亦称前列腺肥大。主要特征是尿潴留

nary retention or difficulty in urination. It is one of the most common conditions in senile men, especially those aged between 50 and 70 years. With the increasing growth of the average life-span in China, the morbidity of prostatic hyperplasia also increases.

和排尿困难。为常见的男性老年病之一，大多数发生在50～70岁之间，近年由于我国平均寿命延长，本病的发病率亦随之增加。

Prostatic hyperplasia belongs to the category of "urinary retention" in Chinese medicine, and is caused by kidney-qi deficiency or liver-qi stagnation.

本病属于中医学"癃闭"范畴。可因肾元亏虚，肝郁气滞致排尿困难或不畅。

1 Clinical manifestation

The syndrome of dampness-heat in the bladder manifests dribbling urination, or scanty hot urine, distension and fullness in the lower abdomen, bitter taste and stickiness in the mouth, red tongue with yellowish greasy coating, and rapid pulse. The syndrome of kidney-qi deficiency manifests dribbling urination, feeble urination, even blockage of urine, pale complexion, soreness and weakness in the loins and knees, pale tongue and deep thready pulse. The syndrome of hyperactive fire due to yin deficiency manifests the desire but inability to urination, dry throat, vexation, heat sensation in the palms and soles, red tongue with less coating, and thready rapid pulse.

1 临床表现

膀胱湿热者，小便点滴不通，或量少而灼热，小腹胀满，口苦口黏，舌质红，苔黄腻，脉数；肾气不足者，小便淋沥不爽，排出无力，甚则点滴不通，面色㿠白，腰膝酸软，舌质淡，脉沉细；阴虚火旺者，时欲小便不得尿，咽干，心烦，手足心热，舌红少苔，脉细数。

2 Treatment

Principal acupoints: Qihai(CV 6), Zhongji(CV 3), Zhibian(BL 54) penetrating to Shuidao(ST 28), Huiyin(CV 1), Sanyinjiao(SP 6), and Lieque(LU 7).

2 治疗

主穴：气海，中极，秩边透水道，会阴，三阴交，列缺。

Supplementary acupoints: In the syndrome of dampness-heat in the bladder, add Yinlingquan(SP 9), Taichong(LR 3), Jinmen(BL 63) and Feiyang (BL 58); in the syndrome of kidney-qi deficiency, add Sanjiaoshu(BL 22) and Weiyang(BL 39); in the

配穴：膀胱湿热加阴陵泉、太冲、金门、飞扬；肾气不足加三焦俞、委阳；阴虚火旺加巨阙、太溪、神门。

syndrome of hyperactive fire due to yin deficiency, add Juque(CV 14), Taixi(KI 3) and Shenmen(HT 7).

In addition, auricular acupuncture and dermal needling therapy can be applied to treat prostatic hyperplasia.

此外，本病还可选择耳针、皮肤针等方法进行治疗。

3　Remarks

Acupuncture is effective for chronic prostatic hyperplasia. When the bladder is full, the acupoints in the lower abdomen should be punctured shallowly or obliquely to avoid injuring the bladder.

3　按语

针灸治疗慢性前列腺肥大有一定效果。膀胱充盈时，下腹部穴位宜浅刺、斜刺。

Appendix 2　Chronic Prostaitis

Chronic prostatitis is one of the most common urological disorders in men aged between 20 to 50 years. It can be divided into bacterial prostatitis and non-bacterial prostatitis. In Chinese medicine, there is no such term as "chronic prostatitis", but it falls into the categories of "stranguria" or "urinary retention" according to its symptoms and signs. This condition may be caused by indulgence in sexual activities, postponing ejaculation, as well as excessive intake of alcohol or fatty diets.

[附 2]　慢性前列腺炎

慢性前列腺炎是泌尿生殖系统最常见的疾病之一，发病年龄在 20～50 岁之间，本病可分为细菌性和无菌性前列腺炎两种。中医学无此病名，根据症状，可归属于"淋浊""癃闭"范畴。本病多因房劳不节，忍精不泄或嗜酒和过食肥甘而发病。

1　Clinical manifestation

Chief symptoms: Turbid urine or incontinent discharge of urine, frequent and urgent urination with burning sensation, dribbling or difficulty in urination, and sexual dysfunction.

1　临床表现

主症：尿道滴白或遗尿，尿频、尿急、尿道灼热，有时有排尿困难，性功能障碍。

The syndrome of spleen-kidney deficiency may be accompanied by difficult bowel movements, soreness and weakness of the lower back and knees, shortness of breath, fatigue, and weak pulse. The syndrome of dampness-heat accumulation may be accompanied by fever, lumbar soreness, pain and distension in the genital area, and wiry rapid pulse.

脾肾虚弱者，兼大便不畅，伴有腰膝酸软、气短体倦、脉多虚弱；湿热蕴结者，兼发热腰酸、下阴胀痛，脉多弦数。

2 Treatment

Principal acupoints: Qihai(CV 6), Guanyuan (CV 4), Taixi(KI 3), Zhongji(CV 3), Yinlingquan (SP 9), Sanyinjiao(Sp 6) and Huiyin (CV 1).

Supplementary acupoints: In the excess syndrome, add Sanjiaoshu(BL 22) and Weiyang(BL 39); in the deficiency syndrome, add Pishu(BL 20) and Shenshu(BL 23). Besides, local hot compress or moxibustion can help improve the clinical symptoms.

3 Remarks

Chronic prostatitis is an intractable disease and does not respond well to drug therapy because of its anatomical structure. Acupuncture has positive effects on chronic prostatitis but requires a long-term treatment.

2 治疗

取穴：气海，关元，太溪，中极，阴陵泉，三阴交，会阴。

配穴：实证加三焦俞、委阳；虚证加脾俞、肾俞。可配合局部热敷或用艾灸，有助于改善症状。

3 按语

前列腺炎是一种较顽固的疾病，由于其病变部位特殊，药物治疗效果不显著。针灸治疗本病有肯定的效果，但需要长期坚持治疗。

Impotence

Impotence refers to inability to engage in sexual intercourse because of inability to have an adequate strong erection in young men, and chiefly results from kidney deficiency, fright or downward accumulation of dampness heat, which cause loosening or flaccidity of penis muscles. In Western medicine, the treatment of impotence in sex neuroasthenia and some chronic diseases can refer to following therapies.

1 Etiology and pathogenesis

Impotence can result from over-indulgence in sexual intercourse, or from frequent masturbation which consumes kidney essence and declines kidney-fire, or from anxiety and emotional depression which impairs the heart and spleen, or from fright impairing kidneys which causes qi-blood deficiency and malnutrition of penis tendons.

阳 痿

阳痿是指青壮年时期，由于虚损、惊恐或湿热等原因，使宗筋失养而弛纵，引起阴茎痿弱不起，临房举而不坚的病证。西医学的性神经衰弱和某些慢性疾病表现以阳痿为主者，可参考本篇施治。

1 病因病机

房劳纵欲过度，或久犯手淫，以致精气虚损，命门火衰；思虑忧郁，伤及心脾；惊恐伤肾，使气血不足，宗筋失养。

2 Syndrome differentiation

Chief symptoms: Inability to have a strong erection, which affects sexual intercourse.

The deficiency syndrome manifests occasional seminal emission, dizziness, tinnitus, palpitations, shortness of breath, aching and weak lower back, aversion to coldness and cold extremities, pale tongue and weak thready pulse. The excess syndrome manifests inadequate erection of short duration, premature emission, damp scrotum with foul odor, dark yellowish urine, yellow greasy coating, and soggy rapid pulse.

2 辨证

主症：阳事不举，不能进行正常性生活。

虚证者，时有滑精，头晕耳鸣，心悸气短，腰酸乏力，畏寒肢冷，舌淡白，脉细弱；实证者，阴茎勃起不坚，时间短暂，每多早泄，阴囊潮湿、臊臭，小便黄赤，舌苔黄腻，脉濡数。

3 Treatment

3.1 Essential treatment

Principal acupoints: Guanyuan(CV 4), Sanyinjiao(SP 6) and Shenshu(BL 23).

Supplementary acupoints: In the syndrome of kidney-yang deficiency, add Mingmen(GV 4); in the syndrome of kidney-yin deficiency, add Taixi (KI 3) and Fuliu(KI 7); in the syndrome of heart-spleen insufficiency, add Xinshu(BL 15), Pishu(BL 20) and Zusanli(ST 36); in the case of fright impairing kidneys, add Zhishi(BL 52) and Danshu(BL 19); in the syndrome of downward dampness-heat, add Huiyin(CV 1) and Yinlingquan(SP 9); in the syndrome of qi stagnation and blood-stasis, add Taichong(LR 3), Xuehai(SP 10) and Geshu(BL 17). In the presence of insomnia or sleepiness, add Neiguan(PC 6), Shenmen(HT 7) and Xinshu(BL 15); in the presence of poor appetite, add Zhongwan(CV 12) and Zusanli(ST 36); in the presence of aching loins, add Mingmen (GV 4) and Yanglingquan(GB 34).

Explanation: Impotence is caused by kidney de-

3 治疗

3.1 基本治疗

主穴：关元，三阴交，肾俞。

配穴：肾阳不足者，加命门；肾阴亏虚者，加太溪、复溜；心脾两虚者，加心俞、脾俞、足三里；惊恐伤肾者，加志室、胆俞；湿热下注者，加会阴、阴陵泉；气滞血瘀者，加太冲、血海、膈俞；失眠或多梦者，加内关、神门、心俞；食欲不振者，加中脘、足三里；腰膝酸软者，加命门、阳陵泉。

方义：本病为肾气虚衰，

ficiency, which fails to nourish the penis muscles and give rise to inadequate erection. Guanyuan(CV 4), where original qi is stored, acts to enrich the original qi and restore the functions of the kidneys. Sanyinjiao(SP 6), a Crossing acupoint of the three foot yin meridians, functions to invigorate the liver, kidney and spleen. Shenshu(BL 23) is used to tonify the kidney-qi.

肾虚宗筋弛缓,阳事不举。关元为元气所居之处,补之使真元得充,恢复肾之作强功能。三阴交为足三阴经交会穴,补益肝肾、健运脾土。肾俞培补肾气。

3.2 Other therapy

Ear acupuncture: Select 3 to 5 acupoints from Kidney(CO 10), Liver(CO 12), Spleen(CO 13), Heart(CO 15), External Genitals(HX 4), Shenmen (TF 4), Endocrine (CO 18) and Subcortex(AT 4). Puncture these acupoints with filiform needles by mild stimulation, once a day or once every other day. These acupoints can also be treated by embedding dermal needles or applying *Semen Vaccaeiae* (Wang Bu Liu Xing).

3.2 其他治疗

耳针: 选肾、肝、心、脾、外生殖器、神门、内分泌、皮质下。每次选3~5穴,针刺施以弱刺激,每日或隔日1次。亦可用耳穴埋针或王不留行贴压。

4 Remarks

Acupuncture therapy works well on primary impotence. As for secondary impotence, it is advisable to treat the underlying diseases. Psychological treatment can be prescribed to soothe the emotion and relieve emotional distress.

4 按语

针灸对原发性阳痿可获满意疗效,对继发性者,应治疗原发病。配合心理治疗,予以精神疏导,消除其紧张心理。

Appendix Sexual Dysfunction

Sexual dysfunction refers to the condition in which sexual intercourse cannot be achieved due to inability to have erection, sexual intercourse and seminal emission in men, and frigidity in women.

[附] 性功能障碍

性功能障碍指男子阴茎勃起、性交、射精或女子性冷淡等性功能障碍,以至于不能进行或无法完成正常性交过程的病证。

1 Clinical manifestation

Chief symptoms Decline or absence of sexual desire, impotence, premature emission or absence of ejaculation.

1 临床表现

主症:性欲低下或无性欲,男子阳痿、早泄、不射精。

The syndrome of kidney-yang deficiency manifests an inability to gain firm erection or premature ejaculation and frequent seminal emission in men, scanty menses and irregular menstruation in women, accompanied by dizziness, soreness and weakness in the loins and knees, cold extremities, pale complexion, pale tongue with whitish coating, and weak, deep and thready pulse. The syndrome of heart-spleen deficiency manifests seminal emission, impotence and premature ejaculation in men, and diminished sexual desire, scanty and light-colored menses in women, accompanied by poor appetite, sallow complexion, pale tongue with whitish coating, and weak thready pulse. The syndrome of fright impairing kidney manifests impotence and premature ejaculation due to excitation, irritability and nervousness in men, and aversion to contact with men partner in women, accompanied by timidness with skepticism, palpitations and irritability, insomnia and sleepiness, thin greasy tongue coating, and thready wiry pulse. The syndrome of downward dampness-heat may manifest impotence, premature ejaculation, seminal emission, accompanied by genital dampness and itchiness, hot sore and heavy sensation in the lower extremities, hot and dark-colored urine, yellow greasy tongue coating, and deep slippery pulse. The syndrome of liver-qi stagnation manifests impotence and absence of ejaculation in men, and irregular menstruation or amenorrhea, and pain and distension in the breasts in women, accompanied by emotional depression, restlessness, irritability, dark tongue and wiry thready pulse.

肾阳不足者，男子临房阴茎不举或早泄、平时有遗精，女子月经稀少、月经不调，兼头晕目眩、腰膝酸软、四肢不温、面色淡白，舌淡，舌苔白，脉沉细而弱；心脾两虚者，男子遗精、阳痿、早泄，女子性欲淡漠、月经稀少色淡，兼胃纳不佳、面色无华，舌淡，苔白，脉细弱无力；惊恐伤肾者，男子常因过于兴奋、激动、紧张以致阳痿、早泄，女子则恐惧异性接触（恐异症），平时胆怯多疑、心悸易惊、失眠多梦，苔薄腻，脉弦细；湿热下注者，男子阳痿、早泄、遗精，兼外阴潮湿、瘙痒，下肢灼热酸沉，小便赤热，苔黄腻，脉沉滑；肝郁气滞者，男子阳痿、不射精，女子经行不畅或闭经、乳房胀痛，兼情志抑郁不舒、心烦易怒，舌质暗淡，脉弦细。

2 Treatment

Principal acupoints: Guanyuan (CV 4), Qihai

2 治疗

主穴：关元，气海，肾俞，

(CV 6), Shenshu(BL 23), Ciliao(BL 32), Zhibian (BL 54) and Sanyinjiao(SP 6).

次髎,秩边,三阴交。

Supplementary acupoints: In the syndrome of kidney-yang deficiency, add Mingmen(GV 4) and Zusanli(ST 36); in the syndrome of heart-spleen deficiency, add Xinshu(BL 15) and Pishu(BL 20); in the syndrome of fright impairing kidney, add Xinshu(BL 15), Danshu(BL 19) and Shenmen(HT 7); in the syndrome of downward dampness-heat, add Qugu(CV 2) and Yinlingquan(SP 9); in the syndrome of liver-qi stagnation, add Taichong(LR 3) and Hegu(LI 4).

配穴:肾阳不足加命门、足三里;心脾两虚加心俞、脾俞;惊恐伤肾加心俞、胆俞、神门;湿热下注加曲骨、阴陵泉;肝郁气滞加太冲、合谷。

3 Remarks

Acupuncture therapy is quite effective against sexual dysfunction, especially against diminished sexual ability due to psychological problems. Combined use of acupuncture and psychological therapy can cure sexual dysfunction. Acupuncture has poor effects on male sexual dysfunction due to organic diseases, so it is necessary to treat the causative factors.

3 按语

针灸治疗本病有较满意的疗效,尤其对精神因素引起的性功能低下有显著的疗效,坚持针灸并配合心理治疗,往往可获痊愈。对由器质性病变引起的男性性功能低下则疗效欠佳,需要同时治疗原发病。

Section 2 Gynecological and Pediatric Diseases

第2节 妇儿科病证

Irregular Menstruation

Irregular menstruation refers to any abnormal change in the menstrual cycle, volume and color of the menses, or any other accompanying symptoms. Irregular menstruation can be classified into advanced menstruation(early periods), delayed menstruation(late periods) and undue menstruation(ir-

月经不调

月经不调是指月经周期、经色、经量、经质等出现异常改变,并伴有其他症状的疾病。月经不调可分为月经先期(经早)、月经后期(经迟)、月经先后无定期(经

regular periods). In Western medicine, the dynamic relationship between the hypothalamus, pituitary and ovary is disturbed, then irregular menstruation results.

乱)。西医认为,如下丘脑-垂体-卵巢三者之间的动态关系失于平衡,则致其功能失常而产生月经不调。

1 Etiology and pathogenesis

Irregular menstruation results from constitutional yang hyperactivity and spicy diets which causes heat accumulation in the thoroughfare vessel and conception vessel, or from emotional depression which transforms into fire and then disturbs the blood vessels, or from endogenous yin-deficiency heat following long-term diseases which disturbs the thoroughfare vessel and conception vessels, or from improper diets and excessive exertion and thinking which injure the spleen failing to control the blood and secure the thoroughfare vessel and conception vessel; all these causes lead to advanced menstruation. Irregular menstruation may also result from contraction of exogenous cold which coagulates the blood, or from yang-deficiency following prolonged diseases which influences blood flow, or from yin-blood deficiency after long-term illnesses, or from improper diets, over-exertion, and over-thinking injures the spleen which fails to produce qi and blood; all these causes lead to delayed menstruation. Irregular menstruation may also result from emotional depression which causes liver-qi stagnation and blood-stasis, or from deficiency kidney-qi failing to store essence and dysfunction of the thoroughfare vessel and conception vessel; all these causes may lead to undue menstruation.

1 病因病机

素体阳盛,过食辛辣,热伏冲任;或情志抑郁,肝郁化火,热扰血海;或久病阴亏,阴虚内热,热扰冲任;或饮食不节,劳倦过度,思虑伤脾,因而统摄无权,冲任不固,可致月经先期。外感寒邪,血为寒凝,或久病伤阳,影响血运,或久病体虚,阴血亏损,或饮食劳倦,思虑伤脾,化源不足,可致月经后期。因情志抑郁,肝气不疏,血为气滞,或肾气亏虚,失其封藏,冲任失调,以致血海溢蓄失常而致月经先后无定期。

2 Syndrome differentiation

2.1 Advanced menstruation

Chief symptoms: Menstruation 7 days or even 10

2 辨证

2.1 月经先期

主症:月经周期提前 7

days earlier than the due date.

日以上,甚至 10 日以上。

The syndrome of excess heat manifests profuse menses with dark red or purple color, stickiness, accompanied by flushed face, dry mouth, vexation heat in the chest, scanty dark urine, dry stools, red tongue with yellowish coating, and rapid pulse. The syndrome of deficiency heat manifests scanty or profuse menses, red color and stickiness, accompanied by flushed cheeks, feverishness in palms and soles, red tongue with less coating, and rapid and thready pulse. The syndrome of qi deficiency manifests profuse thin light-colored menses, listlessness, lassitude, palpitations and shortness of breath, pale tongue and weak thready pulse.

实热者,月经量多,色深红或紫,质黏稠,兼面红口干,心胸烦热,小便短赤,大便干燥,舌红苔黄,脉数;虚热者,月经量少或量多,色红质稠,兼两颧潮红,手足心热,舌红苔少,脉细数;气虚者,月经量多,色淡质稀,兼神疲肢倦、心悸气短、纳少便溏、舌淡、脉细弱。

2.2 Delayed menstruation

Chief symptoms: Menstruation 7 days later than the due date, or even once 40 ~ 50 days.

The syndrome of excess cold manifests dark scanty menses with clots, accompanied by cold pain in the lower abdomen which is alleviated by warmth, cold limbs and aversion to cold, thin whitish tongue coating, and deep tight pulse. The syndrome of deficiency cold manifests late menstruation, scanty light and thin menses, accompanied by dull pain in the lower abdomen, preference for warmth and pressure, pale tongue with whitish coating, and deep slow pulse.

2.2 月经后期

主症:月经推迟 7 日以上,甚至 40~50 日一潮。

寒实者,月经量少色暗,有血块,兼小腹冷痛、得热则减,畏寒肢冷,苔薄白,脉沉紧;虚寒者,月经周期延后,月经色淡而质稀、量少,兼小腹隐隐作痛、喜暖喜按,舌淡苔白,脉沉迟。

2.3 Undue menstruation

Chief symptoms: Menstruation 1 to 2 weeks earlier or later over consecutive two menstrual cycles, with a profuse or scanty menses.

The syndrome of liver stagnation manifests profuse or scanty dark menses with clots, unsmooth menstrual flow, accompanied by distension in the

2.3 月经先后无定期

主症:月经或提前或错后 1~2 周,连续 2 个月经周期以上,经量或多或少。

肝郁者,月经量或多或少,经色紫暗,有块,经行不畅,兼胸胁乳房作胀、少腹胀

hypochondriac regions and breasts, distending fullness in the lower abdomen, frequent sighing, belching, thin whitish tongue coating, and wiry pulse. The syndrome of kidney deficiency manifests scanty, light-colored menses, accompanied by aching waist and knees, dizziness and tinnitus, pale tongue with whitish coating, and deep weak pulse.

痛、时叹息、嗳气不舒、苔薄白、脉弦；肾虚者，经来先后不定，量少，色淡，兼腰骶酸痛、头晕耳鸣、舌淡苔白、脉沉弱。

3 Treatment

3 治疗

3.1 Essential treatment

3.1 基本治疗

3.1.1 Advanced menstruation

3.1.1 月经先期

Principal acupoints: Guanyuan(CV 4), Sanyinjiao(SP 6), and Xuehai(SP 10).

主穴：关元，三阴交，血海。

Supplementary acupoints: In the syndrome of excess heat, add Taichong(LR 3) or Xingjian(LR 2) and Qimen(LR 14); in the syndrome of deficiency heat, add Taixi(KI 3); in the syndrome of qi deficiency, add Zusanli(ST 36) and Pishu(BL 20). In the presence of profuse menses, add Yinbai(SP 1); in the presence of lumbosacral pain, add Shenshu (BL 23) and Ciliao(BL 32); in the presence of restlessness, add Shenmen(HT 7).

配穴：实热证加太冲或行间、期门；虚热证加太溪；气虚证加足三里、脾俞。月经过多加隐白；腰骶疼痛加肾俞、次髎；心烦加神门。

Explanation: Guanyuan(CV 4) is applied to regulate the thoroughfare vessel and conception vessel. Sanyinjiao(SP 6), a key acupoint to regulate menstruation, acts to regulate the liver, spleen and kidney; Xuehai(SP 10) is used to clear blood heat.

方义：关元调理冲任，三阴交调理肝脾肾，为调经要穴，血海清泻血分之热。

3.1.2 Delayed menstruation

3.1.2 月经后期

Principal acupoints: Qihai (CV 6) and Sanyinjiao(SP 6).

主穴：气海，三阴交。

Supplementary acupoints: In the syndrome of excess cold, add Zigong(EX-CA 1), Tianshu(ST 25) and Diji(SP 8); in the syndrome of deficiency cold, add Mingmen(GV 4), Yaoyangguan(GV 3), Guanyuan(CV 4) and Guilai(ST 29).

配穴：寒实证加子宫、天枢、地机；虚寒证加命门、腰阳关、关元、归来。

Explanation: Qihai(CV 6) acts to enrich qi and warm yang, with moxibustion to warm meri-dians and dispel cold; Sanyinjiao(SP 6), the Crossing acupoint of the liver, spleen and kidney meridians, functions to supplement qi of the liver, spleen and kidney meridians, and hence to harmonize blood and regulate menstruation.

方义：气海可益气温阳，温灸更可温经散寒；三阴交为肝脾肾三经交会穴，可调补三阴经经气，从而和血调经。

3.1.3 Undue menstruation

3.1.3 月经先后无定期

Principal acupoints: Guanyuan(CV 4), Sanyinjiao(SP 10), and Ganshu(BL 18).

主穴：关元，三阴交，肝俞。

Supplementary acupoints: In the syndrome of liver stagnation, add Qimen(LR 14) and Taichong (LR 3); in the syndrome of kidney deficiency, add Shenshu(BL 23) and Taixi(KI 3); in the case of distension and pain in the chest and hypochondriac regions, add Zhigou(TE 6), Neiguan(PC 6) and Yanglingquan(GB 34); in the case of lumbosacral pain, add Ciliao(BL 32).

配穴：肝郁加期门、太冲；肾虚加肾俞、太溪；胸胁胀痛加支沟、内关、阳陵泉；腰骶疼痛加次髎；肾虚证加肾俞、太溪。

Explanation: Guanyuan(CV 4) functions to nourish the kidney and replenish the original qi, and regulate the thoroughfare vessel and conception vessel. Sanyinjiao(SP 6) can nourish the spleen and stomach, benefit the liver and kidney, and re-gulate qi and blood. Ganshu(BL 18), the Back-Shu acupoint of the liver, functions to soothe the liver qi. The combined use of these three points may regulate menstrual flow.

方义：关元补肾培元，通调冲任。三阴交补脾胃、益肝肾、调气血。肝俞乃肝之背俞穴，有疏肝理气之作用。三穴共用可调理经血。

3.2 Other therapy

3.2 其他治疗

Ear acupuncture: Select 2 to 4 acupoints from Subcortex(AT 4), Internal Genitals(TF 2), Endocrine(CO 18), Kidney(CO 10), Liver(CO 12), and Spleen(CO 13). Puncture these acupoints with filiform needles by moderate intensity; the treatment is given once a day and the needles are retained for 20

耳针：选皮质下、内生殖器、内分泌、肾、肝、脾。每次选 2～4 穴，毫针刺用捻转法，中等强度刺激，每日 1 次，每次留针 20 分钟。也可用揿针埋藏或用王不留行贴

minutes. Or embed intradermal needles or apply *Semen Vaccariae* (Wang Bu Liu Xing) at these acupoints.

压。

4 Remarks

Usually, acupuncture treatment for this disease starts 5～7 days prior to menstruation, and the same treatment is given at about the same time before the next menstruation; this treatment should be applied for successive 3～5 months till it is resolved. Irregular menstruation caused by organic disorders of the reproductive system need comprehensive treatments as early as possible.

Pay attention to personal hygiene during menstruation; eat fewer cold, raw and spicy foods; harmonize emotion and avoid mental irritation and stress; properly diminish the intensity of physical labor.

4 按语

一般应在经前 5～7 日开始治疗,至下次月经来潮前再治疗,连续治疗 3～5 个月,直到病愈。如系生殖系统器质性病变引起的月经不调,应及早作适当处理。

注意经期卫生,少进生冷及刺激性饮食;调摄情志,避免精神刺激;适当减轻体力劳动强度。

Dysmenorrhea

Dysmenorrhea refers to cold pain in the lower abdomen with possible radiation to the lumbosacral region, sometimes intolerable, occurring during, before or after menstruation. It is often seen in young women.

In Western medicine, dysmenorrhea without organic changes of the genitalia is known as primary or functional dysmenorrhea, and often occurs in girls after menarche or non-pregnant women, which may spontaneously disappear after marriage or labor. Dysmenorrhea due to organic changes of the genitalia is known as secondary dysmenorrhea and is often seen in endometriosis, acute and chronic pelvic inflammation, tumors, and blockage or narrowing of uterine neck.

痛 经

痛经是指妇女在月经期或月经期前后出现小腹冷痛,或痛引腰骶,甚者剧痛难忍的病证。本病以青年妇女为多见。

西医学认为,生殖器官无器质性病变者称为“原发性痛经”或“功能性痛经”,常发生于月经初潮后不久的未婚或未孕的年轻妇女,常于婚后或分娩后自行消失;由于生殖器官器质性病变所引起的痛经称为“继发性痛经”,常见于子宫内膜异位症、急慢性盆腔炎、肿瘤、宫颈口狭窄及阻塞等。

1 Etiology and pathogenesis

Excess syndrome of dysmenorrhea mainly results from emotional irritation and ensuing liver-qi stagnation which impedes blood circulation in the uterus, or from cold-dampness invasion in the uterine by contraction of exogenous coldness and cold be-verages, dwelling in damp places, or exposure to rains or wading in cold water during menstruation. Deficiency syndrome mainly results from spleen-stomach deficiency, or from qi-blood insufficiency after long-term illnesses, or from deficiency of the thoroughfare and conception vessels and uterine malnourishment due to constitutional weakness, liver-kidney insufficiency and essence-blood deficiency.

1 病因病机

实证痛经多因情志不调,肝气郁结,经血阻滞于胞宫,或经期受寒饮冷,坐卧湿地,冒雨涉水,寒湿客于胞宫所致;虚证痛经多因脾胃虚弱,或大病久病,气血虚弱,或禀赋素虚,肝肾不足,精血亏虚,以致冲任不足,胞脉失养而发。

2 Syndrome differentiation

2.1 Excess syndrome

Chief symptoms: Lower abdominal pain and refusal to pressure before and during menstruation, dark-red or purple menses with clots, pain relief after clots discharge.

The syndrome of qi stagnation and blood stasis manifests distension and pain in the breasts before menstruation, petechia tongue and wiry thready pulse. The syndrome of cold accumulation manifests cold pain in the lower abdomen which is alleviated by warmth, scanty dark-purple menses with clots, cold limbs and aversion to cold, whitish greasy tongue coating, and deep tight pulse.

2.2 Deficiency syndrome

Chief symptoms: Dull pain in the lower abdomen after menstruation, preference for pressure, and scanty light-colored menses.

The syndrome of qi-blood deficiency manifests

2 辨证

2.1 实证

主症:多在经前或经期少腹疼痛拒按,经色紫红或紫黑,有血块,下血块后疼痛缓解。

气滞血瘀者,经前兼有乳房胀痛、舌有瘀斑、脉细弦;寒邪凝滞者,腹痛有冷感,得温热疼痛可缓解,月经量少,色紫黑有块,畏寒肢冷,苔白腻,脉沉紧。

2.2 虚证

主症:腹痛多在经后,小腹绵绵作痛,喜按,月经色淡,量少。

气血不足者,兼面色苍

sallow or yellowish complexion, lassitude, vertigo, dizziness, palpitations, pale enlarged tongue with teeth marks, and weak thready pulse. The syndrome of liver-kidney deficiency manifests soreness and weakness in the waist and knees, poor sleep, dizziness, tinnitus, red tongue with scanty coating, and thready pulse.

白或萎黄、倦怠无力、头晕眼花、心悸、舌淡、舌体胖大边有齿痕、脉细弱；肝肾不足者，兼腰膝酸软，夜寐不宁，头晕耳鸣，舌红苔少，脉细。

3 Treatment

3 治疗

3.1 Essential treatment

3.1 基本治疗

3.1.1 Excess syndrome

3.1.1 实证

Principal acupoints: Sanyinjiao(SP 6), Zhongji (CV 3), Ciliao(BL 32), and Diji(SP 8).

主穴：三阴交，中极，次髎，地机。

Supplementary acupoints: In the syndrome of qi stagnation and blood stasis, add Taichong(LR 3) and Yanglingquan(GB 34); in the syndrome of cold accumulation, add Guilai(ST 29).

配穴：气滞血瘀加太冲、阳陵泉；寒邪凝滞加归来。

Explanation: Sanyinjiao(SP 6) can remove the obstruction from the meridians to relieve pains. Zhongji(CV 3) functions to harmonize the thoroghfare and conception vessels, disperse coldness and move qi circulation. Ciliao(BL 32) is an empiric acupoint for treating dysmenorrhea. Diji(SP 8), the Xi-Cleft acupoint of the spleen meri-dian, can regulate spleen qi and relieve pain. The combined use of these four acupoints may promote qi and blood circulation, disperse coldness and relieve pain.

方义：三阴交可通经止痛。中极通调冲任，散寒行气。次髎为治疗痛经的经验穴。地机乃脾经郄穴，能疏调脾经经气而止痛。四穴合用，以行气活血、散寒止痛。

3.1.2 Deficiency syndrome

3.1.2 虚证

Principal acupoints: Guanyuan(CV 4), Qihai (CV 6), Sanyinjiao(SP 6), and Zusanli(ST 36).

主穴：关元，气海，三阴交，足三里。

Supplementary acupoints: In the syndrome of qi-blood deficiency, add Pishu(BL 20) and Weishu (BL 21); in the syndrome of liver-kidney insufficiency, add Taixi(KI 3), Ganshu(BL 18) and Shen-

配穴：气血亏虚加脾俞、胃俞；肝肾不足加太溪、肝俞、肾俞。

shu(BL 23).

Explanation: Guanyuan(CV 4), an acupoint for strengthening the entire body, and Qihai (CV 6) can warm the lower energizer and nourish the thoroughfare and conception vessels. Sanyinjiao(SP 6), a Crossing acupoint of the liver, spleen and kidney meridians, can replenish spleen-qi and benefit liver and kidney to enrich kidney-essence and uterus to harmonize the thoroughfare and conception vessels. Zusanli(ST 36) can supplement qi and blood.

方义：关元为全身强壮要穴，与气海均可暖下焦，温养冲任。三阴交为肝脾肾三经之交会穴，可以健脾益气，调补肝肾，精血充盈，胞脉得养，冲任自调。足三里补益气血。

3.2 Other therapy

Ear acupuncture: Select 2 to 4 acupoints from Uterus, Internal Genitals(TF 2), Sympathesis(AH 6a), Subcortex(AT 4), Endocrine(CO 18), Shenmen(TF 4), Liver(CO 12) and Kidney(CO 10) for each treatment. Puncture these acupoints with filiform needles by moderate intensity of twirling and rotating needles; the needles are retained for 20 to 30 minutes, once a day or every other day. Or embed intradermal needles or apply *Semen Vaccariae* (Wang Bu Liu Xing) at these acupoints, once every 3 to 4 days.

3.2 其他治疗

耳针：选子宫、内生殖器、交感、皮质下、内分泌、神门、肝、肾。每次选2～4穴，毫针刺，中等强度捻转数分钟，每次留针20～30分钟，每日或隔日1次。也可用揿针埋藏或王不留行贴压，每3～4日更换1次。

4 Remarks

The treatment for dysmenorrhea usually begins 3 to 5 days prior to menstruation till the menstruation ends. Generally, treatment should be administered for 2 to 4 consecutive menstrual cycles. For secondary dysmenorrhea, symptoms may be relieved after acupuncture treatment, however, gynecological examination is necessary to make a definite diagnosis and corresponding treatments are prescribed. During menstruation, avoid strong physical labor and violent exercises, and mental irritation; pay attention to personal hygiene, prevent from cold con-

4 按语

针灸治疗宜在月经前3～5日开始，直到月经期末，一般连续治疗2～4个月经周期。对继发性痛经，运用针灸疗法减轻症状后，应确诊原发病，以采取相应治疗。经期避免重体力劳动、剧烈运动和精神刺激，注意经期卫生，防止受凉或过食生冷。

traction and avoid too much raw and cold foods.

Amenorrhea

Amenorrhea refers to the absence of menarche in healthy girls over 18 years old, or suppression of menstruation for longer than three months in succession. The former is called primary amenorrhea and the latter called secondary amenorrhea. No menstruation before puberty or during gestation, lactation, and menopausal period is a physiological phenomenon.

1 Etiology and pathogenesis

Amenorrhea may result from constitutional weakness and kidney-qi insufficiency, or from many deliveries of children and abortions, or from qi-blood exertion following chronic and serious diseases; or from invasion of exogenous cold and cold drinks that impede the blood flow in the thoroughfare and conception vessels; or from the failure of spleen to transform and transport grain and water and resultant dampness-phlegm retention in the thoroughfare and conception vessels; or from emotional impairments and following qi-blood obstruction in the uterus.

2 Syndrome differentiation

Chief symptoms: No coming of menstruation in girls over 18 years old, or delayed menstruation, with decreasing menses and even menstrual suppression longer than three consecutive three months.

The syndrome of liver-kidney deficiency may be accompanied by dizziness and tinnitus, soreness and weakness in the loins and knees, thirstiness and dry

经　闭

经闭又称“闭经”。是指女子年过 18 周岁，月经尚未来潮，或已形成月经周期，但又连续中断 3 个月以上的病证。前者属原发性闭经，后者为继发性闭经。至于青春期前、妊娠期、哺乳期以及绝经期的闭经都属生理现象。

1 病因病机

经闭多因禀赋不足，肾气未充，或多产堕胎，或久病大病，耗伤气血，血海空虚，无血以下而致血枯经闭；或受寒饮冷，血为寒凝，冲任阻滞不通，或脾失健运，痰湿内盛，阻于冲任，或七情内伤，气机不畅，气滞血瘀，胞脉闭阻导致血滞经闭。

2 辨证

主症：女子年过 18 岁而月经尚未来潮，或以往有过正常月经，经期错后，经量逐渐减少，终至经闭，已连续中断 3 个周期以上。

肝肾不足者，兼头晕耳鸣、腰膝酸软、口干咽燥、五心烦热、潮热盗汗、舌红苔

throat, feverish sensation in the soles, palms and chest, tidal fever and night sweating, red tongue with scanty coating, and wiry thready pulse. The syndrome of qi-blood deficiency may be accompanied by dizziness and vertigo, palpitations, shortness of breath, lassitude, poor appetite, pale tongue with whitish coating, and deep slow pulse. The syndrome of qi stagnation and blood stasis may be accompanied by emotional depression, or vexation and irritability, distension and fullness in the chest and hypochondriac regions, distending pain in the lower abdomen with refusal to pressure, dark purple tongue with ecchymosis, and deep wiry pulse. The syndrome of phlegm-dampness accumulation may be accompanied by obese body, fullness and distension in the chest and hypochondriac regions, lassitude, profuse leukorrhea, greasy tongue coating and slippery pulse. The syndrome of cold accumulation may be accompanied by cold pain in the lower abdomen, preference for warmth and pressure, whitish tongue coating and deep slow pulse.

少、脉弦细；气血亏虚者，兼头晕目眩、心悸气短、神疲肢倦、食欲不振、舌淡苔薄白、脉沉缓；气滞血瘀者，兼情志抑郁或烦躁易怒、胸胁胀满、小腹胀痛拒按、舌质紫暗或有瘀斑、脉沉弦；痰湿阻滞者，兼形体肥胖、胸胁满闷、神疲倦怠、白带量多、苔腻、脉滑；寒邪凝滞者，兼小腹冷痛、形寒肢冷、喜温喜按、苔白、脉沉迟。

3 Treatment

3.1 Essential treatment

Principal acupoints: Guanyuan(CV 4), Zusanli (ST 36), and Guilai(ST 29).

Supplementary acupoints: In the syndrome of liver-kidney insufficiency, add Ganshu(BL 18), Shenshu(BL 23), Taichong(LR 3) and Taixi(KI 3); in the syndrome of qi-blood deficiency, add Qihai(CV 6), Pishu(BL 20) and Weishu(BL 21); in the syndrome of qi stagnation and blood stasis, add Hegu(LI 4), Xuehai(SP 10) and Taichong(LR 3); in the syndrome of phlegm-dampness retention, add Yinlingquan(SP 9) and Fenglong(ST 40); in the

3 治疗

3.1 基本治疗

主穴：关元，足三里，归来。

配穴：肝肾不足加肝俞、肾俞、太冲、太溪；气血不足加气海、脾俞、胃俞等；气滞血瘀加合谷、血海、太冲；痰湿阻滞加阴陵泉、丰隆；寒邪凝滞加命门、腰阳关。

syndrome of cold accumulation, add Mingmen(GV 4) and Yaoyangguan(GV 3).

Explanation: Guanyuan (CV 4), the Crossing acupoint of the conception vessel and the three foot-yin meridians, acts to tonify the original qi to produce qi and blood. Zusanli(ST 36) and Guilai(ST 29), two acupoints of the stomach meridian, function to nourish the spleen and stomach to transform qi and blood, thus the sea of blood becomes full to ensure timely menstruation.

方义: 关元为任脉与足三阴经交会穴,可补下焦真元而化生精血。足三里、归来为胃经穴,健脾胃而化生气血,血海充盈,则经自通,月事自能按时而下。

3.2 Other therapy

Ear acupuncture: Select 2 to 4 acupoints from Endocrine(CO 18), Internal Genitals(TF 2), Liver (CO 12), Kidney(CO 10), Ovary, Shenmen(TF 4) for each treatment. Puncture these acupoints with filiform needles by moderate intensity, or embed intradermal needles or apply *Semen Vaccariae* (Wang Bu Liu Xing) at these acupoints, once every 3 to 4 days.

3.2 其他治疗

耳针: 选内分泌、内生殖器、肝、肾、卵巢、神门。每次选2～4穴,毫针用中等刺激,或用揿针埋藏或用王不留行贴压,每3～4日更换1次。

4 Remarks

Maintain a good mood and stay optimistic. Do physical excises to strengthen the constitution. Pay attention to appropriate work and rest, and keep a regimented life. Before acupuncture treatment, a careful examination is required to ascertain the cause and give treatment accordingly.

4 按语

注意情绪调节,保持乐观,加强体育锻炼,增强体质,劳逸结合及生活起居有规律。治疗前必须进行认真检查,明确发病原因,采取相应的治疗。

Uterine Bleeding

Uterine bleeding, known as "Beng Lou" in Chinese medicine, refers to vaginal bleeding beyond the menstrual period. Sudden onset of menstrual flooding is named as "Beng", whilst gradual onset of continuous scanty bleeding is named as "Lou". "Beng"

崩　漏

崩漏是指妇女非周期性子宫出血。其中:发病急骤,暴下如注,大量出血者为"崩";病势缓,出血量少,淋漓不绝者为"漏"。崩与漏虽

and "Lou" differ in the bleeding volume, but they may transform into each other in clinic. Massive bleeding can decrease and then change into mere dripping of blood, whereas long-term bleeding may also progress into heavy bleeding. Therefore, "Beng" and "Lou" are collectively named as "Beng Lou". This disease occurs mostly in pubescent and menopausal women. In Western medicine, uterine bleeding is often seen in dysfunctional uterine bleeding, absent from organic changes in the entire body and reproductive organs. It can be classified into ovulatory and non-ovulatory bleeding.

出血情况不同,但在发病过程中两者常互相转化,如崩血量渐少,可能转化为漏,漏势发展又可能变为崩,故临床多以崩漏并称。青春期和更年期妇女多见。崩漏可见于西医学的功能失调性子宫出血,全身及内外生殖器官无器质性病变存在,可分为排卵性和无排卵性两类。

1 Etiology and pathogenesis

Uterine bleeding often results from exogenous heat factors and liver-depression transforming into fire which impairs the thoroughfare and conception vessels and drive blood out of vessels, or from blood stasis and blood failing to return into the vessels, or spleen-qi deficiency and inability to secure the blood, or from kidney-qi deficiency and inability to store and ensuing insecurity of the thoroughfare and conception vessels and blood flow. This disease may involve in the thoroughfare and conception vessels, as well as the liver, spleen and kidneys.

1 病因病机

常因外感热邪,肝郁化火,损伤冲任,迫血妄行;或瘀血阻滞,血不归经;或脾气虚弱,统摄无权,或肾气亏损,失于封藏,而致冲任不固,经血妄行。本病涉及冲任二脉和肝脾肾三脏。

2 Syndrome differentiation

Chief symptoms: Vaginal bleeding beyond the menstrual period, which is either massive or continuously dripping red blood, or presence of scanty bleeding.

The syndrome of blood heat manifests sticky bright red blood with foul smell, dry mouth and preference for drinking, red tongue with yellowish coating, and slippery rapid pulse. The syndrome of dampness-heat manifests massive viscous purple-red

2 辨证

主症:经血非时而下,量多如崩,或淋漓不断,血色红,或量少,淋漓不净。

血热者,血色深红,质黏稠,气味臭秽,口干喜饮,舌红苔黄,脉滑数;湿热者,出血量多,色紫红而黏腻,带下量多,色黄臭秽,阴痒,苔黄

blood, copious yellow foul leukorrhea, itchiness in the vulva, yellowish greasy coating, and soggy rapid pulse. The syndrome of qi stagnation manifests bleeding with normal color or with clots, irritability, frequent sighing, distending pain in the lower abdomen, thin whitish tongue coating, and wiry pulse. The syndrome of blood stasis manifests persistent dripping of blood or sudden onset of profuse bleeding with dark-colored clots, pain in the lower abdomen which is aggravated by pressure and alleviated after discharge of blood clots, dark purple tongue with petechia, and deep rough pulse. The syndrome of spleen deficiency manifests light red blood, sallow complexion, lassitude, shortness of breath, poor appetite and loose stools, pale plump tongue with whitish coating, and deep weak thready pulse. The syndrome of kidney-yang deficiency manifests profuse bleeding or continuous scanty light-red thin blood, accompanied by cold pain in the lower abdomen, preference for warmth and pressure, cold limbs and aversion to cold, loose stools, pale tongue with whitish coating, and slow deep thready pulse. The syndrome of kidney-yin deficiency manifests scanty or profuse red sticky blood, accompanied by dizziness, tinnitus, restlessness, insomnia, weakness in the waist and knees, red tongue with less coating, and rapid thready pulse.

腻,脉濡数;气郁者,血色正常,或带有血块,烦躁易怒,时欲叹息,小腹胀痛,苔薄白,脉弦;血瘀者,漏下不止,或突然下血甚多,色紫红而黑、有块,小腹疼痛拒按,下血后疼痛减轻,舌质紫暗有瘀点,脉沉涩;脾虚者,血色淡,面色萎黄,神疲肢倦,气短懒言,纳呆便溏,舌质淡而胖,苔白,脉沉细无力;肾阳虚者,出血量多,淋漓不净,色淡质稀,兼少腹冷痛、喜温喜按,形寒畏冷,大便溏薄,舌淡苔白,脉沉细而迟;肾阴虚者,下血量少或多,色红质稠,兼头晕耳鸣、心烦不寐、腰膝酸软、舌红少苔、脉细数者。

3 Treatment

3.1 Essential treatment

Principal acupoints: Guanyuan (CV 4), Gongsun (SP 4), Sanyinjiao (SP 6), and Yinbai (SP 1).

Supplementary acupoints: In the syndrome of blood heat, add Xuehai (SP 10), in the syndrome of dampness-heat accumulation, add Yinlingquan (SP

3 治疗

3.1 基本治疗

主穴: 关元,公孙,三阴交,隐白。

配穴: 血热加血海;湿热者,配阴陵泉;气郁加太冲;血瘀加地机;脾气虚加百会、

9); in the syndrome of qi stagnation, add Taichong (LR 3); in the syndrome of blood stasis, add Diji (SP 8); in the syndrome of spleen-qi deficiency, add Baihui(GV 20) and Zusanli(ST 36); in the syndrome of kidney-yang deficiency, add Yaoyangguan (GV 3) and Mingmen(GV 4); in the syndrome of kidney-yin deficiency, add Rangu(KI 2) and Taixi (KI 3).

足三里;肾阳虚加腰阳关、命门,肾阴虚加然谷、太溪。

Explanation: Guanyuan(CV 4) is the Crossing acupoint of the conception vessel, thoroughfare vessel and the three foot-yin meridians; Gongsun(SP 4) is the Confluent acupoint communicating with the thoroughfare vessel; combined use of these two acupoints can regulate the thoroughfare and conception vessels to stem the menstrual flow. Sanyinjiao(SP 6), the Crossing acupoint of the three foot-yin meridians, serves to eliminate the pathogenic dampness, heat and blood stasis in the three meridians, and soothes the liver-qi to help the spleen secure the blood. Yinbai (SP 1), the Jing-Well acupoint of the spleen meridian, is an empiric acupoint for the treatment of uterine bleeding.

方义: 关元为任脉与冲脉、足三阴经交会穴,公孙通冲脉,二穴配合可通调冲任,固摄经血。三阴交为足三阴经交会穴,可清泻三经之湿、热、瘀等病邪,又可疏肝理气,邪除则脾可统血。隐白为脾经的井穴,是治疗崩漏的经验穴。

3.2 Other therapy

Ear acupuncture: Select Internal Genitals(TF 2), Subcortex(AT 4), Endocrine(CO 18), Kidney(CO 10), Liver(CO 12), Spleen(CO 13) and Ovary. Puncture these acupoints with filiform needles by moderate intensity; the needles are retained for 20 to 30 minutes per treatment. Or embed intradermal needles or apply *Semen Vaccariae* (Wang Bu Liu Xing) at these acupoints, once every 3 to 5 days.

3.2 其他治疗

耳针: 选内生殖器、皮质下、内分泌、肾、肝、脾、卵巢。毫针刺用中等刺激,每次留针20～30分钟。或用揿针埋藏或王不留行贴压,左右两耳交替使用,每3～5日更换1次。

4 Remarks

Acupuncture has certain effects in treating uterine bleeding, however, it takes a relative long

4 按语

针灸治疗本病有一定疗效,但所需疗程较长,应坚持

course of treatment and persistent treatment is necessary. For massive bleeding and blood loss or even collapse, emergency treatments must be prescribed immediately.

治疗。若大量出血，出现虚脱时，应及时抢救，采用综合治疗。

Perimenopausal Syndrome

Before and after menstrual pause, with the menstrual disturbance or pause, there display episode of flush and sweating, feverishness in the soles, palms and chest, vexation and irritability, bad mood, vertigo and tinnitus, palpitation and insomnia, facial edema, or insects cramping sensation on the kin, which is termed as perimenopausal syndrome. In 1994, World Health Organization (WHO) defined perimenopausal syndrome as a group of symptoms marked by neurovegetative disturbance and mental upsets due to endocrine changes such as ovary decline and diminished blood estradiol in women over 40 years. About 75%～85% of perimenopausal women exhibit varying degrees of symptoms, whose severity differs in different women; among which, some 25% women suffer from severe symptoms and their work and life are influenced. The duration of perimenopausal syndrome differs, 1～2 years in the short duration and over 10 years in the long duration.

绝经前后诸证

妇女绝经前后，随着月经紊乱或绝经，出现阵发性烘热汗出、五心烦热、烦躁易怒、情绪不稳、头晕耳鸣、心悸失眠、面浮肢肿或皮肤蚁走样感等症状，称为“绝经前后诸证”，亦称“经断前后诸证”，又称更年期综合征。1994 年 WHO 推荐采用“围绝经期综合征”名称，指妇女在 40 岁以后由于卵巢功能逐渐减退，血中雌二醇水平降低等内分泌改变引起的自主神经系统功能紊乱为主，伴有神经心理症状的症候群。绝经期妇女中有 75%～85%患有不同程度的症状，其严重程度可因人而异，其中约有 25%的妇女因症状严重，影响工作和生活。病程长短不一，短者一二年，长者数年至十余年。

1　Etiology and pathogenesis

Perimenopausal syndrome is in close relation to *Tian Kui*. In perimenopausal women, kidney-qi and *Tian Kui* decrease and essence-blood becomes insufficient, thus yin and yang disharmonize and visceral functions become disordered; or the heart does not

1　病因病机

绝经前后诸证与天癸关系密切。妇女绝经前后，肾气渐亏，天癸将竭，精血不足，以致阴阳失调，脏腑功能失常，或心肾不交，或肝肾阴

coordinate with the kidneys; or liver-kidney yin becomes deficient; or spleen-kidney yang becomes insufficient.

虚，或脾肾阳虚而生诸症。

2 Syndrome differentiation

Chief symptoms: Menstrual suppression or disturbance, mental upsets, flush and sweating, insomnia, palpitation and vertigo.

The syndrome of heart-kidney incoordination manifests palpitation, insomnia and sleepiness, tidal fever and sweating, feverish sensation in the soles, palms and chest, susceptibility to anxiety and worry, aching loin and knees, vertigo and tinnitus, red tongue with less coating, and deep thready pulse. The syndrome of liver-kidney yin deficiency manifests vertigo and dizziness, vexation and irritability, tidal fever and sweating, restless feverish in the soles, palms and chest, distention and fullness in the chest and hypochondriac regions, aching loin and knees, dry mouth, scanty urine, constipation, red tongue with less coating, and deep wiry pulse. The syndrome of spleen-kidney yang deficiency manifests head cloudiness and distention, depression and forgetfulness, abdominal bloating, belching and acid regurgitation, nausea and diminished appetite, fatigue, aching loin and cold limbs, limb edema, loose stools, plump tongue with whitish slippery coating, and deep thready pulse.

2 辨证

主症：绝经或月经紊乱，情绪不稳定，潮热汗出，失眠，心悸，头晕。

心肾不交者，兼心悸怔忡、失眠多梦、潮热汗出、五心烦热、易喜易忧、腰膝酸软、头晕耳鸣、舌红少苔、脉沉细数；肝肾阴虚者，兼头晕目眩、心烦易怒、潮热汗出、五心烦热、胸闷胁胀、腰膝酸软、口干舌燥、尿少、便秘、舌红少苔、脉沉弦细；脾肾阳虚者，兼头昏脑胀、忧郁善忘、脘腹满闷、嗳气吞酸、呕恶食少、神疲倦怠、腰酸肢冷、肢体浮肿、大便稀溏、舌胖大、苔白滑、脉沉细弱。

3 Treatment

3.1 Essential treatment

Principal acupoints: Shenshu(BL 23), Taixi (KI 3), Guanyuan(CV 4), Sanyinjiao(SP 6) and Baihui(GV 20).

Supplementary acupoints: In the syndrome of heart-kidney incoordination, add Xinshu(BL 15),

3 治疗

3.1 基本治疗

主穴：肾俞，太溪，关元，三阴交，百会。

配穴：心肾不交者，加心俞、神门、劳宫、内关。肝肾

Shenmen(HT 7), Laogong(PC 8) and Neiguan(PC 6); in the syndrome of liver-kidney yin deficiency, add Taichong(LR 3), Yongquan(KI 1) and Fengchi (GB 20); in the spleen-kidney yang deficiency, add Zusanli(ST 36), Qihai(CV 6), Pishu(BL 20) and Weishu(BL 21).

阴虚者,加太冲、涌泉、风池。脾肾阳虚者,加灸足三里、气海、脾俞、胃俞。

Explanation: Shenshu(BL 23) and Taixi(KI 3) act to enrich kidney-yin and essence-blood, replenish brain-marrow and strengthen loin and knees; Guanyuan(CV 4) functions to supplement original qi and harmonize the thoroughfare and conception vessels; Sanyinjiao(SP 6) acts to nourish the spleen and soothe the liver, enrich the kidneys, move qi and relieve depression, regulate and enrich the thoroughfare and conception vessels; Baihui (GV 20) serves to ascend clear yang and descend turbidity, pacify the liver and suppress yang, clear and arouse the head and eyes.

方义: 肾俞、太溪补肾滋阴,益精血、益脑髓、强腰膝;关元补益元气、调和冲任;三阴交健脾疏肝益肾,理气开郁,调补冲任;百会可升清降浊,平肝潜阳,清利头目。

3. 2 Other therapy

Ear acupuncture: Select 3 ~ 5 acupoints from Shenmen(TF4), Subcortex(AT4), Endocrine (CO 18), Internal Genitalia (TF 2), Kidney (CO 10), and Sympathesis (AH 6a). Puncture these acupoints with the filiform needles, and retain the needles for 20 minutes; the treatment is given once a day and 10 treatments make up one course. Or apply *Semen Vaccariae* (Wang Bu Liu Xing)at these acupoints, once every 3 to 5 days.

3. 2 其他治疗

耳针: 选神门、皮质下、内分泌、内生殖器、肾、交感。每次选 3～5 穴,毫针刺激,留针 20 分钟。每日 1 次,10 次为 1 个疗程,或用王不留行贴压,3～5 日换穴 1 次。

4 Remarks

Acupuncture has wonderful effects on perimenopausal syndrome. Ask patients to keep optimistic and open-minded, avoid depression, anxiety and irritability; pay attention to dietary regulation and physical exercises.

4 按语

针灸治疗本证具有较好的临床疗效。应嘱患者保持乐观开朗,避免忧郁、焦虑、急躁情绪。注意饮食调节,加强体育锻炼。

Morbid Leukorrhea

Morbid leukorrhea refers to persistent massive vaginal discharge with abnormal color, volume and odor, or accompanied by general and local symptoms. Normal leukorrhea refers to colorless, sticky, odorless, scanty vaginal discharge. Slight increase in the amount of the vaginal discharge during and before menstruation or during the pregnancy is a normal physiological phenomenon. Morbid leukorrhea is often seen in vaginitis, cervicitis and pelvic inflammation in Western medicine.

1 Etiology and pathogenesis

Commonly, morbid leukorrhea results from invasion of exogenous toxic dampness impairing the conception and belt vessels; or from downward dampness heat transformed from emotional depression; or from downward dampness due to improper diet and overexertion impairing the spleen and stomach, or from constitutional kidney-qi and original qi exertion, or from many deliveries of children and over-indulgence in sexual intercourse that consume kidney-qi. All these causes may lead to the dysfunction of belt vessel and inability of the thoroughfare and conception vessels to secure, thus the water and dampness flow downwards.

2 Syndrome differentiation

Chief symptoms: Obviously increased sticky, pus or sputum-liked vaginal discharge.

The syndrome of downward dampness-heat manifests yellowish sticky foul vaginal discharge like pus and tear, vulva itching, pain in the lower abdomen, scanty dark urine, body feverishness, bitter

带下病

带下病是指妇女阴道分泌物明显增多,色、质、气味异常,或伴全身及局部症状的疾患。正常带下是指妇女阴道内流出的一种无色、黏稠、无臭液体,量不多。行经期间、经前或妊娠期带下稍有增多者,属正常生理现象。带下病可见于西医学的阴道炎、宫颈炎、盆腔炎等。

1 病因病机

带下病的常见原因是:外感湿毒,损伤任带二脉;或情志不舒,郁久化热,湿热下注;或饮食劳倦,损伤脾胃,运化失职,湿聚下注;或素体肾气不固,下元亏损;或房劳多产,伤及肾气,而使带脉失约,冲任不固,水湿浊液下注所致。

2 辨证

主症:阴道流出的黏稠液体增多,如涕如脓。

湿热下注者,带下色黄稠黏,如脓如涕,气秽臭,阴中瘙痒,小腹作痛,小便短赤,身热,口苦咽干,舌红,苔

taste in the mouth and dry throat, and red tongue with yellowish coating, and rapid slippery pulse. The syndrome of spleen deficiency manifests whitish or light yellow, odorless and sticky discharge, sallow complexion, poor appetite, loose stools, fatigue and lassitude, pale tongue with whitish greasy coating, and weak soggy pulse. The syndrome of kidney deficiency manifests persistent thin whitish discharge, cold sensation in the lower abdomen, soreness of the lower back, frequent and voluminous urine especially at night, loose stools, pale tongue with thin whitish coating, and deep pulse.

黄，脉滑数；脾虚者，带下色白或淡黄，无臭味，质黏稠，连绵不断，面色萎黄，食少便溏，神疲乏力，舌淡，苔白腻，脉濡弱；肾虚者，带下色白，质清稀，绵绵不断，小腹寒凉，腰部酸痛，小便频数清长，夜间尤甚，大便溏薄，舌淡，苔薄白，脉沉。

3 Treatment

3.1 Essential treatment

Principal acupoints: Daimai (GB 26), Zhongji (CV 3), Baihuanshu (BL 30), and Sanyinjiao (SP 6).

Supplementary acupoints: In the syndrome of downward dampness-heat, add Yinlingquan (SP 9) and Xingjian (LR 2); in the syndrome of spleen deficiency, add Qihai (CV 6), Zusanli (ST 36) and Pishu (BL 20); in the syndrome of kidney deficiency, add Guanyuan (CV 4) and Shenshu (BL 23).

Explanation: Daimai (GB 26) can stem the belt vessel and adjust meridian-qi. Zhongji (CV 3) acts to clear heat, remove dampness and resolve turbidity in the lower energizer. Baihuanshu (BL 30) activates bladder qi to disinhibit dampness in the lower energizer. Sanyinjiao (SP 6) serves to reple-nish the spleen and disinhibit dampness, regulate liver and kidney, stem menstruation and stop leukorrhagia.

3.2 Other therapy

Ear acupuncture: Select 2 to 4 acupoints from Internal Genitalia (TF 2), Endocrine (CO 18),

3 治疗

3.1 基本治疗

主穴：带脉，中极，白环俞，三阴交。

配穴：湿热下注加阴陵泉、行间；脾虚加气海、足三里、脾俞；肾虚加关元、肾俞。

方义：带脉穴固摄带脉，调理经气。中极可清理下焦，利湿化浊。白环俞助膀胱之气化，利下焦之湿邪。三阴交健脾利湿，调理肝肾，固经止带。

3.2 其他治疗

耳针：选内生殖器、内分泌、膀胱、三焦、脾、肾、肝。

Bladder(CO 9), Triple Energizer(CO 17), Spleen (CO 13), Kidney(CO 10), and Liver(CO 12). Puncture these acupoints with filiform needles by moderate intensity and the needles are retained for 20 to 30 minutes per treatment. Or embed intradermal needles or apply *Semen Vaccariae* (Wang Bu Liu Xing) at these acupoints once every 3 to 5 days.

每次选 2～4 穴,毫针用中等强度刺激,每次留针 20～30 分钟。亦可用揿针埋藏法或王不留行贴压法,每3～5 日更换 1 次。

4 Remarks

Acupuncture has good effects in the treatment of morbid leukorrhea. The patient is advised to take regular diets, restrict sexual activities and keep the external genitalia clean.

4 按语

针灸治疗本病疗效较好,应注意饮食调养,节制房事,保持外阴清洁。

Fetal Malposition

Fetal position refers to the positioning relationship between the body of prenatal fetus and the maternal pelvis. The normal fetal position is most occiput anterior. Malposition of the fetus refers to those which are breech, transverse, occiput posterior and facial in presentation found by prenatal examination 30 weeks after conception. The common malposition is the breech presentation. If the malposition is not corrected, during the delivery period, slow cervical dilation, uterine inertia, prolonged delivery process, premature rupture of the fetal membranes, protrusion of the umbilical cord, fetus distress or death, uterine rupture and injury to the birth canal may happen.

胎位不正

胎位是指胎儿先露的指定部位与母体骨盆前、后、左、右的关系,正常胎位多为枕前位。胎位不正是指妊娠 30 周后,经产前检查发现臀位、横位、枕后位、颜面位胎位等,其中以臀位为常见。胎位不正如不纠正,临产时常表现为宫颈扩张缓慢、宫缩不强、产程延长,或胎膜早破、脐带脱出、胎儿窘迫或死亡,有的可发生子宫破裂或产道损伤等。

1 Etiology and pathogenesis

Fetal malposition is usually seen in multiparous women or those with a loose abdominal wall. It is caused by qi-blood deficiency failing to consolidate the fetus in a normal position, or by liver-qi stagna-

1 病因病机

本病多见于经产妇或腹壁松弛的孕妇。常因孕妇气血虚弱,无力安正胎位;或肝气郁结,气机不畅而导致胎

tion which impedes qi movement to correct the fetal position in time.

体不能应时转位。

2 Syndrome differentiation

Chief symptoms: Abnormal position of the fetus 30 weeks after conception, found by prenatal examination, absence of subjective symptoms.

The syndrome of qi-blood deficiency can be accompanied by lassitude and fatigue, shortness of breath, reluctance to speech, palpitation, poor appetite, loose stools, pale tongue with thin whitish coating, and feeble slippery pulse. The syndrome of liver-qi stagnation can be accompanied by emotional depression, vexation and irritability, distension in the chest, belching, thin whitish tongue coating and wiry slippery pulse.

2 辨证

主症：妊娠 30 周后，发现胎位不正。本病在临床上多无自觉症状，可通过妊娠后期妇科检查而发现。

气血虚弱者，兼神疲乏力、少气懒言、心悸气短、食少便溏、舌淡苔薄白、脉滑无力；肝气郁滞者，兼情志抑郁、烦躁易怒、胸胁胀满、嗳气、苔薄白、脉弦滑。

3 Treatment

3.1 Essential treatment

Principal acupoints: Zhiyin(BL 67).

Supplementary acupoints: In the syndrome of qi-blood deficiency, add Zusanli(ST 36), Sanyinjiao (SP 6) and Shenshu(BL 23); in the syndrome of liver-qi stagnation, add Ganshu(BL 18) and Xingjian (LR 2).

Explanation: Blood is the key to women. The abundance of qi and blood in the pregnant woman and the free flow of the qi ensure the normal position of the fetus. The kidney stores the essence and dominates reproduction, while the harmony of kidney-yin and kidney-yang ensures the smooth flow of qi and blood, hence the fetal position is corrected and delivery stays normal. Zhiyin(BL 67), the Jing-Well acupoint of foot-taiyang meridian, connects with the kidney meridian of foot-shaoyin; moxibus-

3 治疗

3.1 基本治疗

主穴：至阴。

配穴：气血虚弱加足三里、三阴交、肾俞；肝气郁滞加肝俞、行间。

方义：妇女以血为本，孕妇气血充沛、气机通畅则胎位正常。肾藏精，主生殖，肾阴、肾阳调和，则气顺血和，胎正产顺。至阴是足太阳经井穴，与足少阴肾经相连，灸之可调理肾经经气、调和冲任，是治疗胎位不正的经验效穴。操作时嘱孕妇平卧位，解松腰带，每次灸双侧

tion at this acupoint can regulate kidney-meridian qi and harmonize the thoroughfare and conception vessels; it is an empirical acupoint for fetal malposition. In the treatment procedure, ask the patient to lie supine and unfasten her belt. Perform moxibustion at bilateral acupoints for 15 to 20 minutes, once or twice a day. Check the patient every three days until the malposition is corrected.

15～20 分钟，每日 1～2 次，3 日后复查，至胎位转正为止。

4 Remarks

Moxibustion at Zhiyin(BL 67) has wonderful effects in correcting malposition of the fetus, with a higher rate than its spontaneous correction. However, proper treatment opportunity is necessary, usually 7 to 8 months(30 to 32 weeks) after conception is the optimum time to correct fetal position.

If this condition is caused by uterine deformity, contracted pelvis, carcinoma, fetal disorders, habitual abortion, or toxemia of pregnancy, moxibustion is contraindicated. They should refer to obstetric measures to prevent from accidents.

4 按语

艾灸至阴穴矫正胎位成功率较高，超过自然恢复率。但应掌握好治疗时机，妊娠 7～8 个月（30～32 妊娠周）是转胎最佳时机。

因子宫畸形、骨盆狭窄、肿瘤，或胎儿本身因素引起的胎位不正，或习惯性早产、妊娠毒血症，不适合针灸治疗，应尽快转产科处理，以免发生意外。

Prolonged Labor

The period from the beginning of labor till the the complete opening of uterine cervix is known as the first stage of labor. If during this period the contraction of the uterus fails to increase gradually, it makes the first stage of labor exceed 24 hours. It is also known as “difficult labor” or “difficult childbirth” in ancient literature. Prolonged labor is seen in uterine inertia in Western medicine.

滞　产

自分娩开始至宫口完全张开为第一产程。在此期间如果子宫收缩不能逐渐增强，使第一产程时间超过 24 小时，称为“滞产”。古代称“产难”“子难”等。滞产见于西医学中的子宫收缩无力。

1 Etiology and pathogenesis

Prolonged labor results from constitutional

1 病因病机

滞产多因孕妇素体虚

weakness and healthy qi deficiency, or from consumption of energy and qi by too early force and exertion, or from qi-blood deficiency due to premature amniorrhea, or from nervousness of the primipara, or from qi-blood stagnation due to excessive quietness and peacefulness, or from contraction of exogenous cold which causes qi stagnation and blood stasis, resulting in prolonged labor.

弱，正气不足；或产时用力过早，耗气伤力；或临产胞水早破，浆血枯干，导致气血虚弱，分娩时久产不下；或临产过度紧张，或产前过度安逸，气不运行，血不流畅，或感受寒邪，血寒凝滞，气机不利，气滞血瘀，而成滞产。

2　Syndrome differentiation

Chief symptoms: Amniotic fluid flowing down during the parturient period while the fetus cannot be delivered for a long time.

The syndrome of qi-blood deficiency manifests mild delivery pains, weak downward distention, or massive light-red blood, sallow complexion, lassitude and limb weakness, palpitations, shortness of breath, pale tongue with whitish coating, and weak thready pulse. The syndrome of qi stagnation and blood stasis manifests severe pain in the abdomen and lower back with refusal to pressure, or massive dark-red blood, nervousness, distension and fullness in the abdomen and chest, dark tongue with ecchymosis, and large wiry or tight rough pulse.

2　辨证

主症：临产浆水已下，胎儿久久不能娩出。

气血虚弱者，兼阵痛微弱、坠胀不甚、或下血量多、色淡、面色苍白、神疲肢软、心悸气短、舌淡苔白、脉沉弱而细；气滞血瘀者，兼腰腹剧痛、拒按，或下血量多，色暗，精神紧张，胸脘胀闷，舌暗或有瘀斑，脉弦大或紧涩。

3　Treatment

3.1　Essential treatment

Principal acupoints: Hegu(LI 4), Sanyinjiao(SP 6), and Zhiyin(BL 67).

Supplementary acupoints: In the syndrome of qi-blood deficiency, add Zusanli(ST 36); in the syndrome of qi stagnation and blood stasis, add Ciliao (BL 32), Xuehai(SP 10) and Taichong(LR 3).

Explanation: Hegu (LI 4), the Yuan-Source acupoint of the hand-yangming meridian, and Sanyinjiao(SP 6), the Crossing acupoint of the three

3　治疗

3.1　基本治疗

主穴：合谷，三阴交，至阴。

配穴：气血虚弱加足三里；气滞血瘀加次髎、血海、太冲。

方义：合谷为手阳明经原穴，三阴交为足三阴经之交会穴，两穴相配可理气行

foot-yin meridians, are combined to promote qi and blood circulation to expel the fetus out. Zhiyin(BL 67), the Jing-Well acupoint of the foot-taiyang meridian, is an empirical acupoint to promote delivery.

血以致胎下。至阴是足太阳经井穴,为催产之经验要穴。

3.2 Other therapies

3.2 其他治疗

Ear acupuncture: Select 2 to 3 acupoints from Internal Genitalia(TF 2), Uterus, Kidney(CO 10), Subcortex(AT 4), Sympathesis(AH 6a), and Endocrine(CO 18). Puncture these acupoints with the filiform needles by moderate intensity, and the needles are rotated once every 3 to 5 minutes until the fetus is delivered.

耳针:选内生殖器、子宫、肾、皮质下、交感、内分泌。每次用2~3穴,毫针用中等刺激,每隔3~5分钟捻转行针1次,直到胎儿娩出为止。

Acupoint application: Shenque(CV 8) and Yongquan(KI 1) are selected. Grind the leaf of eastor and make pastes. Take 2 pieces of *Crotonis Fructus* (Ba Dou) and grind them into powder and make into pastes by adding 0.3 g *Moschus* (She Xiang). Apply the pastes on the acupoints and cover them with gauzes, and the pastes should be removed after delivery.

穴位敷贴:选神阙、涌泉。将蓖麻叶捣烂,做成药饼;或用巴豆2粒去壳,加麝香0.3克,研制成药饼,贴于穴位上再盖上敷料,产后则去除贴药。

4 Remarks

4 按语

Acupuncture is a convenient and effective method for prolonged labor and has mild regulatory effects on the pregnant women and fetus, without any side effects; particularly, acupuncture is quite effective to promote delivery due to uterine inertia and relieve pain. If prolonged labor is caused by uterine deformity and contracted pelvis, other management in obstetric is required.

针灸用于处理滞产,方法简便有效,对孕妇、胎儿的调整作用缓和,无不良影响,且有良好的镇痛作用。针灸对宫缩无力的滞产有催产作用,如因子宫畸形、盆腔狭窄等引起的滞产,应转产科处理。

Insufficient Lactation

乳 少

Insufficient lactation refers to the condition in which a nursing mother's milk is insufficient to feed

乳少是指产后乳汁分泌甚少或全无,不能满足婴儿

the baby or even when there is no secretion of milk at all. It occurs after labor and during the feeding period.

需要。本症状可出现于产后及哺乳期。

1 Etiology and pathogenesis

Insufficient lactation usually results from qi and blood deficiency due to constitutional spleen-stomach weakness failing to transform and generate qi and blood, or from massive loss of qi and blood during delivery and resultant inadequate production of milk, or from emotional upsets after delivery, which gives rise to liver-qi stagnation and impairs or obstructs the free flow of milk.

1 病因病机

乳少常见的原因包括素体脾胃虚弱,生化不足,气血虚弱,或分娩失血过多,气血耗损,乳汁化源不足;或产后七情所伤,情志不调,肝失调达,气机不畅,乳汁运行不畅,甚则乳脉不通所致。

2 Syndrome differentiation

Chief symptoms: Milk secretion after labor is insufficient or absent; or milk secretion decreases or ceases during the feeding period.

The syndrome of qi and blood deficiency manifests insufficient or no milk secretion after labor, thin milk, soft breasts without the full sensation, sallow complexion, lusterless lips and nails, lassitude and fatigue, diminished appetite, loose stools, pale tongue with thin whitish coating, and deficient thready pulse. The syndrome of liver-qi stagnation manifests an absence or insufficiency of milk secretion, distending pain in the breasts, even with mild fever, mental depression, fullness and oppression in the chest and hypochondriac regions, epigastric distention, diminished appetite, red tongue with thin yellowish coating, and wiry pulse.

2 辨证

主症:产后乳汁分泌量过少或无乳汁分泌,或在哺乳期乳汁正行之际,乳汁分泌减少或全无。

气血虚弱者,兼产后乳少、乳汁清稀甚或全无、乳房柔软无胀感、面色苍白、唇甲无华、神疲乏力、食少便溏、舌淡苔薄白、脉虚细;肝气郁滞者,兼产后乳汁不行或乳少、乳房胀满疼痛、甚至身有微热、情志抑郁不乐、胸胁胀闷、脘痞食少、舌红苔薄黄、脉弦。

3 Treatment

3.1 Essential treatment

Principal acupoints: Rugen(ST 18), Danzhong (CV 17) and Shaoze(SI 1).

3 治疗

3.1 基本治疗

主穴: 乳根,膻中,少泽。

Supplementary acupoints: In the syndrome of qi and blood deficiency, add Zusanli(ST 36), Pishu (BL 20) and Weishu(BL 21); in the syndrome of liver-qi stagnation, add Taichong (LR 3) and Neiguan(PC 6).

配穴: 气血不足加足三里、脾俞、胃俞;肝气郁结加太冲、内关。

Explanation: Rugen(ST 18) can regulate qi and blood in the yangming meridians and unblock the breast collaterals. Danzhong(CV 17), the Influential acupoint of qi, serves to regulate qi and remove obstruction from collaterals. Shaoze(SI 1) is the empirical acupoint for promoting the flow of milk. Danzhong(CV 17) is subcutaneously punctured with the needle tip towards the breasts; Rugen(ST 18) is subcutaneously punctured with the needle tip upwards to the breasts and induce the needling sensation to spread towards the breasts.

方义: 乳根可调理阳明气血,疏通乳络。膻中为气会,调气通络。少泽为通乳的经验效穴。应注意针刺的方向:针刺膻中宜向乳房两侧平刺;乳根宜沿乳房向上平刺,使针感向乳房扩散。

3.2 Other therapies

3.2 其他治疗

Ear acupuncture: Select Chest(AH 10), Endocrine(CO 18), Sympathesis(AH 6a), Liver(CO 12), Kidney(CO 10) and Spleen(CO 13). Puncture these acupoints with filiform needles by moderate intensity for 15 to 20 minutes per treatment. Or embed intradermal needles or apply *Semen Vaccariae* (Wang Bu Liu Xing) at these acupoints.

耳针: 选胸、内分泌、交感、肝、肾、脾。毫针用中等刺激,每次15~20分钟。或用揿针埋藏或用王不留行贴压。

Dermal needle therapy: Tap the areas from Feishu(BL 13) to Sanjiaoshu(BL 22) on the back and around the breasts. Tapping intensity depends upon the deficiency or excess condition of insufficient lactation, and generally mild or moderate intensity is applied. The back is tapped with 2 cm apart from the up till down; the bilateral intercostal space may be tapped for 5 to 7 rounds. The areas surrounding the breasts are tapped outwards and the areola mammae is tapped in a circular way. The

皮肤针: 背部从肺俞至三焦俞及乳房周围,叩刺强度根据证候的虚实决定,一般多用轻刺激或中等刺激。背部从上而下每隔2厘米叩打一处,并可沿肋间向左右两侧斜行叩刺,叩打5~7次,乳房周围作放射状叩刺,乳晕部作环形叩刺,每次叩刺10分钟,每日1次。

tapping treatment is given once a day and 10 minutes per treatment.

4 Remarks

Ask the patients to keep a good mood, take high-protein fluid food, adopt correct nursing methods of breast-feeding, avoid overexertion and have adequate sleep. Acupuncture has better effects on the shorter duration of insufficient lactation. Early treatment, within one week of its onset is recommended.

4 按语

哺乳期产妇应保持心情舒畅,多食高蛋白流质食物,掌握正确哺乳方法,避免过度疲劳,保证充足睡眠。缺乳时间越短针灸疗效越好,应在早期,乳少发病不超过 1 周时及时进行治疗。

Infertility

Infertility refers to the inability to conceive after two or more years of a normal sexual life without conception, or the inability to conceive for more than two years after giving birth to a baby or an abortion without using any contraceptive mea-sures. The former is known as primary infertility, and the latter secondary infertility. It is often seen in salpingitis, ovaritis, inflammation of the endometrium, cervicitis and disorders of the endocrine system in Western medicine.

不　孕

不孕症又称“绝子”“无子”,指育龄妇女未避孕,其配偶生殖功能正常,婚后有正常性生活,同居两年以上而未怀孕者,或曾有过生育或流产,而又两年以上未怀孕者;前者称“原发性不孕”,后者为“继发性不孕”。不孕症常见于输卵管炎、卵巢炎、子宫内膜炎、宫颈炎以及内分泌失调等病证。

1 Etiology and pathogenesis

Infertility usually results from deficiency of the thoroughfare and conception vessels due to kidney-qi insufficiency and essence-blood deficiency failing to nourish the uterine collaterals, or from mental upsets and liver-qi stagnation failing to ensure the free flow of qi and blood and mutual nutrition between the thoroughfare vessel and conception vessel, or from obstruction of uterine collaterals by phlegm-blood stagnation and qi depression due to

1 病因病机

本病常因先天肾气不充,精血不足,冲任脉虚,胞脉失养;或因情志不畅,肝气郁结,疏泄失常,气血不和,冲任不能相资;或因脾失健运,痰湿内生,痰瘀互结,气机不畅,胞脉受阻,不能摄精成孕。

spleen dysfunction and following inability to get conceived.

2 Syndrome differentiation

Chief symptoms: Inability to conceive after two or more years of a normal sexual life without contraception, while her husband is healthy in reproductivity.

The syndrome of kidney deficiency manifests delayed menstruation, scanty light-colored menses, dark complexion, asexuality, soreness and weakness of the waist and knees, profuse clear urine, loose stools, pale tongue with whitish coating, and deep thready or deep slow pulse. The syndrome of liver-qi stagnation manifests irregular menstruation, abdominal pain during menstruation, unsmooth flow of scanty menses with dark clots, distending pain in the breasts before menstruation, mental depression, vexation and irritability, normal or dark-red tongue with whitish coating, and wiry pulse. The syndrome of spleen deficiency and dampness retention manifests body obesity, delayed menstruation with clots, even amenorrhea, massive sticky leukorrhea, dizziness and palpitation, fullness in the chest and hypochondria, poor appetite, nausea, white greasy tongue coating and slippery pulse.

2 辨证

主症：育龄妇女未避孕，其配偶生殖功能正常，婚后性生活正常，同居两年以上而未怀孕。

肾虚者，兼见月经后期、量少色淡，面色晦暗，性欲淡漠，腰膝酸软，小便清长，大便不实，舌淡苔白，脉沉细或沉迟；肝气郁结者，兼经期先后不定、经来腹痛、行而不畅、量少色暗有块，经前乳房胀痛，精神抑郁，烦躁易怒，舌质正常或暗红，苔薄白，脉弦；脾虚痰阻者，兼形体肥胖，经行推后而不畅、夹有血块，甚或闭经，带下量多、质黏稠，头晕心悸，胸胁胀满，纳呆泛恶，苔白腻，脉滑。

3 Treatment

3.1 Essential treatment

Principal acupoints: Taixi(KI 3), Shenshu(BL 23), Guanyuan(CV 4), and Sanyinjiao (SP 6).

Supplementary acupoints: In the syndrome of kidney deficiency, add Mingmen(GV 4); in the syndrome of liver-qi depression, add Ganshu(BL 18) and Taichong(LR 3); in the syndrome of spleen deficiency and dampness retention, add Zusanli(ST

3 治疗

3.1 基本治疗

主穴：太溪，肾俞，关元，三阴交。

配穴：肾虚加命门；肝气郁结加肝俞、太冲；脾虚痰阻加足三里、丰隆。

36) and Fenglong(ST 40).

Explanation: Taixi (KI 3), the Yuan-Source acupoint of the kidney meridian, and Shenshu(BL 23) serve to replenish kidney essence and warm original yang. Guanyuan(CV 4) acts to replenish the original qi. Sanyinjiao(SP 6) regulates qi of the three foot-yin meridians, adjusts qi and blood, and nourishes the uterine vessels.

方义：太溪为肾经的原穴，配肾俞补益肾精、温补元阳。关元补益元气。三阴交可调补三阴经气，调气血，益胞脉。

3.2 Other therapy

Ear acupuncture: Select 2 to 4 acupoints from Internal Genitalia(TF 2), Subcortex(AT 4), Kidney(CO 10), Liver(CO 12) and Endocrine(CO 18). Puncture these acupoints with filiform needles by moderate intensity from the twelfth day of the menstrual cycle, once a day for consecutive three days. Acupoints on both ears alternate. Or embed intradermal needles or apply *Semen Vaccariae* (Wang Bu Liu Xing) at these acupoints.

3.2 其他治疗

耳针：内生殖器、皮质下、肾、肝、内分泌，每次2～4穴，两耳交替。毫针刺法在月经周期第 12 日开始。每日 1 次，连续 3 日，中等刺激。或用揿针埋藏或用王不留行贴压。

4 Remarks

There are numerous causative factors for infertility. Examination on the patient's spouse is needed to exclude his reasons and treatment can be treated accordingly. Acupuncture is quite effective in the treatment of infertility due to neuroendocrine dysfunction. During treatment, ask the patient to keep a good mood and heed personal hygiene, control sexual activity and accumulate vitality, master the ovulatory date to help conceive.

4 按语

引起不孕的原因很多，应同时对其配偶进行检查，排除男方因素，以便针对性治疗。针灸主要对神经内分泌功能失调性不孕有良好效果。治疗期间应注意调畅情志及经期卫生，节欲、蓄精，掌握排卵日期，利于受精。

Enuresis

Enuresis refers to involuntary and recurrent urination with repeated attacks during sleep in children aged over 3 years.

遗　尿

遗尿是指 3 周岁以上的小儿，在睡眠中小便不能自行控制而排出，醒后方觉，并反复出现的一种病证。

Western medicine holds that enuresis is caused by immature urinary function. It can be classified into persistent and recurrent types. The former refers to absence of established self-controlled urination; the latter refers to relapse of enuresis 6 months after being cured, which is mostly induced by psychological factors. In addition, urinary abnormality, urinary inflammation and occult cleft spine can cause enuresis as well.

西医学认为本病因患儿控制排尿功能不成熟所致，临床可分为持续型和再发型。前者指从未建立起自觉排尿；后者指患儿已不再遗尿，而间隔一段时间（至少6个月）后又出现遗尿，多由精神因素诱发。另外，泌尿系异常、感染、隐性脊柱裂也可导致遗尿。

1 Etiology and pathogenesis

Enuresis primarily results from weak constitution, or from kidney-qi insufficiency and deficiency cold in the lower energizer after long-term illnesses and ensuing failure of the bladder to control urination, or from spleen-lung qi-deficiency failing to enable the bladder to control urination.

1 病因病机

本病多因禀赋不足，或病后体虚，导致肾气不足，下元虚寒，膀胱约束无权；或因脾肺气虚，不能约束下焦，膀胱约束无权，致使发为遗尿。

2 Syndrome differentiation

Chief symptoms: Involuntary urination during sleep in children over 3 years old. In mild cases, it occurs once in several days; in severe cases, it occurs 1～2 times or more in one night.

The syndrome of kidney-qi insufficiency can be accompanied by frequent, profuse and clear urine, lassitude and fatigue, sallow complexion, cold limbs and aversion to cold, soreness and weakness of the waist and knees, pale tongue and deep slow feeble pulse. The syndrome of lung-spleen qi-deficiency may be accompanied by frequent scanty urine during day time, enuresis aggravated after physical exertion, sallow complexion, shortness of breath and reluctance to speak, poor appetite, loose stools, pale tongue with whitish coating, and weak thready pulse.

2 辨证

主症：3周岁以上小儿在睡眠中小便自遗，醒后方觉。轻者几天一次，重者每夜1～2次或更多。

肾气不足者，兼小便清长而频数、神疲乏力、面色苍白、畏寒肢冷、腰膝酸软、甚则肢冷恶寒、舌淡、脉沉迟无力；肺脾气虚者，兼白天小便频而量少、劳累后遗尿加重、面白无华、少气懒言、食欲不振、大便易溏、舌淡苔白、脉细无力。

3 Treatment

3.1 Essential treatment

Principal acupoints: Guanyuan(CV 4), Zhongji (CV 3), Pangguangshu (BL 28), and Sanyinjiao (SP 6).

Supplementary acupoints: In the syndrome of kidney-qi insufficiency, add Shenshu (BL 23), Mingmen(GV 4) and Taxi(KI 3); in the syndrome of lung-spleen qi-deficiency, add Qihai (CV 6), Feishu(BL 13) and Zusanli(ST 36).

Explanation: Guanyuan (CV 4), the Crossing acupoint of the conception vessel and the three foot-yin meridians, replenishes the original qi, nourishes kidney and consolidates the foundation. Zhongji (CV 3) and Pangguangshu(BL 28), the Front-Mu acupoint and Back-Shu acupoint of the bladder, can promote the bladder to activate qi. Sanyinjiao(SP 6), the Crossing acupoint of the three foot-yin meridians, regulates the qi of the liver, spleen and kidney meridians, and serves to replenish spleen-qi, nourish kidney and consolidate foundation.

3.2 Other therapies

Ear acupuncture: Select 2 to 3 acupoints from Kidney(CO 10), Bladder(CO 9), Subcortex(AT 4), Urethra (HX 3) and Shenmen (TF 4). Puncture these acupoints with filiform needles by mild intensity, once a day; and the needles are retained for 20 minutes per treatment. Or embed intradermal needles or apply *Semen Vaccariae* (Wang Bu Liu Xing) at these acupoints and press these acupoints before sleep.

Dermal needle therapy: Select Jiaji (EX-B 2), Qihai(CV 6), Guanyuan(CV 4), Pangguangshu(BL 28), Baliao(BL 31～34) and Pishu(BL 20). Before

3 治疗

3.1 基本治疗

主穴：关元，中极，膀胱俞，三阴交。

配穴：肾气不足加肾俞、命门、太溪；脾肺气虚加气海、肺俞、足三里。

方义：关元为任脉与足三阴经交会穴，培补元气，益肾固本。中极、膀胱俞为膀胱之俞募配穴，可促进膀胱气化功能。三阴交为足三阴经交会穴，通调肝脾肾三经经气，可健脾益气、益肾固本。

3.2 其他治疗

耳针：选肾、膀胱、皮质下、尿道、神门。每次选2～3穴，毫针刺用轻刺激，每日1次，每次留针20分钟。亦可用揿针埋藏或王不留行贴压，于睡前按压以加强刺激。

皮肤针：选夹脊穴、气海、关元、中极、膀胱俞、八髎、肾俞、脾俞。每晚睡前用

sleep, these acupoints are tapped with dermal needle by mild or moderate intensity for 20 minutes till the skin becomes flushed; cupping therapy may be performed after tapping, once every other day.

皮肤针轻叩或中等强度叩刺,每次 20 分钟,使皮肤微微潮红,也可叩刺后加拔火罐,隔日 1 次。

4 Remarks

Acupuncture has good effects in the treatment of functional enuresis. As for enuresis caused by organic changes, treatment should be given to the primary causes. During acupuncture treatment, children's parents are asked to control the children's intake of fluid before sleep, wake them up to discharge urine regularly in attempt to develop the habit of getting up to urinate.

4 按语

针灸对功能性遗尿疗效较好。但对某些器质性病变引起的遗尿,应治疗其原发病。治疗期间嘱家属密切配合,控制患儿睡前饮水,夜间按时唤醒排尿,逐渐养成自觉起床排尿的良好习惯。

Infantile Anorexia

Infantile anorexia refers to a long-term poor appetite in children. It belongs to the categories of "aversion to diets" and "reluctance to eat" in Chinese medicine.

小儿厌食

小儿厌食系指小儿较长时间的食欲不振。属于中医学"恶食""不嗜食"的范畴。

1 Etiology and pathogenesis

In Chinese medicine, infantile anorexia is caused by tender zang-fu organs and spleen deficiency, or by improper intake of foods, or by improper nursing after diseases impairing the spleen and stomach from reception and process.

1 病因病机

中医学认为,小儿厌食是由小儿脏腑娇嫩,脾常不足,或饮食失调,或病后失养,脾胃功能受损,导致受纳运化功能失常所致。

2 Syndrome differentiation

Chief symptoms: Long-term poor appetite, diminished food intake or even refusal to food, thin body, sallow complexion, and fair spirit. In chronic cases, it can manifest emaciation, loss of weight, lassitude, and decreased body resistance against di-seases.

The syndrome of spleen-stomach deficiency may manifest sallow complexion, lassitude, loose tools with undigested food, pale tongue with thin

2 辨证

主症:长期食欲不振,食欲下降甚至拒食,形体偏瘦,面色少华,但精神尚好。病程日久则形体瘦弱,体重减轻,精神疲惫,抗病能力差。

脾胃虚弱者,面色萎黄,神疲乏力,大便多不成形或夹有不消化食物,舌淡苔薄

whitish coating, and weak pulse. The syndrome of stomach-yin deficiency may manifest sallow complexion, dry mouth, massive drinking, even drinking at every meal, restlessness, dry stools, dark urine, bare tongue with peeling coating, and weak thready pulse. The syndrome of liver-excess and spleen-deficiency may manifest hyperactivity, crying, irritability, chewing during sleep, dry stools, scanty urine, bare tongue without coating, and thready wiry pulse.

白，脉弱无力；胃阴不足者，面色萎黄，口干，多饮甚至每食必饮，烦热不安，便干溲赤，舌光、苔净或花剥，脉细无力；肝旺脾虚者，好动多啼，性躁易怒，睡眠中咬齿磨牙，便干溲少，舌光、苔净，脉弦细。

3 Treatment

3 治疗

3.1 Essential treatment

3.1 基本治疗

Principal acupoints: Zhongwan(CV 12), Jianli (CV 11), Liangmen(ST 21), and Zusanli(ST 36).

主穴：中脘，建里，梁门，足三里。

Supplementary acupoints: The syndrome of spleen-stomach deficiency, add Pishu(BL 20) and Weishu(BL 21); in the syndrome of stomach-yin deficiency, add Sanyinjiao(SP 6) and Neiting(ST 2); in the syndrome of liver-excess and spleen-deficiency, add Taichong(LR 3) and Taibai(SP 3).

配穴：脾胃虚弱加脾俞、胃俞；胃阴不足加三阴交、内庭；肝旺脾虚加太冲、太白。

Explanation: Zhongwan (CV 12), Jianli (CV 11) and Liangmen(ST 21) act to regulate the meridian-qi in the epigastric area to help the stomach in reception and the spleen in transportation; Zusanli (ST 36), the He-Sea acupoint of the stomach, serves to harmonize the stomach and replenish the spleen, supplement qi and blood.

方义：中脘、建里、梁门疏调脘腹经气，以助胃纳和脾之运化；足三里是足阳明胃经合穴，可和胃健脾、补养气血。

3.2 Other therapy

3.2 其他治疗

Ear acupuncture: Select 2 to 3 acupoints from Stomach(CO 4), Spleen(CO 13), Large Intestine (CO 7), Small Intestine(CO 6), Shenmen(TF 4), and Subcortex(AT 4). Puncture these acupoints or apply *Semen Vaccariae* (Wang Bu Liu Xing) at these acupoints and press them 3 to 5 times a day.

耳针：取胃、脾、大肠、小肠、神门、皮质下。每次取2～3穴，用王不留行贴压，每日按揉3～5次。

4 Remarks

Acupuncture is effective in the treatment of infantile anorexia. The causes must be ascertained and treatment is given to the primary cases. Correct bad dietary habit and cultivate good living habit.

4 按语

针灸治疗小儿厌食效果较好,应积极寻找引起厌食的病因,采取相应措施。注意纠正不良饮食习惯,保持良好的生活规律。

Childhood Hyperactivity

Childhood hyperactivity refers to the disease of children with normal intelligence but inability to control their behavior and concentration, excessive activity, difficulty in studying, and failure to control emotions. It is caused by many biological, psychological and sociological factors.

小儿多动症

小儿多动症是指儿童智力正常或接近正常,但有不同程度的自我控制能力差、活动过多、注意力不集中、学习困难、情绪不稳定和行为异常等症状的一种疾病。是由多种生物因素、心理因素及社会因素等作用所致。

1 Etiology and pathogenesis

Chinese medicine believes that childhood hyperactivity is caused by prenatal weakness, kidney-essence deficiency, yin deficiency with yang hyperactivity and endogenous wind stirring, or by marrow deficiency and malnutrition of the spirit, or by heart-spirit undernourishment due to the heart-spleen deficiency and qi-blood insufficiency.

1 病因病机

中医学认为,小儿多动症多由先天禀赋不足,肾精虚衰,阴虚阳亢,虚风内动;或髓海空虚,元神失养所致;或因心脾两虚,气血生化不足,心神失养所致。

2 Syndrome differentiation

Chief symptoms: Emotional upsets, abnormal behavior, excessive activity, poor coordination, and inability to concentrate.

The syndrome of yin deficiency with yang hyperactivity may manifest restlessness and irritability, excessive activity, heat sensation in the chest, soles and palms, night sweats, dreaminess, lusterless hair, dry red tongue, and wiry or thready rapid

2 辨证

主症:情绪不稳定,行为异常,运动过多,动作不协调,注意力不集中。

阴虚阳亢者,兼烦躁易怒、多动多语、五心烦热、盗汗多梦、发枯不荣、舌红而干、脉细数或弦细数;心脾两虚者,兼精神疲倦、记忆力

or pulse. The syndrome of heart-spleen deficiency may manifest fatigue, poor memory, dreaminess and susceptibility to fright, sallow complexion, poor appetite, loose stools, pale tongue with whitish coating, and thready slow pulse.

差、多梦易惊、面色萎黄、纳少便溏、舌淡苔白、脉细缓。

3 Treatment

3 治疗

3.1 Essential treatment

3.1 基本治疗

Principal acupoints: Baihui(CV 20), Yintang(EX-HN 3), Taichong(LR 3), Taixi(KI 3), and Shenmen(HT 7).

主穴：百会，印堂，太冲，太溪，神门。

Supplementary acupoints: In the syndrome of yin deficiency with yang hyperactivity, add Sanyinjiao(SP 6) and Xiaxi(GB 43); in the syndrome of heart-spleen deficiency, add Xinshu(BL 15), Pishu(BL 20) and Zusanli(ST 36).

配穴：阴虚阳亢加三阴交、侠溪；心脾两虚加心俞、脾俞、足三里。

Explanation: Baihui(GV 20) and Yintang(EX-HN 3) are combined to calm the mind and spirit, replenish the brain and enhance intelligence. Taixi (KI 3), the Yuan-Source acupoint of the kidney meridian, serves to supplement yin and suppress yang. Taichong(LR 3) can pacify the liver and suppress yang. Shenmen(HT 7) calm the heart and spirit. Combined use of these acupoints function to harmonize yin and yang, and calm the mind and spirit.

方义：百会、印堂两穴相配可安神定志，益智健脑。太溪为肾经原穴，育阴潜阳。太冲平肝潜阳。神门宁心安神。诸穴合用，使阴阳调和，神安志定。

3.2 Other therapy

3.2 其他治疗

Ear acupuncture: Select 2 to 3 acupoints from Heart(CO 15), Liver(CO 12), Kidney(CO 10), Subcortex(AT 4), Adrenal Grand(TG 2p), Sympathesis(AH 6a), and Occiput(AT 3). Puncture these acupoints with filiform needles by moderate intensity, or embed intradermal needles or apply *Semen Vaccariae* (Wang Bu Liu Xing) at these acupoints.

耳针：选心、肝、肾、皮质下、肾上腺、交感、枕。每次选 2～3 穴，毫针刺用中等刺激，或用揿针埋藏或用王不留行贴压。

4 Remarks

4 按语

Acupuncture is effective for childhood hyperac-

针灸治疗本病疗效较

tivity. Combined use of stomatic acupuncture and auricular acupuncture exerts better effects, and auricular acupuncture is more acceptable to children. Strengthen proper education and induction. If necessary, psychological treatment is given to help the children cultivate a good life style.

好，以体针和耳针配合应用为好，耳穴贴压患儿易于接受。注意加强教育与诱导，配合必要的心理治疗，帮助患儿培养良好的生活习惯。

Infantile Cerebral Palsy

Infantile cerebral palsy is a disease with manifestations of cerebral agenesis, mental retardation, and dyskinesia of the limbs. It is categorized into "five kinds of flaccidity" and "five kinds of retardation". Western medicine holds that it is the sequelae of congenital cerebral agenesis or cerebral impairment caused by various factors.

小儿脑性瘫痪

小儿脑性瘫痪简称"小儿脑瘫"，是以小儿大脑发育不全、智力低下、四肢运动障碍为主要症状的一种疾病。本病属中医儿科的"五软""五迟"范畴。西医学认为，本病是由于先天性大脑发育不良或多种原因引起脑损伤而致的后遗症。

1 Etiology and pathogenesis

Infantile cerebral palsy is mainly caused by constitutional insufficiency and liver-kidney deficiency failing to nourish the tendons and bones, or by inactive kidney-yang failing to warm the muscles and limbs, or by insufficient food or milk and improper nursing, or by malnutrition of tendons and muscles due to qi-blood deficiency following spleen-stomach impairment by long-term or severe diseases, or by undernourishment of tendons due to insufficiency of qi-blood and yin-fluid consumed by heat toxin entering jueyin meridian, or by dysfunction of sinews and vessels due to qi-blood stagnation by obstruction of the wind and phlegm in the collaterals.

1 病因病机

本病多因先天禀赋不足，肝肾亏虚，精血不能注于筋骨；或元阳不振，阳气不能温煦肌肤、营于四末；或平素乳食不足，哺养失调，或久病、大病后失于调养，以致脾胃亏损，气血虚弱，筋骨、肌肉失于滋养；或因感受热毒，内陷厥阴，耗气伤阴，日久气血失调，筋脉失养；或风痰留阻络道，气滞血瘀，筋脉失利。

2 Syndrome differentiation

Chief symptoms: Inability of the limbs to move,

2 辨证

主症：肢体运动功能障

accompanied by mental and developmental retardation.

The syndrome of liver-kidney insufficiency can be accompanied by thin weak bones and tendons, retarded development, obviouslydelayed standing, walking and teeth generation in comparison with healthy children of the same age, glow-lost eyes, sallow complexion, lassitude, preference for lying on bed, retarded intelligence, pale tongue with thin whitish coating, and thready pulse. The syndrome of qi-blood deficiency can be accompanied by atrophic muscles and flaccid sinews, nape weakness, lassitude, dull expression, retarded speech, persistent salivation, diminished appetite, loose stools, pale tongue with whitish coating, and feeble thready pulse. The syndrome of phlegm-blood obstruction in the collaterals can be accompanied by dull reaction, aphasia, dementia, flaccidity and numbness of the limbs, pale purple tongue with petechia on the margins, greasy tongue coating, and wiry slippery or rough pulse.

碍,常伴有智力低下,发育迟缓。

肝肾不足者,兼筋骨瘦弱,发育迟缓,站立、行走或长齿等明显迟于正常同龄小儿,目无神采,面色不华,疲倦喜卧,智力迟钝,舌质淡,苔薄白,脉细;气血虚弱者,兼筋肉痿软,头项无力,精神倦怠、神情呆滞、语言发育迟缓,流涎不禁,食少便溏,舌淡苔白,脉细弱;痰瘀阻络者,兼反应迟钝,失语、痴呆,手足软而不用、肢体麻木,舌淡紫或边有瘀点,苔腻,脉弦滑或涩。

3 Treatment

3.1 Essential treatment

Principal acupoints: Baihui(GV 20), Sishenchong(EX-HN 1), Zusanli(ST 36), and Hegu (LI 4).

Supplementary acupoints: In the syndrome of liver-kidney insufficiency, add Ganshu(BL 18) and Shenshu(BL 23); in the syndrome of qi-blood deficiency, add Xinshu(BL 15) and Pishu(BL 20); in the syndrome of phlegm-blood obstruction in the collaterals, add Geshu(BL 17), Xuehai(SP 10) and Fenglong(ST 40). In the case of difficult speech,

3 治疗

3.1 基本治疗

主穴: 百会,四神聪,足三里,合谷。

配穴: 肝肾不足加肝俞、肾俞;气血虚弱加心俞、脾俞;痰瘀阻络加膈俞、血海、丰隆;语言障碍者,加通里、廉泉、金津、玉液;颈软者,加天柱;上肢瘫者,加肩髃、曲池;下肢瘫者,加环跳、阳陵

add Tongli(HT 5), Lianquan(CV 23), Jinjin(EX-HN 12) and Yuye(EX-HN 13); in the case of weak nape, add Tianzhu(BL 10); in the case of paralysis of the upper limbs, add Jianyu(LI 15) and Quchi(LI 11); in the case of paralysis of the lower limbs, add Huantiao(GB 30) and Yang-lingquan(GB 34); in the case of aching loin, Yaoyangguan(GV 3) and Mingmen(GV 4).

泉;腰部瘫软者,加腰阳关、命门。

Explanation: Baihui(GV 20), the meeting acupoint of yang meridians, is attributed to the governor vessel which enters into the brain, and serves to enrich the brain, regulate the spirit and open the orifices. Sishenchong(EX-HN 1) is an extra acupoint and functions to calm the mind and replenish the intelligence. Zusanli(ST 36) may replenish the postnatal foundation to transform qi and blood, nourish the sinews and brain. Hegu(LI 4), an acupoint of the foot-yangming meridian with abundant qi and blood, serves to regulate qi and blood, resolve blood stasis and unblock collaterals.

方义: 百会属于督脉,为诸阳之会,督脉入络脑,故能健脑调神开窍。四神聪为经外奇穴,有宁神醒脑益智之功。足三里培补后天之本,化生气血,滋养筋骨、脑髓。阳明经多气多血,合谷调理气血、化瘀通络。

3.2 Other therapies

3.2 其他治疗

Scalp acupuncture: Middle Line of Forehead (MS 1), Lateral Line 1 of Vertex(MS 8), Lateral Line 2 of Vertex(MS 9), Middle Line of Vertex(MS 5), Posterior Temporal Line(MS 11) and Lower-lateral Line of the Occiput(MS 14) are selected. Filiform needles of 1.5 cun in length should be inserted into the scalp quickly under the galea aponeurotica. Continuously insert the needles transversely underneath the skin to the due depth, and retain the needles for 2 to 4 hours. During the needle retention, the children may move freely. The treatment is given once every other day.

头针: 选额中线、顶颞前斜线、顶旁1线、顶旁2线、顶中线、颞后线、枕下旁线。用1.5寸毫针迅速刺入帽状腱膜下,然后将针体与头皮平行,推送至所需的刺激区,留针2～4小时,留针时可以自由活动,隔日1次。

Ear acupuncture: Occiput(AT 3), Subcortex(AT

耳针: 选枕、皮质下、心、

4), Heart(CO 15), Kidney(CO 10), Liver(CO 12), Spleen(CO 13) and Shenmen(TF 4) are selected. Puncture 2 to 4 acupoints with filiform needles by moderate intensity, and retain the needles for 20～30 minutes in each treatment. Or apply *Semen Vaccariae* (Wang Bu Liu Xing) at these acupoints, and alternate them every 3 to 5 days.

肾、肝、脾、神门。每次选 2～4 穴,毫针刺,中等强度刺激,每次留针 20～30 分钟。或用王不留行贴压,每3～5 日更换 1 次。

4 Remarks

Acupuncture has certain effects in relieving the symptoms of mild infantile cerebral palsy. Early and persistent treatments are a must for this condition. Ask the children to do functional exercises and intelligence training.

4 按语

针灸治疗轻型小儿脑瘫有一定效果,可改善症状。应重视早期治疗,坚持治疗,并注意加强功能训练和智力培训。

Section 3 External Diseases

第 3 节 外伤科病证

Nettle Rash

Nettle rash is a common allergic skin disease characterized by intense itching and an eruption of patchy wheals. Since it comes and goes, and is apt to appear after exposure to wind, it is also termed "hidden rash" and "wind wheal." Its specific manifestations are eruptions of light-red or pale pruritic pimples on the skin with on-and-off appearance. Nettle rash covers acute and chronic urticaria in Western medicine.

风疹

风疹是以皮肤异常瘙痒,出现成块、成片状风团为主症的常见过敏性皮肤病,因其时隐时现,遇风易发,故又称为"瘾疹""风疹块"。其特征为皮肤上出现淡红色或苍白色瘙痒性疹块,时隐时现。风疹相当于西医学的急慢性荨麻疹。

1 Etiology and pathogenesis

Nettle rash is often due to weak body constitution with loose striae and invasion of exogenous wind which accumulates within the skin, or to accu-

1 病因病机

风疹多由体质虚弱,腠理不固,风邪乘虚而入,遏于肌肤而成;或食用鱼虾荤腥

mulated heat in the stomach and intestine after overeating meat and fish and by intestinal insects, as well as attack of exogenous wind which also accumulates underneath the skin.

食物，以及肠道寄生虫等，导致胃肠积热，复感风邪，使内不得疏泄，外不得透达，郁于肌肤之间而发。

2 Syndrome differentiation

2 辨证

Chief symptoms: Sudden appearance of itching wheals of various sizes and irregular shapes or pimples rising one after another, with clear boundaries that look like those caused by mosquito bites; the wheals are red or white, happen and subside quickly, leaving no scars. Acute cases may be cured in two weeks; while chronic cases may repeat and persists.

主症：发病时在皮肤上突然出现大小不等、形状不一的风团，成块或成片，高起皮肤，边界清楚，有如蚊虫叮咬之疙瘩，其色或红或白，瘙痒异常，发病迅速，消退亦快，消退后不留痕迹。急性患者短期发作后 2 周内多可痊愈；慢性者常反复发作，缠绵难愈。

The syndrome of wind-heat invasion manifests rashes in those exposed areas such as the head, face and limbs, usually triggered by the change in weather, accompanied by symptoms of exogenous factors. The syndrome of heat accumulation in the stomach and intestines may be accompanied by distending pain in the epigastric and abdominal areas, constipation, dark yellow urine, or nausea and vomiting, intestinal gurgling and diarrhea, red tongue with yellow-greasy coating, and slippery rapid pulse; its onset is obviously related to diets. The syndrome of blood deficiency and wind-dryness manifests lingering conditions, accompanied by vexation, thirst, red tongue with less coating, and thin weak pulse.

风邪袭表者，疹块以露出部位（如头面、手足部）为重，发作与天气变化有明显关系，常兼有外感表证；胃肠积热者，兼脘腹胀痛，大便秘结，小便黄赤，或恶心呕吐，肠鸣泄泻，舌质红赤，舌苔黄腻，脉滑数，发作与饮食因素有明显关系；血虚风燥者，病久不愈，兼心烦口干，舌红少苔，脉细无力。

3 Treatment

3 治疗

3.1 Essential treatment

3.1 基本治疗

Principal acupoints: Quchi (LI 11), Hegu (LI 4), Xuehai(SP 10), Geshu(BL 17), and San-yinjiao (SP 6).

主穴：曲池，合谷，血海，膈俞，三阴交。

Supplementary acupoints: In the syndrome of wind-heat invasion, add Dazhui(GV 14), Yuji(LU 10), and Jianyu(LI 15); in the syndrome of heat accumulation in the stomach and intestines, add Zusanli(ST 36), Tianshu(ST 25) and Neiting(ST 44); in the syndrome of blood deficiency and wind-dryness, add Zusanli(ST 36).

配穴：外感风热加大椎、鱼际、肩髃；肠胃积热加足三里、天枢、内庭；血虚风燥加足三里。

Explanation: Quchi(LI 11) and Hegu(LI 4), the acupoints of the hand-yangming meridian, disperse wind and release the exterior, and clear the heat of yangming meridian; therefore, they are effective for nettle rash due to both invasion of exogenous factor and heat accumulation in the stomach and intestines. Xuehai(SP 10) and Sanyinjiao(SP 6), the acupoints of the foot-taiyin meridian, dominate diseases of the blood phase, can regulate the nutrient phase and activate the blood. Geshu(BL 17), the Influential acupoint of blood, is applied to activate blood and disperse wind. The combination of those acupoints function to disperse wind and clear heat, activate blood and regulate nutrient phase.

方义：曲池、合谷同为阳明经穴位，既可疏风解表，又能清泻阳明，故凡风疹无论外邪侵袭还是肠胃蕴热者用之皆有效。血海、三阴交属足太阴经穴，主血分病，调营活血。膈俞为血会，活血祛风。诸穴合用共奏疏风清热、活血调营之功。

3.2 Other therapy

3.2 其他治疗

Flashing cupping: The cup is applied on Shenque(CV 8) and retained for 5 minutes. The treatment is given once a day and 3 treatments constitute a full course.

闪罐：在神阙穴上闪罐之后留罐 5 分钟，每日治疗 1 次，3 次为 1 个疗程。

4 Remarks

4 按语

Acupuncture works well on nettle rash. For patients with chronic condition, acupoints such as Feishu(BL 13), Geshu(BL 17), Ganshu(BL 18) and Pishu(BL 20) are often used to enrich qi and strengthen the exterior, activate the blood and resolve stasis.

针灸治疗风疹疗效较好，对慢性患者则常用肺俞、膈俞、肝俞、脾俞等益气固表、活血化瘀。

Mumps

Mumps refers to an acute infectious disease in lung system characterized by fever and painful swelling in the parotid regions resulting from attack of heat epidemics obstructing the shaoyang meridian. It is known as epidemic parotitis in Western medicine and happens in children and adolescents.

痄 腮

痄腮是常见的中医肺系疫病之一，痄腮是指温热疫毒侵袭，壅遏少阳经脉所致以发热、腮部肿胀疼痛为主要表现的疫病类疾病。本病相当于西医学的流行性腮腺炎，多发于儿童和青少年。

1 Etiology and pathogenesis

Mumps is mainly caused by contraction of the exogenous wind and heat via the mouth and nose, which together with the phlegm-fire obstructs the shaoyang and yangming meridians and accumulates in the parotid regions. Since the shaoyang and jueyin meridians are externally-internally related to each other, and the jueyin meridian winds around the genital organs, mumps may be accompanied by distension in the lateral abdomen and swollen testis in the severe cases. If the warm toxin is potent, it may transform into fire and then disturb the heart and liver, resulting in high fever, convulsions, and coma.

1 病因病机

痄腮多因外感风温邪毒，从口鼻而入，夹痰化火，遏阻少阳、阳明经脉，郁结于腮部所致。少阳与厥阴相表里，足厥阴之脉循少腹络阴器，若受邪较重则常并发少腹痛、睾丸肿胀。若温毒炽盛，热极生风，内窜心肝，则出现高热、昏迷、痉厥等变症。

2 Syndrome differentiation

Chief symptoms: Painful swelling in the parotid regions, difficulty in chewing, and possible fever.

The syndrome of warm toxin in the exterior manifests simple soreness and swelling in the parotid regions, which may subside within a few days. The syndrome of severe warm toxin may start with chills, fever and mild general discomforts. The syndrome of heat-toxin accumulation may manifest fever, red and hot sensation and painful swelling in

2 辨证

主症：耳下腮部肿胀疼痛，咀嚼困难，或伴有发热。

温毒在表者，患者仅觉耳下腮部酸痛肿胀，而无其他见症，可在数日内逐渐肿消痛止；温毒较重者，初起有恶寒、发热、全身轻度不适等症。热毒蕴结者，兼发热、耳下腮部红肿热痛、坚硬拒按、

the parotid regions, hard mass and difficulty in chewing. The syndrome of ingoing heat toxin may be accompanied by high fever, intense thirstiness, or swollen and painful testis, or convulsions and coma.

咀嚼困难；温毒内陷者，兼高热烦渴，或睾丸肿痛，甚则神昏抽搐。

3 Treatment

3 治疗

3.1 Essential treatment

3.1 基本治疗

Principal acupoints: Yifeng (TE 17), Jiaosun (TE 20), Waiguan(TE 5), and Hegu(LI 4).

主穴：翳风，角孙，外关，合谷。

Supplementary acupoints: In the syndrome of warm toxin in the exterior, add Fengchi(GB 20) and Shaoshang(LU 11); in the syndrome of heat-toxin accumulation, add Shangyang(LI 1) and Quchi(LI 11). In the presence of painful and swollen testis, add Taichong(LR 3) and Ququan(LR 8); in the presence of convulsions and coma, add Shuigou (GV 26), Shixuan(EX-UE 11) or the twelve Jing-Well acupoints.

配穴：温毒在表加风池、少商；热毒蕴结加商阳、曲池；睾丸肿痛加太冲、曲泉；神昏抽搐加人中、十宣或十二井穴。

Explanation: Yifeng(TE 17) and Jiaosun(TE 20) are local acupoints and used to disperse local qi and blood. Waiguan(TE 5), the Luo-Connecting acupoint of the hand-shaoyang meridian, and Hegu (LI 4), the Yuan-Source acupoint of the hand-yangming meridian, are distal to the parotid regions and are applied to clear heat toxin in the shaoyang and yangming meridians. Moreover, Waiguan(TE 5) communicates with the yang link vessel, which is indicated for chills and fever. Combined use of Waiguan(TE 5) and Hegu(LI 4), the acupoint indicated for disorders on the face and head, helps disperse wind and relieve the exterior, clear heat and resolve swelling.

方义：近取翳风、角孙宣散患部气血。远取外关、合谷，以清泻少阳、阳明两经之郁热温毒，且外关通阳维脉，主寒热，与擅治头面之疾的合谷同用，更有疏风解表、清热消肿之功。

3.2 Other therapy

3.2 其他治疗

Burning-rush moxibustion: Select Jiaosun(TE 20) on the diseased side only or select both if mumps

灯火灸：选取角孙穴，单侧病者取患侧，双侧病者取

occur on both sides. The hair around the acupoint should be cut short and routinely disinfected. A burning oiled rush is pressed directly on the acupoint, which produces a slapping sound as soon as it is lifted. Usually the mumps is cured by only one treatment. If the swelling is still present, one more treatment is needed next day.

双侧。先剪短穴区头发,穴位常规消毒,取灯心草蘸植物油点燃,迅速触点穴位,并立即提起,可闻及"啪"的一声。一般灸治1次即可。若肿势不退,次日再灸1次。

4 Remarks

Mumps is caused by warm toxin epidemics, so prevention of epidemic transmission is the first choice in the treatment of mumps. Apart from early treatment, exogenous wind and foot intake should be cautious.

4 按语

痄腮属于温毒疫邪致病,故辟邪防传是防治本病的首要措施。本病除了应该及早治疗外,还要注意"避风戒口"。

Breast Abscess

Breast abscess is similar to acute mastitis in Western medicine, characterized by reddened, painful and swollen breast as well as nodules and distending pain in the breasts, accompanied by general discomforts such as fever, chills, aching body and poor appetite.

乳 痈

乳痈相当于西医学的急性乳腺炎,临床以患侧乳房结块、胀痛,局部红、肿、热、痛,并可伴有全身表现(如发热、寒战、浑身酸痛、食欲不振等)为特点。

1 Etiology and pathogenesis

Breast abscess results from obstruction of breast collaterals and milk accumulation by invasion of exogenous factors and weak constitution due to emotional upsets, improper diets, qi and blood deficiency after delivery, inappropriate milk-feeding or nipple rupture and unclean nipple. In women, the nipple is in association with the liver and the breast is in association with the stomach. Therefore, the focus of breast abscess is in the breast, and associates with the liver and stomach. Women after delivery suffer from abrupt deficiency of qi and blood, and

1 病因病机

七情内伤、饮食不节、产后气血不足、哺乳不当及乳头破溃、乳头不净感受外邪导致病邪乘虚而入,乳络不畅,乳汁郁积发而为病。女子乳头属肝,乳房属胃,故本病病位在乳房,与肝胃相关。产后妇人由于气血骤虚,易感外邪和伤于情志,具有多虚、多瘀、多外邪的病理特点。

are susceptible to exogenous factors and emotional disturbances, hence breast abscess possesses the pathological features of deficiency, blood stasis and exogenous pathogens.

2 Syndrome differentiation

Chief symptoms: Breast lumps, redness, swelling and pain.

The syndrome of liver-qi stagnation is accompanied by oppression and distending pain in the chest, nausea, poor appetite, thin tongue coating and wiry pulse. The syndrome of heat accumulation in the stomach is accompanied by thirst, foul breath, constipation, yellow-greasy tongue coating, and wiry rapid pulse.

3 Treatment

3.1 Essential treatment

Principal acupoints: Shaoze (SI 1), Danzhong (CV 17), Rugen (ST 18), Taichong (LR 3), and Jianjing(GB 21).

Supplementary acupoints: In the syndrome of liver-qi stagnation, add Qimen(LR 14) and Xingjian(LR 2); in the syndrome of heat accumulation in the stomach, add Liangqiu (ST 34) and Neiting (ST 44).

Explanation: Shaoze(SI 1) acts to remove the obstruction from breast collaterals and activate qi and blood. Rugen(ST 18) and Danzhong(CV 17) are used to promote qi and blood flow in the local breasts. Taichong(LR 3) can soothe the liver and relieve depression. Jianjing(GB 21) is the empirical acupoint for breast abscess and is the Crossing acupoint of foot-shaoyang, hand-shaoyang, foot-yangming meridians and yang link vessel; these meridians run over the chest and breast, so they can un-

2 辨证

主症: 乳房结块,红肿疼痛。

肝气郁结者,兼胸闷胀痛、呕逆、纳呆、脉弦苔薄;胃热蕴滞者,兼口渴口臭、便秘、苔黄腻、脉弦数。

3 治疗

3.1 基本治疗

主穴: 少泽,膻中,乳根,太冲,肩井。

配穴: 肝气郁结加期门、行间;胃热蕴滞加梁丘、内庭。

方义: 少泽疏通乳腺闭塞、行气活血。乳根、膻中两穴疏通局部气血。太冲疏肝解郁。肩井为治疗乳痈的经验用穴,系手足少阳、足阳明、阳维脉交会穴,所交会之经脉均行胸、乳,故用之可通调诸经之气,使少阳通则郁火散,阳明清则肿痛消。诸穴共奏清热、消肿、散结之功。

block the qi of these meridians to disperse depressed fire in the shaoyang meridians and eliminate swelling and pain in the yangming meridian. Combination of those acupoints acts to clear heat, relieve swelling and resolve masses.

3.2 Other therapy

Blood-letting and cupping: Acupoint Gaohuang (BL 43) in the diseased side is disinfected and tapped with seven-star needle by strong intensity. After slight bleeding, cupping therapy is performed and the cup is retained for 10 minutes. If breast abscess is not cured after one treatment, another treatment should be given on the contralateral Gaohuang(BL 43) with the above-mentioned therapy.

3.2 其他治疗

刺络拔罐: 患侧膏肓俞穴消毒后,用七星针叩刺,采用强刺激手法,皮肤微出血后拔罐,留罐10分钟。1次未愈者,次日取对侧膏肓俞穴,如法施治。

4 Remarks

Breast abscess occurs abruptly, transmits quickly and tends to suppurate, so treatment concentrates on the early stage. Acupuncture has better effects on the early stage of breast abscess. During the pyogenic stage, an incision must be performed to the abscess to drain the pus, and then comprehensive treatments should be prescribed.

4 按语

本病发病急、传变较快,易成脓破溃,治疗贵在"早"。针灸对本病初期有良好的疗效。溃脓期应切开排脓,综合治疗。

Breast Nodules

It refers to the common chromic benign lumps in the breasts, mainly marked by nodular masses in the breast with distension and pain. This disease can be seen in middle and old-aged women. Before Ming Dynasty, breast nodules usually refer to the disease pattern caused by indigested paediatric milk and food stagnation. While after Ming Dynasty, it refers to the woman breast disease. It is frequently seen in hyperplasia of the mammary gland, cystic

乳 癖

指妇女乳房部常见的慢性良性肿块,以乳房肿块和胀痛为主症,常见于中老年妇女。明代以前,乳癖一名,指的多是小儿乳食之积不消而致的病证。而在明代以后,乳癖才用于妇人乳腺疾病之名。本病可见于乳腺小叶增生、乳房囊性增生、乳房

hyperplasia of the breast and mastofibroma. In western medicine, it is believed that mammary hyperplasia is related to ovarian dysfunction, such as the decreased secretion of lutein and relatively increased secretion of estrogen.

纤维瘤等疾病。西医学认为乳腺增生症与卵巢功能失调有关，如黄体素分泌减少、雌激素含量相对增高。

1 Etiology and pathogenesis

Pathologically, breast nodules are of liver-qi depression and dysfunction of the thoroughfare and conception vessels. Breast nodules primarily result from mental depression and anxiety that gives rise to failure of liver-qi to disperse, heart-spleen qi-stagnation and qi-blood disharmony, or from phlegm-dampness retention in the breast collaterals, or from meridian malnutrition due to dysfunctions of the thoroughfare and conception vessels and liver-kidney yin-deficiency. In the clinic, a differential diagnosis should be made to distinguish from mammary cancer.

1 病因病机

肝气郁结、冲任失调为本病的病机特点。乳癖多由于忧郁思虑，肝失调达，心脾郁结，气血失调，痰湿阻滞乳络而成；或因冲任失调，肝肾阴虚，经脉失养而成。临床易与乳腺癌混淆，应注意鉴别。

2 Syndrome differentiation

Chief symptoms: Single or multiple nodular masses of different sizes located unilaterally or bilaterally in the breasts, accompanied by distending pain or tenderness, smooth surface with clear boundaries, slow growth, and hard or cystic texture.

The syndrome of liver-qi stagnation manifests increasing symptoms by anger, accompanied by dizziness and chest fullness, distending pain in the lower abdomen, irregular menstruation, mental depression, vexation and irritability, thin tongue coating and wiry pulse. The syndrome of phlegm-dampness retention is accompanied by vertigo, nausea, chest fullness, poor appetite with loose stools, coughing sputum, greasy tongue coating and slippery pulse.

2 辨证

主症：单侧或双侧乳房发生单个或多个大小不等的肿块，胀痛或压痛，表面光滑，边界清楚，推之可动，增长缓慢，质地坚韧或呈囊性感。

肝郁气滞者，常于生气后加重，兼头晕胸闷、少腹胀痛、月经不调、情志抑郁、心烦善怒、苔薄脉弦；痰浊凝结者，兼眩晕、恶心、胸闷脘痞、食少便溏、咳吐痰涎、苔腻、脉滑；肝肾阴虚者，兼午后潮热、头晕耳鸣、失眠多梦、腰背酸痛、舌淡、脉细数。

The syndrome of liver-kidney yin deficiency is accompanied by afternoon fever, dizziness and tinnitus, insomnia and dreaminess, aching waist, pale tongue and thin rapid pulse.

3 Treatment

3.1 Essential treatment

Principal acupoints: Rugen(ST 18), Wuyi(ST 15), Danzhong(CV 17), Qimen(LR 14), Tianzong (SI 11), and Jianjing (GB 21).

Supplementary acupoints: In the syndrome of liver-qi stagnation, add Ganshu(BL 18) and Taichong(LR 3); in the syndrome of phlegm-dampness retention, add Fenglong(ST 40) and Zhongwan(CV 12); in the syndrome of liver-kidney yin deficiency, add Ganshu(BL 18) and Shenshu(BL 23).

Explanation: Rugen(ST 18) and Wuyi(ST 15) may promote qi flow in yangming meridian and unblock local qi and blood. Danzhong(CV 17), the sea of qi, can move qi by reducing methods; Qimen (LR 14) can soothe liver-qi and regulate the thoroughfare and conception vessels. Jianjing(GB 21) relaxes sinews and activates collaterals, resolves mass and relieves pain; puncturing this acupoint can free qi activity of the triple energizer to manage the root and branch factors of breast nodules. Tianzong(SI 11), an empirical acupoint for treating breast diseases, can relieve swelling and resolve mass, and regulate yin and yang to treat breast nodules.

3.2 Other therapy

Abdominal acupuncture: Puncture Zhongwan (CV 12), Xiawan(CV 10), Qihai(CV 6) and Guanyuan(CV 4) 25 mm to the subcutaneous tissues. Puncture Huaroumen(ST 24) on the diseased side beneath the skin and above the muscle layer,

3 治疗

3.1 基本治疗

主穴：乳根，屋翳，膻中，期门，天宗，肩井。

配穴：肝郁气滞加肝俞、太冲；痰浊凝结加丰隆、中脘；肝肾阴虚加肝俞、肾俞。

方义：乳根、屋翳疏导阳明经经气，疏通局部气血。膻中为气海，泻之以利气机。期门疏肝气，调冲任。肩井舒筋活络、散结止痛，刺之可调畅三焦气化，该穴治疗乳癖具有标本同治之妙。天宗为治疗乳腺疾病之经验穴，对乳房肿块具有消肿散结、调和阴阳的功效。

3.2 其他治疗

腹针：选取患侧中脘、下脘、气海、关元深刺至较深的皮下组织中，深度约 25 毫米；患侧滑肉门浅刺，其深度为穿过皮下，位于脂肪层，在

and rotate the needles; it is unnecessary to induce qi arrival. The needles are retained for 20 minutes to wait for qi arrival. The needle at Huaroumen (ST 24) is rotated every 10 minutes with the needle tip towards the breasts. Treatment is given once a week for total 5 weeks.

肌层之上，只捻转不提插，无需得气感觉。进针后停留 20 分钟谓之候气。每隔 10 分钟在滑肉门调针一次，针尖朝乳腺增生的方向进行捻转。留针 20 分钟。每周 2 次，治疗 5 周。

4 Remarks

Acupuncture works well on breast nodules, but needs a long-course treatment; combined use of herbal medicines can help acupuncture in improving clinical efficacy. There is a tendency to cancer formation in a few cases, if so surgery is recommended.

4 按语

针灸对本病有良好的疗效，但疗程较长，配合中药可增强疗效。少数病例有恶变的可能，必要时应及时进行手术治疗。

Intestinal Abscess

Intestinal abscess refers to an internal abscess in the intestines. It falls into large intestine abscess and small intestine abscess in accordance with the pain foci; the former happens in the lower right abdomen around acupoint Tianshu (ST 25), and the latter happens around Guanyuan (CV 4). Clinically, large intestine abscess is more frequent. Intestinal abscess refers to acute and chronic appendicitis in Western medicine.

肠　痈

肠痈是指发生于肠道的痈肿，属内痈范畴。肠痈按疼痛部位的不同，可分为大肠痈和小肠痈，痛处接近右下腹天枢穴者称“大肠痈”，在关元穴附近者称“小肠痈”。临床以大肠痈为常见。西医的阑尾炎多归属于肠痈范畴。

1 Etiology and pathogenesis

Intestinal abscess usually results from improper diet such as excessive eating and drinking, or from overeating fatty diets, raw and contaminated food that injures the stomach and intestines and then gives rise to dampness-heat retention in the intestines, or from qi-blood stagnation and impaired intestine due to fast walking after meals, or from qi

1 病因病机

多因饮食不节，暴饮暴食，或过食油腻、生冷不洁之物，损伤肠胃，湿热内生蕴于肠间；或因饮食后急剧奔走，导致气滞血瘀，肠络受损；或因寒温不适、跌仆损伤、精神因素等，导致气滞、湿阻、热

stagnation, dampness obstruction, heat accumulation, blood stasis and ensuing intestine erosion due to climate alternation, injuries from falls and mental factors.

壅、瘀阻、积热不散,血腐肉败成痈肿。

2 Syndrome differentiation

Chief symptoms: Paroxysmal progressive abdominal pain in the lower right abdomen with muscular tension and rebounding tenderness.

In mild cases, the paroxysmal dull pain is first located in the upper abdomen or around the umbilicus; and several hours later, it appears in the lower right abdomen with gradual progression, accompanied by chills and fever, nausea and vomiting, constipation, abdominal distension, dark-yellow urine, yellowish greasy tongue coating, and surging pulse. In the severe cases, it is accompanied by fixed and progressive pain, muscular tension and spasm of the abdominal wall, refusal to pressure, possible touched masses and persistent high fever.

2 辨证

主症: 持续伴有阵发性加剧的右下腹疼痛、肌紧张、反跳痛。

轻症者,初起上腹部或脐周作痛,阵发性钝痛,数小时后疼痛转移至右下腹部,逐渐加重,伴有恶寒发热、恶心呕吐、便秘、腹胀、溲赤、苔黄腻、脉洪数;重症者,兼痛处固定不移、痛势加剧,腹肌紧张拘急、拒按,局部可触及肿物,高热不退。

3 Treatment

3.1 Essential treatment

Principal acupoints: Tianshu(ST 25), Shangjuxu (ST 37), Lanwei(EX-LE7), and Ashi acupoint.

Supplementary acupoints: In the presence of fever, add Quchi(LI 11) and Dazhui(GV 14); in the presence of vomiting, add Shangwan(CV 13) and Neiguan(PC 6); in the presence of constipation, add Fujie(SP 14); in the presence of abdominal distension, add Dachangshu(BL 25).

Explanation: Since the disease is located in the large intestine, Tianshu(ST 25), the Front-Mu acupoint of the large intestine, and Shangjuxu(ST 37), and the Lower He-Sea acupoint of the large intestine meridian, are applied to regulate the intestines

3 治疗

3.1 基本治疗

主穴: 天枢,上巨虚,阑尾穴,阿是穴。

配穴: 发热加曲池、大椎;呕吐加上脘、内关;便秘加腹结;腹胀加大肠俞。

方义: 本病病位在大肠,故取大肠募穴天枢、下合穴上巨虚以通调肠腑,清泻肠腑积热。阑尾穴是治疗肠痈的经验效穴。针刺阿是穴可

and purge the accumulated heat in the intestines. Lanwei(EX-LE 7) is an empirical acupoint for intestinal abscess. Puncturing Ashi acupoint can work on the diseased area to promote qi-blood flow and resolve abscess and relieve pain.

直达病所，畅通患部气血，消痈止痛。

3.2 Other therapy

Floating acupuncture: For chronic appendicitis, subcutaneously puncture the points 7 cm bilateral to Ashi acupoint with the needle tips towards the painful sites. When the needles are inserted, shake the needles and press the Ashi acupoint till no pain is felt, then apply plaster to fixate the needles for 24 hours. For acute appendicitis, four floating needles are inserted into Ashi acupoint from above, below, left and right, and then shake the needles more than 10 times till the pain is eased or disappears.

3.2 其他治疗

浮针：慢性阑尾炎在阿是穴左、右侧 7 厘米处分别进针，针尖对准疼痛点方向沿皮下进针，待针全部刺入后，将针尖呈扇形摆动5～7次，再按压阿是穴，反应不痛，即可取出针芯，用胶布固定，24 小时后取出；急性阑尾炎患者在阿是穴的上下左右各刺入一支浮针，扇形摆动针尖 10 次以上，直至压痛明显减轻或消失为止。

4 Remarks

Acupuncture works well on intestinal abscess in the early stage and on some in the suppurative stage in relieving pain instantly. However, it is not so effective against severe abscess. In the treatment of chronic appendicitis with recurrent pain in the lower right abdomen, moxibustion is recommended in combination with acupuncture.

4 按语

针灸对初期或一部分酿脓期患者效果较好，有即刻止痛的作用，但对于重症则疗效较差。对于慢性阑尾炎右少腹经常疼痛者，除针刺外，应配合灸法治疗。

Hemorrhoids

Hemorrhoids, a chronic anorectal disease, refers to venous bulges developing from enlarged veins under the mucosa of the lower rectum and the skin of the anal canal. It may happen in both males and females, and is frequently seen in young adults and

痔　疮

痔疮是发生于肛肠部的慢性疾病，指直肠下端黏膜下和肛管皮下的静脉扩大曲张形成的静脉团块，男女均可发病，以青壮年、经产妇多

multiparous women. In Western medicine, hemorrhoids is classified into internal, external and mixed hemorrhoids according to the location of the lesion.

见。西医学将其分为内痔、外痔和混合痔。

1 Etiology and pathogenesis

Hemorrhoids often results from long-term sitting and standing, carrying heavy loads for long distances, and pregnancy, or from improper diets and over-indulgence in spicy and greasy food that produces internal dryness and heat and then injures the stomach and intestine, or from prolonged diarrhea or dysentery and constipation that bring about accumulation of internal dampness-heat and blood stasis in anal collaterals.

1 病因病机

痔疮发生多因久坐、久站、负重远行、妊娠所致;或因饮食不节,嗜食辛辣厚味,燥热内生,肠胃受损而得,或因久泻、久痢、便秘,以致湿热内生,脉络郁阻,壅结肛肠而致。

2 Syndrome differentiation

Chief symptoms: Sarcoid protuberance in the anorectal area with no symptoms, other than some pain, or only with foreign-body sensation, possible swelling around the anus and bleeding during defecation.

The syndrome of downward dampness-heat may be accompanied by local swelling, pain and damyzness. The syndrome of qi deficiency and collapse may be accompanied by a prolapse of anus and fatigue.

2 辨证

主症:肛门部出现小肉状突出物,无症状或仅有异物感,也可伴有肛门处疼痛、肿胀和大便时出血。

湿热下注者,兼局部肿胀、疼痛、潮湿等;气虚下陷者,兼脱肛、乏力等症状。

3 Treatment

3.1 Essential treatment

Principal acupoints: Chengshan(BL 57), Huiyang (BL 35), Ciliao(BL 32), and Changqiang(GV 1).

Supplementary acupoints: In the syndrome of downward dampness-heat, add Dachangshu(BL 25) and Yinlingquan(SP 9); in the syndrome of qi deficiency and collapse, apply moxibustion on Shenque (CV 8) and Baihui(GV 20); in the presence of constipation, add Zhigou(TE 6) and Tianshu(ST 25).

3 治疗

3.1 基本治疗

主穴:承山,会阳,次髎,长强。

配穴:湿热下注加大肠俞、阴陵泉;气虚下陷加灸神阙、百会;便秘加支沟、天枢。

Explanation: Chengshan(BL 57), Huiyang(BL 35) and Ciliao(BL 32) are acupoints of the foot-taiyang meridian whose meridian divergency derives from the calf, and reaches the popliteal fossa and enters into anus, so these three acupoints are needled with reducing methods to clear dampness-heat in the anus and rectum, activate bladder-meridian qi and resolve blood stasis. The local acupoint Changqiang (GV 1) is used to enhance the therapeutic efficacy.

方义：承山、会阳、次髎均为足太阳经穴，足太阳经别又自腨至腘，别入肛中，故取三穴用泻法，清泻肛肠湿热，疏导膀胱经气而消瘀滞；近取长强以加强其作用。

3.2 Other therapy

3.2 其他治疗

Fire acupuncture: The foli on Yinjiao(GV 28) or just acupoint Yinjiao(GV 28) is pricked with fire needle to make the site scarred.

火针：用火针点刺龈交穴处的滤泡（滤泡不明显时点刺龈交穴），使其形成焦痂。

4 Remarks

4 按语

Acupuncture can relieve pain and swelling instantly when hemorrhoids is in acute attacks. However, specialized treatment is needed for a radical cure. Patients are advised to take fewer spicy foods and maintain normal bowel movements.

痔疮肿痛发作时，用针刺能迅速缓解症状，若求根治则须专科处理。平素少食辛辣刺激性食物，保持大便通畅。

Sprain

扭　伤

Sprain refers to the injury of the soft tissues (muscles, tendons, ligaments, and vessels) of the four extremities and trunk without fractures, dislocations and wounds on the skin. Its cardinal clinical manifestation includes local pain and swelling with limitation of joint movements around the diseased sites, frequently on the loin, ankles, knees, shoulder, wrists, elbows, neck and hips.

扭伤是指四肢关节或躯体部的软组织（如肌肉、肌腱、韧带、血管等）损伤，而无骨折、脱臼、皮肉破损等情况。临床主要表现为损伤部位疼痛肿胀和关节活动受限，多发于腰、踝、膝、肩、腕、肘、颈、髋等部位。

1 Etiology and pathogenesis

1 病因病机

Usually, sprain is caused by violent move-

扭伤起因多为剧烈运动

ments, improper posture when carrying heavy loads, falling down, trauma, over-stretching and over-straining, which bring about spasm and rupture of such soft tissues as muscles, tendons, ligaments and vessels, hence leading to local qi-blood stagnation, swelling and pain, and even limited movement of the joints.

或负重不当,或不慎跌仆、外伤、牵拉和过度扭转等原因,引起肌肉、肌腱、韧带、血管等软组织的痉挛、撕裂,以致气血壅滞局部,导致局部肿胀疼痛,甚至关节活动受限的一种疾病。

2 Syndrome differentiation

2 辨证

Chief symptoms: Pain in the sprained area with restriction or inability of joint movement, followed by swelling, redness or bruising at the injured sites.

主症: 扭伤部位疼痛,关节活动不利,继则出现肿胀,伤处肌肤发红或青紫。

The syndrome of qi-blood stagnation is accompanied by red, bluish or purplish discoloration of the local skin. The syndrome of cold-dampness contraction is accompanied by recurrent pain triggered by climate alternation.

气血阻滞者,兼伤处皮色发红或青或紫;寒湿侵袭者,兼陈伤每遇天气变化而疼痛反复发作。

3 Treatment

3 治疗

3.1 Essential treatment

3.1 基本治疗

Principal acupoints: Loin: Ashi acupoint, Shenshu(BL 23), Yaotong(EX-UE 7), and Weizhong (BL 40).

主穴: 腰部:阿是穴,肾俞,腰痛穴,委中。

Ankle: Ashi acupoint, Shenmai(BL 62), Qiuxu (GB 40), and Jiexi(ST 41).

踝部:阿是穴,申脉,丘墟,解溪。

Knee: Ashi acupoint, Xiyan (EX-LE5), Xiyangguan(GB 33), and Liangqiu(ST 34).

膝部:阿是穴,膝眼,膝阳关,梁丘。

Shoulder: Ashi acupoint, Jianyu(LI 15), Jianliao(TE 14), and Jianzhen(SI 9).

肩部:阿是穴,肩髃,肩髎,肩贞。

Elbow: Ashi acupoint, Quchi(LI 11), Xiaohai (SI 8), and Tianjing(TE 10).

肘部:阿是穴,曲池,小海,天井。

Wrist: Ashi acupoint, Yangxi(LI 5), Yangchi (TE 4), and Yanggu(SI 5).

腕部:阿是穴,阳溪,阳池,阳谷。

Hip: Ashi acupoint, Huantiao(GB 30), Zhibian(BL 54), and Juliao (GB 29).

髋部:阿是穴,环跳,秩边,居髎。

Supplementary acupoints: The distal acupoints

配穴: 可根据受伤部位

of the meridians that travel through the diseased areas can be selected; for example, Shuigou(GV 26) and Houxi(SI 3) can be selected if the sprain experiences in the column of the lumbar region where the governor vessel supplies. The acupoints adjacent to the diseased area along the affected meridian can also be selected; for example, the sprain on the medial side of the knee where the spleen meridian of the foot-taiyin supplies, Xuehai (SP 10) and Yinlingquan(SP 9), apart from Ashi acupoint, can be selected together to unblock qi and blood flow in the spleen meridian.

的经络所属，配合循经远取，如腰部正中扭伤病在督脉，可远取人中、后溪；也可在其上下循经邻近取穴，如膝内侧扭伤病在足太阴脾经者，除用阿是穴外，可在扭伤部位其上取血海、其下取阴陵泉，以疏通脾经气血。

Explanation: Most of the sprains are injuries of the joint tendons which are attributed to "diseases of muscle region". Based on the theory that "when a certain muscle region is injured, the treatment is focused on the corresponding meridian", local acupoints in the sprained area are used as the principal acupoints to unblock meridians and eliminate local qi-blood stagnation for the purpose of achieving the effect of "free flow creates no pain". Moreover, the acupoints bearing the same name on the hand and foot meridians can also be applied; and physical therapy on the sprained area should be combined at the same time. In addition, moxibustion is recommended for the prolonged sprain.

方义：扭伤多为关节伤筋，属经筋病，故治疗时取扭伤部位穴位为主，以疏通经络，散除局部的气血壅滞，达到"通则不痛"的效果。亦可采用手足同名经对应取穴法，同时配合作扭伤部位的活动。兼陈伤者可加灸。

3.2 Other therapy

Blood-letting and cupping: Select Ashi acupoint and tap the painful and swollen area with the dermal needle until the skin is slightly bleeding, followed by cupping. This therapy is applicable to treat acute sprain with remarkable local hematomas and old injury with stagnant blood, or with the invasion of external coldness.

3.2 其他治疗

刺络拔罐：选取阿是穴，用皮肤针叩刺疼痛肿胀处，以微出血为度，再拔火罐。适用于新伤局部血肿明显者或陈伤瘀血久留、寒邪袭络等。

4 Remarks

Acupuncture works well on sprains, and other methods such as massage and fumigating-washing therapy can be applied to enhance therapeutic outcomes. In clinical practice, it is necessary to exclude sprain from fracture, dislocation and ruptured ligaments. The sprained area should be kept warm to avoid invasion of the external wind, cold and dampness.

4 按语

针灸对扭伤疗效较好，可配合推拿、药物熏洗等疗法以增强疗效。治疗时须排除骨折、脱位、韧带断裂等情况。注意患部保暖，避免风寒湿邪的侵袭。

Elbow Strain

Elbow strain belongs to the category of "injury of the tendon". It is usually marked by slow onset, repeated attacks and absence of trauma, and is frequently seen in people who have to rotate their forearms and stretch their elbows in order to work, such as woodworkers, locksmiths, plumbers, electricians, mineworkers as well as tennis players. Elbow strain is commonly known as external humeral epicondylitis, internal humeral epicondylitis and inflammation of the olecranon.

肘 劳

肘劳属“伤筋”范畴，一般起病缓慢，常反复发作，无明显外伤史，多见于从事旋转前臂和屈伸肘关节的劳动者，如木工、钳工、水电工、矿工及网球运动员等。本病常见于肱骨外上髁炎、肱骨内上髁炎和尺骨鹰嘴炎等。

1 Etiology and pathogenesis

Elbow strain is usually caused by chronic injury and overuse of the elbow joint that result in consumption of the qi and blood, and the blood fails to nourish the muscles and tendons. However, the exogenous wind-cold invades the elbow joint and impairs the tendons of the hand three yang meridians, giving rise to elbow strain.

1 病因病机

本病主要由慢性劳损引起，肘关节长期劳作，以致劳伤气血，血不荣筋，筋脉失却濡养，风寒之邪乘虚侵袭肘关节，手三阳经筋受损而发为本病。

2 Syndrome differentiation

Chief symptoms: Localized pain in the lateral elbow that is aggravated by clenching fists, rotating the forearms and stretching the elbow, local tender-

2 辨证

主症：肘关节外侧出现局限性疼痛，用力握拳及前臂作旋前伸肘动作时可加

ness and absence of abnormal appearance.

The syndrome of hand-yangming meridian sinew manifests obvious tender points on the lateral and superior side of the elbow joint(around the external humeral epicondyle). The syndrome of the hand-taiyang meridian sinew manifests obvious tender points on the medial and inferior side of the elbow joint(around the internal humeral epicondyle). The syndrome of the hand-shaoyang meridian sinew manifests obvious tender points on the lateral side of elbow joint(on the olecranon).

3 Treatment

3.1 Essential treatment

Principal acupoints: Ashi acupoint.

Supplementary acupoints: In the syndrome of hand-yangming meridian sinew, add Quchi(LI 11), Shousanli(LI 10) and Hegu(LI 4); in the syndrome of hand-taiyang meridian sinew, add Yanggu(SI 5) and Xiaohai(SI 8); in the syndrome of hand-shaoyang meridian sinew, add Waiguan(TE 5) and Tianjing(TE 10).

Explanation: Ashi acupoints function to promote local qi-blood flow, relax muscles and tendons, unblock collaterals and stop pain.

3.2 Other therapy

Warm acupuncture: Select Zhongzhu(TE 3), Hegu(LI 4), Houxi(SI 3) and Ashi acupoint as the principal acupoints, and Quchi(LI 11), Shousanli(LI 10) and Lieque(LU 7) as the supplementary acupoints. After qi arrives, the ignited moxa sections are inserted into the needle body to perform moxibustion, two sections in one treatment. The treatment is given once every other day, and ten

重,局部有多处压痛,而外观无异常。

手阳明经筋证:肘关节外上方(肱骨外上髁周围)有明显的压痛点。手太阳经筋证:肘关节内下方(肱骨内上髁周围)有明显的压痛点。手少阳经筋证:肘关节外部(尺骨鹰嘴处)有明显的压痛点。

3 治疗

3.1 基本治疗

主穴: 阿是穴。

配穴: 手阳明经筋证加曲池、手三里、合谷;手太阳经筋证加阳谷、小海;手少阳经筋证加外关、天井。

方义: 阿是穴疏通局部经络气血,舒筋通络止痛。

3.2 其他治疗

温针灸: 取中渚、合谷、后溪、阿是穴为主穴,辅以曲池、手三里、列缺。进针得气后将点燃的艾炷套在针柄上,灸2壮。隔日治疗1次,10次为1个疗程。

treatments constitute a full course.

4 Remarks

Acupuncture and moxibustion work excellently on elbow strain. During treatment, the elbow should be kept warm to avoid the invasion of exogenous wind, cold and dampness.

4 按语

针灸治疗肘劳有很好的临床疗效。治疗期间注意局部保暖，尽量避免风寒湿邪的侵袭。

Shoulder Pain

Shoulder pain refers to a group of symptoms characterized by pain and motor dysfunction due to the periarthritis of the shoulder. In a broad sense, shoulder pain includes subacromial bursitis, supraspinatus tendinitis, rotator culf rupture, bicipital tenosynovitis, coracoiditis, frozen shoulder and acromioclavicular articulation diseases; In a narrow sense, it just refers to frozen shoulder or "Shoulders of Fifties", and often experiences abrupt onset of pain and contraction of shoulder joint in middle-aged people.

肩 痛

肩痛是由肩关节周围炎症引起的一组表现为疼痛及运动功能障碍的症候群，广义上包括肩峰下滑囊炎、冈上肌腱炎、肩袖破裂、肱二头肌长头腹及其腹鞘炎、喙突炎、冻结肩、肩锁关节病变等多种疾患；狭义上仅指冻结肩(或称"五十肩")，中年以后突发性的肩关节疼痛及关节挛缩症。

1 Etiology and pathogenesis

Shoulder pain is primarily caused by weak constitution, chronic strain and invasion of exogenous wind-cold that obstruct qi flow in the meridians. Invasion of exogenous wind and cold blocks the flow of qi and blood of the shoulder; over-strain may injure the muscles and tendons and then bring about qi and blood stagnation; in the aged, qi and blood are deficiency and fail to nourish the muscles, tendons and bones. All these causes can affect the flow of qi and blood in the shoulder meridians, leading to shoulder pain.

1 病因病机

本病多因体虚、劳损、风寒侵袭肩部，致使经气不利所致。肩部感受风寒，气血痹阻；或劳作过度，损及筋脉，气滞血瘀；或年老气血不足，筋骨失养，皆可使肩部经络气血不利，不通则痛。

2 Syndrome differentiation

Chief symptoms: Pain, soreness and heavy sen-

2 辨证

主症：肩周疼痛、酸重，

sation around the shoulder joint that worsens at night. It is often triggered or aggravated by the climate alternation and over-strain. Tender points are found in the anterior, posterior and lateral aspects of the shoulder joint. Both active and passive movements of the shoulder joint such as abduction, backward extension and rising of the arm are obviously limited, and muscular atrophy will happen in the late stage.

夜间为甚，常因天气变化及劳累而诱发或加重，患者肩前、后及外侧均有压痛，主动和被动外展、后伸、上举等功能明显受限，后期可出现肌肉萎缩。

The syndrome of invasion of pathogenic cold manifests the pain aggravated by wind and cold, and alleviated by warmth, aversion to wind and cold, with the history of cold contraction. The syndrome of qi and blood stagnation manifests pain aggravated by pressure, dark tongue with possible ecchymosis, rough pulse, with the history of trauma or over-strain. The syndrome of qi and blood deficiency may manifest aches and heaviness in the shoulder aggravated by over-strain, or accompanied by vertigo and dizziness, weakness of the four limbs, pale tongue with thin whitish coating, and thready weak pulse.

寒邪侵袭者，疼痛症状遇风寒则剧，得温则减，畏风恶寒，有明显的受寒病史；气滞血瘀者，疼痛拒按，舌暗或有瘀斑，脉涩，肩部有外伤或劳作过度史；气血虚弱者，肩部酸痛，劳累加重，或兼头晕目眩，四肢乏力，舌淡，苔薄白，脉细弱。

3 Treatment

3.1 Essential treatment

Principal acupoints: Jianyu(LI 15), Jianliao(TE 14), Jianzhen(SI 9), and Ashi acupoint.

Supplementary acupoints: In the syndrome of invasion of pathogenic cold, add Hegu(LI 4) and Fengchi(GB 20); in the syndrome of qi and blood stagnation, add Xuehai(SP 10) and Geshu(BL 17); in the syndrome of qi and blood deficiency, add Zusanli(ST 36) and Qihai(CV 6).

Explanation: All these acupoints are around the shoulder joint, and are applied to promote the flow

3 治疗

3.1 基本治疗

主穴：肩髃，肩髎，肩贞，阿是穴。

配穴：寒邪侵袭加合谷、风池；气滞血瘀加血海、膈俞；气血虚弱加足三里、气海。

方义：诸穴皆在病变局部，可疏通肩部经络气血，活

of qi and blood in the shoulder meridians, activate blood and dispel wind to stop pain.

血祛风而止痛。

3.2 Other therapy

Fire acupuncture: For chronic cases with severe adhesion and inability to move, fire acupuncture may be performed at the most painful site on the shoulder, and passive exercises can be conducted.

3.2 其他治疗

火针：对病程较长、粘连严重而不能活动的患者，可用火针刺肩部最痛点并配合被动运动。

4 Remarks

Acupuncture works well on shoulder pain in the early stage, and massage can be combined in the late stage to enhance the therapeutic outcomes. After shoulder pain is eased and swelling disappears, patients should be instructed to do exercises of the shoulder joint, keep the shoulder warm.

4 按语

本病早期针灸治疗效果较好，后期可配合推拿疗法以提高疗效。肩关节疼痛减缓和肿胀消失后，应在医生指导下坚持关节功能锻炼，并注意肩部保暖。

Cervical Spondylopathy

Cervical spondylopathy refers to a group of symptoms resulting from degenerative changes of the cervical intervertebral discs and its ensuing patho- logical changes in the surrounding tissues. According to the tissues involved and clinical manifestations, cervical spondylopathy may fall into neck spondylosis, cervical spondylotic radiculopathy, cervical spondylotic myelopathy, cervical spondylotic vertebrarteriopathy, and cervical spondylotic sympathy. Its some symptoms can be seen respectively in the diseases of "stiff neck" "cervical muscular spasm" "neck and shoulder pain" "headache" and "vertigo" in Chinese medicine. It is prone to occur in middle-aged and elderly people between the ages of 40 to 60 years.

颈椎病

颈椎病是颈椎间盘组织退行性改变及其继发病理改变累及其周围结构而出现相应的一组临床综合症候群。根据不同组织结构受累出现不同临床表现，将颈椎病分为颈型、神经根型、脊髓型、椎动脉型、交感型等。其部分症状分别见于中医学"项强""颈筋急""颈肩痛""头痛""眩晕"等病证中。好发于40～60岁中老年人，但近年来该病有年轻化的趋势。

1 Etiology and pathogenesis

In Chinese medicine, cervical spondylopathy is

1 病因病机

中医学认为，颈椎病因

caused by undernourishment of tendons and bones due to weak constitution and liver-kidney insufficiency, or by qi consumption and tendon-muscle injury after long-term sitting, or by invasion of exogenous factors into the meridians, or by blood stagnation and meridian obstruction following tendon sprain and contusion.

年老体衰、肝肾不足、筋骨失养；或久坐耗气、劳损筋肉；或感受外邪、客于经脉，或扭挫伤筋、气血瘀滞、经脉闭阻不通所致。

2 Syndrome differentiation

Chief symptoms: Chronic onset of the symptoms, pain in the head, neck, shoulder, upper back and upper limbs; and progressive sensory and motor disturbance of the limbs.

The syndrome of wind-cold obstruction is caused by sleeping with uncovered shoulders at night or lying in damp environments for a long time, manifesting stiff neck and painful spine, aching pain in the shoulders, limited movement of the neck, even numbness and coldness in the arms which are aggravated by exposure to coldness, or accompanied by aversion to cold, aching body, thin white or white greasy tongue coating, and wiry tight pulse. The syndrome of over-strain and blood-stasis manifests pain in the neck, shoulders and arms even radiating to the forearms, numbness in the fingers exacerbated by exertion, stiff or swollen neck, limited movement of the neck, dark purple tongue with petechia, and rough pulse, usually with the history of trauma or the habit of sitting with head bending. The syndrome of liver-kidney yin-deficiency manifests pain in the neck, shoulders and arms, numbness and weakness of the limbs, accompanied by such symptoms as dizziness, blurred vision, tinnitus, aching waist, spermatorrhea, irregular menstruation, red tongue with less coating, and weak

2 辨证

主症：发病缓慢，头枕、颈项、肩背、上肢等部疼痛以及进行性肢体感觉和运动障碍。

风寒闭阻者，夜寐漏肩或久卧湿地而致颈强脊痛，肩痹酸楚，颈部活动受限，甚则手臂麻木发冷，遇寒加重，或伴形寒怕冷、全身酸楚，舌苔薄白或白腻，脉弦紧；劳伤血瘀者，颈项、肩臂疼痛，甚则放射至前臂，手指麻木，劳累后加重，颈部僵直或肿胀，活动不利，舌质紫暗有瘀点，脉涩，常有外伤史或见于久坐低头职业者；肝肾阴亏者，颈项、肩臂疼痛，四肢麻木乏力，兼头晕眼花、耳鸣、腰膝酸软、遗精或月经不调、舌红少苔、脉细弱。

thready pulse.

3 Treatment

3.1 Essential treatment

Principal acupoints: Dazhui(GV 14), Houxi(SI 3), Tianzhu(BL 10), and Cervical Jiaji(EX-B 2).

Supplementary acupoints: In the syndrome of wind-cold obstruction, add Fengmen(BL 12) and Fengfu(GV 16); in the syndrome of over-strain and blood-stasis, add Geshu(BL 17) and Hegu(LI 4); in the syndrome of liver-kidney yin-deficiency, add Ganshu(BL 18), Shenshu(BL 23) and Zusanli(ST 36).

Explanation: Dazhui (GV 14), the acupoint where yang meridians meet, acts to activate qi of the yang meridians, and unblock meridians and collaterals. Tianzhu(BL 10), a local acupoint, and Houxi(SI 3), the Confluent acupoint communicating with the governor vessel, function to regulate the qi of taiyang meridian and the governor vessel, and unblock collaterals to stop pain. Cervical Jiaji (EX-B 2) acupoints have the action of regulating the local qi and blood to stop pain. The combined use of distal and local acupoints together exert the functions of soothing the tendons and activating collaterals, and regulating qi flow to ease pain.

3.2 Other therapy

Electro-acupuncture: Select 2 to 4 acupoints of Cervical Jiaji(EX-B 2), Dazhui(GV 14), Fengchi (GB 20), Jianzhongshu(SI 15), Dazhu(BL 11), and Tianzong(SI 11) each time, and electric stimulation at the frequency of 10~12 Hz is applied for 20 minutes, once a day.

4 Remarks

In acupuncture clinic, cervical spondylotic radicu-

3 治疗

3.1 基本治疗

主穴：大椎，后溪，天柱，颈椎夹脊。

配穴：风寒闭阻者加风门、风府；劳伤血瘀者加膈俞、合谷；肝肾亏虚者加肝俞、肾俞、足三里。

方义：大椎为诸阳之会，能激发诸阳经经气，通经活络。天柱为局部取穴，后溪与督脉相通，二穴配伍可疏调太阳经和督脉经气，通络止痛。颈椎夹脊穴具有疏理局部气血而止痛的作用。诸穴远近配伍，共奏疏筋活络、理气止痛之功。

3.2 其他治疗

电针：选颈部夹脊穴、大椎、风池、肩中俞、大杼、天宗。每次选 2～4 穴，频率 10～12 Hz，每次 20 分钟，每日 1 次。

4 按语

针灸临床多见神经根型

lopathy and cervical spondylotic vertebrarteriopathy are often encountered. Acupuncture is quite effective to relieve stiffness and pain in the neck, shoulder, upper back and limbs, dizziness and headache. Acupuncture can be used alone, but it is more effective in combination with massage. The neck should be kept warm to prevent invasion of exogenous wind and cold.

和椎动脉型颈椎病，针灸治疗对于缓解颈项强痛、肩背痛、上肢痛、头晕头痛等，效果尤为明显，可单用针灸，若配合推拿则疗效更佳。注意颈部保暖，避免风寒之邪侵袭。

Appendix　Stiff Neck

［附］　落枕

Stiff neck refers to a condition marked by stiff pain and limited range of motion of the neck. It often results from invasion of pathogenic cold on neck muscles or over-stretching the neck muscles for long time. This condition occurs mostly in adults. Frequent stiff neck in middle-aged or elderly people usually indicates cervical spondylopathy, and the condition may persist and is prone to recurrence. Chinese medicine holds that the disease is mainly caused by disharmony between the qi and blood, and convulsion of the tendons and vessels in the neck due to awkward sleeping posture and improper height of the pillow. It can also be caused by local meridian-qi obstruction due to invasion of the exogenous wind-cold on the neck and upper back.

落枕是指患者颈项部强痛、活动受限的一种病证。主要由项部肌肉感受寒邪或长时间过分牵拉而发生痉挛所致，好发于青壮年。中老年患者落枕往往是颈椎病变的反应，且易反复发作。中医学认为，本病多由睡眠姿势不当，枕头高低不适，颈部扭伤引起颈部气血不和，筋脉拘急而致病。也可由风寒侵袭项背，局部经气不调而致。

1　Clinical manifestations

The head twisting towards the affected side, limited movement of the neck, and marked tenderness; difficulty in bending and straightening the head in some severe cases, and even rigid neck making the head in an abnormal position towards the diseased side.

1　临床表现

头向患侧倾斜，颈部活动受限，并有明显压痛；严重者俯仰也有困难，甚至头部强直于异常位置，使头偏向患侧。

2　Treatment

Principal acupoints: Ashi acupoint, Houxi (SI 3), Xuanzhong (GB 39), and Luozhenxue (EX-UE 8).

Supplementary acupoints: In the presence of

2　治疗

主穴：阿是穴，后溪，悬钟，落枕穴。

配穴：风寒侵袭加风池、

wind-cold invasion, add Fengchi(GB 20) and Hegu (LI 4); in the presence of shoulder pain, add Jianyu (LI 15) and Waiguan(TE 5); in the presence of back pain, add Jianwaishu(SI 14) and Tianzong(SI 11). Moreover, dermal needle therapy and cupping therapy may be combined.

合谷;肩痛加肩髃、外关;背痛加肩外俞、天宗。此外,还可配合皮肤针、拔罐等方法。

3 Remarks

Acupuncture therapy works quickly and effectively on stiff neck. The key to successful treatment is to select local tender points; the distal acupoints should be given strong stimulation and the patients are asked to move the neck during needling procedure. Another attention should be paid to adopt moderate pillow in sleeping.

3 按语

针灸治疗落枕疗效快而显著。治疗的关键在于局部取穴,强调"以痛为腧",远端穴位要用强刺激,并令患者配合颈项部运动。注意睡眠时枕头高低适中。

Herpes Zoster

Herpes zoster refers to a disease manifested mainly by abrupt onset of a cluster of blisters like a belt along one side of the body, accompanied by scorching and stabbing pain. It often occurs in the spring and autumn and mostly on the waist, abdomen, chest, back and face. As its name suggests, herpes zoster is caused by varicella-herpes zoster virus and often accompanied by neuralgia. The clinical manifestation includes a cluster of blisters on one side of the body in the shape of a belt along the peripheral nerves, especially along the intercostal nerves, accompanied by intense neuralgia and local enlarged lymph nodes, susceptibility to neuralgia sequelae, occasional occurrence on bilateral sides, and less relapse. This disease can be seen in all ages, but mostly in the elderly.

蛇 丹

蛇丹是以突发单侧簇集状水疱,呈带状分布,并伴有烧灼刺痛为主症的病证。好发于春秋两季,多见于腰腹、胸背及颜面部。蛇丹见于带状疱疹,西医学认为本病是由水痘-带状疱疹病毒所致,多伴有神经痛。临床表现为聚集成簇的水疱沿体表一侧的皮肤周围神经呈带状分布,好发部位为肋间神经分布区域,常伴剧烈的神经痛及局部淋巴结肿痛,易发生后遗神经痛,一般很少见到双侧发病,亦少有复发。本病各年龄段均可见发病,中老年发病率更高。

1 Etiology and pathogenesis

Herpes zoster is primarily caused by emotional disturbances, or by excessive liver-gallbladder fire and accumulated dampness-heat in the spleen meridian due to improper diets in combination with exogenous heat toxin, which obstructs the meridians and congeals in the skin and collaterals.

1 病因病机

蛇丹起病多因情志内伤，或因饮食失节而致肝胆火盛，脾经湿热内蕴，复又外感火热时邪，毒热交阻经络，凝结于肌肤、脉络而成。

2 Syndrome differentiation

Chief symptoms: Scorching, stabbing pain and redness of the diseased skin in the early stage, followed by a millet-sized cluster of eruptions, distributed like a belt along one side of the body, mainly on the waist and the flank. Pain may leave after the disappearance of the eruptions.

The syndrome of liver-gallbladder fire-toxin manifests bright red eruptions with scorching pain, tense eruptions, bitter taste in the mouth, vexation and irritability, and wiry rapid pulse. The syndrome of dampness-heat in the spleen and stomach manifests light red eruptions and yellowish-whitish blisters with thin permeable walls, liquid exudation and erosion, body heaviness and abdominal distension, yellowish and greasy tongue coating, and slippery rapid pulse. If the pain remains after the disappearance of eruptions, it is attributed to the syndrome of residual pathogen and blood-collateral obstruction.

2 辨证

主症：初起时先觉发病部位皮肤灼热刺痛，皮色发红，继则出现簇集性粟粒大小丘状疱疹，多呈带状排列，多发生于身体一侧，以腰胁部为最常见。疱疹消失后可遗留疼痛感。

肝胆火毒者，疱疹色鲜红，灼热疼痛，疱壁紧张，口苦，心烦，易怒，脉弦数；脾胃湿热者，疱疹色淡红，起黄白水疱，疱壁易于穿破，渗水糜烂，身重腹胀，苔黄腻，脉滑数。疱疹消失后遗留疼痛者，证属余邪留滞、血络不通。

3 Treatment

3.1 Essential treatment

Principal acupoints: Ashi acupoint, Jiaji (EX-B2) on the corresponding diseased area, Hegu(LI 4), and Quchi(LI 11).

Supplementary acupoints: In the syndrome of liver-gallbladder fire-toxin, add Taichong (LR 3)

3 治疗

3.1 基本治疗

主穴：阿是穴，病变相应部位夹脊穴，合谷，曲池。

配穴：肝胆火盛加太冲、支沟；脾胃湿热加血海、阴陵

and Zhigou(TE 6); in the syndrome of dampness-heat in the spleen and stomach, add Xuehai(SP 10) and Yinlingquan(SP 9).

泉。

Explanation: Circular needling or pricking with cupping on the local Ashi acupoint acts to drain the fire-toxin out of the body. The disease is caused by herpes viruses infringing on the nerve roots, so the corresponding Jiaji (EX-B 2) are needled directly at the toxin to purge the fire and relieve the toxin, free the collaterals from pain. Combined use of Hegu(LI 4) and Quchi(LI 11) can unblock the yangming meridian-qi to remove the pathogenic toxin.

方义：局部阿是穴围针刺或点刺拔罐可引火毒外出。本病是疱疹病毒侵害神经根所致，取相应的夹脊穴，直针毒邪所留之处，可泻火解毒、通络止痛。合谷、曲池合用疏导阳明经气，以清解邪毒。

3.2 Other therapy

Shallow acupuncture with fire needle: The two ends and mid-point of the cluster of blisters are selected and disinfected, and then needled in sequence. Insert the needles vertically to the bottom of blisters and withdraw directly. The early blisters are needled first. After the blisters are punctured, the pus and fluids are squeezed completely with disinfectant cotton, and cupping therapy is performed for 5～10 minutes. Then same performance is conducted at the mid-point and the other end of the blister. The treatments are given once a day respectively on the first, second, third, fifth, seventh and ninth days, no more than six treatments in all.

3.2 其他治疗

火针赞刺：在疱疹起止两端及中间选定好针刺部位，消毒后以疱疹簇为单位，呈“品”字形依次点刺。直入直出，深度以透入疱疹皮肤达到其基底部。先刺早发的疙疹。刺后用消毒棉球挤净脓液，再选用适当大小的火罐吸拔，并留罐5～10分钟。继而在皮损中间部、尾端行同样治疗。于就诊第1、第2、第3日每日治疗1次，以后隔日(第5、第7、第9日)治疗1次，总共治疗不超过6次。

4 Remarks

Acupuncture and moxibustion are quite effective in curing herpes zoster. Needling has better effects on shortening the pain duration.

4 按语

针刺治疗带状疱疹有较高的痊愈率；针刺对缩短带状疱疹患者的疼痛持续时间有较好疗效。

Neurodermatitis

Neurodermatitis is a common chronic skin disease due to dysfunction of the skin nerves, characterized by intense itching and lichenoid skin changes. It is mostly seen in adults. The skin lesion is usually localized in one site, mostly in the neck, cubital fossa, axillary fossa, popliteal fossa, pudendum and pars sacralis; occasionally, it may scatter through the body with bilateral symmetrical distribution.

1　Etiology and pathogenesis

In the early stage, neurodermatitis is caused by wind-heat obstruction in the skin or mechanical irritation by tough collar, or by undernourishment of the skin due to yin-fluid consumption and yin-blood insufficiency and ensuing wind dryness in long-term illnesses, or by liver-fire accumulation due to emotional upsets and depression, or by qi and blood obstruction in the skin due to over-strain and up-flaring heart fire. All these factors may be important contributions to the onset of the disease and can also lead to its relapse. In general, the emotional impairment and invasion of pathogenic wind are the evoked factors for the disease; nutrient-blood disharmony and qi-blood coagulation are the pathogenic mechanism of the disease.

2　Etiology and pathogenesis

Chief symptom: Lichenoid skin with paroxysmal intense itching.

The syndrome of wind-heat is often seen in the early stage and manifests simple pruritus without skin rash, or papules with normal skin in color or red, ag-

神经性皮炎

神经性皮炎是一种慢性常见的皮肤神经功能障碍性皮肤病，以剧烈瘙痒及皮肤局限性苔藓样变为特征。成年人多发。多局限于某处，如颈项、肘窝、腋窝、腘窝、阴部、骶部等，偶可见散发全身，双侧对称分布。本病属中医学“顽癣”“牛皮癣”“摄领疮”等范畴。

1　病因病机

初起为风热之邪阻滞肌肤或硬领等外来机械刺激所引起；病久耗伤阴液，营血不足，血虚风燥，皮肤失去濡养而成；或肝火郁滞，情志不遂，郁闷不舒，或紧张劳累，心火上炎，以致气血运行失职，凝滞肌肤，每易成为诱发的重要因素，且致病情反复。总之，情志内伤、风邪侵扰是神经性皮炎发病的诱发因素，营血失和、气血凝滞为其病机。

2　辨证

主症：皮肤损害呈苔藓样改变，阵发性剧痒。

风热者，常见于发病初期，仅有瘙痒而无皮疹，或丘疹呈正常皮色或红色，食辛

gravated by taking spicy and pungent food, accompanied by scanty dark urine, thin yellowish tongue coating, and wiry rapid pulse. The syndrome of liver depression transforming into fire manifests symptoms triggered or aggravated by vexation and irritability; the syndrome of blood-deficiency and wind-dryness manifests fused papules with lichenified, thickened, leathery and dry skin, or covered by small number of scales, pruritus aggravated at night.

辣食物加重,伴小便短赤,苔薄黄,脉弦数;肝郁化火者,每因心烦发怒,情志不畅而诱发或加重;血虚风燥者,病久丘疹融合成片,皮肤增厚,干燥如皮革样,或有少量灰白鳞屑,而成苔藓化,夜间瘙痒加剧。

3 Treatment

3 治疗

3.1 Essential treatment

3.1 基本治疗

Principal acupoints: Ashi acupoint, Hegu(LI 4), Quchi(LI 11), Xuehai(SP 10), and Geshu(BL 17).

主穴: 阿是穴,合谷,曲池,血海,膈俞。

Supplementary acupoints: In the syndrome of wind-heat, add Taiyuan(LU 9) and Fengchi(GB 20); in the syndrome of liver depression transforming into fire, add Ganshu(BL 18) and Taichong(LR 3); in the syndrome of blood-deficiency and wind-dryness, add Pishu(BL 20) and Zusanli(ST 36).

配穴: 风热加太渊、风池;肝郁化火加肝俞、太冲;血虚风燥加脾俞、足三里。

Explanation: Treatment at Ashi acupoint can work directly on diseased location, and cannot only disperse accumulated wind-heat and also frees the qi-blood flow in obstructed meridians to nourish the muscles and skin. Hegu(LI 4) and Quchi(LI 11) dispel the wind and arrest itching. Xuehai(SP 10) and Geshu(BL 17) are used to activate blood flow and enrich the blood.

方义: 取阿是穴可直刺病所,既可散局部的风热郁火,又能疏通患部的经络气血,使患部肌肤得以濡养。合谷、曲池祛风止痒。取血海、膈俞活血养血。

3.2 Other therapy

3.2 其他治疗

Dermal needle therapy: Ashi acupoint are used for dermal needle treatment. Initially, gently tap the surrounding area of Ashi acupoint and then heavily tap the Ashi acupoint till slight bleeding is seen, followed by cupping or moxibustion with a

皮肤针: 取阿是穴,先轻叩皮损周围,再重叩患处阿是穴以少量出血为度,同时可配合拔罐或艾条灸。

moxa stick.

4 Remarks

Acupuncture has certain effects on neurodermatitis, and the treatment mainly concentrates on the skin lesion and corresponding Jiaji(EX-B 2). Neurodermatitis is difficult to be cured and persistent treatment is necessary. During treatment, heart-spirit-calming acupoints may be added to enhance clinical efficacy and reduce relapse; patients are advised to avoid fish and shrimp, spicy food, wine or liquor, as well as abstinence from anger.

4 按语

针灸治疗本病有一定疗效，以皮肤针叩刺局部及相应夹脊穴较为多用。本病较难痊愈，须坚持治疗。治疗时可适当增加宁心安神的穴位，以提高治疗效果，减少复发。治疗期间忌食鱼虾、辛辣、饮酒，忌恼怒。

Acne

Acne is a common chronic disease of the hair follicle and sebaceous gland in males and females during adolescence. Acne frequently occurs on the face, chest and upper back, and is manifested by lesions such as black-headed acne, papules, pustules, nodules and cysts, and is often accompanied by an exodus of seborrhea. Most cases can heal by themselves or are relieved after adolescence.

1 Etiology and pathogenesis

Chinese medicine holds that the vitality is vigorous in adolescence; acne results from weak constitution and lung-meridian blood-heat accumulation in the skin that fumigates the face, or by disharmony between the thoroughfare vessel and conception vessel failing to ensure the qi-blood flow to the muscles and skin, or by upward fumigation of accumulated stomach-intestine heat to the face, chest and back due to over indulgence in fatty and spicy diets and following spleen-stomach dysfunction and dampness-heat retention.

痤　疮

痤疮又称“粉刺”“青春痘”，是青春期男女常见的一种毛囊及皮脂腺的慢性炎症。好发于颜面、胸背等处，可形成黑头粉刺、丘疹、脓疱、结节、囊肿等损害，常伴有皮脂溢出。青春期以后，大多可自然痊愈或减轻。

1 病因病机

中医学认为，人在青春期生机旺盛，由于先天禀赋的原因，使肺经血热郁于肌肤，熏蒸面部而发为痤疮；或冲任不调，肌肤疏泄失畅而致；或恣食膏粱厚味、辛辣之品，使脾胃运化失常，湿热内生，蕴于肠胃，不能下达，上蒸头面、胸背而成。

2 Syndrome differentiation

Chief symptoms: In the beginning, acne usually manifests comedo or black-headed eruptions that produce whitish powder-like substance when squeezed; the skin lesion is usually symmetrically distributed.

The syndrome of wind-heat in the lung meridian manifests papules, with possible pustules, nodules and cysts, thin yellowish tongue coating, and rapid pulse. The syndrome of dampness-heat in the spleen and stomach mainly manifests greasiness on the face, skin rash with pustules, nodules and cysts, usually accompanied by constipation, yellow greasy tongue coating, and soggy rapid pulse. The syndrome of dysfunction of the Thoroughfare and Conception Vessels is related to the menstrual cycle, and may be accompanied by irregular menstruation, menstrual cramps, dark red tongue with thin yellowish coating, and wiry, thready and rapid pulse.

3 Treatment

3.1 Essential treatment

Principal acupoints: Hegu (LI 4), Quchi (LI 11), Neiting(ST 44), Yangbai(GB 14), and Sibai (ST 2).

Supplementary acupoints: In the syndrome of wind-heat in the lung meridian, add Shaoshang(LU 11), Chize(LU 5) and Fengmen(BL 12) to clear the lung heat; in the syndrome of dampness-heat in the spleen and stomach, add Zusanli(ST 36), Sanyinjiao(SP 6) and Yinlingquan(SP 9) to clear heat and rcsolvc dampness; in the syndrome of dysfunction of the thoroughfare and conception vessels, add Xuehai(SP 10), Geshu(BL 17) and Sanyinjiao(SP 6) to harmonize the thoroughfare and conception

2 辨证

主症：初起为粉刺，有的为黑头丘疹，可挤出乳白色粉质样物，常呈对称分布。

肺经风热者，多以丘疹损害为主，可有脓疱、结节、囊肿等，苔薄黄，脉数；脾胃湿热者，多有颜面油腻不适，皮疹有脓疱、结节、囊肿等，伴有便秘，苔黄腻，脉濡数；冲任不调者，病情与月经周期有关，可伴有月经不调、痛经，舌暗红，苔薄黄，脉弦细数。

3 治疗

3.1 基本治疗

主穴：合谷，曲池，内庭，阳白，四白。

配穴：肺经风热加少商、尺泽、风门清泻肺热；脾胃湿热加足三里、三阴交、阴陵泉清热化湿；冲任不调加血海、膈俞、三阴交调和冲任。

vessels.

Explanation: Yangming meridians are rich in qi and blood and go up to the face; in addition, the hand-yangming meridian is interiorly-exteriorly related to the lung meridian, while the lung governs the skin and body hair. Hegu(LI 4), Quchi(LI 11) and Neiting(ST 44) are used to clear heat in the yangming meridians; Sibai(ST 2) and Yangbai(GB 14) are selected to promote the flow of local qi and blood, and restore the normal function of the skin to disperse and release.

方义: 阳明经多气多血，其经脉上走于面，又手阳明大肠经与肺经相表里，肺主皮毛，取合谷、曲池、内庭清泻阳明邪热；四白、阳白可疏通局部气血，使肌肤疏泄功能得以调畅。

3.2 Other therapies

Scraping therapy: Scrape the five lines of the governor vessel and bladder meridian on the back, from Yamen(GV 15) to Yaoshu(GV 2) of the governor vessel, and from Tianzhu(BL 10) to Dachangshu(BL 25) and from Fufen(BL 41) to Baohuang (BL 53) of the bladder meridians.

Blood-letting and cupping therapy: The Back-Shu acupoints, frequently Dazhui(GV 14), Feishu (BL 13) and Weishu(BL 21) are usually pricked and cupped, twice a week, and the volume of blood should be 2～3 ml in the cups.

3.2 其他治疗

刮痧: 取项背部督脉、膀胱经共 5 线，督脉从哑门刮至腰俞以下，两侧膀胱经则分别从天柱至大肠俞以下，从附分至胞肓。

刺络拔罐: 以背俞穴为主，常用穴位有大椎、肺俞、胃俞等，每周 2 次，每次罐内出血量为 2～3 毫升。

4 Remarks

Acupuncture therapy is fairly effective for acne and even cures it in some cases. In mild cases, it is sufficient to keep the face clean and clear. The patients are advised to avoid spicy, fatty and sweet diets, and take fresh vegetables and fruits to keep the bowels open.

4 按语

针灸对本病有一定的疗效，部分患者可达到治愈目的。轻症注意保持面部清洁卫生即可。忌食辛辣、油腻及糖类食品，多食新鲜蔬菜及水果，保持大便通畅。

Section 4 Diseases of the Sensory Organs

第4节 五官科病证

Reddened Swollen and Painful Eyes

Reddened, swollen and painful eyes is an acute manifestation seen in various eye disorders and is characterized by conjunctival redness, increased eye discharge, alternate pain and itching of the eyes. It is frequently seen in such diseases as acute conjunctivitis, pseudo-membranous conjunctivitis and epidemic keratoconjunctivitis in Western medicine.

1 Etiology and pathogenesis

This disease is mainly caused by invasion and accumulation of exogenous wind-heat into the eyes, or by predominant fire in the liver and gallbladder which flares up along the meridians to block the meridians and bring about qi-blood stagnation, hence giving rise to sudden onset of redness, swelling and pain of the eyes.

2 Syndrome differentiation

Chief symptoms: Redness, swelling and pain of the eyes, photophobia, lacrimation and increased eye discharge.

The syndrome of wind-heat invasion is accompanied by headache, fever, and floating rapid pulse. The syndrome of predominant fire in the liver and gallbladder fire is accompanied by bitter taste in the mouth, vexation and feverish sensation, constipation and wiry slippery pulse.

目赤肿痛

目赤肿痛为多种眼部疾患中的一个急性症状，以白睛红赤、眵多黏稠、痒痛交作为主要特征。常见于西医学的急性结膜炎、假性结膜炎以及流行性角膜炎等疾病。

1 病因病机

本病多因外感风热时邪，风热相搏，侵袭目窍，郁而不宣；或因肝胆火盛，循经上扰，以致经脉闭阻，血壅气滞，骤然发生目赤肿痛。

2 辨证

主症：目赤肿痛，畏光，流泪，眵多。

外感风热者，兼头痛、发热、脉浮数；肝胆火盛者，兼口苦、烦热、便秘、脉弦滑。

3 Treatment

3.1 Essential treatment

Principal acupoints: Hegu(LI 4), Taichong(LR 3), Fengchi(GB 20), Jingming(BL 1), and Taiyang (EX-HN 5).

Supplementary acupoints: In the syndrome of wind-heat invasion, add Shaoshang (LU 11) and Shangxing(GV 23); in the syndrome of predominant fire in the liver and gallbladder, add Xingjian (LR 2) and Xiaxi(GB 43).

Explanation: The liver opens into the eyes, and the shaoyang, yangming and taiyang meridians all run over the eyes. Hegu(LI 4) is used to regulate qi circulation of the yangming meridian to eliminate wind-heat. Taichong(LR 3) and Fengchi(GB 20) respectively belong to the liver and gallbladder meridians, and they can conduct the liver-gallbladder fire downwards. Jingming(BL 1), the Crossing acupoint of the taiyang and yangming meridians, is used to purge local accumulated heat. Taiyang(EX-HN 5), an extra acupoint, can clear heat and brighten eyes when it is pricked to bleed.

3.2 Other therapies

Ear acupuncture: Puncture acupoints Eye (LO 5), Liver(CO 12), Lung(CO 14), Eye1 and Eye2 with filiform needles. The needles are retained for 20 minutes and rotated intermittently, and the treatment is applied once daily. Also, the Ear Apex (HX 6,7i) or vein behind the ear can be pricked to bleed.

Pricking therapy: The pricking therapy is applied to the sensitive points on the scapular region or the sites 0.5 cun bilateral to Dazhui(GV 14). This therapy is indicated for acute conjunctivitis.

3 治疗

3.1 基本治疗

主穴: 合谷，太冲，风池，睛明，太阳。

配穴: 风热证加少商、上星；肝胆火盛加行间、侠溪。

方义: 目为肝之窍，阳明、太阳、少阳经脉均循行目系。合谷调阳明经气以泻风热。太冲、风池分属肝胆两经，上下相应，导肝胆之火下行。睛明为足太阳、足阳明经交会穴，可宣泄患部之郁热。太阳为经外奇穴，点刺出血可泻热明目。

3.2 其他治疗

耳针: 选眼、肝、肺、目1、目2穴。毫针刺，留针20分钟，间歇捻转，每日1次。亦可在耳尖或耳后静脉点刺出血。

挑刺: 在肩胛间按压过敏点，或大椎两旁0.5寸处选点挑刺。本法适用于急性结膜炎。

Bloodletting and cupping therapy: Prick Taiyang (EX-HN 5) to cause bleeding, followed by cupping. The treatment can be prescribed once daily.

刺血拔罐：在太阳穴处点刺出血后拔罐，每日1次。

4 Remarks

Acupuncture is very effective for reddened, swollen and painful eyes, and can shorten the course of treatment. In needling intraorbital acupoints, the needles should be inserted and withdrawn slowly, with a slight rotation, but without any lifting-thrusting of the needle, and the needling sites are pressed with cotton ball for several seconds to avoid bleeding. During the treatment period, patients are advised to take sufficient rest and have adequate sleep, refrain from straining the eyes, avoid getting angry, abstain frequent sexual intercourse and eating spicy foods.

4 按语

针刺治疗目赤肿痛疗效显著，缓解病情快，可明显缩短病程。取眼眶内穴位时，进出针须缓慢，轻捻转不宜提插，出针时用棉球按压数秒钟，以防止出血。患病期间应注意休息，睡眠充分，减少视力活动，忌发怒，戒房劳，忌辛辣食物。

Stye

Stye is an ophthalmologic condition characterized by small wheat pellet-like pustule on the inner border or rims of the eyelid. It is usually reddened, swollen, itchy and painful, and is prone to be purulent. In Western medicine, it is an acute suppurative inflammatory condition caused by infection of the ciliary glands of the eye, and it can be classified into two types, namely internal and external style. An infection in the hair follicle of the eyelash or an accessory glandula sebacea causes external stye, while infection in the glandulae tarsales is internal stye.

麦粒肿

麦粒肿是指胞睑内面或边缘生小疖肿，形似麦粒，红肿痒痛，易于溃脓的眼病，又称“针眼”“眼丹”等。西医学认为，本病是指眼皮脂腺受感染而引起的一种急性化脓性炎症，可分为内、外麦粒肿。凡睫毛毛囊或附属皮脂腺感染称外麦粒肿；而睑板腺感染称内麦粒肿。

1 Etiology and pathogenesis

Stye is mainly caused by invasion of wind heat, or accumulated heat in the spleen and stomach, or

1 病因病机

本病多因风热之邪外侵或脾胃蕴热，或心火上炎，又

up-flaming of the heart fire. All these factors, in the contraction of exogenous wind-heat, cause qi and blood stagnation and accumulate fire heat in the eyelids, manifesting redness and swelling, and even pustules.

复外感风热，积热与外风相搏，气血瘀阻，火热结聚于胞睑，以致眼睑红肿，熟腐化为脓液。

2 Syndrome differentiation

2 辨证

Chief symptoms: In the beginning, there is a confined, red and swollen nodule at the rim of the eyelid with pain and tenderness. Subsequently, the redness and swelling of the nodule gradually increase. Several days later, the nodule starts to produce yellowish pus and exudate.

主症：始则睑缘局限性红肿硬结、疼痛和触痛，继则红肿渐扩大；数日后硬结顶端出现黄色脓点，溃破后脓自流出。

The syndrome of wind-heat invasion manifests slight swelling and itching pain in the stye, accompanied by headache, fever, general discomforts, thin whitish tongue coating, and floating rapid pulse. The syndrome of heat accumulation in the spleen and stomach manifests redness, swelling and burning pain at the local area, accompanied by thirst, foul breath, constipations, yellowish tongue coating and rapid pulse.

外感风热者，局部微肿痒痛，伴有头痛、发热、全身不适、苔薄白、脉浮数；脾胃蕴热者，局部红肿灼痛，伴有口渴口臭、便秘、苔黄、脉数。

3 Treatment

3 治疗

3.1 Essential treatment

3.1 基本治疗

Principal acupoints: Taiyang (EX-HN 5), Yuyao(EX-HN 4), and Fengchi(GB 20).

主穴：太阳，鱼腰，风池。

Supplementary points: In the syndrome of wind-heat invasion, add Cuanzhu(BL 2), Hegu(LI 4), Sizhukong(TE 23), and Xingjian(LR 2); in the syndrome of heat accumulation in the spleen and stomach, add Quchi (LI 11), Neiting(ST 44), Erjian(LI 2), and Yinlingquan(SP 9).

配穴：外感风热加攒竹、合谷、丝竹空、行间；脾胃蕴热加曲池、内庭、二间、阴陵泉。

Explanation: Pricking Taiyang (EX-HN 5) to bleed can clear heat and relieve toxicity, and activate blood and resolve stasis. Yuyao (EX-HN 4),

方义：太阳点刺出血，可清热解毒、活血散结。鱼腰疏调眼部气血，为治疗眼病

an effective acupoint for eye disorders, is used to regulate qi and blood flow of the eyes. Fengchi(GB 20), the Crossing acupoint of the foot-shaoyang meridian and yang link vessel, can disperse wind and clear heat in the head and face.

常用的有效奇穴。风池为足少阳经与阳维脉之交会穴，可泻头面之风热。

3.2 Other therapies

Ear acupuncture: Select Eye(LO 5), Liver(CO 12), Spleen(CO 13) and Ear Apex (HX 6,7i). Ear Apex (HX 6,7i) is pricked for bleeding, while the other acupoints are punctured with filiform needles for 20 minutes, and the needles are rotated intermittently. The treatment is given once a day.

Pricking therapy: The light-red papules bilateral to the first till seventh thoracic vertebrae are searched and pricked with a three-edged needle, and small amount of blood or viscous fluid is squeezed out; the procedure can be repeated 3 to 5 times. Sometimes the white fibers underneath the papules are broken by pricking with a three-edge needle, 2 to 3 fibers are pricked each time. The treatment is usually conducted once every other day.

3.2 其他治疗

耳针：选眼、肝、脾、耳尖穴。耳尖点刺出血，余穴毫针刺，留针 20 分钟，间歇捻转，每日 1 次。

挑刺：在肩胛间探寻第 1～7 胸椎旁淡红色疹点，三棱针点刺，挤出少量血液或黏液，可反复挤 3～5 次；或挑断疹下白色纤维组织，每次挑断 2～3 根，隔日 1 次。

4 Remarks

Patients are suggested to keep proper local hygiene and avoid pressing the papule, otherwise the pus-toxin may be spread and result in serious consequences. Patients should avoid spicy, carbonized, sweet and fatty foods.

4 按语

嘱患者注意眼睑局部卫生，切忌挤压，以免脓毒扩散，造成严重后果。忌辛辣、焦燥、肥甘之品。

Myopia

Myopia is an eye condition characterized by ability to clearly see near objects and inability to clearly see distant objects. It is one of the ametropic diseases.

近　视

近视是以视近清楚、视远模糊为主症的眼病。为眼科屈光不正疾病之一。

In Western medicine, myopia can be classified into light, medium and severe myopia; myopia with a diopter lower than −3.0D is known as low myopia, below diopter −6.0D as moderate myopia, and above diopter −6.0 as high myopia.

西医学将近视分为低、中、高度，凡屈光度 −3.0D 以下者为低度近视，−6.0D 以下者为中度近视，−6.0D 以上者为高度近视。

1 Etiology and pathogenesis

1 病因病机

Myopia is generally attributed to congenital insufficiency, postnatal maldevelopment and heart-spirit over-exertion, which consume qi, blood, the yin and yang of the heart, liver and kidney, resulting in abnormal shape of the eyeballs. In addition, myopia is also due to bad habit of using one's eyes, which causes blood stagnation in the eye collaterals and malnutrition of the eyes.

本病多因先天禀赋不足、后天发育不良、劳心伤神等，使心、肝、肾气血阴阳受损，睛珠形态异常；或因用眼不当，使目络瘀阻，目失所养，导致本病。

2 Syndrome differentiation

2 辨证

Chief symptoms: Normal near-sightedness, and inability to clearly see the distant objects.

主症：视近物正常，视远物模糊不清。

The syndrome of liver-kidney deficiency is usually accompanied by insomnia, forgetfulness, aching loins, dry eyes, red tongue and thready pulse. The syndrome of heart-spleen deficiency is accompanied by lassitude, poor appetite, loose stools, dizziness and palpitations, lusterless complexion, white tongue and thready pulse.

肝肾不足者，兼失眠健忘、腰酸、目干涩、舌红、脉细；心脾两虚者，兼神疲乏力、纳呆便溏、头晕心悸、面色不华、舌淡、脉细。

3 Treatment

3 治疗

3.1 Essential treatment

3.1 基本治疗

Principal acupoints: Chengqi (ST 1), Jingming (GB 1), Fengchi (GB 20), Yiming (EX-HN 13), and Guangming (GB 37).

主穴：承泣，睛明，风池，翳明，光明。

Supplementary acupoints: In the syndrome of liver-kidney deficiency, add Ganshu (BL 18) and Shenshu (BL 23); in the syndrome of heart-spleen deficiency, add Xinshu (BL 15), Pishu (BL 20) and Zusanli (ST 36).

配穴：肝肾不足加肝俞、肾俞；心脾两虚加心俞、脾俞、足三里。

Explanation: Chengqi(ST 1) and Jingming(GB 1) are local acupoints and function to regulate qi circulation in the meridians around the eyes. Fengchi(GB 20), the Crossing acupoint of foot-shaoyang meridian and yang link vessel, can regulate qi and blood around the eyes. Yiming (EX-HN 13) and Guangming(GB 37) are empirical acupoints effective for myopia.

方义: 承泣、睛明为局部选穴,可疏通眼部经络。风池为足少阳经与阳维脉之交会穴,可疏通眼部气血。翳明、光明为治疗眼病的经验效穴。

3.2 Other therapies

Ear acupuncture: Select Eye(LO 5), Liver(CO 12), Eyel and Eye2. Puncture 2 to 3 acupoints each time with filiform needles for 20～60 minutes, and the needles are rotated intermittently; or apply intradermal needles or *Semen Vaccariae* (Wang Bu Liu Xing) at these acupoints, which are replaced once every 3 to 5 days; ask patients to press these acupoints several times a day.

Dermal needle therapy: Tap the acupoints around the eyes and Fengchi(GB 20) by mild or moderate intensity, once a day.

3.2 其他治疗

耳针: 选眼、肝、目 1、目 2。毫针刺,每次 2～3 穴,留针 20～60 分钟,间歇捻转;或行埋针或王不留行贴压,3～5 日更换 1 次,嘱患者每日按压数次。

皮肤针: 轻度或中度叩刺眼周穴位及风池穴,每日 1 次。

4 Remarks

Acupuncture is fairly effective for myopia, especially for pseudomyopia. Instruct the patients to use their eyes in a scientific way, persistently do eye exercises, and massage the meridians and acupoints around the eyes.

4 按语

针刺治疗本病有一定效果,尤以假性近视为佳。嘱患者科学用眼,坚持做眼保健操及经络穴位按摩等。

Optic Atrophy

Optic atrophy is a common cataract ophthalmic disorder characterized by normal appearance of the eye, light-colored optic disk, decreasing vision, and even blindness. Optic atrophy can be classified into three types, namely primary, secondary and ascend-

视神经萎缩

视神经萎缩是指眼外观正常、视盘色淡、视力渐降,甚至盲无所见的内障眼病。分为原发性、继发性、上行性三种,是一种严重影响视力

ing optic atrophy. It is a chronic fundus disorder that seriously affects the vision. It belongs to "glaucoma" in traditional Chinese medicine.

的慢性眼底病，也为致盲率较高的一种眼病。属于中医学"青盲"范畴。

1 Etiology and pathogenesis

Optic atrophy results from eye malnutrition and blockage due to weak constitution and liver-kidney deficiency, or from meridian obstruction and vision decrease due to emotional upsets and liver-qi depression, or from blood-stasis in eye collaterals and vision loss due to maltreatment and trauma on the head and eyes.

1 病因病机

本病或因禀赋不足，肝肾精血亏虚，不得荣目，目窍萎闭；或情志抑郁，肝气不舒，经络郁滞，目窍郁闭；或眼疾失治，头眼外伤致脉络瘀阻，目窍闭塞而神光泯灭所致。

2 Syndrome differentiation

Chief symptoms: Decreasing eyesight, or narrowing visual field, progressive condition, eventual loss of eyesight.

The syndrome of liver-kidney deficiency manifests dryness of the eyes, dizziness, tinnitus, palpitations, aching loin and knees, red tongue with whitish coating, and thready rapid pulse. The syndrome of qi-blood stagnation manifests history of head and eye injuries, headache, vertigo, poor memory, dark purplish tongue and rough pulse. The syndrome of liver-qi depression manifests flank distention and pain, bitter taste in the mouth, red tongue with thin whitish or yellowish coating, and wiry or thready pulse.

2 辨证

主症：视力渐降，或视野窄小，逐渐加重，终致失明。

肝肾亏虚者，兼双目干涩、头晕耳鸣、心悸、腰膝酸软、舌红、苔薄白、脉细数；气血瘀滞者，常有头及眼部外伤史，可见头痛、眩晕、健忘、舌暗有瘀斑、脉涩；肝气郁结者，兼胸胁胀痛、口苦咽干、舌红、苔薄白或薄黄、脉弦或细弦。

3 Treatment

3.1 Essential treatment

Principal acupoints: Chengqi (ST 1), Jingming (BL 1), and Qiuhou(EX-HN 7).

Supplementary acupoints: In the syndrome of liver-kidney deficiency, add Ganshu(BL 18), Shenshu(BL 23), Taixi(KI 3) and Guangming(GB 18); in the syndrome of qi-blood stagnation, add Hegu

3 治疗

3.1 基本治疗

主穴：承泣，睛明，球后。

配穴：肝肾亏虚加肝俞、肾俞、太溪、光明；气血瘀阻加合谷、三阴交、膈俞；肝气郁结加行间、侠溪、太冲。

(LI 4), Sanyinjiao (SP 6) and Geshu(BL 17); in the syndrome of liver-qi depression, add Xingjian (LR 2), Xiaxi(GB 43) and Taichong(LR 3).

Explanation: Chengqi(ST 1), Jingming(BL 1) and Qiuhou(EX-HN 7) are all located near the eyes and function to regulate qi and blood circulation, move qi and activate blood.

方义：承泣、睛明、球后皆位于眼部，可疏通眼部经络、行气活血。

3.2 Other therapies

3.2 其他治疗

Dermal needle therapy: Select the surrounding areas of eyes, bilateral sides of the fifth till twelfth thoracic vertebrae, Fengchi(GB 20) and Geshu(BL 17). Gently tap the surrounding areas of eyes, and tap the other acupoints with moderate intensity. The treatment is applied once every other day.

皮肤针：在眼眶周围、胸椎5～12两侧、风池、膈俞。眼区轻度叩刺，其余部位及经穴中度叩刺，隔日1次。

Ear acupuncture: Select auricular points Eye1 (LO 5), Eye2(LO 5), Liver(CO 12), kidney(CO 10), Spleen(CO 13), Subcortex(AT 4) and Qcciput (AT 3). Intradermal needles or *Semen Vaccariae* (Wang Bu Liu Xing) may be applied at these acupoints, which are replaced every 3 to 5 days. Patients are asked to press these acupoints several times a day.

耳针：选目1、目2、肝、肾、脾、皮质下、枕区。埋针或王不留行贴压，3～5日更换1次，嘱患者每日按压数次。

Scalp acupuncture: Select Lateral Line 2 of Forehead(MS 3), Upper-middle Line of Occiput (MS 12), and Upper-lateral Line of Occiput(MS 13). After qi arrives, the needles are swiftly rotated at the frequency of 200 times per minute. The needles are retained for 30 to 60 minutes and manipulated intermittently. The treatment is applied once a day or once every other day, with 10 to 15 treatments in a full treatment course.

头针：选额旁2线、枕上正中线、枕上旁线。针刺得气后快速捻转，200次/分钟，留针30～60分钟，间隔运针。每日或隔日1次，10～15次为1个疗程。

4 Remarks

4 按语

Acupuncture can produce short-term clinical results on optic atrophy, help control its progression,

针灸治疗本病有一定的近期疗效，可控制病情发展，

improve eyesight and delay occurrence of blindness.

提高视力，延缓致盲。

Tinnitus and Deafness

Tinnitus and deafness are hearing disturbances. Tinnitus is characterized by a ringing in the ears sounding like the chirping of a cicada and the ocean tide, which disturbs the hearing. Deafness refers to decreasing hearing or complete hearing loss. Deafness often evolves from tinnitus. Tinnitus and deafness are often coexistent. Due to the similarities in etiology and acupuncture treatment of these two conditions, they are discussed together. In Western medicine, deafness is caused by the injury of the auditory nerves due to inner ear diseases and some medications or congenital auditory defects, whereas tinnitus is caused by the spasms of blood vessels supplying the inner ear.

耳鸣、耳聋

耳聋、耳鸣都是听觉异常。耳鸣是以自觉耳内鸣响为主症，如蝉如潮，妨碍听觉；耳聋则以听力喊退或听力丧失为主症，耳聋往往由耳鸣发展而来。两者常常同时存在，且在病因病机及针灸治疗方面大致相同，故合并论述。西医学认为内耳疾病、某些药物等导致听神经等损伤或先天听觉障碍可致耳聋，而内耳的血管痉挛常是耳鸣发生的重要原因。

1　Etiology and pathogenesis

The cause of tinnitus and deafness falls into two types, internal and external causes. The internal cause usually involves anger and fright and subsequent upward adversity of liver-gallbladder wind-fire, which blocks the shaoyang meridians; or the accumulated phlegm-heat obstructs the ear orifices; or kidney-qi deficiency and liver-kidney insufficiency fail to nourish the ears. The external cause usually refers to the invasion of exogenous wind which blocks the ear orifices, or sometimes sudden explosion or loud noise can directly damage the ears.

1　病因病机

耳鸣、耳聋的发生，可分为内因外因。内因多由恼怒、惊恐，肝胆风火上逆，以致少阳经气闭阻；或痰热郁结，壅遏清窍；或肾虚气弱，肝肾亏虚，精气不能上濡于耳而成。外因多由风邪侵袭，壅遏清窍，亦有因突然暴响震伤耳窍引起者。

2　Syndrome differentiation

Chief symptoms: Loss of hearing, or conti-nuous ringing in the ears sound like the chirping of a cicada, or the blowing of the wind, or the sound of

2　辨证

主症：耳聋，或耳中鸣响，如蝉鸣、如风声、如雷鸣、如哨声等。

thunder or a whistling sound.

The syndrome of predominant liver-gallbladder fire manifests distending headache, flushed face, dry throat, irritability, and wiry pulse. The syndrome of phlegm-heat accumulation manifests chest fullness, copious sputum, and rapid slippery pulse. The syndrome of exogenous wind invasion manifests chills and fever, and floating pulse. The syndrome of kidney-qi deficiency manifests vertigo, aching loin and knees, lassitude, and weak thready pulse. The syndrome liver-kidney deficiency manifests vexing heat in the chest, palms and soles, night sweats, tinnitus especially at night, red tongue with scanty coating, and thready rapid pulse.

肝胆火盛者,兼头胀、面赤、咽干、烦躁善怒、脉弦;痰热郁结者,兼胸闷痰多、脉滑数;外感风邪者,兼畏寒、发热、脉浮;肾气亏虚者,兼头晕、腰膝酸软、乏力、脉细弱;肝肾亏虚者,兼五心烦热、盗汗,耳鸣夜间尤甚,舌红少津,脉细数。

3 Treatment

3.1 Essential treatment

Principal acupoints: Yifeng(TE 17), Tinghui(GB 2), Xiaxi(GB 43), and Zhongzhu(TE 3).

Supplementary acupoints: In the syndrome of predominant liver-gallbladder fire, add Taichong(LR 3) and Qiuxu(GB 40); in the syndrome of phlegm-heat accumulation, add Fenglong(ST 40) and Laogong(PC 8); in the syndrome of exogenous wind invasion, add Waiguan(TE 5), Hegu(LI 4) and Fengchi(GB 20); in the syndrome of kidney-qi deficiency, add Shenshu(BL 23), Zhaohai(KI 6), and Qihai(CV 6); in the syndrome of liver-kidney deficiency, add Shenshu(BL 23), Ganshu(BL 18), and Taixi(KI 3).

Explanation: The shaoyang meridians of the hand and foot travel around the ears, so Zhongzhu(TE 3) and Yifeng(TE 17), the acupoints of hand-shaoyang meridian, and Tinghui(GB 2) and Xiaxi(GB 43), the acupoints of foot-shaoyang meridian,

3 治疗

3.1 基本治疗

主穴: 翳风,听会,侠溪,中渚。

配穴: 肝胆火盛加太冲、丘墟;痰热郁结加丰隆、劳宫;外感风邪加外关、合谷、风池;肾气亏虚加肾俞、照海、气海;肝肾亏虚加肾俞、肝俞、太溪。

方义: 手足少阳两经经脉均循耳之前后,因此取手少阳经中渚、翳风,足少阳经听会、侠溪,诸穴相配通上达下,疏通少阳经气而宣通耳

are used to communicate the upper body and lower body, unblock shaoyang meridians to free ear orifices.

窍。

3.2 Other therapies

Ear acupuncture: Select acupoints Heart (CO 15), Liver(CO 12), Kidney(CO 10), Internal Ear (LO 6) and Subcortex (AT 4). Puncture these acupoints with filiform needles by moderate intensity. Or apply intradermal needles at these acupoints. For sudden onset of deafness, strong stimulation is given.

Scalp acupuncture: Select bilateral Posterior Temporal Line (MS 11). Puncture the acupoint with a filiform needle, rotate the needle intermittently, and retain the needle for 20 minutes. The treatment is conducted once a day or every other day.

3.2 其他治疗

耳针：选心、肝、肾、内耳、皮质下，毫针中等刺激，亦可埋针。暴聋者，毫针强刺激。

头针：选两侧颞后。毫针刺，间歇捻转，留针 20 分钟，每日或隔日 1 次。

4 Remarks

Acupuncture has certain effects on tinnitus and deafness. However, it is not effective for complete hearing loss caused by damage to the ear drum.

4 按语

针灸治疗耳鸣、耳聋有一定疗效，但对鼓膜损伤致听力完全丧失者疗效不佳。

Nasosinusitis

Nasosinusitis is characterized by discharge of thick stinking snivels, nasal obstruction, and loss of smelling. It is usually seen in acute and chronic rhinitis, acute and chronic nasosinusitis, and accessory nasosinusitis.

鼻　渊

鼻渊是以鼻流腥臭浊涕、鼻塞、嗅觉丧失等为主症。重者称为“脑漏”。鼻渊常见于西医学的急慢性鼻炎、急慢性鼻窦炎和副鼻窦炎等疾病。

1 Etiology and pathogenesis

The nose is the external orifice of the lung, so nasosinusitis is closely associated with the invasion of exogenous pathogens in the lung meridian. Nasosinusitis is primarily caused by exogenous wind-heat,

1 病因病机

鼻为肺之外窍，因此鼻渊的发生，与肺经受邪有关。多因感受风热邪毒，或因风寒袭肺，蕴而化热，乃致肺失

or wind-cold transforming into heat, which disturbs the function of lung to depurate and goes up to affect the nose. When the wind is resolved, the residual heat condenses the body fluids into thick discharges, which block the noses and transforms into purulent snivels; it can also be caused by exuberant live-gallbladder fire, which rises to affect the nose orifices.

清肃，客邪上干清窍而致鼻塞流涕。风邪解后，郁热未清，酿为浊液，壅于鼻窍，化为脓涕，迁延而发鼻渊；亦有因肝胆火盛，上犯清窍，引起鼻渊者。

2 Syndrome differentiation

Chief symptoms: Yellowish, thick and stinking nasal discharges, and nasal obstruction.

The syndrome of wind-heat accumulation in the lung meridian manifests copious thick snivels, accompanied by headache, fever, cough, red tongue with yellowish coating, and floating rapid pulse. The syndrome of dampness-heat obstruction manifests lingering and recurrent onset, vertigo, distending pain in the forehead, red tongue with greasy coating, and wiry slippery pulse. The syndrome of exuberant liver-gallbladder fire manifests headache, vertigo, bitter taste in the mouth, thirst, red tongue with yellowish coating, and wiry pulse.

2 辨证

主症：鼻流浊涕，色黄腥秽，鼻塞不闻香臭。

肺经风热者，病变初发，兼鼻涕量多，或伴头痛、发热、咳嗽，舌红，苔黄，脉浮数等症；湿热阻窍者，经久不愈，反复发作，兼见头昏、眉额胀痛，舌红，苔腻，脉弦滑；肝胆火盛者，兼头痛目眩、口苦咽干，舌红，苔黄，脉弦。

3 Treatment

3.1 Essential treatment

Principal acupoints: Lieque(LU 7), Hegu(LI 4), Yingxiang(LI 20), Yintang(EX-HN 3), and Shangxing(GV 23).

Supplementary acupoints: In the syndrome of wind-heat accumulation in the lung meridian, add Shaoshang(LU 11) and Waiguan(TE 5); in the syndrome of dampness-heat obstruction, add Quchi(LI 11) and Yinlingquan(SP 9); in the syndrome of exuberant liver-gallbladder fire, add Taichong (LR 3) and Fengchi(GB 20).

3 治疗

3.1 基本治疗

主穴：列缺，合谷，迎香，印堂，上星。

配穴：肺经风热加少商、外关；湿热阻窍加曲池、阴陵泉；肝胆火旺加太冲、风池。

Explanation: The nose is the outer orifice of the lung. The hand-yangming meridian is exteriorly-interiorly related to the hand-taiyin meridian, and runs to the sides of the nose. Lieque(LU 7) is the Luo-Connecting acupoint of the hand-taiyin meridian, and Hegu(LI 4) is the Yuan-Source acupoint of the hand-yangming meridian; combination of these two acupoints is the combination of acupoints of the exteriorly-interiorly paired meridians, and acts to disperse wind and clear heat, release lung and unblock noses. Yingxiang(LI 20) is located beside the nose and Yintang(EX-HN 3) is located at the root of the nose; combination of these two acupoints with Shangxing(GV 23) functions to activate blood and unblock collaterals to free the nose.

方义：鼻为肺窍，手阳明经与手太阴经相为表里，其脉上夹鼻孔。取手太阴经络穴列缺，手阳明经原穴合谷，属远部表里配穴，可疏风清热、宣肺开窍。迎香夹于鼻旁，印堂位于鼻根，远近相配，更配督脉之上星，活血通络而利鼻窍。

3. 2　Other therapies

3. 2　其他治疗

Ear acupuncture: Select acupoints Internal Ear (LO 6), Lower Tragus(TG 2), Forehead(AT 1), and Lung(CO 14). Puncture these acupoints with the filiform needles, manipulate the needles intermittently, and retain the needles for 20 minutes. The treatment is applied once per day or every other day. Intradermal needles can also be applied once a week.

耳针：选内耳、下屏、额、肺。毫针刺，间歇捻转，留针 20 分钟，每日或隔日 1 次。或埋针 1 周。

Acupoints massage: Self-massage is applied at Yingxiang(LI 20) and Hegu(LI 4) for 5 to 10 minutes, 1 to 2 times every day. Or rub both sides of Yingxiang(LI 20) up and down with the great thenar eminence until heat penetrates deep into the manipulated area, several times a day.

穴位按摩：选取迎香、合谷。自我按摩，每次5～10分钟，每日 1～2 次。或用两手大鱼际，沿两侧迎香穴上下按摩至发热，每日数次。

4　Remarks

4　按语

Acupuncture is effective for nasosinusitis. But it is less effective for accessory nasosinusitis, and just serves as a supplementary treatment method.

针刺治疗鼻窦炎有一定疗效，对副鼻窦炎效果较差，可作为辅助治疗。嘱患者锻

Patients should be asked to engage in regular exercises to enhance body constitution, avoid spicy food, and abstain from smoking and alcohol.

炼身体，增强体质，禁食辛辣刺激食物，戒除烟酒。

Toothache

Toothache refers to the pain in the teeth caused by various reasons, and it is one of the common symptoms in stomatopathy. Toothache can be triggered or aggravated by some noxious irritations such as cold, hot, acid and sweet foods. This disease is frequently seen in dental caries, pulpitis, apicitis, periodontitis and hypersensitive teeth.

牙 痛

牙痛是指牙齿因各种原因引起的疼痛而言，为口腔疾患中常见的症状之一，遇冷、热、酸、甜等刺激时牙痛发作或加重。属中医学“牙宣”“牙槽风”范畴。牙痛常见于西医学的龋齿、牙髓炎、根尖炎、牙周炎和牙本质过敏等疾病。

1 Etiology and pathogenesis

Toothache is closely related to the hand and foot yangming meridians as well as the kidney meridian. The hand and foot yangming meridians respectively go into the lower and upper gums. Toothache may be caused by accumulated heat in the stomach and intestine, or by invasion of exogenous wind into yangming meridian that transforms into fire and goes up to affect the teeth. The kidney governs the bone while the teeth are the surplus of the bones. Kidney-yin deficiency may induce deficiency fire that flares up to cause toothache. Sometimes, toothache results from over-intake of sweet or sour foods, poor oral hygiene and dental caries.

1 病因病机

牙痛主要与手足阳明经和肾经有关。手足阳明经脉分别入下齿、上齿，大肠、胃腑积热，或风邪外袭经络，郁于阳明而化火，火邪循经上炎而发牙痛。肾主骨，齿为骨之余，肾阴不足，虚火上炎亦可引起牙痛。亦有多食甘酸之物，口齿不洁，垢秽蚀齿而作痛者。

2 Syndrome differentiation

Chief symptoms: Pain in the teeth.

The syndrome of yangming fire manifests severe toothache with foul breath, thirst, constipation, and surging pulse. The syndrome of wind fire

2 辨证

主症：牙齿疼痛。

阳明郁火者，牙痛甚剧，兼有口臭、口渴、便秘，脉洪；风火牙痛者，痛甚而龈肿，兼

manifests severe toothache with swollen gums, accompanied by chills and fever, and floating rapid pulse. The syndrome of kidney deficiency manifests on-and-off dull pain in the teeth, or loose teeth, absence of foul breath, red tongue, and thready pulse.

形寒身热,脉浮数;肾虚牙痛者,兼见隐隐作痛,时作时止,或牙齿浮动,口不臭,舌尖红,脉细。

3 Treatment

3 治疗

3.1 Essential treatment

3.1 基本治疗

Principal acupoints: Hegu(LI 4), Jiache(ST 6), and Xiaguan(ST 7).

主穴: 合谷,颊车,下关。

Supplementary acupoints: In the syndrome of wind fire, add Waiguan(TE 5) and Fengchi(GB 20); in the syndrome of stomach fire, add Neiting (ST 44) and Erjian(LI 2); in the syndrome of kidney deficiency, add Taixi (KI 3) and Xingjian(LR 2).

配穴: 风火牙痛加外关、风池;胃火牙痛加内庭、二间;肾虚牙痛加太溪、行间。

Expianation: Hegu(LI 4), a key acupoint for toothache and distal to the teeth, acts to unblock yangming meridian and clear heat in the stomach, disperse wind and unobstruct collaterals; the contralateral Hegu(LI 4) is often used. Jiache(ST 6) and Xiaguan(ST 7), two local acupoints, are used to unblock yangming meridians, unobstruct collaterals and relieve pain.

方义: 合谷为治疗牙痛之要穴,为远端取穴,可疏通阳明经络、清阳明之热,兼有祛风通络作用,循经远取可左右交叉取穴。颊车、下关为近部选穴,疏通足阳明经气、通络止痛。

3.2 Other therapy

3.2 其他治疗

Ear acupuncture: Upper Jaw (LO 3), Lower Jaw(LO 3), Shenmen(TF 4), Upper Tragus (TG 1), and Toothache point are selected. Puncture 2～3 acupoints with the filiform needles by strong intensity, and retain the needles for 20～30 minutes. The treatment is applied once a day.

耳针: 选上颌、下颌、神门、上屏尖、牙痛点。每次取2～3 穴,毫针刺,强刺激,留针 20～30 分钟,每日 1 次。

4 Remarks

4 按语

Acupuncture is quite effective for the common toothache, but can just produce temporary pain relief for toothache caused by dental caries.

针刺对一般牙痛效果良好,但对龋齿所致牙痛只能暂时止痛。

Sore Throat

Sore throat is a common cardinal symptom of oral-pharyngeal and laryngeal-pharyngeal disorders, characterized by swelling, pain and foreign-body sensation in the throat, and throat discomforts in swallowing. It is often seen in acute tonsillitis, acute pharyngitis, simple laryngitis, and purulent tonsils in Western medicine.

咽喉肿痛

咽喉肿痛是口咽和喉咽部病变的主要症状，以咽喉部红肿疼痛、异物感、吞咽不适为特征，中医学称之为“喉痹”。咽喉肿痛常见于西医学的急性扁桃体炎、急性咽炎和单纯性喉炎、扁桃体周围脓肿等疾病。

1 Etiology and pathogenesis

The pharynx connects with the esophagus and stomach, and the larynx connects with the trachea and lung. Sore throat is caused by exogenous wind-heat that scorches the lung system, or by accumulated heat in the lung and stomach meridians that burns the throat in combination with exogenous factors. Also, sore throat may result from up-flaring of deficiency fire and kidney-yin deficiency failing to moisten the throat.

1 病因病机

咽接食管，通于胃；喉接气管，通于肺。可因外感风热之邪熏灼肺系，或肺胃二经蕴热，复感外邪，内外邪热搏结，熏灼咽喉而为病；如肾阴不能上润咽喉，虚火上炎，亦可致咽喉肿痛。

2 Syndrome differentiation

Chief symptoms: Swelling and pain in the throat.

The syndrome of exogenous wind-heat manifests red, swollen and painful throat, difficulty in swallowing and coughing, accompanied by fever and chills, headache, and floating rapid pulse. The syndrome of lung-stomach heat manifests swelling and pain in the throat, thirst, constipation, yellow urine, red tongue with yellowish coating, and surging pulse. The syndrome of intense deficiency fire mani-fests slightly swollen and painful throat, dryness of the throat, discomforts in swallowing aggra-

2 辨证

主症：咽喉肿痛。

外感风热者，兼咽喉红肿疼痛、吞咽困难、咳嗽，伴寒热头痛、脉浮数；肺胃实热者，兼咽部红肿疼痛、口渴、便秘、尿黄、舌红、苔黄、脉洪大；阴虚火旺者，兼咽喉微肿、疼痛；或咽干喉燥、吞咽时觉痛楚，入夜则见症较重，舌红、脉细数。

vated at night, red tongue, and thready rapid pulse.

3 Treatment

3.1 Essential treatment

Principal acupoints: Shaoshang(LU 11), Hegu (LI 4), Lieque(LU 7), and Zhaohai(KI 6).

Supplementary acupoints: In the syndrome of exogenous wind-heat, add Fengchi (GB 20) and Waiguan(TE 5); in the syndrome of lung-stomach heat, add Chize(LU 5), Shangyang(LI 1) and Neiting(ST 44); in the syndrome of intense deficiency fire, add Taixi(KI 3) and Yuji(LU 10).

Explanation: Shaoshang (LU 11) is the Jing-Well acupoint of the hand-taiyin meridian, and pricking it to bleed can clear heat in the lung. Thus, Shaoshang(LU 11) is the essential acupoint in the treatment of throat diseases. Hegu (LI 4), the Yuan-Source acupoint of the large intestine meridian, can clear the accumulated heat of the yangming meridian. Lieque(LU 7) and Zhaohai(KI 6) are the Confluent acupoints and are specifically effective for sore throat.

3.2 Other therapy

Ear acupuncture: Select Pharynx Larynx (TG 3), Lung(CO 14), Heart(CO 15), Adrenal Gland (TG 2p), Tonsil(LO 7,8,9), Helix 1～4 (HX 9～12), Helix 5, and Helix 6. Puncture these acupoints with the filiform needles by moderate intensity and retain the needles for 1 hour.

4 Remarks

Acupuncture is quite effective for sore throat. However, attention should be paid to the treatment of primary diseases. If an abscess has formed, surgery is necessary. Patients are advised to avoid spicy food and refrain from smoking and drinking alcohol.

3 治疗

3.1 基本治疗

主穴：少商，合谷，列缺，照海。

配穴：外感风热加风池、外关；肺胃实热加尺泽、商阳、内庭；阴虚火旺加太溪、鱼际。

方义：少商系手太阴经井穴，点刺出血，可清泻肺热，为治疗喉证的主穴。合谷为手阳明经原穴，善清泻阳明积热。列缺与照海相配，为八脉交会配穴，专治咽喉疾病。

3.2 其他治疗

耳针：选咽喉、肺、心、下屏尖、扁桃体、轮 1～6。毫针刺，中强刺激，每次留针 1 小时。

4 按语

针刺治疗咽喉肿痛效果好。但应注意对原发病的治疗。如已成脓则转科处理。忌食辛辣等刺激性食物，力戒烟酒。

Canker Sore

Canker sore is a commonly seen disease of the mucous membrane of the mouth. It mostly occurs in the lips, cheeks and tongue margins. The typical manifestations include single or multiple round or oval ulcers, which are prone to recurrence. Canker sore is often seen in recurrent aphthous stomatitis and periglandular canker sore in Western medicine.

1 Etiology and pathogenesis

The mouth associates with the spleen, and the tongue associates with the heart. Canker sore results from accumulated heat in the heart and spleen that goes upwards to cause swelling and sore in the mouth and the tongue; or it is caused by an inherent effulgent fire due to yin deficiency or after illnesses which flares upwards to damage the oral mucous membranes; or it is caused by spleen-kidney yang-deficiency failing to warm and transform body fluids, which congeal cold and dampness in the mouth can cause erosion in the membranes.

2 Syndrome differentiation

Chief symptoms: Recurrent circular or elliptical ulcers in the mouth with clear boundaries.

The syndrome of accumulated heat in the heart and spleen manifests white-yellow ulcers, congestion and swelling, burning pain, thirst, constipation, red tongue with yellowish and greasy coating, and rapid pulse. The syndrome of effulgent deficiency fire manifests grayish-white or grayish-yellow ulcers, with slightly swollen and congested mucous membrane, small ulcers, lingering recurrence, red tongue with less coating, and thready rapid pulse.

口　疮

口疮是口腔黏膜病中最常见的一种疾病。好发于唇、颊、舌缘等处。典型表现为圆形或椭圆形溃疡，可单发或多发，反复发作。常见于西医学的复发性阿弗他溃疡及腺周口疮等疾病。

1 病因病机

口属脾，舌属心，心脾俱蕴热毒，不得发散，攻冲上焦，令口舌生疮肿痛；或因素体阴亏，病后劳伤，真阴耗损，虚火内旺，上炎口舌而生疮；或脾肾阳虚，温化失调，津液停滞，寒湿困于口腔，黏膜溃烂而成疮。

2 辨证

主症：反复出现圆形或椭圆形口腔溃疡，边缘整齐。

心脾蕴热者，溃疡呈黄白色、周围红肿，灼热作痛，口干，便秘，舌红，苔黄腻，脉数；阴虚火旺者，口疮灰白或灰黄、周围黏膜微红肿，溃疡面较小而少，此愈彼起，反复绵延，舌红，苔少，脉细数；脾肾阳虚者，溃点紫暗色、四周苍白、不红不肿，舌淡，苔白

The syndrome of spleen-kidney yang-deficiency manifests dark purple ulcers with pale margins, absence of congestion and swelling, pale tongue with whitish slippery or whitish greasy coating, and deep weak pulse.

滑或白腻，脉沉弱。

3 Treatment

3.1 Essential treatment

Principal acupoints: Lianquan(CV 23), Dicang (ST 4), Hegu(LI 4), and Laogong(PC 8).

Supplementary acupoints: In the syndrome of accumulated heat in the heart and spleen, add Tongli(HT 5) and Xuehai(SP 10); in the syndrome of effulgent deficiency fire, add Zhaohai(KI 6) and Taixi (KI 3); in the syndrome of spleen-kidney yang-deficiency, add Guanyuan(CV 4) and Qihai (CV 6); in the presence of severe pain, prick Jinjin (EX-HN 12) and Yuye(EX-HN 13) to bleed.

Explanation: Lianquan(CV 23), the Crossing acupoint of the yin link vessel and conception vessel, connects with the tongue and can regulate meridian qi in the mouth. Dicang(ST 4) is the Crossing acupoint of the hand and foot-yangming meridians and yang heel vessel, and Hegu(LI 4) is the Yuan-Source acupoint of the hand-yangming meridian; combination of these two acupoints can purge heat in the yangming meridians. Laogong(PC 8), the Ying-Spring acupoint of hand-jueyin meridian, can purge heart fire and relieve pain.

3.2 Other therapies

Ear acupuncture: Select Heart(CO 15), Mouth (CO 1), Spleen(CO 13), Stomach(CO 14) and Triple Energizer (CO 17). Apply *Semen Vaccariae* (Wang Bu Liu Xing) at these acupoints, once 3 to 5 days on alternate ears every time.

3 治疗

3.1 基本治疗

主穴：廉泉，地仓，合谷，劳宫。

配穴：心脾蕴热加通里、血海；阴虚火旺加照海、太溪；脾肾阳虚加关元、气海；痛甚者点刺金津、玉液出血。

方义：廉泉为阴维、任脉之会，联系舌本，可疏通口腔气机。地仓为手足阳明经与阳蹻脉之会，合谷为手阳明经原穴，二穴相配以泻阳明经之热。劳宫为手厥阴经荥穴，可清心火而止痛。

3.2 其他治疗

耳针：选心、口、脾、胃、三焦等穴。采用王不留行贴压，3～5 日更换 1 次，双耳交替。

Pricking therapy: Select Dazhui (GV 14) and the sites 1.5 ~ 2 cm lateral to Dazhui (GV 14). These areas are pricked with a three-edged needle to cut 2 to 3 fibers of the subcutaneous tissues, followed by squeezing a few drops of blood out, twice a week.

挑刺：选大椎及大椎旁开1.5～2厘米处。三棱针划断皮下纤维组织2～3根，挤压针孔，令少许出血，每周2次。

4 Remarks

Acupuncture has certain effects on canker sore. During the acute stage of the disease, patients are advised to take liquid or semi-liquid diets, and avoid spicy, salty and hard foods.

4 按语

针刺治疗口疮有一定疗效。发作期应选流质或半选流质饮食，避免过热、过咸及粗硬食物。

Section 5 Emergency Conditions

第5节 急 症

Syncope

Syncope refers to sudden and temporary loss of consciousness and movement, characterized by abrupt vertigo, weak limbs, quick loss of consciousness and fainting, and recovery of consciousness in several seconds to several minutes. Syncope is frequently seen in transient ischemic attacks in Western medicine.

晕 厥

晕厥是指骤起短暂的意识和行动丧失。其特征为突感眩晕、行动无力，迅速失去知觉而昏倒，数秒至数分钟后恢复清醒。属于中医学“厥证”范畴。晕厥常见于西医学的一过性脑缺血发作。

1 Etiology and pathogenesis

Syncope is mostly caused by weak original qi, qi and blood deficiency after diseases, heavy bleeding during labor, over-strain, and sudden standing up or movement, in which the qi and blood fail to ascend in time to nourish the brain and the yang qi fails to reach the limbs; it may also be due to emotional fluctuation or post-traumatic violent headache,

1 病因病机

晕厥多由元气虚弱，病后气血未复，产后失血过多，每因操劳过度、骤起骤立等致使经气紊乱，气血不能上充于头，阳气不能通达于四末而致；或因情志异常波动，或因外伤剧烈疼痛，以致气

which causes the adversity of qi-blood flow and then disturbs the clear orifices(brain), resulting in sudden fainting.

血运行逆乱，清窍受扰而突然昏倒。

2 Syndrome differentiation

Chief symptoms: Subjective dizziness and vertigo, weakness and lassitude, nausea and vomiting, followed by collapse and unconsciousness.

The excess syndrome is usually seen in strong people with sudden loss of consciousness and fainting due to trauma and anger, shortness of breath, locked jaw, pale tongue with thin whitish coating, and wiry deep pulse. The deficiency syndrome is usually seen in weak people with sudden loss of consciousness and fainting due to poor constitution, over- strain and fright, sallow complexion, cold limbs, shortness of breath and dizziness, spontaneous sweating, pale tongue and weak thready pulse.

2 辨证

主症：自觉头晕乏力，眼前发黑，泛泛欲吐，继则突然昏倒不省人事。

实证者，素体健壮，偶因外伤、恼怒等致突然昏仆，不省人事，呼吸急促，牙关紧闭，舌淡薄白，脉沉弦；虚证者，素体虚弱，疲劳惊恐而致昏仆，面色苍白，四肢厥冷，气短眼花，汗出，舌淡，脉细缓无力。

3 Treatment

3.1 Essential treatment

Principal acupoints: Shuigou(GV 26), Neiguan (PC 6), Zhongchong(PC 9), Yongquan(KI 1), and Zusanli(ST 36).

Supplementary acupoints: In the excess syndrome, add Hegu(LI 4) and Taichong(LR 3); in the deficiency syndrome, add Qihai (CV 6), Guanyuan(CV 4), and Baihui(GV 20).

Explanation: Shuigou (GV 26) is at the site where the meridian qi flows from the governor vessel to the conception vessel. The governor vessel enters the brain and runs to the vertex of the head and controls all yang meridians, therefore Shuigou(GV 26) functions to open orifices and arouse consciousness. Neiguan(PC 6), the Luo-Connecting acupoint of the hand-jueyin pericardium meridian, acts to

3 治疗

3.1 基本治疗

主穴：水沟，内关，中冲，涌泉，足三里。

配穴：实证加合谷、太冲；虚证加气海、关元、百会。

方义：水沟居任督脉交接之处，督脉入脑上巅，又总督诸阳，取之有开窍醒神之功；内关为手厥阴心包经络穴，可醒脑宁心。二穴相配，有苏厥开窍之功。中冲为心包经井穴，刺之能调阴阳经气之逆乱，为治疗晕厥之要

waken brain and calm mind. Combined use of Shuigou(GV 26) and Neiguan(PC 6) can arouse consciousness and open orifices. Zhongchong(PC 1), the Jing-Well acupoint of the pericardium meridian, can correct the adversity of qi flow in the yin and yang meridians and is an essential acupoint for the treatment of syncope. Yongquan(KI 1) can activate qi in the kidney meridian and restores consciousness, thus it is indicated for severe syncope. Zusanli(ST 36) is applied to enrich qi and blood and harmonize the middle energizer, and nourish the brain.

穴。涌泉可激发肾经之气，最能醒神开窍，多用于晕厥之重证。足三里可补益气血而和中，以滋养神窍。

3.2 Other therapy

Blood-letting therapy: Select the twelve Jing-Well acupoints, Shixuan(EX-EU 11), and Dazhui(GV 14). Prick these acupoints with filiform needles to let out several drops of blood. This therapy is applicable for the excess syndrome.

3.2 其他治疗

刺络放血：选十二井穴、十宣、大椎，毫针刺，出血数滴，适用于实证。

4 Remarks

In managing syncope cases, let the patient lie flat at once, unbutton the clothes and yet keep the patient warm. Acupuncture works well on syncope, especially on that caused by emotional upsets and and traumatic injury. Meanwhile, a detailed examination should be given to ascertain the cause of the syncope so that treatment can be adopted accordingly.

4 按语

迅速使患者平卧，解开衣扣，并注意保暖。针灸对情绪激动、外伤疼痛引起的晕厥治疗效果良好。在急救同时，应查明晕厥原因，注意原发病的治疗。

Collapse

Collapse is a critical condition characterized by pallid complexion, apathy, or unconsciousness, clod limbs and sweating, and drop in blood pressure. It corresponds to shock due to various reasons in Western medicine.

虚 脱

虚脱是以面色苍白、神情淡漠或昏迷；肢冷汗出；血压下降为特征的危重证候。属于中医学“脱证”范畴。可常见于西医学各种原因引起的休克病证。

1 Etiology and pathogenesis

Collapse is mostly caused by heavy hemorrhage, violent vomiting and diarrhea, or attacks by six exogenous factors, emotional injury, drug hypersensitivity or toxicosis, or consumption of qi, blood and body fluids after long-term diseases. All these factors may cause the dysfunction of the zang-fu organs and the failure of qi and blood to nourish the body, even resulting in the critical condition of yin-yang exhaustion and depletion.

2 Syndrome differentiation

Chief symptoms: Pale or purple complexion, apathy, dull expression and reaction, occasional coma, or irritability, scanty urine, shortness of breath with mouth open, spontaneous sweating, coldness in the limbs and skin, drop in blood pressure, feeble thready or hollow pulse.

The syndrome of yang depletion manifests feeble breathing, purple lips, enlarged tongue, and thin weak pulse. The yin depletion syndrome manifests thirst, irritability, dry and red tongue, and thready rapid pulse. If the disease deteriorates, the critical condition of yin-yang collapse may happen.

3 Treatment

3.1 Essential treatment

Principal acupoints: Suliao (GV 25), Shuigou (GV 26), and Neiguan(PC 6).

Supplementary acupoints: In the presence of coma, add Zhongchong(PC 9) and Yongquan(KI 1); in the presence of cold limbs and feeble pulse, add Guanyuan (CV 4), Shenque(CV 8) and Baihui(GV 20).

Explanation: Suliao(GV 25) is an acupoint of the governor vessel, and functions to ascend yang

1 病因病机

本病多由大量失血、大吐大泻,或因六淫邪毒,情志内伤,药物过敏或中毒,久病虚衰等严重损伤气血津液,致脏腑阴阳失调,气血不能供养全身所致。甚者导致阴阳衰竭,出现亡阳亡阴之危候。

2 辨证

主症:面色苍白或紫绀,神情淡漠,反应迟钝,昏迷或烦躁不安,尿量减少,张口,自汗,肢冷肤凉,血压下降,脉微细或芤大无力。

亡阳者,兼呼吸微弱、唇发紫、舌胖、脉细无力;亡阴者,兼口渴、烦躁不安、唇舌干红、脉细数无力。若病情恶化可导致阴阳俱脱之危候。

3 治疗

3.1 基本治疗

主穴:素髎,水沟,内关。

配穴:神志昏迷加中冲、涌泉;肢冷脉微加关元、神阙、百会。

方义:素髎属督脉,有升阳救逆、开窍醒神之功,急刺

and rectify adversity, open orifices and arouse consciousness; in emergency, puncturing this acupoint can elevate the blood pressure. Shuigou(GV 26) is an essential acupoint to induce resuscitation, and can restore yang and arrest collapse in emergency needling. Neiguan(PC 6), the Luo-Connecting acupoint of the pericardium meridian, can reinforce heart-qi and promote the flow of qi and blood to calm the heart spirit. The combination of these three acupoints can restore yang and arrest collapse.

可使血压回升。水沟为苏厥救逆之要穴,急刺可回阳固脱。内关属心包经,可调补心气,助气血之运行以宁心安神。三穴合用,回阳固脱。

3. 2 Other therapy

Moxibustion: Select acupoints Baihui(GV 20), Danzhong(CV 17), Shenque(CV 8), Guanyuan (CV 4) and Qihai(CV 6). Direct moxibustion with moxa cones is applied on 2 to 3 acupoints each time until the limbs turn warm, the pulse recovers and the sweating is arrested.

3. 2 其他治疗

艾灸: 选百会、膻中、神阙、关元、气海。艾炷直接灸,每次选 2～3 穴,灸至肢温、脉复、汗收为止。

4 Remarks

Collapse can be caused by various factors, with sudden onset and complicated condition, and should be rescued in time. Acupuncture can be employed as one of the emergency measures. However, the underlying causes must be ascertained and treated accordingly; some rescuing therapies in Western medicine should be considered if necessary.

4 按语

虚脱可由多种原因引起,发病突然,病情复杂,应及时抢救,针灸可作为抢救措施之一,但必须对虚脱的原发病进行治疗,必要时配合西医抢救方法。

High Fever

High fever refers to high body temperature over 39 ℃. It may be seen in acute infections, acute contagious diseases, heatstroke, rheumatic fever, tuberculosis, and malignant tumors in Western medi-cine.

高 热

高热是体温超过 39 摄氏度的急性症状。属于中医学“壮热”“日晡潮热”的范畴。高热可见于西医学的急性感染性疾病、急性传染病,以及中暑、风湿热、结核病、恶性肿瘤等疾病。

1 Etiology and pathogenesis

The exogenous wind-heat attacks body from the mouth and nose, makes the defensive qi failing to release and disperse and the lung failing to depurate; warm epidemic toxin invades the body and scorches qi or involves nutrient and blood phase, giving rise to high fever. It may also result from exogenous summer-heat disturbs the pericardium.

1 病因病机

外感风热之邪从口鼻而入，卫失宣散，肺失清肃；或温邪疫毒侵袭人体，燔灼气分，或内陷营血引起高热。也有因外感暑热之邪，内犯心包而致者。

2 Syndrome differentiation

Chief symptoms: High fever over 39 ℃.

The syndrome of exogenous wind-heat manifests high fever and chills, dry throat, headache, coughing, red tongue with yellowish coating, and floating rapid pulse. The syndrome of lung heat manifests coughing with yellow thick sputum, dry throat, thirst, and rapid pulse. The syndrome of heat in qi phase manifests high fever, sweating, extreme thirst with desire to drink, red tongue and surging pulse. The syndrome of heat phase in blood manifests high fever at night, papules, vomiting of blood, bloody stools or nosebleed, vexation, crimson tongue, and even coma, delirium and convulsions.

2 辨证

主症：体温升高，超过 39 摄氏度。

风热表证者，兼高热恶寒、咽干、头痛、咳嗽、舌红苔黄、脉浮数；肺热证者，兼咳嗽、痰黄而稠、咽干、口渴、脉数；热在气分者，兼高热汗出、烦渴引饮、舌红、脉洪数；热入营血者，兼高热夜甚，斑疹隐隐，吐血、便血或衄血，心烦，舌绛，甚则出现神昏谵语，抽搐。

3 Treatment

3.1 Essential treatment

Principal acupoints: Dazhui(GV 14), the twelve Jing-Well acupoints, Shixuan(EX-UE 11), Quchi(LI 11), and Hegu(LI 4).

Supplementary acupoints: In the syndrome of exogenous wind-heat, add Yuji(LU 10) and Waiguan(TE 5); in the syndrome of lung heat, add Chize(LU 5); in the syndrome of heat in qi phase,

3 治疗

3.1 基本治疗

主穴：大椎，十二井穴，十宣，曲池，合谷。

配穴：风热加鱼际、外关；肺热加尺泽；气分热盛加内庭；热入营血加内关、血海；抽搐加太冲；神昏加水

add Neiting(ST 44); in the syndrome of heat in blood phase, add Neiguan(PC 6) and Xuehai(SP 10). In the presence of convulsion, add Taichong (LR 3); in the presence of coma, add Shuigou(GV 26) and Neiguan(PC 6).

沟、内关。

Explanation: Dazhui(GV 14), an acupoint of the governor vessel where the yang meridians meet, functions to disperse heat in the yang meridians. The twelve Jing-Well acupoints and Shixuan(EX-UE 11) are located at the distal ends of the four extremities where the yin meridians connect with the yang meridians. Pricking these acupoints can relieve heat obviously. Quchi(LI 11), the He-Sea acupoint of the hand-yangming meridian, can clear the excess heat in the yangming meridians in combination with Hegu(LI 4).

方义: 大椎属督脉,为诸阳之会,能宣散一身阳热之气。十二井穴、十宣穴皆在四末,为阴阳经交接之处。三穴点刺,具有明显的退热作用。曲池为阳明经合穴,配合谷清泻阳明经实热。

3.2 Other therapy

Scraping therapy: Scrape the areas besides the spinal column and the Back-Shu acupoints with specially-made plate or porcelain spoon by cooking oil or water till the skin turns flushed.

3.2 其他治疗

刮痧: 选脊柱两侧和背俞穴,用特制刮痧板或瓷汤匙蘸食油或清水,刮脊柱两侧和背俞穴,刮至皮肤红紫色为度。

4 Remarks

Acupuncture works quite well in decreasing body temperature and can be used as one therapy against high fever. At the same time, the underlying causes must be ascertained and treated accordingly.

4 按语

针灸退热有很好的效果,可以作为处理高热的措施之一。但在针刺治疗同时,须查明原因,明确诊断,针对病因进行治疗。

Convulsion

Convulsion refers to violent and involuntary muscular contraction or spasm of the limbs, or accompanied by stiff neck, opisthotonos and lockjaw.

抽　搐

抽搐是指四肢不随意的肌肉抽动,或兼有颈项强直、角弓反张、口噤不开等。引

Convulsion is caused by many reasons, and can be divided into two types depending on where fever is accompanied or not. In Western medicine, it occurs in such diseases as high fever, tetanus, epilepsy, craniocerebral trauma and hysteria, etc.

起抽搐的原因很多,临床根据有无发热分为发热性抽搐和无发热性抽搐两类。抽搐常见于西医学的高热惊厥、破伤风、癫痫、颅脑外伤和癔病等疾病。

1　Etiology and pathogenesis

Convulsion can be caused by exogenous seasonal factors that stagnate in the body and then transform into heat or fire, or by tendon dysfunctions resulting from heat and liver-wind due to improper diets and dampness-heat, or by brain obstruction of phlegm heat due to spleen deficiency and dampness accumulation, or by undernourishment of the tendons and endogenous wind due to constitutional spleen-stomach deficiency and qi-blood insufficiency.

1　病因病机

抽搐多为感受时邪,郁闭于内,化热化火;或饮食不节,湿热壅滞,郁久化火,上扰神明,热极引动肝风,经筋功能失常而致;或因脾虚湿盛,聚液成痰,痰热互结,上蒙清窍而致;或因平素脾胃素虚、气血不足而致虚风内动。

2　Syndrome differentiation

Chief symptoms: Muscular spasms of the limbs, possible temporary loss of consciousness, upturned eyes or deviated vision, lockjaw, or foaming at the mouth, and urinary and fecal incontinence. Severe cases may be accompanied by coma and fainting.

The syndrome of extreme heat engendering wind may manifest exterior condition, sudden onset, possible sweating, headache and coma. The syndrome of phlegm-heat transforming into wind manifests high fever, vexation and agitation, sputum rattling in the throat and lockjaw. The syndrome of deficient blood generating wind manifests absence of fever, muscular spasms of limbs, exposure of the eyeballs, and weak thready pulse.

2　辨证

主症: 四肢抽搐,或有短时间的意识丧失,两目上翻或斜视,牙关紧闭或口吐白沫,二便失禁,严重者伴有昏迷。

热极生风者,兼见表证,起病急骤,有汗或无汗,头痛,神昏;痰热化风者,兼壮热烦躁、喉间痰鸣、牙关紧闭;血虚生风者,多无发热,兼手足抽搦、露睛、脉细无力。

3　Treatment

3.1　Essential treatment

Principal acupoints: Shuigou(GV 26), Neiguan

3　治疗

3.1　基本治疗

主穴: 水沟,内关,合谷,

(PC 6), Hegu(LI 4), and Taichong(LR 3).

Supplementary acupoints: In the syndrome of extreme heat engendering wind, add Laogong(PC 9), Quchi(LI 11) and Zhongchong(PC 8); in the syndrome of phlegm-heat transforming into wind, add Fenglong(ST 40) and Yinlingquan(SP 9); in the syndrome of deficient blood generating wind, add Xuehai(SP 10) and Zusanli(ST 36). In the presence of fever, add Dazhui(GV 14) and Quchi (LI 11); in the presence of coma, add Shixuan (EX-UE 11) and Yongquan (KI 1).

Explanation: Shuigou(GV 26), an important acupoint of the governor vessel which enters the brain, can arouse the brain and open the orifices, regulate spirit and conduct qi. Neiguan(PC 6), the Luo-Connecting acupoint of the pericardium meridian, can regulate heart-qi and activate blood, and help Shuigou(GV 26) to arouse consciousness. Hegu (LI 4) and Taichong(LR 4) are collectively known as "Four Passes"; needling these two acupoints functions to extinguish wind and relieve spasms. In the light of the general therapeutic principle of "treating the branches first in an emergent condition", the wind-extinguishing and spasm-relieving therapy is applied first and then the underlying causes should be identified and treated accordingly.

3.2 Other therapies

Ear acupuncture: Select Subcortex(AT 4), Liver(CO 12), Kidney(CO 10), Shenmen(TF 4), Heart(CO 15) and Brain Stem(AT 3, 4i). Each time, puncture 3～4 acupoints with filiform needles by strong stimulation.

Electro-acupuncture: Select Neiguan (PC 6), Sishencong(EX-HN 1), Hegu(LI 4), Taichong (LR

太冲。

配穴：热极生风加劳宫、曲池、中冲；痰热化风加丰隆、阴陵泉；血虚生风加血海、足三里；发热加大椎、曲池；神昏加十宣、涌泉。

方义：水沟为督脉要穴，督脉入络脑，可醒脑开窍、调神导气。内关为手厥阴心包经穴，可调理心气、活血通络，助水沟醒脑开窍。合谷、太冲相配，称为开"四关"，为熄风止痉之首选穴。根据急则治标的原则，先宜熄风止痉，然后对因治疗。

3.2 其他治疗

耳针：选皮质下、肝、肾、神门、脑干、心。每次选3～4穴，毫针刺，强刺激。

电针：选内关、四神聪、合谷、太冲、神门等穴。毫针

3) and Shenmen(HT 7). When the needles are inserted and connected with electricity by the stimulation intensity at the patients' tolerance. Electro-acupuncture is given for 10 to 30 minutes. This therapy is advisable to treat an acute paroxysm of convulsion.

刺后通脉冲电，刺激强度以患者能忍受为度。每次通电10～30 分钟。用于急性发作患者。

4 Remarks

In the treatment of paroxysmal convulsion, intense acupuncture techniques should be given to relieve the limb spasms. When the convulsion stops, the underlying causes should be identified as early as possible to give appropriate management.

4 按语

发作期治疗时，务必要求重手法(强针感，以使痉挛抽搐的肢体得到缓解)。抽搐停止之后必须查明病因，及早作出诊断，采取针对病因的治疗措施。

Angina Pectoris

Angina pectoris refers to abrupt onset of squeezing, dull and suffocative pain in the left chest, oppression in the chest and shortness of breath. It is the cardinal manifestation of coronary artery disease, and a syndrome caused by acute transient myocardial ischemia and anoxia due to inadequate blood supply to the coronary arteries. It is often triggered by tiredness, over-excitement, over-eating, catching cold, etc.

心绞痛

心绞痛以左侧胸部心前区突然发作的压榨性、闷胀性或窒息性疼痛及胸闷、气短为特征，是冠心病的主要临床表现，是因冠状动脉供血不足，心肌急剧短暂的缺血缺氧所引起的综合征。常因劳累、情绪激动、饱食、受寒等因素诱发。心绞痛属于中医学“胸痹”“心痛”“厥心痛”“真心痛”等范畴。

1 Etiology and pathogenesis

Angina pectoris primarily results from healthy qi deficiency, internal invasion of pathogenic coldness and ensuing chest-yang impediment, or from emotional depression and qi-blood stagnation, or from excessive intake of foods and alcohol, and internal phlegm accumulation that causes heart vessel obstruc-

1 病因病机

本病多因正气内虚、寒邪内侵，胸阳闭阻；或情志郁结，气滞血瘀；或饮食无度，痰浊内生，导致阴寒、气滞、血瘀、痰浊闭阻心络，不通则痛；或劳逸失度，年迈肾虚，

tion by yin cold, qi stagnation, blood stasis and phlegm, or from over-exertion, kidney deficiency in the elderly, ying-blood consumption, heart-yang inactivity and malnutrition of heart vessels.

营血亏耗,心阳不振,心脉失养,发为本病。

2 Syndrome differentiation

2 辨证

Chief symptoms: Sudden angina in the left chest, chest oppression, palpitation, shortness of breath, even pain radiating to the back, panting and inability to lie flat.

主症:突发左胸心前区绞痛,胸闷,心悸,气短,甚至心痛彻背、喘息不得平卧。

The syndrome of qi-stagnation and blood stasis manifests fixed stabbing pain in the chest aggravated at night, dark purple tongue with possible ecchymosis, and rough or knotted pulse. The syndrome of cold coagulation manifests chest pain radiating to the back which is aggravated by the cold and relieved by the warmth, limb coldness, and tight wiry or slow deep pulse. The syndrome of phlegm-damp obstruction in the chest manifests chest fullness and pain, poor appetite and abdominal bloating, dark purple tongue with greasy coating, and deep slippery pulse. The syndrome of yang deficiency manifests chest oppression, shortness of breath, coldness of the body and limbs, aching loin, sallow complexion, purplish or pale lips and nails, light red tongue with tooth-marks, whitish tongue coating, and feeble thready or deep thin pulse.

气滞血瘀者,胸膺刺痛,痛处固定不移,入夜更甚,舌紫黯或有瘀斑,脉涩或结代;寒邪凝滞者,心痛彻背,遇寒痛剧,得热痛减,四肢不温,脉弦紧或沉迟;痰湿闭阻者,胸闷痞满而痛,纳呆脘胀,舌紫暗、苔浊腻,脉沉滑;阳气虚衰者,胸闷气短,形寒肢厥,腰酸乏力,面色淡白,唇甲青紫或淡白,舌淡红有齿痕,苔白,脉沉细或沉微欲绝。

3 Treatment

3 治疗

3.1 Essential treatment

3.1 基本治疗

Principal acupoints: Xinshu(BL 15), Jue-yinshu (BL 14), Neiguan (PC 6), Yinxi (HT 6), and Danzhong(CV 17).

主穴:心俞,厥阴俞,内关,阴郄,膻中。

Supplementary acupoints: In the syndrome of qi-stagnation and blood stasis, add Xuehai(SP 10) and Taichong(LR 3); in the syndrome of cold coagula-

配穴:气滞血瘀加血海、太冲;寒邪凝滞加神阙、关元;痰湿闭阻加中脘、丰隆;

tion, add Shenque(CV 8) and Guanyuan(CV 4); in the syndrome of phlegm-damp obstruction in the chest, add Zhongwan(CV 12) and Feng-long(ST 40); in the syndrome of yang depletion, add Shuigou(GV 26) and Baihui(GV 20).

阳气欲脱配水沟、百会。

Explanation: Xinshu(BL 15) and Jueyinshu (BL 14) are the Back-Shu acupoints of the heart and the pericardium. According to the therapeutic principle that the disorders of the zang-organ should be treated by the Back-Shu acupoints, these two acupoints are selected to move yang and activate blood. Neiguan(PC 6), the Luo-Connecting acupoint of the pericardium meridian of hand jueyin and the Confluent acupoint communicating with the yin link vessel, can regulate heart-qi, activate blood and unblock collaterals; it is the specific acupoint for angina pectoris. Yinxi(HT6), the Xi-Cleft acupoint of the heart meridian, is used to relieve and stop pain. Danzhong(CV 17), the Front-Mu acupoint of the pericardium and the Influential acupoint of qi, can regulate qi activity to treat heart and chest disorders.

方义：心俞、厥阴俞为手少阴心经和手厥阴心包经之背俞穴，根据脏病多取背俞的原则，取两穴通阳活血。内关为心包经络穴及八脉交会穴之一，可调理心气、活血通络，为治疗心胶痛的特效穴。阴郄为心经郄穴，可缓急止痛。膻中为心包经募穴，又为气之会穴，可疏调气机，治心胸疾患。

3.2 Otther therapy

Warm acupuncture: Puncture Jueyinshu(BL 14), Xinshu(BL 15), Geshu(BL 17), Danzhong (CV 17) and Neiguan (PC 6). When qi arrives, even reinforcing-reducing techniques are performed till local numbness or pain appears, then moxibustion is applied at these acupoints. The treatment is given once a day and 6 treatments a week.

3.2 其他治疗

温针灸：取厥阴俞、心俞、膈俞、膻中、内关，针刺得气后行平补平泻手法，至局部麻胀或胀痛感，在所有穴位施以温针灸。每日 1 次，每周治疗 6 次。

4 Remarks

Angina pectoris is a critical condition that needs immediate rescue and prudent management. Acupuncture is helpful in relieving angina pectoris and

4 按语

心绞痛病情危急，必须及时救治，慎重处理。针灸对减轻和缓解心绞痛、心律

arrhythmias, and myocardial infarction as well. Pay attention to healthy diets and good living habits, such as taking bland diets, avoiding fatty and sweet foods, and refraining from smoking and alcohol.

不齐疗效确切，对心肌梗死也有一定疗效。注意饮食起居，饮食宜清淡，忌肥甘厚味，力戒烟酒。

Acute Cholecystitis and Cholelithiasis

Acute cholecystitis manifests persistent colic in the upper right abdomen and is characterized by paroxysmal aggravation. The painful site cannot be touched, pressed and percussed. The pain often radiates to the right scapular area, and is accompanied by nausea and vomiting, obvious tenderness around the gallbladder area and myotonia. Some patients may experience jaundice and high fever or palpable gallbladder.

Cholelithiasis refers to stone formation in any parts of the gallbladder tract. Its clinical presentations depend on the position and shape of stones, and its complications such as gallbladder colic, present with violent pain, nausea and vomiting, jaundice and high fever. Paroxysm of gallbladder colic generally lasts a short time, or several hours in some cases. Cholecystitis and cholelithiasis can exist simultaneously and affect each other.

急性胆囊炎、胆石症

急性胆囊炎以右上腹胁肋区绞痛，呈持续性，并阵发性加剧为主要特征。其疼痛部位拒按、压痛或叩击痛，常放射至右肩胛区，伴有恶心、呕吐，右上腹胆囊区明显压痛和肌紧张。部分患者可出现黄疸和高热，或触及肿大的胆囊。

胆石症是指胆道系统的任何部位发生结石的疾病。其临床表现决定于结石的部位、形状和并发症，主要为胆绞痛，其疼痛剧烈，恶心呕吐，并可有不同程度的黄疸和高热。胆绞痛发作一般时间短暂，也有延及数小时者。胆囊炎、胆石症可同时存在，相互影响。

1 Etiology and pathogenesis

These diseases may be caused by emotional distress, liver-gallbladder qi-stagnation, improper diets impairing the spleen and stomach, and accumulated phlegm-dampness that transforms into fire and then scorchcs body fluids to stones.

1 病因病机

本病的发生多与情绪不遂、肝胆气滞，饮食不节、伤及脾胃、痰湿壅盛，化热或煎熬成石有关。

2 Syndrome differentiation

Chief symptoms: Abrupt persistent colic in the

2 辨证

主症：突发性右上腹剧

upper right abdomen that worsens in a paroxysmal manner.

痛，持续性绞痛，阵发性加剧。

The syndrome of liver-gallbladder qi stagnation manifests colic which is triggered by emotional fluctuation, accompanied by nausea and vomiting, poor appetite, vexation, irritability and wiry tense pulse. The syndrome of liver-gallbladder dampness-heat manifests chills with high fever, bitter taste in the mouth, dry throat, nausea and vomiting, even jaundiced eyes and body, bright yellow urine, yellowish tongue coating, and rapid wiry pulse.

肝胆气滞者，绞痛常因情绪波动而发作，伴见恶心呕吐、纳差、心烦易怒，脉弦紧；肝胆湿热者，伴见寒战高热、口苦咽干、恶心呕吐，甚者目黄、身黄、小便黄，舌苔黄腻，脉弦数。

3 Treatment

3 治疗

3.1 Essential treatment

3.1 基本治疗

Principal acupoints: Danshu(BL 19), Ganshu (BL 18), Riyue(GB 24), Qimen(LR 14), Yanglingquan(GB 34), and Dannang EX-LE 6).

主穴：胆俞，肝俞，日月，期门，阳陵泉，胆囊穴。

Supplementary acupoints: In the syndrome of liver-gallbladder qi stagnation, add Taichong(LR 3) and Xiaxi(GB 43); in the syndrome of liver-gallbladder dampness-heat, add Sanyinjiao(SP 6) and Yinlingquan(SP 9). In the presence of nausea and vomiting, add Neiguan(PC 6) and Zusanli(ST 36); in the presence of dampness-heat jaundice, add Zhiyang(GV 9) and Yinlingquan(SP 9); in the presence of fever, add Dazhui(GV 14) and Quchi (LI 11).

配穴：肝胆气滞加太冲、侠溪；肝胆湿热加三阴交、阴陵泉；恶心呕吐加内关、足三里；湿热发黄加至阳、阴陵泉；发热加曲池、大椎。

Explanation: Danshu(BL 19) and Riyue(GB 24), Ganshu(BL 18) and Qimen(LR 14) are two paired combination of the Back-Shu and Front-Mu acupoints. One group of acupoints in the right side are used in each time. These two groups of acupoints act to soothe the liver and gallbladder and ease pain. Yanglingquan(GB 34), the Lower He-Sea acupoint of the gallbladder, is applied to treat

方义：胆俞配日月，肝俞配期门为俞募配穴，每次用一组，选取右侧，以疏肝利胆而止痛。阳陵泉为胆之下合穴，胆腑有病，首选阳陵泉。胆囊穴为治疗胆腑疾病的经验效穴。

any gallbladder diseases. Dannang(EX-LE 6) is an empirical acupoint for gallbladder diseases.

3.2 Other therapy

Ear acupuncture: Select Liver(CO 12), Pancreas and Gallbladder(CO 11), Sympathesis(AH 6a), Shenmen(TF 4) and Root of the Ear Vagus(R 2). In the acute onset, puncture these acupoints with filiform needles by strong stimulation via continuous rotation of needles for 30 to 60 minutes each time. After pain relief, apply *Semen Vaccariae* (Wang Bu Liu Xing) at these acupoints; the two ears are used alternately.

3.2 其他治疗

耳针：选肝、胰胆、交感、神门、耳迷根。急性发作时用毫针刺，强刺激，持续捻针，每次留针 30～60 分钟；剧痛缓解后再行耳穴压丸法，两耳交替进行。

4 Remarks

Acupuncture has excellent pain-easing effects on this disease. If the pain does not respond to acupuncture, the underlying causes should be further ascertained and treatment should be given accordingly.

4 按语

针灸对本病有良好的镇痛作用。若经治疗疼痛不能缓解者，应查明原因，给予相应的处理。

Heatstroke

Heatstroke refers to shock due to high temperature in summer, characterized by dysfunction of thermoregulatory center, functional failure of sweat glands, and excessive loss of water and electrolytes. It is a clinical emergency condition. If it is not rescued in time, the life will be endangered.

中 暑

中暑是夏季由于高温环境而引起的，以体温调节中枢功能障碍、汗腺功能衰竭和水、电解质丢失过多而引起休克为特点的疾病。临床发病多为急症，如不及时抢救可危及生命安全。

1 Etiology and pathogenesis

Heatstroke results from high temperature in summer or working under scorching sun, or from summer heat and dampness in clammy hot environment that attack the zang-fu organs and block the heart-spirit, or from stirring liver-wind by heat con-

1 病因病机

此病是因夏季在高温或烈日下劳作，或处于气候炎热湿闷的环境，暑热或暑湿秽浊之邪卒中脏腑，热闭心神，或热盛津伤，引动肝风，

suming body fluids, or from summer heat blocking qi activity.

或暑闭气机所致。

2 Syndrome differentiation

Chief symptoms: High fever, vertigo, headache, vexation and thirst, lassitude, chest distress, nausea, aching and distending loin and back, body heaviness, even coma and convulsion, red tongue with thin whitish or yellowish-greasy coating.

2 辨证

主症：表现为壮热，头晕，头痛，烦躁口渴，疲乏无力，胸闷，恶心，腰背酸胀，身重，甚则神昏，抽搐，舌红，苔薄白或黄腻。

3 Treatment

3.1 Essential treatment

Principal acupoints: Zhongwan(CV 12), Shixuan(EX-UE 11), and Dazhui(GV 14).

Supplementary acupoints: In the presence of fever and thirst, add Quchi(LI 11); Shuigou(GV 26) is added to waken the brain and arouse consciousness; Hegu(LI 4) and Zusanli(ST 36) are added to enhance the stress capacity of the body.

Explanation: Summer heat is often mingled with dampness. Dampness encumbers the spleen and stomach, and results in failure to ascend and descend, displaying summer-heat symptoms. Therefore, treatment aims to nourish the spleen and stomach, and resolve dampness; Zhongwan (CV 12), an acupoint of the conception vessel, is the first-choice acupoint in the relief of summer heat. Pricking Shixuan(EX-UE 11) can communicate yin and yang, regulate qi activity, open orifice and waken brain, free qi and induce resuscitation. Needling Dazhui(GV 14) can promote sweating and relieve exterior, and clear pathogenic heat.

3 治疗

3.1 基本治疗

主穴：中脘，十宣，大椎。

配穴：发热口渴加曲池；醒脑开窍加水沟；合谷、足三里增加机体应激能力。

方义：暑多夹湿，湿困脾胃，中洲失运，以致升降失司，出现伤暑之症，故当急补脾胃、健运化湿。因此任脉之中脘在解暑穴中名列诸穴之首，刺十宣可以交通阴阳、调理气机、开窍醒脑、顺气苏厥，刺大椎可发汗解表、清除热邪。

3.2 Other therapy

Pricking and cupping therapy: Select Dazhui (GV 14), Feishu(BL 13) to Xinshu(BL 15), Ganshu(BL 18) to Danshu(BL 19). In each treatment,

3.2 其他治疗

刺络拔罐：取大椎，肺俞至心俞，肝俞至胆俞。每次取 3～5 个穴位，消毒后用七

3～5 acupoints are tapped with a seven-star needle till the local skin turns flushed and slightly bleeds. Then cupping is performed for 5～15 minutes, with bleeding volume of 5～15 ml from each acupoint. The treatment is given once a day and 3 treatments make up one full course.

星针叩刺皮肤至局部潮红，少量渗血为度，拔罐 5～15 分钟，每穴拔罐出血量5～15毫升，每日 1 次，3 次为 1 个疗程。

4 Remarks

Severe heatstroke should be rescued in time by combined Chinese and Western medicine to avoid delaying the condition.

4 按语

重症中暑应及时采取中西医结合治疗，以免延误病情。

Renal Colic

Renal colic refers to a paroxysm of severe pain in the loin or lateral abdomen radiating up or down along the ureters, accompanied by painful urination and bloody urine.

肾绞痛

肾绞痛以阵发性剧烈腰部或侧腹部绞痛并沿输尿管向上或向下放射，伴有不同程度的尿痛、尿血为主要特征。属于中医学“腰痛”“石淋”“砂淋”“血淋”范畴。

1 Etiology and pathogenesis

Renal colic is mostly caused by the calculus in the urinary system due to irregular food intake and dampness-heat accumulation in the lower energizer. Colic experiences when the moving stones stimulate the urinary organs, and bloody urine happens when the moving stones injure the mucous membranes or the capillaries of organs.

1 病因病机

本病多因饮食不节、下焦湿热而致泌尿系结石引起。结石排出过程中刺激脏腑组织则发生绞痛；伤及脏腑组织黏膜、血络则出现尿血。

2 Syndrome differentiation

Chief symptoms: Paroxysmal severe pain in the waist or lateral abdomen that radiates up or down along the ureters, accompanied by painful urination and bloody urine.

The urine is dark and yellow, with blood in the urine, or with stone discharge, painful and obstruc-

2 辨证

主症：阵发性剧烈腰部或侧腹部绞痛并沿输尿管向下或向上放射，常伴有尿痛、尿血。

小便黄赤浑浊或尿血或有砂石排出，溺时涩痛，淋沥

ted urination, red tongue with yellowish or yellow-greasy coating, and wiry tense or wiry rapid pulse.

不畅，舌红，苔黄或黄腻，脉弦紧或弦数。

3 Treatment

3 治疗

3.1 Essential treatment

3.1 基本治疗

Principal acupoints: Shenshu (BL 23), Sanjiaoshu(BL 22), Guanyuan(CV 4), Yinlingquan (SP 9), and Sanyinjiao(SP 6).

主穴：肾俞，三焦俞，关元，阴陵泉，三阴交。

Supplementary acupoints: In the presence of bloody urine, add Xuehai(SP 10) and Taichong (LR 3); in the presence of marked dampness heat, add Weiyang(BL 40) and Hegu(LI 4).

配穴：血尿加血海、太冲；湿热重加委阳、合谷。

Explanation: Shenshu (BL 23) and Sanjiaoshu (BL 22) are located in the kidney area, and are also the acupoints of the bladder meridian of foot-taiyang. They can regulate the qi activity of the bladder in combination with Guanyuan(RN 4). Yinlingquan (SP 9) and Sanyinjiao(SP 6), distal to the loin, can clear heat and disinhibit dampness, promote urination and relieve pain.

方义：肾俞、三焦俞位于肾区，又为足太阳膀胱经穴，配关元疏利膀胱气机。远取三阴交、阴陵泉以清利湿热、通淋止痛。

3.2 Other therapy

3.2 其他治疗

Pricking and blood-letting therapy: The purplish vessels near Weizhong(BL 40) are quickly pricked with a three-edged needle to let out black blood. Disinfected cotton may be used to press the upper end of the vessels to help discharge the blood. When the bleeding stops, the disinfected cotton may be used again to press the pricking hole.

刺络放血：用三棱针对准委中部青紫脉络处，斜刺入脉中后迅速将针退出，使瘀血流出。可用消毒棉球轻轻按压静脉上端，以助瘀血排出。待出血自行停止后，再用消毒棉球按压针孔。

4 Remarks

4 按语

Acupuncture has positive effects on renal colic by strong stimulation. In order to enhance the clinical efficacy, the patients should be instructed to drink plenty of water and do jumping exercises during treatment procedure.

针灸在治疗肾绞痛方面，疗效肯定，多采用强刺激手法。为增强治疗作用，治疗期间宜多饮水，多做跑跳类运动。

Section 6 Other Disorders

第 6 节 其他病证

Postoperative Gastrointestinal Dysfunction

Postoperative gastrointestinal dysfunction refers to a group of symptoms of gastrointestinal dysfunction such as abdominal bloating and pain, nausea and vomiting, difficulty in gas passage and defecation or diarrhea, which develops due to operative anesthesia and injury, postoperative fasting, long-term bedding, electrolyte disturbance, intra-abdominal inflammation and blood, mechanical stimulation of draining-tube, deterioration of primary diseases and advanced ages. It is a frequent postoperative complication in general surgery.

术后胃肠功能紊乱

术后胃肠运动功能紊乱是指由于手术麻醉、创伤、术后禁食、长时间卧床、电解质紊乱、腹腔内炎症、残留积血或引流管的机械刺激，以及患者原发病恶化、高龄等综合因素的作用，导致术后出现腹胀腹痛、恶心呕吐、排气排便困难或腹泻等胃肠运动功能障碍的一系列症状。它是普通外科手术后常见的并发症。

1 Etiology and pathogenesis

Postoperative gastrointestinal dysfunction is attributed to the disturbance of qi activities of the zang-fu organs. Operation itself and anesthesia may disturb the qi activity of the spleen and stomach, which further slows down the conveyance of the large intestine; then the qi stagnates in the middle energizer, bringing about failure of the clear qi to ascend and the turbid qi to descend, and subsequent bowels movement dysfunction.

1 病因病机

术后胃肠功能紊乱责之于脏腑气机逆乱。由于手术和麻醉的原因，常可导致脾胃气机紊乱，大肠传导失司，气滞于中，清气不得上升，浊气不得下降，上下不通，腑失通降功能。

2 Syndrome differentiation

Chief symptoms: Epigastric discomforts, dull pain, obvious fullness in the upper abdomen, vomiting with acid materials, bile or foods, abdominal pain, diarrhea with thin stools in the early stage and

2 辨证

主症：上腹部不适、隐痛、饱胀明显，呕吐，吐出物为酸水、胆汁或食物，腹痛、腹泻，初为稀便，重者呈水样

watery stools in the late stage.

The syndrome of qi stagnation and blood stasis manifests paroxysmal abdominal pain and rumbling, abdominal lumps, difficulty in defecation or constipation, dark tongue with petechia, yellowish tongue coating, and wiry rough pulse. The syndrome of liver depression and spleen deficiency manifests flank pain, headache, dizziness, bitter taste in the mouth, dryness in the throat, lassitude, diminished appetite, irregular menstruation in women, pale tongue with whitish coating, and rapid wiry pulse. The syndrome of spleen-yang deficiency may manifest loss of appetite after surgery, abdominal fullness after meals, lassitude and weakness, cold limbs and body, sallow complexion, thin body, loose stools, abdominal fullness, belching with acid regurgitation, stomachache with preference for pressure and hot drinks, pale tongue with whitish coating, and thready pulse.

便。

气滞血瘀者，腹痛阵作，腹胀、腹鸣，或腹中包块，大便不畅或秘结，舌质暗，有瘀点，舌苔黄，脉弦涩；肝郁脾虚者，兼两胁作痛，头痛，目眩，口苦咽干，神疲食少，女子出现月经不调，舌淡苔薄白，脉弦数；脾阳亏虚者，术后不思饮食，兼食后作胀、倦怠无力、形寒肢冷、面色萎黄、消瘦便溏、胃脘满闷、嗳气吞酸、胃痛喜按、喜热饮、舌淡、苔白、脉细。

3　Treatment

Principal acupoints: Zusanli(ST 36), Neiguan (PC 6), Hegu(LI 4), Shangjuxu(ST 37), and Tianshu(ST 25).

Supplementary acupoints: In the syndrome of qi stagnation and blood stasis, add Taichong(LR 3) and Xuehai(SP 10); in the syndrome of liver depression and spleen deficiency, add Taichong(LR 3) and Sanyinjiao(SP 6); in the syndrome of spleen-yang deficiency, add Pishu(BL 20) and Guanyuan (CV 4).

Explanation: Zusanli(ST 36), the He-Sea acupoint of the stomach meridian of foot yangming, harmonizes the stomach and nourishes the spleen, moves the bowels and resolves phlegm, and frees qi

3　治疗

主穴：足三里，内关，合谷，上巨虚，天枢。

配穴：气滞血瘀加太冲、血海；肝郁脾虚加太冲、三阴交；脾阳亏虚加脾俞、关元。

方义：足三里为足阳明胃经的合穴，有和胃健脾、通腑化痰、升降气机的功能。内关为手厥阴心包经穴位，

activities. Neiguan(PC 6), an acupoint of the pericardium meridian of hand-jueyin, calms the heart and spirit, soothes the liver, harmonizes the stomach and alleviates pain. The combination of these two acupoints may nourish the spleen and stomach, regulate qi and relieve pain. Hegu(LI 4) is the Yuan-Source acupoint of the large intestine meridian of hand yangming, Shangjuxu(ST 37) is the Lower He-Sea acupoint of the large intestine, and Tianshu(ST 25) is the Front-Mu acupoint of the large intestine, thus these three acupoints can regulate the qi activities of the bowels.

具有宁心安神、疏肝和胃、止痛之功效。两穴相配，共奏健脾和胃、理气止痛之功。合谷为手阳明大肠经原穴，上巨虚为大肠下合穴，天枢为大肠募穴，均有调理肠腑气机的作用。

4 Remarks

Hand acupuncture prefers to shorten the time of first gas passage, improve defecation and advance the time of taking fluid foods. While, electro-acupuncture prefers to improve intestinal gurgling, relieve abdominal distention and gastrointestinal reactions.

4 按语

手针在整体调节首次排气排便时间，改善排便质量，促使患者提前恢复流质饮食方面较有优势，而电针在改善和促进肠鸣音恢复、减轻腹胀和胃肠反应方面较有优势。

Radiochemical Adverse Reactions

Radiochemical adverse reactions refer to the side reactions in cancer patients undergoing radiotherapy and chemotherapy, including digestive tract conditions, bone marrow suppression, general fatigue and inflammatory reactions.

放化疗反应

放化疗反应是癌症患者在接受放疗、化疗后出现的各种不同程度的副作用，多表现为消化道、骨髓抑制、机体衰弱和炎性反应等。

1 Etiology and pathogenesis

In the treatment of malignant tumors, radiotherapy and chemotherapy may consume qi and blood, and impair the functions of the spleen and stomach, giving rise to disturbance of qi activities of the spleen and stomach and inadequate production

1 病因病机

放疗、化疗治疗恶性肿瘤，会损伤气血，又会影响脾胃功能，使脾胃升降失常，气血生化不足，加上患者久病脾胃虚弱，肝肾亏损，致使血

of qi and blood; in addition, the chronic cases are deficient in the spleen and stomach, the liver and kidney, resulting in insufficiency of essence-blood and body fluids.

亏精少,阴津亏耗。

2 Syndrome differentiation

Chief symptoms: Nausea and vomiting, poor appetite, lack of strength, dry mouth, distention and fullness in the epigastric area, constipation or loose stools and even watery diarrhea.

The syndrome of qi-blood deficiency may manifest fatigue and lassitude, reluctance to speech, shortness of breath, vertigo and dizziness, pale complexion, stomach distention after meals, loose stools, diminished count of white blood cells, reduced platelets or red blood cells, pale tongue with thin coating, and weak thready pulse. The syndrome of yin-liquid deficiency manifests dryness in the mouth and throat, feverishness in the palms and soles, dry stools, dark urine, red tongue with thin coating, and rapid thready pulse. The syndrome of liver-kidney deficiency may manifest tinnitus, aching loin and knees, seminal emission, pale tongue and deep thready pulse.

2 辨证

主症:恶心呕吐,纳差,乏力,口干舌燥,脘腹胀满,大便秘结或稀溏,甚则水泻。

气血两虚者,兼倦怠乏力、少气懒言、头晕目眩、面色苍白、食后胃胀、大便溏薄、白细胞计数降低、血小板及红细胞计数减少、舌质淡、苔薄、脉细弱;阴津亏耗者,兼口干、咽干、手足心热、大便结、尿黄、舌红苔薄、脉细数;肝肾亏损者,兼耳鸣、腰膝酸软、遗精、舌淡、脉沉细。

3 Treatment

Principal acupoints: Zusanli (ST 36), Sanyinjiao(SP 6), Quchi(LI 11), Hegu(LI 4), Neiguan (PC 6), Zhongwan(CV 12), Pishu(BL 20) and Weishu(BL 21).

Supplementary acupoints: In the syndrome of qi-blood deficiency, add Qihai(CV 6) and Geshu(BL 17); in the syndrome of yin-liquid deficiency, add Zhaohai(KI 6) and Shenshu(BL 23); in the syndrome of liver-kidney deficiency, add Taixi(KI 3), Ganshu(BL 18) and Shenshu(BL 23).

3 治疗

主穴:足三里,三阴交,曲池,合谷,内关,中脘,脾俞,胃俞。

配穴:气血两虚加气海、膈俞;阴津亏耗加照海、肾俞;肝肾亏损加太溪、肝俞、肾俞。

Explanation: Zusanli(ST 36), the He-Sea acupoint of the stomach, acts to regulate the qi activities in the stomach and intestines. Sanyinjiao(SP 6) functions to harmonize yin and yang. Quchi (LI 11), Hegu(LI 4) and Neiguan(PC 6) are used to harmonize the stomach and descend qi adversity. Zhongwan(CV 12), Pishu(BL 20) and Weishu(BL 21) are used to nourish the spleen and enrich qi.

方义：根据"肚腹三里留""合治内腑"的理论，选用足三里以调节胃肠道气机。三阴交协调阴阳。曲池、合谷、内关和胃降逆。中脘、脾俞、胃俞健脾益气。

4 Remarks

Acupuncture is quite effective for nausea and vomiting, fatigue, dry mouth and persistent hiccup following radiochemical therapy.

4 按语

针灸在减轻放化疗引起的恶心、呕吐、疲劳、口干及缓解持续性呃逆等方面具有较好的作用。

Chronic Fatigue Syndrome

Chronic fatigue syndrome refers to severe lassitude over six months, as well as general discomforts, aching muscles and knees, insomnia, poor memory, concentration deficiency, absence of spirit, and low efficiency at work, which cannot be alleviated by rest. No abnormalities are found in the physical examination and laboratory investigations.

慢性疲劳综合征

慢性疲劳综合征是以持续半年以上严重疲乏无力，休息后不能缓解为突出表现，出现全身不适、肌肉关节酸痛、失眠、记忆力减退、注意力不集中、精神萎靡、工作效率低等症状的一组症候群。体检和常规实验室检查一般无异常发现。

1 Etiology and pathogenesis

Chronic fatigue syndrome principally results from over-exertion, excessive contemplation, emotional disturbance, and contraction of exogenous factors, giving rise to functional disturbance of the liver, spleen and kidney. When the liver qi is depressed, the liver fails to free qi and store blood, and the tendons are not nourished, resulting in a variety of symptoms in the nervous, cardiovascular

1 病因病机

慢性疲劳综合征的发生主要与劳役思虑过度、情志内伤或复感外邪，致肝脾肾功能失调有关。肝气不疏，失于条达，肝不藏血，筋无所主，则出现神经、心血管、运动系统的各种症状；脾气虚弱，失于健运，精微不布，则

and musculoskeletal systems. When the spleen qi is deficient, the spleen loses its function of transportation and transformation, and the essence and nutrients cannot be distributed properly, bringing about weakness of muscles and limbs. When the kidney-essence is deficient, the bones are flaccid and spirit is absent.

肌肉疲惫、四肢倦怠无力；肾精不足则骨软无力，精神萎靡。

2 Syndrome differentiation

Chief symptoms: Continual or recurrent onset of severe fatigue, vertigo and dizziness, insomnia, poor memory, depression, anxiety, mental fluctuation, poor concentration, muscular weakness and pain, sore throat, and lymphadenextasis around the neck with mild fever.

2 辨证

主症：持续或反复发作的严重疲劳，头晕目眩，失眠健忘，精神抑郁，焦虑，情绪不稳定，注意力不集中，肌肉疲乏无力或疼痛，咽痛不适，颈前后部或咽峡部淋巴结肿大，轻度发热。

3 Treatment

3.1 Essential treatment

Principal acupoints: Baihui (GV 20), Yintang (EX-HN 3), Shenmen (HT 7), Taixi (KI 3), Taichong (LR 3), Sanyinjiao (SP 6), and Zusanli (ST 36).

Supplementary acupoints: In the presence of vertigo and poor concentration, add Sishencong (EX-HN 1) and Xuanzhong (GB 39); in the presence of palpitation and anxiety, add Xinshu (BL 15) and Neiguan (PC 6); in the presence of insomnia and sleepiness, add Anmian (EX-UE) and Neiguan (PC 6).

Explanation: Baihui (GV 20) and Yintang (EX-HN 3) act to clear the mind and brighten vision, nourish brain and benefit wisdom. Shenmen (HT 7) is the Yuan-Source acupoint of the heart meridian, and Taixi (KI 3) is the Yuan-Source acupoint of the kidney meridian; combination of these two acu-

3 治疗

3.1 基本治疗

主穴：百会，印堂，神门，太溪，太冲，三阴交，足三里。

配穴：头晕、注意力不集中加四神聪、悬钟；心悸、焦虑加心俞、内关；失眠、多梦易醒加安眠、内关。

方义：百会、印堂清利头目、健脑益智。神门为心经原穴，太溪为肾经原穴，二穴相配交通心肾。太冲、三阴交、足三里疏肝理气、恢复体力。

points can coordinate the heart with kidney. Taichong(LR 3), Sanyinjiao(SP 6) and Zusanli(ST 36) are selected to soothe the liver, regulate qi and restore body vitality.

3.2 Other therapy

Cupping therapy: Perform flame-flashing or moving cupping method on the back along the two lines of the bladder meridian until the local skin turns flushed. The cup may be retained for 5～10 minutes.

3.2 其他疗法

拔罐：选足太阳膀胱经背部第1、第2侧线，用火罐行走罐法或闪罐法，以背部潮红为度。亦可留罐5～10分钟。

4 Remarks

Acupuncture is obviously effective to relieve subjective fatigue, boost patients' moods and improve sleep.

4 按语

针灸治疗本病可明显缓解躯体疲劳的自觉症状，调节患者情绪，改善睡眠。

Depression

Depression is a mental disorder characterized by low spirit, negative mood and pessimism, despair and sadness, apathy, accompanied by headache, restlessness, fatigue, diarrhea, and nightmares. In severe cases, the patients feel very pessimistic or even commit suicide. This disease is closely related to patients' personality, including introversion, unsociability, sentimentality, and dependence.

抑郁症

抑郁症是以情绪抑郁为主要症状的一种心理病证。本症的特点为忧郁和厌世心理。患者有凄凉感，常唉声叹气，对人和事物失去兴趣，伴头痛、心烦、乏力、腹泻，常梦中惊恐。严重者强烈厌世，甚至有自杀念头。抑郁症与患者性格密切相关，患者多性格内向、孤僻，多愁善感，依赖性强。

1 Etiology and pathogenesis

Depression is usually caused by remarkable emotional trauma, including unfortunate lot in life, setback in career, unregardedness and disharmony of personal relationship, causing excessive stimulation on cerebral cortex and functional imbalance be-

1 病因病机

抑郁症发生的病因，一般以明显的精神创伤为诱因，如生活中的不幸遭遇、事业上的挫折、不受重用、人际关系不和等，导致大脑皮质受过度刺

tween the cortex and subcortex.

激而致皮质和皮质下相应关系的功能失调、障碍。

2 Syndrome differentiation

Chief symptoms: Depressed mood, sadness, irascibility, susceptibility to anger and cry, insomnia and dreaminess, and poor appetite.

The syndrome of liver-qi stagnation manifests distention and fullness in the chest and hypochondriac regions, abdominal bloating, belching, irregular bowel movements, thin whitish coating, and wiry pulse. The syndrome of fire transformed from depressed qi manifests vexation and irritability, bitter taste and dryness in the mouth, headache and reddened eyes, constipation, red tongue with yellowish coating, and wiry rapid pulse. The syndrome of qi-phlegm accumulation manifests foreign-body sensation in the throat that cannot be swallowed or spit out, greasy coating, and wiry slippery pulse. The syndrome of heart-spleen deficiency manifests excessive anxiety and worry, palpitation, fright, insomnia and forgetfulness, poor appetite, dim complexion, pale tongue and thready pulse. The syndrome of liver-kidney deficiency manifests dizziness, tinnitus, dry eyes, photophobia, palpitation, restlessness, vexing heat in the chest, palms and soles, night sweats, dry mouth and throat, dry tongue with less coating, and thready rapid pulse.

2 辨证

主症：精神抑郁，善忧，情绪不宁或易怒易哭，失眠多梦，不思饮食。

肝气郁结者，兼胸胁胀满、脘闷嗳气、大便不调、舌苔、薄白、脉弦；气郁化火者，兼急躁易怒、口苦口干、头痛目赤、大便秘结、舌红、苔黄、脉弦数；痰气郁结者，兼咽中如物梗阻、吞之不下、咯之不出、苔白腻、脉弦滑；心脾两虚者，兼多思善虑、心悸胆怯、失眠健忘、纳差、面色不华、舌淡、脉细；肝肾亏虚者，兼眩晕耳鸣、目干畏光、心悸不安、五心烦热、盗汗、口咽干燥、舌干少津、脉细数。

3 Treatment

3.1 Essential treatment

Principal acupoints: Baihui (GV 20), Shuigou (GV 26), Shenmen(HT 7), Neiguan(PC 6), and Taichong(LR 3).

Supplementary acupoints: In the syndrome of liver-qi stagnation, add Danzhong(CV 17) and Qi-

3 治疗

3.1 基本治疗

主穴：百会，水沟，神门，内关，太冲。

配穴：肝气郁结加膻中、期门；气郁化火加行间、侠

men(LR 14); in the syndrome of fire transformed from depressed qi, add Xingjian(LR 2) and Xiaxi (GB 43); in the syndrome of qi-phlegm accumulation, add Fenglong(ST 40), Yinlingquan(SP 9) and Tiantu(CV 22); in the syndrome of heart-spleen deficiency, add Xinshu(BL 15), Pishu(BL 20) and Zusanli(ST 36); in the syndrome of liver-kidney deficiency, add Ganshu(BL 18), Shenshu(BL 23) and Taixi(KI 3).

溪;痰气郁结加丰隆、阴陵泉、天突;心脾两虚加心俞、脾俞、足三里;肝肾亏虚加肝俞、肾俞、太溪。

Explanation: The brain houses the original spirit. The governor vessel enters the brain. Baihui(GV 20) and Shuigou(GV 26) can waken brain and regulate spirits, and clear head and eyes. Shenmen(HT 7) is the Yuan-Source acupoint of the heart meridian, and Neiguan(PC 6) is the Luo-Connecting acupoint of pericardium meridian. These two acupoints can regulate the heart and calm spirit. Neiguan(PC 6) can also loosen the chest and regulate qi. Taichong(LR 3) can soothe the liver and relieve depression.

方义: 脑为元神之府,督脉入络脑,百会、水沟可醒脑调神、清利头目。神门为心之原穴,内关为心包经络穴,二穴相配可调心安神。内关又可宽胸理气。太冲疏肝解郁。

3.2 Other therapy

Intradermal needle therapy: Select bilateral Xinshu(BL 15) and Ganshu(BL 18). After sterilization, the intradermal needles are horizontally inserted into these two acupoints with the needle tips towards the spine; two days later, the needles are withdrawn. The treatment is given twice a week, with more than 48 hours apart, for total 12 weeks.

3.2 其他治疗

皮内针: 取双侧心俞和肝俞,使用麦粒型皮内针。消毒后,由外侧向脊柱方向,沿皮下横向平刺,留置 2 日后取出。每周 2 次,每次治疗间隔时间大于 48 小时,共治疗 12 周。

4 Remarks

Acupuncture therapy has good effects on depression, and it is recommended to combine with psychotherapy.

4 按语

针灸治疗本病具有较好的临床疗效,但是应结合心理安慰疗法。

Male Infertility

Male infertility is caused by hypospermia, azospermatism, necrospermia, uncolliquation of semen, anejaculation and retrogressive spermatism. Male infertility is a condition in which the female fails to get pregnant via normal intercourse for a period of over two years without adopting any contraceptive methods.

男性不育症

男性不育症多见于精子减少症、无精子症、死精子症、精液不化症、不射精症、逆行性射精等。男性不育症系指育龄夫妇共同生活 2 年(WHO 规定为 1 年)以上,未采取任何避孕措施,由于男方生殖功能障碍导致女方不能受孕。

1 Etiology and pathogenesis

Male infertility is in close relationship with the kidney, heart and spleen, especially with the kidney. It is due to oligospermatism, asthenospermia, thin and stagnated sperm resulting from kidney-essence deficiency, qi-blood insufficiency, qi-blood stagnation, and downward flow of dampness-heat.

1 病因病机

不育与肾、心、肝、脾有关,尤其与肾的关系最密切。多由于肾精亏虚、气血不足、气滞血瘀和湿热下注等因素导致精少、精弱、精薄、精瘀等引起不育。

2 Syndrome differentiation

Chief symptoms: Inability to make his wife conceive.

The syndrome of kidney-yang deficiency manifests aching loin and cold abdomen, sexual hypoesthesia, impotence, thin spermatorrhea, pale tongue with thin whitish coating, and deep weak thready pulse. The syndrome of qi-blood deficiency manifests sallow complexion, lassitude and reluctance to speech, fatigue, dizziness, palpitations, decline of sexual desire, scanty semen, pale tongue with less coating, deep and thready pulse. The syndrome of qi-blood stagnation manifests distention and fullness in the chest and flanks, sinking and distending sensation in the testes, varicocele of the spermatic veins, dark purple tongue with possible petechia,

2 辨证

主症: 不能孕育。

肾阳虚者,兼腰酸腹冷、畏寒、性欲淡漠、阳痿、滑精清稀、舌淡、苔薄白、脉沉细弱;气血虚弱者,兼面色萎黄、少气懒言、体倦乏力、头晕心悸、性欲低下、精子稀少、舌淡、少苔、脉沉细;气滞血瘀者,兼胸胁胀闷不舒、睾丸坠胀、精索曲张、舌质暗或有瘀斑、脉弦涩;痰湿阻滞者,兼形体肥胖,面色皖白,纳呆,大便溏薄,舌胖色淡、舌边有齿痕,苔白腻,脉滑;湿

wiry and rough pulse. The syndrome of phlegm-dampness obstruction manifests obesity, sallow complexion, poor appetite, loose stools, pale enlarged tongue with teeth marks and whitish greasy coating, and slippery pulse. The syndrome of down-pouring dampness heat manifests flank pain, bitter taste in the mouth, clammy and hyperhidrotic scrotum, swelling and itching of the external genitals, oligouresis, impotence, premature ejaculation, scanty urine, red tongue with yellowish greasy coating, and rapid slippery pulse.

热下注者,兼胁痛口苦、阴囊潮湿多汗、阴肿阴痒、死精过多、阳痿早泄、小便短少、舌红、苔黄腻、脉滑数。

3 Treatment

3 治疗

Principal acupoints: Shenshu(BL 23), Guanyuan (CV 4), Ciliao(BL 32), Zhibian(BL 54) and Sanyinjiao(SP 6).

主穴: 肾俞,关元,次髎,秩边,三阴交。

Supplementary acupoints: In the syndrome of kidney-yang deficiency, add Mingmen(GV 4) and Shenque(CV 8) with moxibustion; in the syndrome of qi-blood deficiency, add Qihai(CV 6), Xuehai (SP 10) and Zusanli(ST 36); in the syndrome of qi-blood stagnation, add Taichong(LR 3) and Geshu (BL 17); in the syndrome of phlegm-dampness obstruction, add Fenglong(ST 40) and Yinlingquan (SP 9); in the syndrome of down-pouring dampness heat, add Zhongji(CV 3) and Yinlingquan(SP 9).

配穴: 肾阳虚加灸命门、神阙;气血虚弱加气海、血海、足三里;气滞血瘀加太冲、膈俞;痰湿阻滞加丰隆、阴陵泉;湿热下注加中极、阴陵泉。

Explanation: Shenshu(BL 23), Ciliao(BL 32) and Zhibian(BL 54), located in the lumbar area and the sacrum, can nourish the kidney and replenish essence to help conceive. Guanyuan(CV 4), an acupoint of the conception vessel, regulates the thoroughfare and conception vessels. Sanyinjiao(SP 6), the Crossing acupoint of the three yin meridians of the foot, invigorates the spleen to resolve dampness, soothes the liver-qi and removes blood stasis,

方义: 肾俞、次髎、秩边位于腰骶部,调补下元、益肾填精、调经助孕。关元属任脉,调理冲任。三阴交为足三阴经交会穴,既能健脾化湿导滞,又能疏肝理气行瘀,还能益肾、调和冲任。

nourishes the kidney and regulates the thoroughfare and conception vessels.

4 Remarks

Acupuncture works well on infertility caused by male sexual dysfunction.

4 按语

针灸治疗男子性功能障碍所引起的不育症疗效较为显著。

Smoking Withdrawal Syndrome

Smoking withdrawal syndrome develops when the smokers quit smoking after a long-term inhalation of cigarettes and manifests low spirit, restlessness and irritability, dizziness, headache, fatigue, coughing, excessive sweating, low heart rate, nausea, vomiting, muscular spasms, and hypoesthesia.

戒烟综合征

戒烟综合征是有较长吸烟史者在戒断时产生的一系列瘾癖症状，可出现精神萎靡，情绪烦躁，头晕头痛，疲倦乏力，咳嗽多汗，心率下降，恶心呕吐，甚至出现肌肉抖动、感觉迟钝等症状。

1 Etiology and pathogenesis

In long-term smoking, a great amount of nicotine is inhaled and combined with the cerebral opioid receptors in the human body, bringing about the suppression of endogenous opiod secretion. Therefore, once a person quits smoking, the secretion of endogenous opioids cannot meet the needs of the body, hence leading to a series of unbearable withdrawal symptoms.

1 病因病机

长期吸烟，大量的尼古丁进入人体内，与中枢内阿片类受体相结合，致使体内内源性阿片类物质的分泌受到抑制。一旦外源性尼古丁停止供应，内源性阿片类物质的分泌不能满足人体需要，则诱发出现一系列难以忍受的戒断现象。

2 Syndrome differentiation

Chief symptoms: A long history of smoking, 10 to 20 or over 20 cigarettes a day. The withdrawal symptoms develop when smoking is quit, including low spirit, tastelessness, continuous yawning, dizziness, headache, fatigue, cough and massive sweating, and even slowed heart rate, nausea and vomiting, restlessness and irritability, insomnia and an-

2 辨证

主症：有较长吸烟史，每日吸烟 10～20 支或 20 支以上，中断吸烟后出现精神萎靡，口淡无味，呵欠连连，头晕头痛，疲倦乏力，咳嗽多汗。严重者可见心率下降，恶心呕吐，情绪烦躁，失眠忧

xiety in severe cases.

虑。

3 Treatment

3 治疗

3.1 Essential treatment

3.1 基本治疗

Principal acupoints: Chize (LU 5), Fenglong (ST 40), Hegu(LI 4), Baihui(GV 20), Shenmen (HT 7), and Tianmei(EX-LE) [the midpoint of the line between Lieque(LU 7) and Yangxi(LI 5)].

主穴: 尺泽,丰隆,合谷,百会,神门,甜美穴(列缺与阳溪连线的中点)。

Explanation: Smoking is primarily related to the lung. Chize(LU 5), the He-Sea acupoint of the lung meridian, is used to release the lungs to relieve coughing. Fenglong (ST 40), the Luo-Connecting acupoint of the stomach meridian, is used to resolve phlegm. Hegu(LI 4) and Baihui(GV 20) serve to regulate qi activity in the head, and harmonize qi and blood as well. Shenmen(HT 7) calms the mind to relieve restlessness. Tianmei acupoint is an empirical acupoint for quitting smoking; it can transfer the pleasant taste in smoking to bitter taste in the mouth, dry throat and nausea, consequently resulting in an aversion to cigarettes.

方义: 吸烟主要与肺的关系密切,故取肺之合穴尺泽,宣肺止咳。胃经络穴丰隆豁痰。合谷、百会疏调头部气机,调和气血。神门宁心安神除烦。甜美穴为戒烟的经验穴,能改变吸烟时的欣快感而使其产生口苦、咽干、恶心欲呕等不适感,导致对香烟产生厌恶感而达到戒烟目的。

3.2 Other therapy

3.2 其他治疗

Ear acupuncture: Select 2 to 3 acupoints from Lung(CO 14), Mouth(CO 1), Internal Nose(TG 4), Subcortex(AT 4), Sympathesis(AH 6a), and Shenmen(TF 4). Puncture these acupoints with filiform needles and retain the needles for 20 minutes; the treatment is given once a day, and 10 treatments constitute a course of treatment. The above acupoints can also be treated by ear-pressure with *Semen Vaccariae* (Wang Bu Liu Xing), and replaced once every 3 to 5 days.

耳针: 选肺、口、内鼻、皮质下、交感、神门。每次选2~3穴,毫针刺激,留针20分钟,每日1次,10次为1个疗程;或用王不留行贴压,3~5日换穴1次。

4 Remarks

4 按语

The smokers' smoking-quitting expectation is the necessary prerequisite for good long-term re-

吸烟者自身的戒烟愿望是获得远期戒断疗效的必要

sults. The result is also related to smoking years, specifically, the smoking year is longer and the result is worse.

条件，且烟龄与疗效关系密切，即烟龄越长，疗效越差。

Drug Withdrawal Syndrome

Drug withdrawal syndrome develops when addicts quit after long-term abuse and cravings for opium, displaying symptoms such as nausea or vomiting, myalgia, sniveling and tear-shedding, platycoria, upright hair, excessive sweating, diarrhea, yawning, fever, and insomnia. These symptoms vary in intensity and often occur in 8 to 12 hours after quitting, reach their peak intensity within 36 to 72 hours, and gradually vanish in 7 to 10 days after discontinuation of drug use.

戒毒综合征

戒毒综合征是指吸毒者因长期吸食毒品成瘾，戒断时出现的渴求使用阿片、恶心或呕吐、肌肉疼痛、流泪流涕、瞳孔扩大、毛发竖立或出汗、腹泻、呵欠、发热、失眠等瘾癖症候群。戒毒综合征有轻有重，一般发生于停药8～12小时，通常在36～72小时内达到高峰，大部分症状在7～10日内消失。

1　Etiology and pathogenesis

In long-term drug abuse, lots of opioids are combined with the cerebral opioid receptors in the human body, causing the inhibition of the secretion of endogenous opioids. Therefore, once drug abuse is discontinued, the secretion of endogenous opioids cannot meet the body's needs, thereby leading to a series of unbearable withdrawal symptoms.

1　病因病机

长期吸毒，大量的阿片类进入人体内，与中枢内阿片类受体相结合，致使体内内源性阿片类物质的分泌受到抑制。一旦外源性阿片类药物停止供应，内源性阿片类物质的分泌不能满足人体需要，则诱发出现一系列难以忍受的戒断现象。

2　Syndrome differentiation

Chief symptoms: Initial symptoms showing yawning, tearing and nasal discharge, sweating, followed by platycoria, sneezing, chills, hypertension, and muscular spasms.

The syndrome of stirring liver-wind manifests restlessness and irritability, clonic convulsions,

2　辨证

主症：最初表现为呵欠、流泪、流涕、出汗，继而出现瞳孔扩大，打喷嚏、寒战、血压升高，肌肉抽动。

肝风内动者，兼性情暴躁、烦躁不安、抽搐谵言、毁

damaging objects, complete insomnia, bloodshot eyes, bitter taste in the mouth, tearing and nasal discharge, abdominal pain and diarrhea, red tongue with yellowish coating, and wiry slippery and rapid pulse. The syndrome of spleen-kidney insufficiency manifests fatigue, weak limbs, low spirit, drooling, poor appetite, dizziness and insomnia, palpitations and breathlessness, abdominal pain and diarrhea, sweating, tearing, muscular spasms, collapse, inability to stand, fecal incontinence and enuresis, pale tongue with whitish coating, and deep, weak and thready pulse. The syndrome of heart-kidney incoordination manifests absent-mindedness, restlessness, insomnia, dizziness, palpitations, tastelessness in mouth, poor appetite, weak limbs, red tongue with whitish coating, and wiry thready pulse.

3 Treatment

3.1 Essential treatment

Principal acupoints: Shuigou(GV 26), Fengchi (GB 20), Baihui (GV 20), Neiguan(PC 6), Laogong(PC 8), and Fenglong(ST 40).

Supplementary acupoints: In the syndrome of stirring liver-wind, add Taichong(TR 3), Xingjian (LR 2) and Xiaxi(GB 43); in the syndrome of spleen-kidney insufficiency, add Pishu(BL 20), Shenshu(BL 23) and Sanyinjiao(SP 6); in the syndrome of heart-kidney incoordination, add Xinshu (BL 15), Shenshu(BL 23) and Taixi(KI 3).

Explanation: Shuigou(GV 26) and Baihui(GV 20) are both located on the governor vessel, which enters into the brain; Fengchi(GB 20), located on the back of the occipital bone, is also linked with the brain; combination of these three acupoints may

衣损物、碰伤头身、彻夜不眠、眼红口苦、涕泪齐下、腹痛腹泻、舌红、苔黄、脉弦滑数；脾肾两虚者，兼精神疲乏、肢体困倦、萎靡不振、口流涎沫、不思饮食、头晕不寐、心慌气促、腹痛腹泻、汗出流泪、肌肉震颤甚或发抖、虚脱、卧床不起、遗屎遗尿、舌淡、苔白、脉沉细弱；心肾不交者，兼精神恍惚、烦扰不安、眠而易醒、头晕心悸、口淡乏味、不思饮食、四肢无力、舌红、苔白、脉弦细。

3 治疗

3.1 基本治疗

主穴：水沟，风池，百会，内关，劳宫，丰隆。

配穴：肝风内动加太冲、行间、侠溪；脾肾两虚加脾俞、肾俞、三阴交；心肾不交加心俞、肾俞、太溪。

方义：水沟、百会为督脉经穴，督脉内通于脑，风池位于枕后，内络于脑，三穴醒脑开窍、安神；内关为心包经络穴，劳宫为心包经荥穴，合用

a waken the brain, open orifice and calm the mind. Neiguan(PC 6), the Luo-Connecting acupoint of the pericar-dium meridian, and Laogong(PC 8), the Ying-Spring acupoint of the pericardium meridian, may quieten heart and spirit, and clear heart fire to eliminate vexation. Fenglong(ST 40), an essential acupoint to resolve phlegm, invi-gorates the spleen to dissolve phlegm, extinguish wind and unblock the collaterals.

可宁心安神、清心除烦；丰隆为豁痰要穴，健脾化痰、熄风通络。

3.2 Other therapy

Ear acupuncture: Select 3 to 5 acupoints from Lung(CO 14), Mouth(CO 1), Heart(CO 15), Spleen(CO 13), Liver(CO 12), Kidney(CO 10), Shenmen(TF 4), Subcortex(AT 4), Endocrine(CO 18), and Sympathesis(AH 6a). Puncture these acupoints with filiform needles and retain the needles for 20 minutes. The treatment is given once a day and 10 treatments make up one course. Or *Semen Vaccariae*(Wang Bu Liu Xing) is applied at these acupoints, which are replaced once every 3 to 5 days.

3.2 其他治疗

耳针：选肺、口、心、脾、肝、肾、神门、皮质下、内分泌、交感。每次选 3～5 穴，毫针刺激，留针 20 分钟，每天 1 次，10 次为 1 个疗程；或用王不留行贴压，3～5 日换穴 1 次。

4 Remarks

In detoxification stage, acupuncture can be used as an adjunct method; while in convalescence stage, acupuncture is used to fight against withdrawal symptoms and promote the addicts' recovery.

4 按语

针灸在脱毒期作为辅助治疗，而在康复期用于抗稽延性症状，促进成瘾者康复。

Obesity

Obesity develops when the body takes in more calories than needed for a long period of time and then the fat accumulates inside the body, manifesting body weight exceeding standard body by over 20%. Obesity is classified into primary and secon-

肥胖症

肥胖症是指由于机体能量摄入长期超过消耗量，从而导致体内脂肪积聚过多，体重超过标准体重 20%以上的一种疾病证状。肥胖症分

dary conditions. Primary obesity refers to being overweight with a metabolic disorder without any morphological and functional changes in the nervous and endocrine systems, which is more commonly seen. Secondary obesity refers to being overweight caused by diseases of the nervous, endocrine or metabolic systems, or by acquired genetic diseases or medicine.

为单纯性肥胖和继发性肥胖两类。单纯性肥胖是指不伴有显著的神经、内分泌形态及功能变化，但可伴有代谢调节过程障碍，这一类在临床多见。继发性肥胖是指由于神经、内分泌及代谢疾病，或遗传、药物等因素引起的肥胖。

1 Etiology and pathogenesis

Obesity results from qi-blood imbalance and yin-yang disharmony due to the dysfunction of the spleen and stomach and kidney deficiency, or from accumulation of dampness and phlegm due to spleen-stomach deficiency, or from turbid fat condensed from body fluids by stomach heat, or from retention of phlegm and dampness beneath the muscles due to kidney-qi failing to activate the body fluids.

1 病因病机

脾胃功能失常，肾元虚惫引起气血偏盛偏衰、阴阳失调，导致肥胖。脾胃虚弱则水湿不化，痰浊内生；胃肠腑热则食欲偏旺，水谷精微反被炼成浊脂；真元不足则气不行水，凝津成痰，遂致痰湿浊脂滞留肌肤而形成肥胖。

2 Syndrome differentiation

Chief symptoms: Plumpness in the face, neck, shoulder, back, waist and buttocks.

The syndrome of stomach-intestine heat manifests swift digestion and rapid hungering, bulimia, dry mouth with desire to drink, aversion to heat, massive sweating, abdominal distention, constipation, scanty dark urine, red tongue with yellowish greasy coating, and forceful slippery pulse. The syndrome of spleen-stomach deficiency manifests poor appetite, fatigue, palpitation and shortness of breath, sleepiness, reluctance to speech, lusterless complexion and pale tips, loose stools, scanty urine, body edema, pale tongue with tooth marks and thin-whitish coating, and feeble thready pulse.

2 辨证

主症：面肥颈壅，项厚背宽，腹大腰粗，臀丰腿圆。

胃肠腑热者，兼消谷善饥、食欲亢进、口干欲饮、怕热多汗、腹胀便秘、小便短黄、舌质红、苔黄腻、脉滑有力；脾胃虚弱者，兼食欲不振、神疲乏力、心悸气短、嗜睡懒言、面唇少华、大便溏薄、尿少身肿、舌淡边有齿印、苔薄白、脉细缓无力；真元不足者，兼畏寒怕冷、腰膝酸软、耳鸣、神疲乏力、月经不调或阳痿早泄、面色㿠白、

The syndrome of kidney-qi deficiency manifests aversion to cold, aching loin and knees, tinnitus, fatigue, irregular menstruation or impotence and premature ejaculation, sallow complexion, tender tongue with tooth marks and thin-whitish coating, and deep slow pulse.

舌质嫩边有齿印、苔薄白、脉沉细迟缓。

3 Treatment

3 治疗

3.1 Essential treatment

3.1 基本治疗

Principal acupoints: Zhongwan(CV 12), Tianshu(ST 25), Daheng(SP 15), Quchi(LI 11), Yinlingquan(SP 9), Fenglong(ST 40), and Shangjuxu (ST 37).

主穴: 中脘,天枢,大横,曲池,阴陵泉,丰隆,上巨虚。

Supplementary acupoints: In the syndrome of stomach-intestine heat, add Hegu(LI 4) and Neiting(ST 44); in the syndrome of spleen-stomach deficiency, add Pishu(BL 20) and Zusanli(ST 36); in the syndrome of kidney-qi deficiency, add Shen-shu (BL 23) and Guanyuan(CV 4).

配穴: 胃肠腑热加合谷、内庭;脾胃虚弱加脾俞、足三里;真元不足加肾俞、关元。

Explanation: Obesity is closely related to the dysfunction of the spleen, stomach and intestine. Zhongwan(CV 12) is the Front-Mu acupoint of the stomach and the Confluent acupoint of fu-organ; Quchi(LI 11) is the He-Sea acupoint of the large intestine meridian; Tianshu(ST 25) is the Front-Mu acupoint of the large intestine; Shangjuxu(ST 37) is the Lower He-Sea acupoint of the large intestine. Combination of these four acupoints may move the bowels, descend the turbidity and eliminate the fat. Daheng(SP 15) helps invigorate the spleen to dissolve dampness. Fenglong(ST 40) and Yinlingquan (SP 9) act to disinhibit dampness, and resolve phlegm turbidity.

方义: 肥胖之症,多责之于脾胃肠腑,中脘乃胃募、腑会,曲池为大肠经的合穴,天枢为大肠募穴,上巨虚为大肠的下合穴,四穴共用可通利肠腑、降浊消脂。大横健脾助运。丰隆、阴陵泉分利水湿、蠲化痰浊。

3.2 Other therapy

3.2 其他治疗

Ear acupuncture: Select three or four acupoints

耳针: 选口、胃、脾、肺、

from Mouth(CO 1), Stomach(CO 4), Spleen(CO 13), Lung (CO 14), Triple Energizer (CO 17), Shenmen(TF 4), Endocrine(CO 18) and Subcortex (AT 4). Puncture these acupoints with filiform needles and retain the needles for 20 minutes; the treatment is given once a day, and 10 treatments constitute a full course. The above acupoints can also be applied with *Semen Vaccariae*(Wang Bu Liu Xing), which are replaced once every 3 to 5 days.

三焦、神门、内分泌、皮质下。每次选 3～4 穴，毫针刺激，留针 20 分钟，每日 1 次，10 次为 1 个疗程；或用王不留行贴压，3～5 日换穴 1 次。

4 Remarks

Acupuncture works well on simple obesity. However, it is necessary to receive 1 ～ 2 more treatment courses after expected therapeutic results have been achieved to avoid weight gain.

4 按语

针灸治疗单纯性肥胖具有较好的临床疗效，但应在取得疗效后宜巩固治疗 1～2 个疗程，以防体重反弹。

图书在版编目(CIP)数据

中国针灸:英汉对照/张海蒙,沈雪勇主编. —上海:上海浦江教育出版社有限公司,2017.9

(精编实用中医文库/陈凯先,李其忠,何星海主编)

ISBN 978-7-81121-527-4

Ⅰ.①中… Ⅱ.①张… ②沈… Ⅲ.①针灸学—英、汉 Ⅳ.①R245

中国版本图书馆 CIP 数据核字(2017)第245108号

上海浦江教育出版社出版

社址:上海海港大道 1550 号上海海事大学校内　　邮政编码:201306

分社:上海蔡伦路 1200 号上海中医药大学内　　邮政编码:201203

电话:(021)38284910(12)(发行)　38284923(总编室)　38284916(传真)

E-mail: cbs@shmtu. edu. cn　URL: http://www. pujiangpress. cn

上海盛通时代印刷有限公司印装　上海浦江教育出版社发行

幅面尺寸:170 mm×240 mm　印张:35　字数:666 千字

2017 年 9 月第 1 版　2018 年 4 月第 1 次印刷

责任编辑:黄　健　封面设计:赵宏义

定价:120.00 元